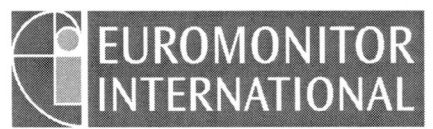

D1121046

World Health Databook

World Health Databook

2006

1st edition

Euromonitor International plc, 60-61 Britton Street, London EC1M 5UX

World Health Databook 2006

1st edition

Researched and published by:

Euromonitor International Plc
60-61 Britton Street
London EC1M 5UX
United Kingdom
Tel: +44 207-251-8024
Fax: +44 207-608-3149

Euromonitor International Inc
122 South Michigan Avenue
Suite 810
Chicago
Illinois 60603, USA
Tel: + 1 312 922 1115
Fax: +1 312 922 1157

Euromonitor International (Asia) Pte Ltd
3 Lim Teck Kim Road
#08-02 Singapore Technologies Building
Singapore 088934
Tel: + 65 6429 0590
Fax: + 65 6324 1855

Euromonitor International (Shanghai) Co. Ltd
Bund Centre, Level 41, Unit 5A
222 Yan An Road (East)
Shanghai 200002
China
Tel: 86 21 6335 2808
Fax: 86 21 6335 2801

Euromonitor International (Eastern Europe) UAB
Jogailos Street 4,
Vilnius
LT-01116
Lithuania
tel: +370 5 243 1577
Fax: +370 5 243 1599

E-mail: info@euromonitor.com

http://www.euromonitor.com

British Library Cataloguing in Publication Data

A CIP catalogue record for this book is available from the British Library

Printed in Great Britain

Euromonitor International is a member of the Data Publishers Association and the European Association of Directory Publishers

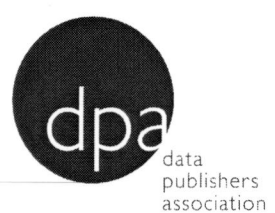

ISBN: 184264 3959

Disclaimer
This edition of the World Health Databook has been prepared with painstaking care but the editors cannot accept responsibility for any errors which may have occurred during its compilation. We would welcome comments and feedback about the contents to assist in the compilation of subsequent editions.

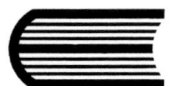

Printed in Great Britain

Summary of Contents

Table of Contents

Section 3
World Health Rankings 129

Section 4
Country Snapshots 147

Introduction

Introduction

Scope of the Databook

World Health Databook is a brand new title from Euromonitor International and presents a wealth of up-to-date statistical information on health across 71 countries worldwide. The databook aims to provide insight into the health of each nation and includes detailed data on life expectancy, health expenditure, healthcare infrastructure and services, incidence of infectious diseases and immunisation, causes of death, and lifestyle health issues such as obesity, nutrition and prevalence of smoking.

The data contained in this publication are presented in spreadsheet form and arranged in four sections covering socio-economic parameters, comparative world rankings, and cross-country and country-specific trends.

Value data in the rankings and cross-country sections are presented in US dollars in order to facilitate comparisons and the easy identification of trends and developments. Exchange rates used for converting national currencies are shown in the following table.

Exchange rates against US$ 1998-2004

Table: 0.1

National currency per US$

	1998	1999	2000	2001	2002	2003	2004
Algeria	58.74	66.57	75.26	77.22	79.68	77.39	72.06
Argentina	1.00	1.00	1.00	1.00	3.06	2.90	2.92
Australia	1.59	1.55	1.72	1.93	1.84	1.54	1.36
Austria	0.89	0.94	1.09	1.12	1.06	0.89	0.81
Azerbaijan	3,869.00	4,120.17	4,474.15	4,656.58	4,860.82	4,910.73	4,913.48
Belarus	46.13	249.29	876.75	1,390.00	1,790.92	2,051.27	2,160.26
Belgium	0.89	0.94	1.09	1.12	1.06	0.89	0.81
Bolivia	5.51	5.81	6.18	6.61	7.17	7.66	7.94
Brazil	1.16	1.81	1.83	2.36	2.92	3.08	2.93
Bulgaria	1.76	1.84	2.12	2.18	2.08	1.73	1.58
Canada	1.48	1.49	1.49	1.55	1.57	1.40	1.30
Chile [a]	460.29	508.78	539.59	634.94	688.94	691.43	609.37
China [a]	8.28	8.28	8.28	8.28	8.28	8.28	8.28
Colombia	1,426.04	1,756.23	2,087.90	2,299.63	2,504.24	2,877.65	2,628.61
Croatia	6.36	7.11	8.28	8.34	7.87	6.70	6.04
Czech Republic [a]	32.28	34.57	38.60	38.04	32.74	28.21	25.70
Denmark	6.70	6.98	8.08	8.32	7.89	6.59	5.99
Ecuador	1.00	1.00	1.00	1.00	1.00	1.00	1.00
Egypt [a]	3.39	3.40	3.47	3.97	4.50	5.85	6.20
Estonia	14.07	14.68	16.97	17.48	16.61	13.86	12.60
Finland	0.89	0.94	1.09	1.12	1.06	0.89	0.81
France	0.89	0.94	1.09	1.12	1.06	0.89	0.81
Germany	0.89	0.94	1.09	1.12	1.06	0.89	0.81
Greece	0.89	0.94	1.09	1.12	1.06	0.89	0.81
Hong Kong, China	7.75	7.76	7.79	7.80	7.80	7.79	7.79
Hungary	214.40	237.15	282.18	286.49	257.89	224.31	202.75
India	41.26	43.06	44.94	47.19	48.61	46.58	45.32
Indonesia	10,013.60	7,855.15	8,421.77	10,260.80	9,311.19	8,577.13	8,938.85
Ireland	0.89	0.94	1.09	1.12	1.06	0.89	0.81
Israel	3.80	4.14	4.08	4.21	4.74	4.55	4.48
Italy	0.89	0.94	1.09	1.12	1.06	0.89	0.81
Japan	130.91	113.91	107.77	121.53	125.39	115.93	108.19
Jordan	0.71	0.71	0.71	0.71	0.71	0.71	0.71
Kazakhstan	78.30	119.52	142.13	146.74	153.28	149.58	136.04
Kuwait	0.30	0.30	0.31	0.31	0.30	0.30	0.29
Latvia	0.59	0.59	0.61	0.63	0.62	0.57	0.54
Lithuania	4.00	4.00	4.00	4.00	3.68	3.06	2.78
Malaysia	3.92	3.80	3.80	3.80	3.80	3.80	3.80
Mexico	9.14	9.56	9.46	9.34	9.66	10.79	11.29
Morocco	9.60	9.80	10.63	11.30	11.02	9.57	8.87
Netherlands	0.89	0.94	1.09	1.12	1.06	0.89	0.81
New Zealand	1.87	1.89	2.20	2.38	2.16	1.72	1.51
Nigeria [a]	86.00	92.34	101.70	111.23	120.58	129.22	132.89
Norway	7.55	7.80	8.80	8.99	7.98	7.08	6.74
Pakistan	45.05	49.50	53.65	61.93	59.72	57.75	58.26
Peru	2.93	3.38	3.49	3.51	3.52	3.48	3.41
Philippines	40.89	39.09	44.19	50.99	51.60	54.20	56.04
Poland	3.48	3.97	4.35	4.09	4.08	3.89	3.66
Portugal	0.89	0.94	1.09	1.12	1.06	0.89	0.81
Romania [a]	8,875.58	15,332.80	21,708.70	29,060.80	33,055.40	33,200.10	32,636.60
Russia	9.71	24.62	28.13	29.17	31.35	30.69	28.81
Saudi Arabia	3.75	3.75	3.75	3.75	3.75	3.75	3.75
Singapore	1.67	1.69	1.72	1.79	1.79	1.74	1.69
Slovakia [a]	35.23	41.36	46.04	48.35	45.33	36.77	32.26
Slovenia	166.13	181.77	222.66	242.75	240.25	207.11	192.38
South Africa [a]	5.53	6.11	6.94	8.61	10.54	7.56	6.46
South Korea	1,401.44	1,188.82	1,130.96	1,290.99	1,251.09	1,191.61	1,145.32
Spain	0.89	0.94	1.09	1.12	1.06	0.89	0.81
Sweden	7.95	8.26	9.16	10.33	9.74	8.09	7.35
Switzerland	1.45	1.50	1.69	1.69	1.56	1.35	1.24
Taiwan	33.43	32.22	33.50	32.85	34.57	34.46	33.60
Thailand	41.36	37.81	40.11	44.43	42.96	41.48	40.22
Tunisia	1.14	1.19	1.37	1.44	1.42	1.29	1.25
Turkey	260,724.00	418,783.00	625,218.00	1,225,590.00	1,507,230.00	1,500,890.00	1,425,540.00
Turkmenistan	4,890.17	5,200.00	5,200.00	5,200.00	5,200.00	5,200.00	5,172.67
Ukraine	2.45	4.13	5.44	5.37	5.33	5.33	5.32
United Arab Emirates	3.67	3.67	3.67	3.67	3.67	3.67	3.67
United Kingdom	0.60	0.62	0.66	0.69	0.67	0.61	0.55
USA	1.00	1.00	1.00	1.00	1.00	1.00	1.00
Venezuela	547.56	605.72	679.96	723.67	1,160.95	1,606.96	1,891.33
Vietnam	13,268.00	13,943.20	14,167.70	14,725.20	15,279.50	15,509.60	16,235.50

Source: *International Monetary Fund (IMF)/Euromonitor International research*
Note: (a) Principal rate

Following this introductory section, World Health Databook contains four main data sections, as follows:

Section One: Socio-Economic Parameters
This section provides some context to the health datasets by presenting those background parameters that are relevant to the health of a nation. These include population and age profile; fertility, birth and death rates; household characteristics; and consumer expenditure.

Section Two: World Health Trends
Data are presented in standardised units within 63 statistical tabulations grouped under 11 health topics. This allows for the easy identification of trends and quick comparisons across countries. Each table presents comparative statistics for the time series 1998-2004 or for the latest year for which data are available.

The health topics covered in this section are life expectancy, sanitation, health expenditure, healthcare infrastructure and services, immunisation, infectious diseases, causes of death, smoking, nutrition and obesity, over-the-counter (OTC) healthcare, and health and wellness.

Section Three: World Health Rankings
The standardisation of units allows for the unique compilation of a series of health rankings showing the relative position of each of the 71 countries. Rankings have been put together for around half of the 63 statistical tabulations.

Section Four: Country Snapshots
Using the same standardised approach followed in Sections One and Two, this section deals with each of the 71 countries in turn, presenting socio-economic and health data under a series of standard headings. This allows for a review of health datasets at national level.

Quality and availability of data vary considerably country by country. Where possible, therefore, Euromonitor International has sought to overcome any shortfalls by providing informed estimates based on country knowledge combined with government statistics.

Definitions

- **Life expectancy at birth**
Indicates the number of years a newborn infant would live if prevailing patterns of mortality at the time of its birth were to remain the same throughout its life.

- **Public Health Expenditure (PHE)**
The sum of outlays on health paid for by taxes, social security contributions and external resources (without double-counting the government transfers to social security and extra-budgetary funds).

- **Public expenditure on pharmaceuticals and other medical non-durables**
Data comprise pharmaceuticals such as medicinal preparations, branded and generic medicines, drugs, patent medicines, serums and vaccines, vitamins and minerals, and oral contraceptives.

- **Consumer expenditure on health goods and medical services**
Expenditure on pharmaceutical products, medical appliances and equipment, outpatient and hospital services. This division also includes health services purchased from school and university health centres.

- **In-patient beds**
Beds accommodating patients who are formally admitted to a hospital or other institution providing in-patient care and who stay for a minimum of one night. In-patient care is delivered in hospitals, other nursing and residential care facilities or in establishments, which are classified according to their focus of care under the ambulatory care industry but perform in-patient care as a secondary activity.

- **Hospital admissions**
Admission is the hospitalisation of a patient in an in-patient facility normally involving a stay of at least 24 hours. In the case of death or discharge to another health establishment, the actual stay may be shorter than 24 hours. These cases are registered as a one-day hospitalisation. Discharge is the conclusion of a period of in- patient care, whether the patient returned to his home, was transferred to another in- patient facility or died. The number of admissions/discharges excludes: a transfer from one department to another one at the same hospital; day-cases of day patients; weekend leave when the patient has been released temporarily and the hospital bed is still reserved; cases where treatment is provided by hospital personnel at the patient's home. Newborns are not included.

- **In-patient surgical procedures**
All invasive therapies performed as in-patient surgery, where in-patient surgery is defined as a surgical operation or procedure that is performed with an overnight stay in an in-patient institution.

- Out-patient contacts

  The total number of primary healthcare (PHC) or ambulatory care contacts divided by the population. An out-patient contact is one episode of examination/consultation performed by a physician or by a nurse in the presence of a physician, in relation to one out-patient at one time and location, normally at the physician's office or the patient's home. The number of out-patient contacts includes: patient's visit to physician's office; physician's visit to patient's home or other place; call for ambulance; day-patient cases. The number of out-patient contacts excludes: telephone calls for consultation purposes; visits for prescribed laboratory tests; contacts to perform prescribed and scheduled treatment procedures, e.g. injections, physiotherapy etc.; visits to dentist. Definition of out-patient: A person attending a PHC unit or out- patient department in an out-patient establishment or hospital and who makes use of the diagnostic or therapeutic service but does not occupy a regular hospital bed.

- Doctors

  The number of physicians, general practitioners and specialists (including self- employed) who are actively practising medicine in public and private institutions. The data should exclude dentists, stomatologists, qualified physicians who are working abroad, working in administration, research and industry positions. Data should include foreign physicians licensed to practice and actively practising medicine in the country.

- Nurses

  The data refer to the total number of nurses certified/registered and actively practising in public and private hospitals, clinics and other health facilities, including self- employed. Nursing assistants and midwives should be included. Data should exclude nurses who are working abroad, in administrative, research and industry positions.

- Consultations with general practitioners

  Consultations include visits of patients to the physician's office, telephone contacts made in lieu of visits and visits made to the patient's home.

- Active pharmacists

  Number of pharmacists (self-employed or employed by other). The data exclude full- time salaried pharmacists working in hospitals and in pharmaceutical manufacturing corporations as well as pharmacists working abroad.

- Dentists

  Number of dentists (self-employed or employed by other). The data exclude qualified dentists working abroad, but includes foreign dentists licensed to practice.

- Causes of death

  Number of deaths and age-standardised death rate. Age-standardised death rates per 100,000 population are calculated by the OECD Secretariat, using the total OECD population for 1980 as the reference population. The causes of death are grouped according to the tenth revision of the International Classification of Diseases (ICD).

- Average supply of calories, protein and fat per day

  Per capita food supplies available for human consumption in terms of calorific value, protein content and fat content. Figures represent only the average supply of food available for the population and do not necessarily indicate what is actually consumed by individuals.

- Over-the-counter (OTC) healthcare

  This is the aggregation of analgesics, cough, cold and allergy remedies, digestive remedies, medicated skin care, vitamins & dietary supplements, smoking cessation aids, eye care, ear care, adult mouthcare, calming and sleeping aids and wound treatments. It refers to medicines and healthcare products that are available to buy in a retail outlet without the need for a prescription.

- Organic packaged food

  Packaged food that is certified organic by an approved certification body, such as the Soil Association in the UK. To be included, the organic aspect needs to form part of the positioning/marketing of the product. Organic food production is based on a system of farming that maintains and replenishes soil fertility without the use of toxic and persistent pesticides and fertilisers. Organic foods are minimally processed without artificial ingredients, preservatives, or irradiation to maintain the integrity of the food. The use of GMOs (Genetically Modified Organisms) is prohibited.

- Fortified/functional food

  Generally food products which are enhanced due to fortification with vitamins or minerals, and/or the addition of a functional ingredient. Enhancement must be over and above any level, which can be considered as industry standard.

- **Packaged food for food intolerance**
Packaged foods that have been specifically manufactured for those who are diabetic, or gluten or lactose intolerant. Foodstuffs that are naturally sugar-, gluten-, or lactose- free are excluded.

Country Coverage

World Health Databook includes a total of 71 countries around the world as follows:

Algeria	Egypt	Lithuania	Slovenia
Argentina	Estonia	Malaysia	South Africa
Australia	Finland	Mexico	South Korea
Austria	France	Morocco	Spain
Azerbaijan	Germany	Netherlands	Sweden
Belarus	Greece	New Zealand	Switzerland
Belgium	Hong Kong, China	Nigeria	Taiwan
Bolivia	Hungary	Norway	Thailand
Brazil	India	Pakistan	Tunisia
Bulgaria	Indonesia	Peru	Turkey
Canada	Ireland	Philippines	Turkmenistan
Chile	Israel	Poland	Ukraine
China	Italy	Portugal	United Arab Emirates
Colombia	Japan	Romania	United Kingdom
Croatia	Jordan	Russia	USA
Czech Republic	Kazakhstan	Saudi Arabia	Venezuela
Denmark	Kuwait	Singapore	Vietnam
Ecuador	Latvia	Slovakia	

Sources and Methodology

World Health Databook is based on an extensive ongoing programme of research into the health of nations around the world. A team of researchers with extensive country- specific knowledge was employed both in the relevant countries as well as in London. Research was conducted using a combination of both international and national sources in order to achieve the best and most accurate coverage of datasets.

The principal sources used are as follows:

- **National Statistical Offices**
- **International and European organisations, including the following:**
  - Council of Europe
  - Eurostat
  - International Obesity Taskforce
  - Organisation for Economic Co-operation and Development (OECD)
  - UNAIDS
  - United Nations (UN)
  - UN Food and Agriculture Organisation (FAOSTAT)
  - World Bank
  - World Health Organisation (WHO)

On completion of the research phase, findings were thoroughly examined. Tables were standardised for inclusion in the cross-country comparable database. In order to ensure international comparability, definitions were authenticated, supplementary research was conducted as necessary and at times broader breakdowns were applied in order to ensure complete accuracy and comparability. This process ensures that, as far as possible, there is international comparability across the database.

Disclaimer

The compilation of a reference volume of this type involves extracting complex statistical data from numerous sources in different languages. The editors have made every effort to ensure accuracy but the publishers cannot be held responsible for any errors that may have occurred.

Socio-Economic Parameters

■ Population

Total population (national estimates at January 1st) 1998-2004

Table: 1.1

'000 / % change

	1998	1999	2000	2001	2002	2003	2004	% change 1998-2004
Algeria	29,075	29,534	30,005	30,495	31,005	31,532	32,068	10.30
Argentina	35,156	35,519	35,881	36,260	36,632	37,001	37,368	6.29
Australia	18,711	18,926	19,153	19,413	19,663	19,820	20,015	6.97
Austria	7,977	7,992	8,012	8,032	8,053	8,079	8,105	1.61
Azerbaijan	7,991	8,057	8,123	8,191	8,261	8,333	8,408	5.22
Belarus	10,093	10,051	10,019	9,990	9,951	9,899	9,858	-2.33
Belgium	10,192	10,214	10,239	10,263	10,310	10,355	10,393	1.97
Bolivia	7,899	8,066	8,233	8,398	8,562	8,726	8,890	12.54
Brazil	165,688	167,910	170,143	172,386	174,633	176,876	179,114	8.10
Bulgaria	8,211	8,131	8,055	7,986	7,891	7,846	7,768	-5.40
Canada	30,157	30,404	30,689	31,021	31,362	31,630	31,932	5.88
Chile	14,822	15,018	15,211	15,402	15,589	15,774	15,956	7.65
China	1,248,100	1,258,540	1,268,240	1,276,291	1,285,536	1,295,229	1,304,130	4.49
Colombia	40,338	41,053	41,764	42,472	43,175	43,874	44,567	10.48
Croatia	4,501	4,554	4,474	4,437	4,439	4,441	4,442	-1.31
Czech Republic	10,256	10,241	10,228	10,217	10,206	10,203	10,199	-0.55
Denmark	5,295	5,314	5,330	5,349	5,368	5,386	5,404	2.06
Ecuador	11,923	12,123	12,321	12,517	12,712	12,905	13,097	9.84
Egypt	60,839	61,994	63,254	64,466	65,584	66,698	67,798	11.44
Estonia	1,393	1,379	1,372	1,367	1,361	1,356	1,351	-3.05
Finland	5,147	5,160	5,171	5,181	5,195	5,206	5,213	1.28
France	58,299	58,497	58,749	59,038	59,344	59,663	59,979	2.88
Germany	82,057	82,037	82,163	82,260	82,440	82,546	82,636	0.71
Greece	10,511	10,522	10,554	10,585	10,609	10,629	10,646	1.28
Hong Kong, China	6,544	6,607	6,665	6,725	6,787	6,878	6,958	6.33
Hungary	10,135	10,092	10,222	10,200	10,175	10,139	10,097	-0.37
India	974,493	991,634	1,008,549	1,025,166	1,041,471	1,057,505	1,073,345	10.14
Indonesia	204,469	207,320	210,149	212,957	215,743	218,507	221,247	8.21
Ireland	3,694	3,735	3,777	3,826	3,883	3,931	3,973	7.55
Israel	5,971	6,125	6,289	6,439	6,570	6,731	6,890	15.40
Italy	57,563	57,613	57,680	57,844	58,009	58,143	58,251	1.19
Japan	126,479	126,686	126,929	127,291	127,435	127,594	127,738	1.00
Jordan	4,665	4,814	4,961	5,108	5,255	5,400	5,542	18.79
Kazakhstan	16,086	15,887	15,715	15,585	15,500	15,450	15,417	-4.16
Kuwait	2,129	2,274	2,228	2,243	2,302	2,357	2,414	13.37
Latvia	2,421	2,399	2,382	2,364	2,346	2,331	2,319	-4.21
Lithuania	3,562	3,536	3,512	3,487	3,468	3,447	3,426	-3.81
Malaysia	22,180	22,712	23,495	24,014	24,527	25,049	25,581	15.33
Mexico	95,066	96,620	98,163	99,694	101,210	102,710	104,193	9.60
Morocco	27,957	28,411	28,874	29,346	29,827	30,318	30,814	10.22
Netherlands	15,654	15,760	15,864	15,987	16,105	16,192	16,274	3.96
New Zealand	3,816	3,836	3,859	3,880	3,939	3,976	4,012	5.13
Nigeria	107,125	110,157	113,213	116,284	119,366	122,459	125,562	17.21
Norway	4,418	4,445	4,478	4,503	4,524	4,556	4,582	3.71
Pakistan	133,591	137,199	140,835	144,465	148,093	151,743	155,446	16.36
Peru	24,897	25,322	25,743	26,156	26,564	26,966	27,366	9.92
Philippines	73,148	74,746	76,504	78,055	79,612	81,168	82,716	13.08
Poland	38,660	38,667	38,654	38,644	38,632	38,622	38,589	-0.18
Portugal	10,108	10,150	10,198	10,263	10,336	10,394	10,445	3.34
Romania	22,526	22,489	22,455	22,430	22,375	22,316	22,255	-1.21
Russia	146,739	146,328	145,559	144,819	143,954	143,097	142,411	-2.95
Saudi Arabia	19,842	20,338	20,847	21,556	22,289	22,944	23,597	18.92
Singapore	3,175	3,222	3,263	3,319	3,378	3,430	3,478	9.56
Slovakia	5,368	5,372	5,377	5,379	5,379	5,375	5,371	0.06
Slovenia	1,985	1,978	1,988	1,990	1,994	1,996	1,998	0.68
South Africa	42,130	43,054	43,852	44,820	45,654	46,430	47,550	12.87
South Korea	45,434	45,714	45,985	46,253	46,542	46,819	47,085	3.63
Spain	39,388	39,519	39,733	40,122	40,409	40,593	40,748	3.46
Sweden	8,848	8,854	8,861	8,883	8,909	8,940	8,971	1.39
Switzerland	7,096	7,124	7,164	7,204	7,261	7,292	7,316	3.10
Taiwan	21,929	22,092	22,277	22,406	22,521	22,628	22,734	3.67
Thailand	58,086	58,797	58,876	59,362	59,891	60,580	61,249	5.45
Tunisia	9,248	9,358	9,465	9,570	9,675	9,779	9,884	6.87
Turkey	65,157	66,288	67,419	68,527	69,625	70,712	71,790	10.18
Turkmenistan	4,439	4,523	4,603	4,681	4,756	4,830	4,902	10.43
Ukraine	50,245	49,851	49,456	49,053	48,241	47,788	47,339	-5.78
United Arab Emirates	2,834	3,033	3,247	3,488	3,754	3,966	4,180	47.50
United Kingdom	58,305	58,481	58,643	59,051	59,229	59,427	59,613	2.24
USA	270,248	272,691	275,135	277,504	279,807	282,068	284,322	5.21
Venezuela	23,083	23,561	24,038	24,514	24,988	25,462	25,933	12.35
Vietnam	75,580	76,598	77,620	78,666	79,736	80,827	81,928	8.40

Source: *Euromonitor International from national statistics/UN*

Population aged 0-14 (as at January 1st) 1998-2004

Table: 1.2

% of total

	1998	1999	2000	2001	2002	2003	2004
Algeria	37.2	36.4	35.5	34.7	33.9	33.1	32.3
Argentina	28.9	28.8	28.6	28.3	28.0	27.8	27.6
Australia	21.0	20.9	20.7	20.5	20.3	19.8	19.5
Austria	17.4	17.2	17.0	16.8	16.6	16.5	16.3
Azerbaijan	33.0	32.5	31.9	31.2	30.5	29.6	28.8
Belarus	20.4	19.6	18.9	18.3	17.5	16.9	16.2
Belgium	17.7	17.7	17.6	17.6	17.5	17.4	17.3
Bolivia	40.2	40.0	39.7	39.4	39.1	38.8	38.4
Brazil	30.0	29.4	28.9	28.5	28.0	27.6	27.3
Bulgaria	16.8	16.3	15.9	15.5	15.0	14.6	14.2
Canada	19.8	19.5	19.2	18.9	18.6	18.3	18.0
Chile	28.8	28.6	28.5	28.1	27.7	27.3	27.0
China	24.3	23.9	23.5	22.6	21.3	20.5	19.5
Colombia	33.6	33.3	32.9	32.6	32.3	31.9	31.6
Croatia	19.9	19.8	17.1	17.0	16.9	16.8	16.7
Czech Republic	17.4	17.0	16.6	16.2	15.9	15.6	15.3
Denmark	18.0	18.2	18.4	18.6	18.7	18.8	18.9
Ecuador	35.3	34.8	34.3	33.8	33.4	32.9	32.4
Egypt	37.4	37.2	36.7	36.2	35.2	34.2	33.2
Estonia	19.6	18.9	18.3	17.7	17.2	16.6	16.0
Finland	18.7	18.4	18.2	18.1	17.9	17.8	17.6
France	19.0	18.9	18.9	18.8	18.7	18.7	18.7
Germany	16.0	15.8	15.7	15.5	15.3	15.1	14.8
Greece	15.8	15.4	15.2	14.9	14.8	14.6	14.5
Hong Kong, China	17.7	17.5	16.9	16.4	16.1	15.8	15.5
Hungary	17.5	17.3	16.9	16.6	16.3	16.1	15.8
India	35.0	34.7	34.3	33.9	33.5	33.1	32.6
Indonesia	32.1	31.6	31.1	30.6	30.2	29.7	29.3
Ireland	22.7	22.2	21.9	21.5	21.2	21.0	21.0
Israel	28.9	28.7	28.6	28.5	28.4	28.3	28.2
Italy	14.6	14.5	14.4	14.4	14.4	14.4	14.3
Japan	15.1	14.8	14.6	14.4	14.2	14.1	14.0
Jordan	39.9	39.5	39.1	38.7	38.2	37.8	37.4
Kazakhstan	28.9	28.5	28.0	27.3	26.5	25.6	24.7
Kuwait	26.5	25.6	25.9	25.6	25.3	25.0	24.9
Latvia	19.4	18.7	18.0	17.3	16.6	16.0	15.4
Lithuania	21.1	20.7	20.2	19.7	19.0	18.3	17.7
Malaysia	34.0	33.5	34.1	33.8	33.5	33.2	32.9
Mexico	34.9	34.5	34.0	33.6	33.1	32.6	32.0
Morocco	34.6	33.9	33.3	32.6	32.1	31.5	31.0
Netherlands	18.4	18.5	18.6	18.6	18.6	18.6	18.6
New Zealand	23.0	22.9	22.8	22.6	22.3	22.1	21.8
Nigeria	45.5	45.3	45.1	44.9	44.7	44.5	44.3
Norway	19.8	19.9	20.0	20.0	20.0	20.0	19.8
Pakistan	42.7	42.4	42.2	41.9	41.6	41.4	41.1
Peru	35.5	35.1	34.7	34.3	33.9	33.4	32.9
Philippines	37.4	37.1	36.8	36.5	36.2	35.9	35.5
Poland	21.1	20.3	19.6	18.8	18.2	17.6	17.0
Portugal	16.7	16.4	16.1	16.0	16.0	16.0	16.0
Romania	19.2	19.0	18.5	18.0	17.5	16.9	16.4
Russia	19.8	19.0	18.3	17.6	16.8	16.2	15.6
Saudi Arabia	40.3	40.3	40.3	40.3	40.3	40.0	39.8
Singapore	22.1	21.8	21.5	21.2	21.0	20.6	19.9
Slovakia	21.0	20.4	19.8	19.4	18.7	18.1	17.5
Slovenia	17.0	16.6	16.1	15.7	15.4	15.0	14.6
South Africa	33.5	33.1	32.6	32.1	31.6	31.3	30.8
South Korea	21.4	21.2	21.0	20.7	20.5	20.3	20.1
Spain	15.4	15.1	14.9	14.7	14.6	14.6	14.6
Sweden	18.7	18.6	18.5	18.4	18.2	18.0	17.7
Switzerland	17.6	17.5	17.4	17.3	17.1	17.0	16.7
Taiwan	22.0	21.4	21.1	20.8	20.4	19.9	19.5
Thailand	23.8	23.5	23.3	23.0	22.6	22.4	22.1
Tunisia	32.5	31.6	30.7	29.8	29.0	28.1	27.3
Turkey	30.6	30.3	30.0	29.7	29.6	29.4	29.2
Turkmenistan	38.3	37.5	36.8	36.0	35.1	34.2	33.3
Ukraine	19.2	18.5	17.8	17.2	16.5	15.7	15.1
United Arab Emirates	25.7	25.6	25.4	25.3	25.2	25.0	24.9
United Kingdom	19.4	19.3	19.1	18.8	18.6	18.3	18.1
USA	21.5	21.4	21.3	21.2	21.1	21.0	20.9
Venezuela	35.1	34.7	34.2	33.8	33.3	32.8	32.3
Vietnam	35.3	34.5	33.8	33.0	32.2	31.3	30.5

Source: *Euromonitor International from national statistics/UN*

Population aged 15-64 (as at January 1st) 1998-2004

Table: 1.3

% of total

	1998	1999	2000	2001	2002	2003	2004
Algeria	58.8	59.6	60.4	61.2	61.9	62.7	63.4
Argentina	61.5	61.5	61.6	61.8	62.1	62.2	62.5
Australia	66.7	66.8	66.9	66.9	67.1	67.6	67.7
Austria	67.2	67.4	67.5	67.7	67.9	68.1	68.1
Azerbaijan	61.7	62.1	62.6	63.1	63.6	64.1	64.7
Belarus	66.4	67.1	67.8	68.2	68.7	69.1	69.5
Belgium	65.8	65.7	65.6	65.6	65.6	65.7	65.8
Bolivia	55.7	55.8	56.0	56.2	56.5	56.8	57.1
Brazil	65.2	65.7	66.1	66.4	66.8	67.0	67.2
Bulgaria	67.6	67.9	67.9	68.1	68.1	68.4	68.9
Canada	67.9	68.1	68.3	68.5	68.7	68.9	69.2
Chile	64.2	64.3	64.4	64.6	64.9	65.2	65.4
China	68.3	68.4	69.1	69.7	70.6	71.4	72.4
Colombia	61.8	62.0	62.3	62.6	62.9	63.1	63.4
Croatia	67.8	67.9	67.0	66.9	66.7	66.6	66.5
Czech Republic	69.0	69.3	69.6	69.9	70.2	70.5	70.9
Denmark	67.1	66.9	66.8	66.6	66.5	66.4	66.3
Ecuador	60.1	60.5	60.9	61.3	61.7	62.0	62.4
Egypt	58.4	58.9	59.4	59.9	60.8	61.7	62.7
Estonia	65.9	66.3	66.8	67.0	67.3	67.5	67.9
Finland	66.7	66.9	66.9	66.9	66.9	66.9	66.8
France	65.2	65.2	65.1	65.1	65.0	65.1	65.2
Germany	68.2	68.2	68.1	67.8	67.6	67.6	67.5
Greece	67.7	67.7	67.6	67.4	67.4	67.2	67.1
Hong Kong, China	71.7	71.8	72.1	72.4	72.4	72.6	72.8
Hungary	68.1	68.2	68.1	68.3	68.4	68.6	68.9
India	60.2	60.5	60.8	61.1	61.5	61.8	62.2
Indonesia	63.4	63.7	64.1	64.5	64.8	65.1	65.4
Ireland	66.0	66.5	66.9	67.3	67.7	67.9	68.1
Israel	61.2	61.5	61.6	61.7	61.8	61.8	61.9
Italy	68.0	67.8	67.6	67.4	67.3	67.2	67.1
Japan	68.7	68.5	68.1	67.7	67.3	67.1	66.9
Jordan	57.5	57.8	58.2	58.5	58.8	59.2	59.5
Kazakhstan	64.2	64.7	65.2	65.7	66.2	66.7	67.2
Kuwait	72.1	73.0	72.7	72.8	73.1	73.3	73.3
Latvia	66.2	66.7	67.2	67.4	67.8	68.2	68.5
Lithuania	65.8	65.9	66.0	66.2	66.5	66.9	67.3
Malaysia	62.2	62.7	62.0	62.2	62.5	62.7	62.9
Mexico	60.6	60.9	61.2	61.6	62.0	62.4	62.8
Morocco	61.3	61.9	62.5	63.1	63.6	64.1	64.5
Netherlands	68.1	68.0	67.9	67.8	67.7	67.8	67.8
New Zealand	65.4	65.4	65.5	65.5	65.8	66.1	66.4
Nigeria	51.5	51.7	51.8	52.0	52.2	52.4	52.6
Norway	64.6	64.7	64.8	64.9	65.0	65.2	65.4
Pakistan	53.7	54.0	54.2	54.4	54.7	54.9	55.1
Peru	60.0	60.3	60.6	60.9	61.2	61.6	61.9
Philippines	58.9	59.1	59.3	59.5	59.8	60.0	60.3
Poland	67.2	67.8	68.4	68.9	69.3	69.7	70.2
Portugal	67.8	67.8	67.8	67.6	67.5	67.4	67.3
Romania	68.0	68.1	68.3	68.5	68.8	69.2	69.5
Russia	67.7	68.4	69.2	69.8	70.3	70.6	70.8
Saudi Arabia	56.7	56.7	56.7	56.7	56.7	56.9	57.2
Singapore	71.0	71.1	71.2	71.4	71.5	71.8	72.1
Slovakia	67.7	68.3	68.8	69.3	69.9	70.5	71.2
Slovenia	69.7	69.8	70.0	70.1	70.1	70.3	70.5
South Africa	61.6	62.0	62.5	63.0	63.4	63.7	64.1
South Korea	71.9	71.9	71.7	71.6	71.5	71.4	71.4
Spain	68.4	68.4	68.4	68.4	68.3	68.4	68.4
Sweden	63.9	64.0	64.2	64.4	64.6	64.8	65.1
Switzerland	67.4	67.3	67.3	67.3	67.4	67.6	67.8
Taiwan	69.8	70.1	70.3	70.4	70.6	70.9	71.2
Thailand	70.4	70.4	70.6	70.6	70.7	70.8	70.9
Tunisia	62.2	62.9	63.7	64.5	65.2	66.0	66.7
Turkey	64.1	64.4	64.7	64.8	64.9	65.0	65.1
Turkmenistan	57.5	58.2	58.9	59.7	60.4	61.2	62.0
Ukraine	66.8	67.6	68.3	68.8	69.1	69.1	69.2
United Arab Emirates	73.3	73.4	73.6	73.7	73.9	74.0	74.2
United Kingdom	64.7	64.9	65.0	65.4	65.5	65.7	65.8
USA	65.8	65.9	66.1	66.3	66.5	66.7	66.9
Venezuela	60.6	61.0	61.3	61.7	62.1	62.5	63.0
Vietnam	59.5	60.2	60.9	61.7	62.5	63.3	64.1

Source: *Euromonitor International from national statistics/UN*

Population aged 65+ (as at January 1st) 1998-2004

Table: 1.4

% of total

	1998	1999	2000	2001	2002	2003	2004
Algeria	4.0	4.0	4.1	4.1	4.2	4.2	4.3
Argentina	9.6	9.7	9.8	9.9	9.9	10.0	10.0
Australia	12.2	12.3	12.4	12.5	12.7	12.6	12.7
Austria	15.4	15.4	15.4	15.5	15.5	15.4	15.6
Azerbaijan	5.3	5.4	5.5	5.7	5.9	6.2	6.5
Belarus	13.2	13.3	13.3	13.5	13.8	14.0	14.3
Belgium	16.5	16.6	16.8	16.9	16.9	16.9	16.9
Bolivia	4.2	4.2	4.3	4.3	4.4	4.4	4.5
Brazil	4.8	4.9	5.0	5.1	5.2	5.3	5.5
Bulgaria	15.6	15.9	16.2	16.3	16.9	17.0	16.9
Canada	12.3	12.5	12.6	12.6	12.7	12.8	12.8
Chile	7.0	7.1	7.2	7.3	7.4	7.5	7.6
China	7.4	7.6	7.4	7.7	8.2	8.2	8.0
Colombia	4.6	4.7	4.7	4.8	4.9	4.9	5.0
Croatia	12.3	12.4	15.9	16.1	16.4	16.6	16.8
Czech Republic	13.6	13.7	13.8	13.9	13.9	13.9	13.8
Denmark	14.9	14.9	14.8	14.8	14.8	14.8	14.8
Ecuador	4.6	4.7	4.8	4.9	5.0	5.1	5.2
Egypt	4.2	3.9	3.8	3.9	4.0	4.1	4.1
Estonia	14.5	14.8	15.0	15.2	15.5	15.9	16.1
Finland	14.6	14.7	14.8	15.0	15.2	15.3	15.5
France	15.7	15.9	16.0	16.1	16.2	16.2	16.1
Germany	15.8	15.9	16.2	16.6	17.1	17.3	17.7
Greece	16.5	16.9	17.3	17.6	17.9	18.1	18.4
Hong Kong, China	10.6	10.7	10.9	11.2	11.4	11.6	11.7
Hungary	14.4	14.5	15.0	15.1	15.3	15.3	15.3
India	4.7	4.8	4.9	5.0	5.0	5.1	5.2
Indonesia	4.5	4.7	4.8	4.9	5.0	5.2	5.3
Ireland	11.4	11.3	11.2	11.2	11.2	11.1	11.0
Israel	9.9	9.8	9.8	9.8	9.9	9.9	9.9
Italy	17.4	17.7	18.0	18.2	18.3	18.4	18.6
Japan	16.2	16.7	17.4	18.0	18.5	18.9	19.0
Jordan	2.6	2.7	2.8	2.9	2.9	3.0	3.1
Kazakhstan	6.9	6.8	6.8	7.0	7.3	7.7	8.1
Kuwait	1.4	1.4	1.5	1.6	1.6	1.7	1.8
Latvia	14.4	14.7	14.8	15.2	15.5	15.9	16.2
Lithuania	13.2	13.5	13.7	14.1	14.4	14.7	15.0
Malaysia	3.7	3.8	4.0	4.0	4.1	4.1	4.2
Mexico	4.5	4.6	4.7	4.8	4.9	5.0	5.1
Morocco	4.2	4.2	4.2	4.3	4.4	4.4	4.5
Netherlands	13.5	13.5	13.6	13.6	13.7	13.6	13.7
New Zealand	11.6	11.7	11.8	11.9	11.9	11.8	11.8
Nigeria	3.0	3.0	3.0	3.1	3.1	3.1	3.1
Norway	15.7	15.5	15.3	15.1	14.9	14.8	14.7
Pakistan	3.6	3.6	3.6	3.6	3.7	3.7	3.7
Peru	4.5	4.6	4.7	4.8	4.9	5.0	5.1
Philippines	3.8	3.8	3.9	4.0	4.0	4.1	4.2
Poland	11.7	11.9	12.1	12.3	12.5	12.7	12.8
Portugal	15.5	15.8	16.1	16.4	16.5	16.6	16.7
Romania	12.7	13.0	13.2	13.5	13.7	13.9	14.1
Russia	12.5	12.5	12.5	12.6	12.9	13.3	13.6
Saudi Arabia	3.0	3.0	3.0	3.0	3.0	3.0	3.1
Singapore	6.9	7.1	7.3	7.4	7.5	7.7	8.0
Slovakia	11.2	11.3	11.4	11.3	11.4	11.3	11.3
Slovenia	13.2	13.6	13.9	14.1	14.5	14.7	14.8
South Africa	4.8	4.8	4.8	4.9	5.0	5.0	5.1
South Korea	6.7	7.0	7.3	7.6	7.9	8.2	8.6
Spain	16.2	16.5	16.8	16.9	17.1	17.0	17.0
Sweden	17.4	17.4	17.3	17.2	17.2	17.2	17.2
Switzerland	15.0	15.2	15.3	15.4	15.5	15.5	15.5
Taiwan	8.3	8.4	8.6	8.8	9.0	9.1	9.3
Thailand	5.8	6.0	6.1	6.4	6.6	6.9	7.1
Tunisia	5.4	5.5	5.6	5.7	5.8	5.9	6.0
Turkey	5.2	5.3	5.4	5.4	5.5	5.6	5.7
Turkmenistan	4.2	4.3	4.3	4.4	4.5	4.6	4.7
Ukraine	14.0	13.9	13.8	14.0	14.5	15.2	15.7
United Arab Emirates	1.0	1.0	1.0	1.0	1.0	1.0	0.9
United Kingdom	15.9	15.8	15.8	15.9	15.9	16.0	16.1
USA	12.7	12.7	12.6	12.5	12.4	12.3	12.3
Venezuela	4.3	4.4	4.4	4.5	4.6	4.7	4.8
Vietnam	5.2	5.3	5.3	5.4	5.4	5.4	5.4

Source: *Euromonitor International from national statistics/UN*

Male population (as at January 1st) 1998-2004

% of total

	1998	1999	2000	2001	2002	2003	2004
Algeria	50.5	50.5	50.5	50.5	50.5	50.5	50.5
Argentina	48.7	48.7	48.7	48.7	48.7	48.7	48.7
Australia	49.7	49.6	49.6	49.6	49.6	49.8	49.8
Austria	48.3	48.3	48.4	48.4	48.4	48.5	48.5
Azerbaijan	48.8	48.8	48.8	48.8	48.8	48.7	48.7
Belarus	46.9	47.0	46.9	46.9	46.9	46.9	46.8
Belgium	48.9	48.9	48.9	48.9	48.9	48.9	48.9
Bolivia	49.7	49.7	49.8	49.8	49.8	49.8	49.8
Brazil	49.4	49.3	49.3	49.3	49.3	49.2	49.2
Bulgaria	48.9	48.9	48.8	48.8	48.7	48.6	48.6
Canada	49.5	49.5	49.5	49.5	49.5	49.5	49.5
Chile	49.5	49.5	49.5	49.5	49.5	49.5	49.5
China	50.9	50.9	51.2	51.2	51.1	51.1	51.0
Colombia	49.4	49.4	49.4	49.4	49.4	49.4	49.4
Croatia	48.1	48.1	48.1	48.1	48.1	48.1	48.1
Czech Republic	48.7	48.7	48.7	48.7	48.7	48.7	48.7
Denmark	49.4	49.4	49.4	49.4	49.4	49.5	49.5
Ecuador	50.2	50.2	50.2	50.2	50.2	50.2	50.2
Egypt	50.8	51.2	51.2	51.2	51.1	51.1	51.1
Estonia	46.2	46.1	46.1	46.1	46.1	46.1	46.1
Finland	48.7	48.8	48.8	48.8	48.8	48.9	48.9
France	48.6	48.6	48.6	48.6	48.6	48.6	48.6
Germany	48.7	48.8	48.8	48.8	48.9	48.9	48.9
Greece	49.3	49.3	49.3	49.3	49.3	49.3	49.3
Hong Kong, China	49.7	49.4	49.2	48.9	48.6	48.3	48.0
Hungary	47.8	47.7	47.6	47.6	47.5	47.5	47.5
India	51.6	51.6	51.6	51.6	51.6	51.5	51.5
Indonesia	50.0	50.0	50.0	50.0	50.0	50.0	50.0
Ireland	49.6	49.6	49.7	49.7	49.7	49.7	49.7
Israel	49.3	49.3	49.3	49.3	49.3	49.3	49.3
Italy	48.6	48.5	48.5	48.6	48.6	48.5	48.5
Japan	49.0	48.9	48.9	48.9	48.8	48.8	48.8
Jordan	52.2	52.2	52.1	52.1	52.1	52.1	52.0
Kazakhstan	48.4	48.3	48.2	48.1	48.1	48.0	48.0
Kuwait	60.6	61.1	60.8	60.4	60.3	60.2	60.1
Latvia	46.1	46.1	46.1	46.1	46.0	46.0	46.0
Lithuania	46.9	46.9	46.8	46.8	46.7	46.7	46.7
Malaysia	51.2	51.2	50.9	50.9	50.9	50.9	50.9
Mexico	49.2	49.2	49.2	49.1	49.1	49.1	49.1
Morocco	50.1	50.1	50.1	50.1	50.1	50.1	50.1
Netherlands	49.4	49.4	49.5	49.5	49.5	49.5	49.5
New Zealand	49.2	49.1	49.1	49.0	49.1	49.1	49.1
Nigeria	50.3	50.3	50.3	50.3	50.3	50.4	50.4
Norway	49.5	49.5	49.5	49.5	49.6	49.6	49.6
Pakistan	51.2	51.2	51.2	51.2	51.2	51.2	51.2
Peru	50.3	50.3	50.3	50.3	50.3	50.3	50.3
Philippines	50.4	50.4	50.4	50.3	50.3	50.3	50.3
Poland	48.6	48.6	48.6	48.6	48.6	48.6	48.6
Portugal	48.2	48.2	48.2	48.3	48.3	48.3	48.3
Romania	49.0	48.9	48.9	48.9	48.9	48.8	48.8
Russia	46.9	46.9	46.9	46.8	46.7	46.7	46.6
Saudi Arabia	54.3	54.3	54.3	54.3	54.3	54.2	54.1
Singapore	50.1	50.0	50.0	49.9	49.8	49.8	49.7
Slovakia	48.6	48.6	48.6	48.6	48.6	48.6	48.7
Slovenia	48.8	48.7	48.8	48.9	48.9	48.9	48.9
South Africa	48.3	48.3	48.1	47.8	47.8	47.7	47.6
South Korea	50.2	50.2	50.2	50.1	50.2	50.2	50.2
Spain	48.9	48.9	48.9	48.9	48.9	49.0	49.0
Sweden	49.4	49.4	49.4	49.5	49.5	49.5	49.5
Switzerland	48.8	48.8	48.9	48.9	48.9	48.9	48.9
Taiwan	51.3	51.2	51.1	51.1	51.0	51.0	50.9
Thailand	49.7	49.5	49.5	49.5	49.4	49.4	49.4
Tunisia	50.4	50.4	50.4	50.4	50.4	50.4	50.3
Turkey	50.5	50.5	50.5	50.5	50.5	50.5	50.5
Turkmenistan	49.5	49.5	49.5	49.5	49.5	49.5	49.5
Ukraine	46.5	46.5	46.5	46.4	46.3	46.2	46.2
United Arab Emirates	67.1	67.2	67.4	67.6	67.7	67.8	67.9
United Kingdom	48.6	48.6	48.6	48.8	48.8	48.8	48.9
USA	48.9	48.9	48.9	48.9	48.9	48.9	49.0
Venezuela	50.4	50.3	50.3	50.3	50.3	50.3	50.3
Vietnam	49.8	49.8	49.8	49.8	49.8	49.8	49.8

Source: *Euromonitor International from national statistics/UN*

Female population (as at January 1st) 1998-2004

Table: 1.6

% of total

	1998	1999	2000	2001	2002	2003	2004
Algeria	49.5	49.5	49.5	49.5	49.5	49.5	49.5
Argentina	51.3	51.3	51.3	51.3	51.3	51.3	51.3
Australia	50.3	50.4	50.4	50.4	50.4	50.2	50.2
Austria	51.7	51.7	51.6	51.6	51.6	51.5	51.5
Azerbaijan	51.2	51.2	51.2	51.2	51.2	51.3	51.3
Belarus	53.1	53.0	53.1	53.1	53.1	53.1	53.2
Belgium	51.1	51.1	51.1	51.1	51.1	51.1	51.1
Bolivia	50.3	50.3	50.2	50.2	50.2	50.2	50.2
Brazil	50.6	50.7	50.7	50.7	50.7	50.8	50.8
Bulgaria	51.1	51.1	51.2	51.2	51.3	51.4	51.4
Canada	50.5	50.5	50.5	50.5	50.5	50.5	50.5
Chile	50.5	50.5	50.5	50.5	50.5	50.5	50.5
China	49.1	49.1	48.8	48.8	48.9	48.9	49.0
Colombia	50.6	50.6	50.6	50.6	50.6	50.6	50.6
Croatia	51.9	51.9	51.9	51.9	51.9	51.9	51.9
Czech Republic	51.3	51.3	51.3	51.3	51.3	51.3	51.3
Denmark	50.6	50.6	50.6	50.6	50.6	50.5	50.5
Ecuador	49.8	49.8	49.8	49.8	49.8	49.8	49.8
Egypt	49.2	48.8	48.8	48.8	48.9	48.9	48.9
Estonia	53.8	53.9	53.9	53.9	53.9	53.9	53.9
Finland	51.3	51.2	51.2	51.2	51.2	51.1	51.1
France	51.4	51.4	51.4	51.4	51.4	51.4	51.4
Germany	51.3	51.2	51.2	51.2	51.1	51.1	51.1
Greece	50.7	50.7	50.7	50.7	50.7	50.7	50.7
Hong Kong, China	50.3	50.6	50.8	51.1	51.4	51.7	52.0
Hungary	52.2	52.3	52.4	52.4	52.5	52.5	52.5
India	48.4	48.4	48.4	48.4	48.4	48.5	48.5
Indonesia	50.0	50.0	50.0	50.0	50.0	50.0	50.0
Ireland	50.4	50.4	50.3	50.3	50.3	50.3	50.3
Israel	50.7	50.7	50.7	50.7	50.7	50.7	50.7
Italy	51.4	51.5	51.5	51.4	51.4	51.5	51.5
Japan	51.0	51.1	51.1	51.1	51.2	51.2	51.2
Jordan	47.8	47.8	47.9	47.9	47.9	47.9	48.0
Kazakhstan	51.6	51.7	51.8	51.9	51.9	52.0	52.0
Kuwait	39.4	38.9	39.2	39.6	39.7	39.8	39.9
Latvia	53.9	53.9	53.9	53.9	54.0	54.0	54.0
Lithuania	53.1	53.1	53.2	53.2	53.3	53.3	53.3
Malaysia	48.8	48.8	49.1	49.1	49.1	49.1	49.1
Mexico	50.8	50.8	50.8	50.9	50.9	50.9	50.9
Morocco	49.9	49.9	49.9	49.9	49.9	49.9	49.9
Netherlands	50.6	50.6	50.5	50.5	50.5	50.5	50.5
New Zealand	50.8	50.9	50.9	51.0	50.9	50.9	50.9
Nigeria	49.7	49.7	49.7	49.7	49.7	49.6	49.6
Norway	50.5	50.5	50.5	50.5	50.4	50.4	50.4
Pakistan	48.8	48.8	48.8	48.8	48.8	48.8	48.8
Peru	49.7	49.7	49.7	49.7	49.7	49.7	49.7
Philippines	49.6	49.6	49.6	49.7	49.7	49.7	49.7
Poland	51.4	51.4	51.4	51.4	51.4	51.4	51.4
Portugal	51.8	51.8	51.8	51.7	51.7	51.7	51.7
Romania	51.0	51.1	51.1	51.1	51.1	51.2	51.2
Russia	53.1	53.1	53.1	53.2	53.3	53.3	53.4
Saudi Arabia	45.7	45.7	45.7	45.7	45.7	45.8	45.9
Singapore	49.9	50.0	50.0	50.1	50.2	50.2	50.3
Slovakia	51.4	51.4	51.4	51.4	51.4	51.4	51.3
Slovenia	51.2	51.3	51.2	51.1	51.1	51.1	51.1
South Africa	51.7	51.7	51.9	52.2	52.2	52.3	52.4
South Korea	49.8	49.8	49.8	49.9	49.8	49.8	49.8
Spain	51.1	51.1	51.1	51.1	51.1	51.0	51.0
Sweden	50.6	50.6	50.6	50.5	50.5	50.5	50.5
Switzerland	51.2	51.2	51.1	51.1	51.1	51.1	51.1
Taiwan	48.7	48.8	48.9	48.9	49.0	49.0	49.1
Thailand	50.3	50.5	50.5	50.5	50.6	50.6	50.6
Tunisia	49.6	49.6	49.6	49.6	49.6	49.6	49.7
Turkey	49.5	49.5	49.5	49.5	49.5	49.5	49.5
Turkmenistan	50.5	50.5	50.5	50.5	50.5	50.5	50.5
Ukraine	53.5	53.5	53.5	53.6	53.7	53.8	53.8
United Arab Emirates	32.9	32.8	32.6	32.4	32.3	32.2	32.1
United Kingdom	51.4	51.4	51.4	51.2	51.2	51.2	51.1
USA	51.1	51.1	51.1	51.1	51.1	51.1	51.0
Venezuela	49.6	49.7	49.7	49.7	49.7	49.7	49.7
Vietnam	50.2	50.2	50.2	50.2	50.2	50.2	50.2

Source: *Euromonitor International from national statistics/UN*

Median age of population 1998-2004

years

	1998	1999	2000	2001	2002	2003	2004
Algeria	20.6	21.0	21.4	21.8	22.2	22.5	22.9
Argentina	27.3	27.4	27.5	27.7	27.8	28.0	28.1
Australia	34.8	35.1	35.4	35.7	35.9	36.0	36.3
Austria	37.4	37.7	38.1	38.6	39.0	39.3	39.6
Azerbaijan	24.9	25.2	25.5	25.7	26.0	26.3	26.5
Belarus	35.6	36.0	36.3	36.6	36.9	37.1	37.4
Belgium	38.2	38.5	38.7	39.0	39.3	39.5	39.7
Bolivia	19.8	19.9	20.0	20.2	20.3	20.5	20.6
Brazil	24.9	25.3	25.6	25.9	26.2	26.6	26.9
Bulgaria	38.7	38.9	39.1	39.3	40.1	40.4	40.5
Canada	36.0	36.4	36.8	37.2	37.6	37.9	38.2
Chile	27.8	28.1	28.3	28.6	28.8	29.1	29.4
China	30.5	31.1	31.2	32.1	33.1	33.5	33.9
Colombia	23.4	23.6	23.9	24.1	24.4	24.7	25.0
Croatia	35.9	36.0	39.1	39.3	39.5	39.7	39.9
Czech Republic	36.8	37.1	37.3	37.6	37.9	38.2	38.4
Denmark	37.9	38.1	38.2	38.4	38.6	38.8	39.0
Ecuador	21.9	22.2	22.5	22.8	23.1	23.4	23.7
Egypt	21.5	20.8	20.9	21.2	21.5	21.8	22.2
Estonia	37.1	37.5	37.8	38.1	38.3	38.5	38.7
Finland	38.6	38.9	39.2	39.5	39.8	40.1	40.5
France	37.0	37.3	37.5	37.8	38.0	38.2	38.4
Germany	39.1	39.4	39.8	40.2	40.6	40.8	41.1
Greece	38.2	38.5	38.8	39.1	39.4	39.7	40.0
Hong Kong, China	35.2	35.7	36.2	36.8	37.5	37.7	38.2
Hungary	37.9	38.0	38.5	38.6	38.7	38.8	38.9
India	22.9	23.1	23.3	23.5	23.7	23.9	24.1
Indonesia	23.8	24.1	24.4	24.7	25.0	25.4	25.7
Ireland	31.6	31.8	31.9	32.1	32.2	32.3	32.5
Israel	27.3	27.4	27.6	27.7	27.9	28.1	28.3
Italy	39.3	39.7	40.0	40.3	40.5	40.8	41.0
Japan	40.7	41.0	41.5	41.8	42.1	42.2	42.3
Jordan	19.4	19.7	19.9	20.2	20.5	20.7	21.0
Kazakhstan	27.5	27.6	27.7	27.9	28.2	28.5	28.8
Kuwait	28.7	29.0	28.8	29.0	29.3	29.6	30.0
Latvia	37.1	37.5	37.9	38.3	38.5	38.8	39.0
Lithuania	35.0	35.4	35.8	36.2	36.6	36.9	37.3
Malaysia	23.1	23.3	23.3	23.5	23.6	23.8	24.0
Mexico	22.0	22.3	22.6	23.0	23.4	23.7	24.1
Morocco	22.1	22.4	22.7	23.1	23.4	23.8	24.1
Netherlands	36.7	37.0	37.3	37.6	37.8	38.1	38.4
New Zealand	33.6	34.0	34.3	34.7	34.9	35.0	35.2
Nigeria	17.0	17.0	17.1	17.2	17.3	17.4	17.5
Norway	36.5	36.6	36.7	36.9	37.1	37.3	37.6
Pakistan	18.4	18.5	18.6	18.7	18.8	18.9	19.0
Peru	22.0	22.3	22.6	22.8	23.1	23.4	23.7
Philippines	21.1	21.2	21.4	21.6	21.7	21.9	22.1
Poland	34.6	34.8	35.1	35.4	35.7	35.9	36.2
Portugal	36.8	37.2	37.7	38.1	38.3	38.6	38.8
Romania	34.3	34.3	34.4	34.4	34.7	35.2	35.6
Russia	36.1	36.5	36.8	37.1	37.4	37.5	37.7
Saudi Arabia	20.1	20.1	20.1	20.1	20.1	20.2	20.3
Singapore	33.2	33.7	34.2	34.6	35.0	35.4	35.8
Slovakia	33.3	33.6	33.9	34.1	34.4	34.7	35.0
Slovenia	36.9	37.4	37.8	38.2	38.6	39.0	39.3
South Africa	23.1	23.2	23.3	23.5	23.6	23.8	24.0
South Korea	31.0	31.5	32.0	32.5	33.0	33.6	34.1
Spain	36.6	37.0	37.4	37.7	38.0	38.3	38.6
Sweden	38.9	39.1	39.3	39.4	39.6	39.7	39.9
Switzerland	37.9	38.2	38.5	38.8	39.1	39.3	39.6
Taiwan	31.2	31.6	32.1	32.6	33.1	33.5	34.0
Thailand	28.8	29.2	29.7	30.2	30.7	31.2	31.6
Tunisia	23.4	23.8	24.2	24.6	25.0	25.5	26.0
Turkey	24.4	24.7	25.0	25.4	25.7	26.0	26.4
Turkmenistan	20.8	21.1	21.4	21.7	22.0	22.4	22.7
Ukraine	36.8	37.1	37.4	37.7	38.3	38.7	39.0
United Arab Emirates	27.7	27.8	28.0	28.2	28.3	28.5	28.6
United Kingdom	37.2	37.4	37.7	37.9	38.2	38.4	38.7
USA	35.2	35.5	35.7	36.0	36.1	36.3	36.4
Venezuela	22.4	22.7	22.9	23.2	23.5	23.8	24.1
Vietnam	22.1	22.5	22.9	23.3	23.6	24.0	24.4

Source: *UN/Eurostat/Euromonitor International*

Population living below international poverty line (US$2 per day) 1998-2002

Table: 1.8

% of people

	1998	1999	2000	2001	2002
Algeria					
Argentina				14.3	
Australia					
Austria					
Azerbaijan					
Belarus			2.0		
Belgium					
Bolivia		34.3			
Brazil				22.4	
Bulgaria				16.2	
Canada					
Chile			9.6		
China				46.7	
Colombia		22.6			
Croatia			2.0		
Czech Republic					
Denmark					
Ecuador	40.8				
Egypt			43.9		
Estonia	5.2				
Finland					
France					
Germany					
Greece					
Hong Kong, China					
Hungary	7.3				
India			79.9		
Indonesia					52.4
Ireland					
Israel					
Italy					
Japan					
Jordan					
Kazakhstan				8.4	
Kuwait					
Latvia	8.3				
Lithuania			13.7		
Malaysia					
Mexico			26.3		
Morocco		14.3			
Netherlands					
New Zealand					
Nigeria					
Norway					
Pakistan	65.6				
Peru			37.7		
Philippines			46.4		
Poland		2.0			
Portugal					
Romania			20.5		
Russia			23.8		
Saudi Arabia					
Singapore					
Slovakia					
Slovenia	2.0				
South Africa					
South Korea	2.0				
Spain					
Sweden					
Switzerland					
Taiwan					
Thailand			32.5		
Tunisia			6.6		
Turkey			10.3		
Turkmenistan	44.0				
Ukraine		45.6			
United Arab Emirates					
United Kingdom					
USA					
Venezuela	32.0				
Vietnam	63.7				

Source: Euromonitor International from national statistics

▪ Births

Fertility rates 1998-2004

Table: 1.9

children born per female

	1998	1999	2000	2001	2002	2003	2004
Algeria	2.59	2.53	2.49	2.47	2.48	2.50	2.52
Argentina	2.43	2.40	2.37	2.35	2.33	2.31	2.29
Australia	1.76	1.75	1.75	1.73	1.71	1.69	1.67
Austria	1.37	1.34	1.36	1.33	1.40	1.37	1.37
Azerbaijan	1.89	1.72	1.71	1.60	1.67	1.78	1.90
Belarus	1.26	1.29	1.31	1.27	1.24	1.22	1.21
Belgium	1.59	1.61	1.66	1.64	1.63	1.62	1.61
Bolivia	3.78	3.74	3.69	3.65	3.60	3.56	3.53
Brazil	2.53	2.52	2.51	2.49	2.47	2.45	2.44
Bulgaria	1.11	1.23	1.30	1.24	1.21	1.21	1.23
Canada	1.60	1.60	1.60	1.56	1.57	1.55	1.54
Chile	2.33	2.26	2.22	2.18	2.16	2.16	2.14
China	2.06	1.96	1.90	1.84	1.79	1.76	1.74
Colombia	2.27	2.30	2.29	2.19	2.06	2.02	2.01
Croatia	1.45	1.38	1.40	1.38	1.38	1.38	1.35
Czech Republic	1.16	1.13	1.14	1.14	1.16	1.15	1.15
Denmark	1.72	1.73	1.77	1.74	1.74	1.73	1.71
Ecuador	2.77	2.96	2.94	2.90	2.85	2.81	2.78
Egypt	3.25	3.20	3.24	3.17	3.18	3.18	3.17
Estonia	1.21	1.28	1.39	1.34	1.37	1.38	1.40
Finland	1.70	1.74	1.73	1.73	1.72	1.72	1.72
France	1.76	1.79	1.89	1.90	1.92	1.92	1.91
Germany	1.36	1.36	1.38	1.42	1.42	1.41	1.41
Greece	1.29	1.28	1.29	1.27	1.27	1.26	1.25
Hong Kong, China	0.99	0.96	1.02	0.93	0.96	0.95	0.96
Hungary	1.32	1.28	1.32	1.31	1.30	1.29	1.30
India	3.19	3.14	3.09	3.02	2.95	2.88	2.81
Indonesia	2.57	2.54	2.52	2.49	2.46	2.44	2.41
Ireland	1.94	1.90	1.88	1.97	1.98	2.01	2.03
Israel	2.68	2.65	2.67	2.62	2.62	2.59	2.57
Italy	1.20	1.22	1.24	1.23	1.25	1.27	1.29
Japan	1.45	1.40	1.36	1.33	1.32	1.32	1.31
Jordan	3.30	3.27	3.24	3.19	3.13	3.07	3.00
Kazakhstan	1.68	1.79	1.89	1.95	1.97	1.96	1.94
Kuwait	2.45	2.31	2.38	2.34	2.35	2.35	2.34
Latvia	1.10	1.18	1.24	1.21	1.24	1.23	1.24
Lithuania	1.46	1.46	1.39	1.30	1.24	1.23	1.24
Malaysia	2.87	2.80	2.76	2.72	2.69	2.67	2.65
Mexico	2.78	2.71	2.59	2.53	2.48	2.44	2.41
Morocco	2.79	2.74	2.70	2.67	2.64	2.64	2.61
Netherlands	1.63	1.65	1.72	1.71	1.71	1.69	1.66
New Zealand	1.98	2.04	2.01	1.97	1.93	1.92	1.90
Nigeria	4.06	4.02	3.97	3.93	3.89	3.85	3.81
Norway	1.81	1.84	1.85	1.78	1.77	1.73	1.72
Pakistan	3.57	3.54	3.51	3.49	3.49	3.49	3.49
Peru	2.81	2.76	2.71	2.66	2.62	2.58	2.55
Philippines	2.78	2.71	2.66	2.65	2.61	2.58	2.54
Poland	1.44	1.37	1.34	1.29	1.27	1.26	1.26
Portugal	1.47	1.50	1.55	1.46	1.48	1.49	1.50
Romania	1.32	1.30	1.31	1.24	1.25	1.24	1.23
Russia	1.25	1.17	1.21	1.25	1.31	1.29	1.31
Saudi Arabia	3.99	3.96	3.94	3.90	3.90	3.90	3.90
Singapore	1.47	1.47	1.59	1.41	1.37	1.34	1.33
Slovakia	1.38	1.33	1.29	1.20	1.18	1.17	1.16
Slovenia	1.23	1.21	1.26	1.21	1.19	1.18	1.17
South Africa	1.88	1.82	1.84	1.66	1.53	1.52	1.52
South Korea	1.92	1.85	1.88	1.70	1.56	1.68	1.64
Spain	1.16	1.20	1.24	1.26	1.27	1.29	1.30
Sweden	1.50	1.50	1.54	1.57	1.57	1.58	1.60
Switzerland	1.47	1.48	1.50	1.41	1.38	1.37	1.36
Taiwan	1.74	1.79	1.88	1.67	1.60	1.51	1.51
Thailand	1.98	1.82	1.97	1.92	1.90	1.89	1.87
Tunisia	2.29	2.19	2.21	2.19	2.17	2.19	2.22
Turkey	2.63	2.60	2.52	2.50	2.46	2.43	2.38
Turkmenistan	2.73	2.55	2.43	2.40	2.44	2.55	2.66
Ukraine	1.19	1.10	1.10	1.09	1.04	1.03	1.03
United Arab Emirates	2.20	2.14	2.15	2.11	2.05	2.01	2.00
United Kingdom	1.71	1.68	1.65	1.63	1.63	1.65	1.65
USA	2.02	1.99	1.99	1.99	1.99	1.99	1.99
Venezuela	2.65	2.72	2.74	2.64	2.45	2.40	2.36
Vietnam	2.29	2.16	2.09	2.08	2.12	2.21	2.30

Source: National statistical offices/UN/Euromonitor International

Birth rates 1998-2004

Table: 1.10

number per '000 inhabitants

	1998	1999	2000	2001	2002	2003	2004
Algeria	20.9	20.3	19.9	19.7	19.8	20.0	20.2
Argentina	19.1	18.8	18.5	18.2	18.3	18.1	17.9
Australia	13.3	13.2	12.9	12.7	12.5	12.3	12.1
Austria	10.2	9.8	9.8	9.4	9.7	9.4	9.4
Azerbaijan	15.5	14.5	14.3	13.4	13.7	14.8	16.0
Belarus	9.2	9.3	9.4	9.2	8.9	8.7	8.6
Belgium	11.2	11.1	11.2	11.1	11.0	10.9	10.8
Bolivia	32.8	32.4	31.9	31.5	31.0	30.6	30.3
Brazil	20.3	20.2	20.1	19.9	19.7	19.5	19.4
Bulgaria	8.0	8.9	9.2	8.6	8.5	8.2	8.4
Canada	11.5	11.2	11.0	10.6	10.7	10.5	10.4
Chile	18.3	17.6	17.2	16.8	16.6	16.6	16.4
China	15.6	14.6	14.0	13.4	12.9	12.6	12.4
Colombia	17.7	18.0	17.9	16.9	15.6	15.2	15.1
Croatia	10.4	10.0	9.8	9.2	9.2	9.2	8.9
Czech Republic	8.8	8.7	8.9	8.9	9.1	9.0	9.0
Denmark	12.5	12.4	12.6	12.2	12.2	12.1	11.9
Ecuador	22.7	24.6	24.4	24.0	23.5	23.1	22.8
Egypt	27.5	27.0	27.4	26.7	26.8	26.8	26.7
Estonia	8.9	9.1	9.6	9.3	9.6	9.7	9.9
Finland	11.1	11.1	11.0	10.8	10.7	10.7	10.7
France	12.6	12.7	13.2	13.1	13.3	13.3	13.2
Germany	9.6	9.4	9.3	8.9	8.9	8.8	8.8
Greece	9.6	9.6	9.6	9.4	9.4	9.3	9.2
Hong Kong, China	8.1	7.8	8.1	7.2	7.1	7.0	7.1
Hungary	9.5	9.2	9.6	9.5	9.5	9.3	9.4
India	26.9	26.4	25.9	25.2	24.5	23.8	23.1
Indonesia	18.7	18.4	18.2	17.9	17.6	17.4	17.1
Ireland	14.5	14.4	14.3	15.0	15.1	15.4	15.6
Israel	21.8	21.5	21.7	21.2	21.2	20.9	20.7
Italy	9.0	9.3	9.4	9.2	9.3	9.3	9.3
Japan	9.5	9.3	9.4	9.2	9.1	9.1	9.0
Jordan	28.0	27.7	27.4	26.9	26.3	25.7	25.0
Kazakhstan	11.8	12.9	13.9	14.5	14.7	14.6	14.4
Kuwait	19.5	18.1	18.8	18.4	18.5	18.5	18.4
Latvia	7.6	8.1	8.5	8.3	8.6	8.5	8.6
Lithuania	10.4	10.3	9.8	9.1	8.7	8.5	8.6
Malaysia	23.7	23.0	22.6	22.2	21.9	21.7	21.5
Mexico	22.8	22.1	20.9	20.3	19.8	19.4	19.1
Morocco	22.9	22.4	22.0	21.7	21.4	21.4	21.1
Netherlands	12.7	12.7	13.0	12.7	12.7	12.5	12.2
New Zealand	14.9	15.1	14.7	14.1	13.7	13.6	13.4
Nigeria	35.6	35.2	34.7	34.3	33.9	33.5	33.1
Norway	13.2	13.3	13.2	12.6	12.5	12.1	12.0
Pakistan	30.7	30.4	30.1	29.9	29.9	29.9	29.9
Peru	21.1	20.6	20.1	19.6	19.2	18.8	18.5
Philippines	22.3	21.6	23.1	21.5	21.1	20.8	20.4
Poland	10.2	9.9	9.8	9.5	9.3	9.2	9.2
Portugal	11.2	11.4	11.7	10.9	11.1	11.2	11.3
Romania	10.5	10.4	10.4	10.2	10.2	10.1	10.0
Russia	8.8	8.3	8.7	9.1	9.7	9.5	9.7
Saudi Arabia	34.9	34.6	34.4	34.0	34.0	34.0	34.0
Singapore	13.1	12.8	13.7	11.8	11.4	11.1	11.0
Slovakia	10.7	10.5	10.3	9.5	9.3	9.2	9.1
Slovenia	9.0	8.8	9.1	8.8	8.6	8.5	8.4
South Africa	13.8	13.2	13.4	11.6	10.3	10.2	10.2
South Korea	14.2	13.5	13.8	12.0	10.6	11.8	11.4
Spain	9.3	9.6	10.0	10.0	10.1	10.3	10.4
Sweden	10.1	10.0	10.2	10.3	10.3	10.4	10.6
Switzerland	11.1	11.0	10.9	10.2	9.9	9.8	9.7
Taiwan	12.4	12.9	13.8	11.7	11.0	10.1	10.1
Thailand	14.8	13.2	14.7	14.2	14.0	13.9	13.7
Tunisia	17.9	16.9	17.1	16.9	16.7	16.9	17.2
Turkey	23.0	22.6	22.1	21.6	21.2	20.9	20.4
Turkmenistan	22.3	20.5	19.3	19.0	19.4	20.5	21.6
Ukraine	8.4	7.8	7.8	7.7	7.2	7.1	7.1
United Arab Emirates	17.0	16.4	16.5	16.1	15.5	15.1	15.0
United Kingdom	10.9	10.6	10.3	10.1	10.1	10.3	10.3
USA	14.6	14.3	14.3	14.3	14.3	14.3	14.3
Venezuela	21.5	22.2	22.4	21.4	19.5	19.0	18.6
Vietnam	17.9	16.6	15.9	15.8	16.2	17.1	18.0

Source: National statistical offices/UN/Euromonitor International

Number of live births 1998-2004

Table: 1.11

'000

	1998	1999	2000	2001	2002	2003	2004
Algeria	613.6	604.1	602.8	605.3	617.6	636.1	653.7
Argentina	677.3	674.6	671.7	670.3	669.7	668.9	668.3
Australia	249.5	250.0	248.0	247.3	246.2	243.1	241.7
Austria	81.2	78.1	78.3	75.5	78.4	76.2	75.8
Azerbaijan	124.0	117.5	117.0	110.4	113.4	123.6	134.9
Belarus	92.6	93.0	93.7	91.7	88.4	85.6	84.9
Belgium	114.3	113.5	114.9	114.2	113.8	113.0	112.1
Bolivia	262.0	263.7	265.4	266.9	267.7	269.5	271.8
Brazil	3,367.1	3,389.4	3,411.4	3,428.2	3,439.8	3,447.8	3,470.6
Bulgaria	65.4	72.3	73.7	68.2	66.5	64.1	64.9
Canada	344.1	338.3	336.9	327.1	332.8	331.5	330.7
Chile	270.6	263.9	261.6	258.8	259.2	261.2	261.6
China	19,427.7	18,348.6	17,725.4	17,022.9	16,472.5	16,261.5	16,131.5
Colombia	721.0	746.2	752.8	724.3	678.4	671.8	679.4
Croatia	47.1	45.2	43.7	41.0	41.0	40.9	39.7
Czech Republic	90.5	89.5	90.9	90.7	92.8	91.8	92.2
Denmark	66.2	66.2	67.1	65.5	65.4	65.0	64.7
Ecuador	272.9	300.7	303.0	302.2	301.1	300.5	300.1
Egypt	1,689.0	1,690.8	1,749.8	1,736.2	1,772.9	1,801.8	1,823.4
Estonia	12.3	12.5	13.1	12.6	13.0	13.1	13.3
Finland	57.1	57.6	56.7	56.2	55.6	55.7	55.6
France	738.1	744.8	774.8	774.8	789.9	793.0	794.4
Germany	785.0	770.7	767.0	730.0	736.1	730.2	724.4
Greece	100.9	100.6	101.0	100.0	99.6	99.2	97.5
Hong Kong, China	53.0	51.3	54.1	48.2	48.2	48.0	49.2
Hungary	97.3	94.6	97.6	96.8	96.8	94.5	95.0
India	26,421.3	26,403.7	26,291.8	26,067.1	25,727.8	25,324.2	24,952.5
Indonesia	3,845.9	3,845.8	3,843.8	3,838.2	3,829.0	3,817.2	3,804.3
Ireland	54.0	53.9	54.2	57.9	58.8	60.9	62.5
Israel	130.1	131.9	136.4	136.6	139.5	141.0	142.6
Italy	515.4	537.2	543.0	533.7	538.6	541.0	541.1
Japan	1,203.1	1,177.7	1,190.5	1,170.7	1,153.9	1,161.4	1,153.4
Jordan	132.7	135.5	137.8	139.4	140.2	140.5	140.4
Kazakhstan	188.8	204.0	217.3	225.0	227.2	225.5	221.5
Kuwait	41.4	41.1	41.8	41.2	42.6	43.6	44.4
Latvia	18.4	19.4	20.2	19.7	20.0	19.8	19.9
Lithuania	37.0	36.4	34.1	31.5	30.0	29.4	29.5
Malaysia	524.8	521.9	530.0	534.1	537.1	544.2	551.1
Mexico	2,186.5	2,154.6	2,071.2	2,043.7	2,014.1	2,004.7	2,001.5
Morocco	645.8	642.1	641.0	642.7	644.3	654.3	654.3
Netherlands	199.4	200.4	206.6	203.1	205.8	202.2	198.9
New Zealand	56.9	57.9	56.6	54.7	54.0	53.8	53.6
Nigeria	3,863.8	3,926.1	3,986.6	4,045.8	4,103.3	4,159.0	4,212.8
Norway	58.4	59.3	59.2	56.7	56.6	55.2	55.2
Pakistan	4,157.8	4,220.1	4,293.5	4,380.0	4,479.7	4,588.2	4,697.5
Peru	530.7	525.9	521.3	517.5	514.4	512.0	510.3
Philippines	1,632.9	1,613.3	1,766.4	1,679.8	1,683.8	1,686.7	1,688.6
Poland	395.6	382.0	378.3	368.2	357.4	355.7	354.6
Portugal	113.4	116.0	120.0	112.8	114.5	116.7	118.3
Romania	237.3	234.6	234.5	229.2	227.1	225.2	222.6
Russia	1,283.3	1,214.7	1,266.8	1,311.6	1,397.0	1,362.9	1,380.9
Saudi Arabia	692.4	703.7	717.2	733.2	757.8	782.8	807.6
Singapore	41.6	41.2	44.7	39.2	38.5	38.2	38.2
Slovakia	57.6	56.2	55.2	51.1	50.3	49.5	48.9
Slovenia	17.9	17.5	18.2	17.5	17.2	17.0	16.8
South Africa	581.4	568.3	587.6	519.9	470.2	473.6	486.0
South Korea	643.0	616.3	636.8	557.2	494.6	554.1	536.2
Spain	365.2	380.1	397.6	403.9	408.6	418.9	426.0
Sweden	89.0	88.2	90.4	91.5	91.6	93.3	95.3
Switzerland	78.9	78.4	78.5	73.5	72.3	71.7	71.1
Taiwan	271.4	283.7	305.3	260.3	247.5	227.1	229.9
Thailand	862.3	774.3	867.4	841.8	840.5	840.5	839.1
Tunisia	166.5	159.0	162.7	162.6	162.4	166.3	171.2
Turkey	1,498.4	1,501.1	1,488.7	1,483.3	1,478.6	1,475.1	1,463.5
Turkmenistan	99.9	93.3	89.5	89.5	93.2	99.6	106.7
Ukraine	419.2	389.2	385.1	376.5	345.2	339.8	335.0
United Arab Emirates	48.1	49.7	53.7	56.1	58.1	60.0	62.6
United Kingdom	635.9	621.9	604.4	594.6	596.1	610.5	612.8
USA	3,938.5	3,911.9	3,933.4	3,960.5	3,993.5	4,031.4	4,073.2
Venezuela	501.8	527.9	544.4	529.6	492.7	487.4	488.0
Vietnam	1,360.1	1,282.6	1,241.2	1,248.1	1,304.0	1,393.2	1,487.1

Source: *National statistical offices/UN/Euromonitor International*

Infant mortality rates 1998-2004

Table: 1.12

number per '000 live births

	1998	1999	2000	2001	2002	2003	2004
Algeria	48.8	47.5	46.1	44.5	42.8	41.7	40.4
Argentina	21.5	21.2	20.8	20.4	20.0	19.7	19.3
Australia	5.4	5.3	5.3	5.2	5.2	5.2	5.1
Austria	5.3	5.2	5.0	4.9	4.7	4.7	4.6
Azerbaijan	32.0	31.4	30.8	30.1	29.3	28.9	28.5
Belarus	12.5	12.5	12.5	12.5	12.5	12.3	12.1
Belgium	4.4	4.3	4.3	4.3	4.2	4.2	4.2
Bolivia	64.0	62.2	60.2	58.0	55.6	54.0	52.2
Brazil	41.5	40.8	40.1	39.2	38.3	37.6	36.8
Bulgaria	15.2	15.2	15.2	15.2	15.2	15.0	14.8
Canada	5.5	5.5	5.4	5.4	5.4	5.3	5.3
Chile	12.6	12.4	12.1	11.9	11.6	11.4	11.2
China	40.7	39.8	38.8	37.7	36.5	35.9	35.1
Colombia	29.3	28.5	27.6	26.6	25.6	25.0	24.4
Croatia	9.8	9.4	9.0	8.6	8.1	8.0	7.9
Czech Republic	5.7	5.7	5.6	5.5	5.4	5.3	5.2
Denmark	5.8	5.6	5.5	5.3	5.0	5.0	5.0
Ecuador	44.9	44.2	43.3	42.4	41.5	40.8	40.1
Egypt	49.2	47.3	45.2	43.0	40.5	39.2	37.8
Estonia	10.9	10.7	10.4	10.1	9.7	9.6	9.4
Finland	4.3	4.2	4.2	4.1	4.0	4.0	3.9
France	5.4	5.3	5.2	5.1	5.0	5.0	4.9
Germany	4.9	4.9	4.8	4.7	4.6	4.5	4.5
Greece	6.6	6.5	6.4	6.4	6.3	6.3	6.2
Hong Kong, China	4.2	4.2	4.1	4.1	4.1	4.0	4.0
Hungary	9.5	9.3	9.1	8.9	8.7	8.6	8.5
India	71.3	69.9	68.3	66.6	64.7	63.5	62.1
Indonesia	47.0	45.4	43.6	41.7	39.5	38.4	37.2
Ireland	6.5	6.4	6.3	6.1	6.0	5.9	5.9
Israel	6.3	6.2	6.1	6.0	5.9	5.9	5.8
Italy	5.5	5.5	5.5	5.4	5.4	5.3	5.3
Japan	3.5	3.5	3.4	3.4	3.3	3.3	3.3
Jordan	26.0	25.3	24.4	23.6	22.6	22.1	21.5
Kazakhstan	44.3	43.8	43.3	42.7	42.1	41.3	40.4
Kuwait	12.1	11.8	11.5	11.2	10.8	10.7	10.5
Latvia	15.3	14.9	14.5	14.1	13.6	13.4	13.1
Lithuania	10.4	10.1	9.7	9.4	8.9	8.9	8.8
Malaysia	11.4	11.2	10.9	10.6	10.3	10.1	9.9
Mexico	30.5	30.0	29.5	28.9	28.2	27.8	27.3
Morocco	50.6	48.8	46.7	44.5	42.1	41.0	39.7
Netherlands	4.6	4.6	4.5	4.5	4.5	4.5	4.5
New Zealand	6.5	6.5	6.4	6.3	6.2	6.1	6.1
Nigeria	86.6	84.8	82.9	80.8	78.5	77.0	75.3
Norway	4.7	4.7	4.6	4.6	4.5	4.5	4.4
Pakistan	93.9	92.3	90.6	88.6	86.5	85.1	83.6
Peru	43.8	42.4	40.9	39.2	37.4	36.4	35.4
Philippines	33.5	32.5	31.5	30.3	29.0	28.3	27.6
Poland	9.9	9.7	9.5	9.3	9.1	8.9	8.8
Portugal	6.5	6.4	6.3	6.2	6.1	6.0	6.0
Romania	22.1	22.1	22.1	22.1	22.1	21.5	20.9
Russia	16.7	16.7	16.8	16.8	16.8	16.6	16.3
Saudi Arabia	24.3	23.5	22.6	21.6	20.6	20.0	19.4
Singapore	4.8	4.8	4.7	4.6	4.6	4.6	4.5
Slovakia	8.5	8.4	8.2	8.1	8.0	7.9	7.8
Slovenia	6.0	5.9	5.8	5.7	5.6	5.5	5.4
South Africa	58.3	58.5	58.7	59.0	59.2	58.7	58.1
South Korea	7.8	7.6	7.5	7.3	7.1	7.0	6.8
Spain	5.7	5.6	5.5	5.4	5.3	5.3	5.3
Sweden	3.5	3.5	3.5	3.4	3.4	3.4	3.4
Switzerland	5.0	5.0	4.9	4.8	4.8	4.7	4.7
Taiwan	9.5	9.1	8.6	8.3	8.1	7.9	7.7
Thailand	24.7	23.8	22.9	21.9	20.8	20.4	19.9
Tunisia	29.5	28.7	27.7	26.7	25.5	24.8	24.0
Turkey	44.6	43.3	41.9	40.3	38.5	37.7	36.7
Turkmenistan	53.8	52.7	51.5	50.1	48.6	47.9	47.2
Ukraine	15.3	15.3	15.3	15.3	15.3	15.1	14.8
United Arab Emirates	11.8	11.6	11.4	11.2	10.9	10.8	10.6
United Kingdom	5.8	5.7	5.6	5.5	5.4	5.3	5.3
USA	7.5	7.4	7.2	7.0	6.8	6.7	6.6
Venezuela	20.6	20.2	19.8	19.4	18.9	18.6	18.2
Vietnam	39.1	37.9	36.6	35.1	33.6	32.8	32.0

Source: *Euromonitor International from UN/national statistical offices/Eurostat*

Number of legal abortions 1998-2004

Table: 1.13

number

	1998	1999	2000	2001	2002	2003	2004
Algeria							
Argentina							
Australia	90,854	87,605	85,194	88,008	87,467	85,657	85,789
Austria	18,286	14,403	11,769	10,033	9,372	8,772	8,018
Azerbaijan	24,914	20,878	17,501	18,332	16,606	16,618	16,137
Belarus							
Belgium	11,999	12,734	13,762	14,775	15,798	16,819	17,785
Bolivia							
Brazil							
Bulgaria	79,842	72,382	61,378	51,165	50,824	50,735	49,841
Canada	110,331	105,666	105,427	106,418	106,950	107,378	107,163
Chile							
China	7,176,304	6,633,516	7,026,421	5,771,199	5,429,508	5,008,346	4,511,625
Colombia							
Croatia	8,907	8,064	7,534	6,574	6,191	5,802	5,409
Czech Republic	42,959	39,382	34,623	32,528	31,142	29,137	27,543
Denmark	16,592	16,271	15,681	15,315	14,790	14,264	13,747
Ecuador							
Egypt							
Estonia	15,798	14,503	12,743	11,653	10,834	9,815	8,898
Finland	10,744	10,819	10,930	10,694	10,908	10,811	10,876
France							
Germany	131,360	133,524	134,609	134,964	130,387	128,030	127,241
Greece	14,675	15,056	15,448	15,680	16,417	16,581	16,929
Hong Kong, China							
Hungary	68,971	65,981	59,249	56,404	56,075	52,303	47,377
India							
Indonesia							
Ireland							
Israel							
Italy	123,617	138,708	132,685	129,871	126,164	129,215	129,484
Japan							
Jordan							
Kazakhstan							
Kuwait							
Latvia	19,964	18,031	17,240	15,647	14,685	13,819	12,885
Lithuania	21,022	18,846	16,259	13,677	12,495	11,302	10,831
Malaysia							
Mexico							
Morocco							
Netherlands	23,163	23,819	24,494	24,524	24,764	25,117	25,505
New Zealand	13,446	13,379	12,816	13,836	13,974	14,146	14,454
Nigeria	640,701	618,732	610,800	589,457	573,633	561,790	545,505
Norway	14,028	14,251	14,635	13,867	13,557	13,888	13,945
Pakistan							
Peru							
Philippines							
Poland	276	215	151	123	159	160	162
Portugal							
Romania	271,496	259,888	257,865	254,855	247,608	245,337	240,142
Russia	2,346,138	2,181,153	2,138,750	2,014,710	1,782,266	1,687,151	1,573,242
Saudi Arabia							
Singapore	11,398	10,847	10,280	9,652	10,067	9,498	9,154
Slovakia	21,109	19,949	18,468	18,026	17,382	16,552	15,637
Slovenia	9,041	8,486	7,979	7,353	6,791	6,231	5,682
South Africa	30,089	28,626	24,916	26,766	26,262	24,527	23,503
South Korea	111,440	102,495	106,049	111,624	122,085	120,104	123,275
Spain	53,847	58,399	63,756	61,144	63,395	66,661	68,845
Sweden	31,008	30,712	30,980	31,658	33,365	33,838	34,528
Switzerland	11,543	10,461	9,835	10,198	9,825	9,771	9,491
Taiwan							
Thailand							
Tunisia	17,481	17,051	17,319	17,823	18,005	18,501	18,728
Turkey	375,534	389,691	396,248	384,100	380,933	381,163	375,044
Turkmenistan	33,636	32,544	32,095	31,249	30,622	29,825	29,196
Ukraine	525,300	495,800	546,218	535,477	505,927	522,085	524,035
United Arab Emirates							
United Kingdom	187,402	183,250	185,375	186,274	185,260	185,690	183,899
USA	884,273	861,789	857,475	866,907	864,307	856,528	845,393
Venezuela							
Vietnam	1,583,747	1,600,961	1,626,027	1,648,636	1,671,442	1,684,083	1,718,771

Source: *Council of Europe/National Statistics/Euromonitor International*

■ **Deaths**

Number of deaths 1998-2004

Table: 1.14

'000

	1998	1999	2000	2001	2002	2003	2004
Algeria	143.2	121.8	99.6	80.2	75.1	81.5	94.7
Argentina	281.8	289.0	281.6	275.6	280.7	283.3	287.5
Australia	127.8	128.2	129.2	129.2	134.8	135.5	135.3
Austria	78.3	78.2	76.8	74.8	76.1	72.3	71.7
Azerbaijan	46.3	46.3	46.7	45.3	45.4	51.7	58.4
Belarus	137.3	142.0	134.9	140.3	146.5	132.9	130.1
Belgium	104.6	104.9	104.9	104.3	103.9	104.4	104.9
Bolivia	71.5	71.7	71.9	72.2	73.6	75.0	75.7
Brazil	1,109.8	1,122.3	1,136.5	1,152.1	1,170.5	1,188.1	1,220.8
Bulgaria	118.2	111.8	115.1	112.4	112.6	112.7	114.1
Canada	240.2	217.6	217.2	219.1	222.8	227.6	225.6
Chile	80.3	82.0	79.1	81.6	80.6	85.0	87.1
China	8,074.2	8,096.4	8,148.9	8,180.7	8,210.7	8,118.9	8,097.1
Colombia	175.4	183.6	187.4	191.5	187.9	181.4	188.8
Croatia	52.3	52.0	50.2	49.6	44.3	43.2	40.3
Czech Republic	109.5	109.8	109.0	107.8	108.2	105.5	103.1
Denmark	58.5	59.2	58.0	58.3	58.7	58.4	58.3
Ecuador	54.1	55.0	55.9	57.3	58.8	61.6	65.6
Egypt	399.2	400.8	402.3	409.7	415.0	420.3	425.6
Estonia	19.4	18.4	18.4	18.5	18.4	18.5	19.5
Finland	49.3	49.3	49.3	48.5	49.4	49.9	50.4
France	534.0	537.7	535.1	528.0	534.5	538.0	544.6
Germany	852.4	846.3	838.8	821.2	783.0	764.9	747.3
Greece	102.7	103.3	103.0	101.1	100.1	99.3	97.3
Hong Kong, China	32.8	33.3	33.8	33.4	34.3	34.7	35.5
Hungary	140.9	143.2	135.6	132.2	132.8	130.9	128.7
India	8,946.3	9,144.7	9,320.6	9,398.8	9,322.4	9,102.5	8,831.1
Indonesia	855.2	871.0	883.5	892.7	899.6	906.6	913.9
Ireland	31.6	32.6	31.1	29.8	32.0	33.9	34.3
Israel	37.0	37.2	37.6	37.2	38.2	39.6	40.1
Italy	574.2	565.8	560.0	549.2	550.1	549.1	546.6
Japan	936.5	982.0	961.7	970.3	982.4	1,006.1	1,013.4
Jordan	18.1	19.4	21.5	23.5	25.8	28.1	30.7
Kazakhstan	223.3	224.4	225.5	226.6	227.7	226.7	225.7
Kuwait	4.2	4.2	4.2	4.4	4.6	4.8	5.0
Latvia	34.2	32.8	32.2	33.0	32.5	30.6	30.5
Lithuania	40.8	40.0	38.9	40.4	41.1	40.6	40.7
Malaysia	98.3	99.2	104.9	108.1	110.4	111.3	119.8
Mexico	418.3	415.5	422.1	418.7	425.1	435.1	452.7
Morocco	173.3	173.3	173.2	173.1	173.0	177.6	175.1
Netherlands	137.5	140.5	140.5	140.4	145.8	145.4	145.1
New Zealand	27.0	28.0	26.5	28.1	28.1	28.7	29.2
Nigeria	809.0	847.9	893.0	940.4	988.6	1,034.5	1,078.4
Norway	44.1	45.2	44.0	44.0	42.5	40.8	40.6
Pakistan	943.9	952.4	961.0	969.5	1,011.9	1,016.8	1,021.6
Peru	107.6	108.2	108.8	109.3	109.9	109.7	107.6
Philippines	353.0	348.0	366.9	352.7	353.4	359.8	371.0
Poland	375.4	381.4	368.0	363.2	353.3	344.4	342.5
Portugal	106.2	107.9	105.4	105.1	108.1	110.7	112.7
Romania	269.2	265.2	255.8	267.3	267.6	266.6	264.0
Russia	1,988.7	2,144.3	2,225.3	2,254.9	2,332.3	2,104.2	2,128.4
Saudi Arabia	113.1	116.0	109.1	102.5	95.8	99.0	100.5
Singapore	14.6	14.5	14.7	14.6	14.9	15.3	15.8
Slovakia	53.2	52.4	52.7	52.0	51.7	51.4	51.1
Slovenia	19.0	18.9	18.6	18.4	17.4	17.2	16.9
South Africa	223.3	223.9	228.0	228.6	232.8	234.0	235.1
South Korea	248.4	246.5	247.3	242.7	246.5	248.3	249.9
Spain	360.5	371.1	359.1	358.9	380.0	394.5	405.7
Sweden	93.3	94.7	93.5	93.8	93.8	94.7	95.9
Switzerland	62.6	62.5	62.5	61.3	62.0	62.5	62.3
Taiwan	123.2	126.1	126.0	127.6	128.6	130.8	134.3
Thailand	344.2	315.6	322.8	330.2	333.5	341.8	349.4
Tunisia	52.1	53.6	53.3	52.9	56.4	56.5	56.7
Turkey	464.7	469.7	481.2	487.8	488.8	495.9	515.0
Turkmenistan	29.3	29.8	30.3	30.8	31.4	31.9	32.4
Ukraine	720.0	739.2	758.1	746.0	714.5	705.1	694.4
United Arab Emirates	5.0	5.2	5.4	5.8	6.0	7.3	8.7
United Kingdom	555.0	556.1	535.7	530.4	522.6	540.1	538.9
USA	2,344.6	2,328.4	2,409.7	2,489.9	2,560.5	2,613.1	2,652.5
Venezuela	98.6	101.9	103.3	107.9	105.4	107.5	106.9
Vietnam	308.3	227.5	162.7	144.8	181.7	259.9	351.8

Source: National statistical offices/UN/Euromonitor International

Death rates 1998-2004

Table: 1.15

number per '000 inhabitants

	1998	1999	2000	2001	2002	2003	2004
Algeria	4.9	4.1	3.3	2.6	2.4	2.6	2.9
Argentina	8.0	8.1	7.8	7.6	7.7	7.7	7.7
Australia	6.8	6.8	6.7	6.7	6.9	6.8	6.8
Austria	9.8	9.8	9.6	9.3	9.5	8.9	8.8
Azerbaijan	5.8	5.7	5.7	5.5	5.5	6.2	6.9
Belarus	13.6	14.2	13.5	14.1	14.8	13.5	13.2
Belgium	10.3	10.3	10.2	10.1	10.1	10.1	10.1
Bolivia	9.0	8.8	8.6	8.5	8.5	8.5	8.4
Brazil	6.7	6.7	6.7	6.7	6.7	6.7	6.8
Bulgaria	14.5	13.8	14.3	14.2	14.3	14.4	14.8
Canada	8.0	7.2	7.1	7.1	7.1	7.2	7.1
Chile	5.4	5.5	5.2	5.3	5.2	5.4	5.5
China	6.5	6.5	6.5	6.4	6.4	6.3	6.2
Colombia	4.3	4.4	4.5	4.5	4.3	4.1	4.2
Croatia	11.6	11.5	11.3	11.2	10.0	9.7	9.1
Czech Republic	10.7	10.7	10.7	10.6	10.6	10.3	10.1
Denmark	11.0	11.1	10.9	10.9	10.9	10.8	10.8
Ecuador	4.5	4.5	4.5	4.5	4.6	4.7	5.0
Egypt	6.5	6.4	6.3	6.3	6.3	6.2	6.2
Estonia	14.0	13.4	13.4	13.6	13.5	13.7	14.5
Finland	9.6	9.6	9.5	9.4	9.5	9.6	9.7
France	9.1	9.2	9.1	8.9	9.0	9.0	9.1
Germany	10.4	10.3	10.2	10.0	9.5	9.3	9.0
Greece	9.8	9.8	9.7	9.5	9.4	9.3	9.1
Hong Kong, China	5.0	5.0	5.1	5.0	5.0	5.1	5.1
Hungary	13.7	14.0	13.3	13.0	13.1	12.9	12.7
India	9.1	9.1	9.2	9.1	8.9	8.5	8.2
Indonesia	4.2	4.2	4.2	4.2	4.1	4.1	4.1
Ireland	8.5	8.7	8.2	7.7	8.2	8.6	8.6
Israel	6.2	6.1	6.0	5.8	5.8	5.9	5.8
Italy	10.0	9.8	9.7	9.5	9.5	9.4	9.4
Japan	7.4	7.8	7.6	7.6	7.7	7.9	7.9
Jordan	3.8	4.0	4.3	4.5	4.8	5.1	5.5
Kazakhstan	14.0	14.2	14.4	14.6	14.7	14.7	14.7
Kuwait	2.0	1.8	1.9	1.9	2.0	2.0	2.1
Latvia	14.2	13.7	13.6	14.0	13.9	13.2	13.2
Lithuania	11.5	11.4	11.1	11.6	11.9	11.8	11.9
Malaysia	4.4	4.4	4.5	4.5	4.5	4.4	4.7
Mexico	4.4	4.3	4.3	4.2	4.2	4.2	4.3
Morocco	6.2	6.1	6.0	5.9	5.8	5.8	5.6
Netherlands	8.8	8.9	8.8	8.7	9.0	9.0	8.9
New Zealand	7.1	7.3	6.9	7.2	7.1	7.2	7.3
Nigeria	7.4	7.6	7.8	8.0	8.2	8.3	8.5
Norway	10.0	10.1	9.8	9.7	9.4	8.9	8.8
Pakistan	7.0	6.9	6.7	6.6	6.7	6.6	6.5
Peru	4.3	4.2	4.2	4.1	4.1	4.0	3.9
Philippines	4.8	4.7	4.8	4.5	4.4	4.4	4.5
Poland	9.7	9.9	9.5	9.4	9.1	8.9	8.9
Portugal	10.5	10.6	10.3	10.2	10.4	10.6	10.8
Romania	12.0	11.8	11.4	11.9	12.0	12.0	11.9
Russia	13.6	14.7	15.3	15.6	16.2	14.7	15.0
Saudi Arabia	5.7	5.7	5.2	4.8	4.3	4.3	4.2
Singapore	4.6	4.5	4.5	4.4	4.4	4.5	4.6
Slovakia	9.9	9.8	9.8	9.7	9.6	9.6	9.5
Slovenia	9.6	9.5	9.3	9.3	8.7	8.6	8.5
South Africa	5.3	5.2	5.2	5.1	5.1	5.0	4.9
South Korea	5.5	5.4	5.4	5.2	5.3	5.3	5.3
Spain	9.1	9.4	9.0	8.9	9.4	9.7	9.9
Sweden	10.5	10.7	10.5	10.5	10.5	10.6	10.7
Switzerland	8.8	8.7	8.7	8.5	8.5	8.6	8.5
Taiwan	5.6	5.7	5.7	5.7	5.7	5.8	5.9
Thailand	5.9	5.4	5.5	5.6	5.6	5.6	5.7
Tunisia	5.6	5.7	5.6	5.5	5.8	5.8	5.7
Turkey	7.1	7.1	7.1	7.1	7.0	7.0	7.2
Turkmenistan	6.5	6.5	6.5	6.5	6.5	6.6	6.6
Ukraine	14.4	14.9	15.4	15.3	14.9	14.8	14.7
United Arab Emirates	1.8	1.7	1.7	1.7	1.6	1.8	2.1
United Kingdom	9.5	9.5	9.1	9.0	8.8	9.1	9.0
USA	8.7	8.5	8.8	9.0	9.2	9.3	9.3
Venezuela	4.2	4.3	4.3	4.4	4.2	4.2	4.1
Vietnam	4.1	2.9	2.1	1.8	2.3	3.2	4.3

Source: *National statistical offices/UN/Euromonitor International*

■ **Household Characteristics**

Number of households 1998-2004

Table: 1.16

'000

	1998	1999	2000	2001	2002	2003	2004
Algeria	4,426.5	4,560.6	4,696.8	4,840.6	4,982.1	5,132.6	5,285.6
Argentina	9,698.1	9,819.1	9,933.7	10,075.8	10,171.4	10,268.8	10,362.2
Australia	6,719.3	6,835.9	6,956.5	7,072.2	7,184.1	7,304.5	7,420.7
Austria	3,228.0	3,269.3	3,302.5	3,339.7	3,373.3	3,407.0	3,440.8
Azerbaijan	3,045.9	3,103.1	3,174.3	3,218.9	3,277.6	3,332.0	3,385.2
Belarus	3,830.1	3,855.0	3,898.7	3,909.4	3,931.2	3,940.1	3,950.9
Belgium	4,178.7	4,209.1	4,237.8	4,277.7	4,319.0	4,361.9	4,397.6
Bolivia	1,790.5	1,851.5	1,916.1	1,977.7	2,036.4	2,094.3	2,152.7
Brazil	45,187.2	46,306.3	47,376.7	48,473.1	49,510.1	50,558.0	51,604.6
Bulgaria	2,934.9	2,930.4	2,924.8	2,921.9	2,918.4	2,915.1	2,912.0
Canada	11,101.4	11,242.5	11,394.5	11,566.0	11,696.1	11,824.7	11,936.4
Chile	3,768.7	3,856.0	3,943.4	4,033.5	4,141.4	4,229.1	4,316.8
China	349,085.2	344,298.9	348,370.0	356,495.8	364,329.8	371,632.1	378,092.1
Colombia	9,002.7	9,420.7	9,854.5	10,297.1	10,760.8	11,194.1	11,604.4
Croatia	1,496.8	1,490.1	1,482.2	1,477.4	1,472.2	1,465.9	1,461.4
Czech Republic	3,870.0	3,851.1	3,836.5	3,827.7	3,817.1	3,804.3	3,791.6
Denmark	2,407.0	2,423.2	2,434.1	2,444.7	2,456.1	2,466.7	2,473.0
Ecuador	2,434.3	2,476.3	2,509.1	2,538.0	2,566.0	2,594.2	2,618.9
Egypt	13,328.1	13,653.1	13,995.7	14,356.2	14,730.8	15,127.0	15,535.5
Estonia	550.6	563.7	582.1	580.2	578.2	576.5	574.7
Finland	2,355.0	2,365.0	2,382.0	2,382.0	2,396.2	2,404.1	2,413.5
France	23,476.4	23,808.1	24,044.0	24,277.6	24,477.9	24,690.7	24,883.6
Germany	37,532.0	37,795.0	38,124.0	38,456.0	38,720.0	38,930.9	39,166.1
Greece	3,540.6	3,579.2	3,627.6	3,664.4	3,706.5	3,746.4	3,786.0
Hong Kong, China	1,931.5	1,971.7	2,011.2	2,053.4	2,085.9	2,116.9	2,154.2
Hungary	3,735.2	3,729.0	3,783.3	3,720.7	3,714.4	3,711.0	3,697.2
India	180,148.4	184,329.3	188,332.3	191,963.9	195,687.2	199,404.1	202,876.1
Indonesia	49,346.6	50,634.6	52,008.3	53,455.0	55,041.0	56,245.2	57,411.1
Ireland	1,172.2	1,198.8	1,225.5	1,255.8	1,288.0	1,316.7	1,343.1
Israel	1,650.6	1,699.5	1,752.3	1,815.3	1,849.8	1,902.7	1,956.6
Italy	21,669.3	21,918.5	22,226.0	22,445.9	22,642.2	22,839.7	23,026.3
Japan	45,653.0	46,228.1	46,782.4	47,265.6	47,683.6	48,081.2	48,480.0
Jordan	804.3	833.5	862.5	891.1	920.2	948.7	976.7
Kazakhstan	4,103.9	4,152.7	4,161.5	4,235.0	4,299.8	4,335.7	4,358.7
Kuwait	280.5	302.6	322.3	339.0	353.4	365.8	377.7
Latvia	802.8	802.8	802.8	798.5	794.1	790.9	788.5
Lithuania	1,335.8	1,342.0	1,349.0	1,356.8	1,357.0	1,361.7	1,363.9
Malaysia	4,563.5	4,725.8	4,910.9	5,054.6	5,195.7	5,329.1	5,456.0
Mexico	21,295.1	21,771.9	22,268.9	22,756.4	23,220.0	23,690.4	24,158.4
Morocco	4,947.0	5,146.5	5,354.0	5,496.0	5,637.8	5,783.0	5,918.3
Netherlands	6,655.9	6,745.4	6,801.0	6,867.0	6,934.3	7,002.0	7,058.0
New Zealand	1,381.4	1,400.4	1,422.4	1,440.5	1,458.4	1,481.5	1,502.2
Nigeria	22,149.5	22,794.7	23,447.2	24,120.7	24,766.6	25,448.2	26,100.5
Norway	1,901.3	1,922.6	1,946.4	1,961.5	1,978.7	1,998.0	2,015.9
Pakistan	18,673.6	19,136.3	19,492.2	19,755.0	20,430.5	21,069.2	21,532.9
Peru	5,232.9	5,335.4	5,436.0	5,516.1	5,596.0	5,665.9	5,737.3
Philippines	14,519.3	14,901.3	15,271.5	15,645.0	16,009.8	16,391.5	16,758.8
Poland	12,885.9	13,006.8	13,123.1	13,239.3	13,337.0	13,425.9	13,511.2
Portugal	3,480.6	3,534.5	3,592.4	3,650.8	3,707.8	3,757.9	3,808.8
Romania	6,950.5	7,036.1	7,131.1	7,222.9	7,320.2	7,458.9	7,553.8
Russia	50,464.0	51,019.5	51,653.3	52,266.3	52,707.0	52,663.4	52,874.6
Saudi Arabia	3,250.0	3,330.0	3,430.0	3,570.0	3,710.0	3,860.0	3,990.0
Singapore	868.2	896.5	923.3	947.1	968.5	988.8	1,007.2
Slovakia	1,994.3	2,019.6	2,045.4	2,072.0	2,092.4	2,110.7	2,128.5
Slovenia	662.7	667.1	671.6	676.1	684.8	689.5	694.3
South Africa	9,861.7	10,291.1	10,728.5	11,205.7	11,568.2	11,917.5	12,238.4
South Korea	15,172.8	15,442.3	15,765.3	16,081.0	16,489.1	16,755.7	17,034.9
Spain	13,383.2	13,635.1	13,930.2	14,270.1	14,562.9	14,815.6	15,037.6
Sweden	4,076.7	4,092.9	4,104.5	4,127.5	4,152.9	4,175.3	4,196.8
Switzerland	3,126.6	3,152.0	3,181.6	3,208.0	3,245.7	3,270.4	3,289.3
Taiwan	6,140.9	6,310.1	6,495.0	6,636.7	6,777.9	6,912.3	7,038.1
Thailand	15,099.6	15,480.6	15,662.3	15,953.4	16,249.2	16,578.9	16,895.6
Tunisia	1,910.9	1,971.2	2,026.6	2,077.0	2,124.0	2,167.8	2,210.1
Turkey	13,476.7	13,761.2	14,034.8	14,304.0	14,582.6	14,862.3	15,133.9
Turkmenistan	1,185.0	1,223.1	1,266.6	1,287.9	1,337.4	1,387.7	1,438.7
Ukraine	19,412.0	19,546.6	19,640.1	19,750.7	19,668.2	19,730.9	19,763.8
United Arab Emirates	476.0	505.2	536.0	559.0	584.9	618.5	652.2
United Kingdom	24,093.5	24,286.1	24,469.4	24,761.7	24,929.0	25,095.7	25,262.7
USA	101,139.0	102,191.3	105,780.1	107,049.9	108,297.4	109,282.8	110,242.3
Venezuela	4,836.2	4,982.2	5,131.9	5,261.2	5,397.5	5,530.5	5,661.4
Vietnam	20,069.8	20,706.8	21,628.5	22,071.0	22,950.1	23,803.1	24,674.2

Source: *National statistical offices/Euromonitor International*

Average number of occupants per household 1998-2004

Table: 1.17

persons

	1998	1999	2000	2001	2002	2003	2004
Algeria	6.57	6.48	6.39	6.30	6.22	6.14	6.07
Argentina	3.63	3.62	3.61	3.60	3.60	3.60	3.61
Australia	2.78	2.77	2.75	2.75	2.74	2.71	2.70
Austria	2.47	2.44	2.43	2.40	2.39	2.37	2.36
Azerbaijan	2.62	2.60	2.56	2.54	2.52	2.50	2.48
Belarus	2.64	2.61	2.57	2.56	2.53	2.51	2.50
Belgium	2.44	2.43	2.42	2.40	2.39	2.37	2.36
Bolivia	4.41	4.36	4.30	4.25	4.20	4.17	4.13
Brazil	3.67	3.63	3.59	3.56	3.53	3.50	3.47
Bulgaria	2.80	2.77	2.75	2.73	2.70	2.69	2.67
Canada	2.72	2.70	2.69	2.68	2.68	2.67	2.68
Chile	3.93	3.89	3.86	3.82	3.76	3.73	3.70
China	3.58	3.66	3.64	3.58	3.53	3.49	3.45
Colombia	4.48	4.36	4.24	4.12	4.01	3.92	3.84
Croatia	3.01	3.06	3.02	3.00	3.02	3.03	3.04
Czech Republic	2.65	2.66	2.67	2.67	2.67	2.68	2.69
Denmark	2.20	2.19	2.19	2.19	2.19	2.18	2.19
Ecuador	4.90	4.90	4.91	4.93	4.95	4.97	5.00
Egypt	4.56	4.54	4.52	4.49	4.45	4.41	4.36
Estonia	2.53	2.45	2.36	2.36	2.35	2.35	2.35
Finland	2.19	2.18	2.17	2.18	2.17	2.17	2.16
France	2.48	2.46	2.44	2.43	2.42	2.42	2.41
Germany	2.19	2.17	2.16	2.14	2.13	2.12	2.11
Greece	2.97	2.94	2.91	2.89	2.86	2.84	2.81
Hong Kong, China	3.39	3.35	3.31	3.27	3.25	3.25	3.23
Hungary	2.71	2.71	2.70	2.74	2.74	2.73	2.73
India	5.41	5.38	5.36	5.34	5.32	5.30	5.29
Indonesia	4.14	4.09	4.04	3.98	3.92	3.88	3.85
Ireland	3.15	3.12	3.08	3.05	3.01	2.99	2.96
Israel	3.62	3.60	3.59	3.55	3.55	3.54	3.52
Italy	2.66	2.63	2.60	2.58	2.56	2.55	2.53
Japan	2.77	2.74	2.71	2.69	2.67	2.65	2.63
Jordan	5.80	5.78	5.75	5.73	5.71	5.69	5.67
Kazakhstan	3.92	3.83	3.78	3.68	3.60	3.56	3.54
Kuwait	7.59	7.51	6.91	6.62	6.51	6.44	6.39
Latvia	3.02	2.99	2.97	2.96	2.95	2.95	2.94
Lithuania	2.67	2.64	2.60	2.57	2.56	2.53	2.51
Malaysia	4.86	4.81	4.78	4.75	4.72	4.70	4.69
Mexico	4.46	4.44	4.41	4.38	4.36	4.34	4.31
Morocco	5.65	5.52	5.39	5.34	5.29	5.24	5.21
Netherlands	2.35	2.34	2.33	2.33	2.32	2.31	2.31
New Zealand	2.76	2.74	2.71	2.69	2.70	2.68	2.67
Nigeria	4.84	4.83	4.83	4.82	4.82	4.81	4.81
Norway	2.32	2.31	2.30	2.30	2.29	2.28	2.27
Pakistan	7.15	7.17	7.23	7.31	7.25	7.20	7.22
Peru	4.76	4.75	4.74	4.74	4.75	4.76	4.77
Philippines	5.04	5.02	5.01	4.99	4.97	4.95	4.94
Poland	3.00	2.97	2.95	2.92	2.90	2.88	2.86
Portugal	2.90	2.87	2.84	2.81	2.79	2.77	2.74
Romania	3.24	3.20	3.15	3.11	3.06	2.99	2.95
Russia	2.91	2.87	2.82	2.77	2.73	2.72	2.69
Saudi Arabia	6.11	6.11	6.08	6.04	6.01	5.94	5.91
Singapore	3.66	3.59	3.53	3.50	3.49	3.47	3.45
Slovakia	2.69	2.66	2.63	2.60	2.57	2.55	2.52
Slovenia	3.00	2.97	2.96	2.94	2.91	2.90	2.88
South Africa	4.27	4.18	4.09	4.00	3.95	3.90	3.89
South Korea	2.99	2.96	2.92	2.88	2.82	2.79	2.76
Spain	2.94	2.90	2.85	2.81	2.77	2.74	2.71
Sweden	2.17	2.16	2.16	2.15	2.15	2.14	2.14
Switzerland	2.27	2.26	2.25	2.25	2.24	2.23	2.22
Taiwan	3.57	3.50	3.43	3.38	3.32	3.27	3.23
Thailand	3.85	3.80	3.76	3.72	3.69	3.65	3.63
Tunisia	4.84	4.75	4.67	4.61	4.56	4.51	4.47
Turkey	4.83	4.82	4.80	4.79	4.77	4.76	4.74
Turkmenistan	3.75	3.70	3.63	3.63	3.56	3.48	3.41
Ukraine	2.59	2.55	2.52	2.48	2.45	2.42	2.40
United Arab Emirates	5.95	6.00	6.06	6.24	6.42	6.41	6.41
United Kingdom	2.42	2.41	2.40	2.38	2.38	2.37	2.36
USA	2.67	2.67	2.60	2.59	2.58	2.58	2.58
Venezuela	4.77	4.73	4.68	4.66	4.63	4.60	4.58
Vietnam	3.77	3.70	3.59	3.56	3.47	3.40	3.32

Source: National statistics/UN//Euromonitor International

Household facilities 2002

% of total number of households

	Flush toilet	Water supply
Algeria		
Argentina	61.0	98.6
Australia		
Austria		
Azerbaijan	89.3	93.6
Belarus	97.1	98.8
Belgium		
Bolivia	48.2	86.9
Brazil	53.5	89.2
Bulgaria		
Canada		
Chile	88.7	98.6
China		97.4
Colombia	94.0	98.1
Croatia		
Czech Republic		
Denmark	99.9	
Ecuador	67.5	88.4
Egypt	35.3	92.2
Estonia	93.2	97.3
Finland	95.7	98.2
France		
Germany		
Greece		100.0
Hong Kong, China		
Hungary	80.1	88.3
India		
Indonesia	57.5	18.3
Ireland		99.5
Israel		
Italy		
Japan	83.7	
Jordan	92.0	86.5
Kazakhstan	49.4	52.4
Kuwait		
Latvia	74.7	82.2
Lithuania	91.0	93.0
Malaysia		
Mexico	88.0	96.2
Morocco		
Netherlands		
New Zealand		
Nigeria	13.6	7.3
Norway		
Pakistan		
Peru	78.3	78.3
Philippines		
Poland	93.2	98.9
Portugal	98.5	99.8
Romania		
Russia	74.0	75.3
Saudi Arabia		
Singapore		
Slovakia	55.7	82.3
Slovenia		98.9
South Africa		
South Korea		
Spain		
Sweden		
Switzerland		
Taiwan		
Thailand		
Tunisia		99.0
Turkey		
Turkmenistan	79.3	88.1
Ukraine	52.4	54.9
United Arab Emirates		
United Kingdom		
USA		
Venezuela	86.7	91.0
Vietnam	82.1	75.9

Source: Euromonitor International from national statistics

■ **Consumer Expenditure**

Per capita trends in total consumer expenditure 1998-2004

Table: 1.19

US$ per capita

	1998	1999	2000	2001	2002	2003	2004
Algeria	955.78	919.03	822.37	858.42	889.59	965.06	1,107.04
Argentina	5,958.44	5,726.32	5,604.76	5,197.86	1,752.90	1,728.06	1,642.68
Australia	11,573.75	12,424.78	11,772.77	11,055.64	12,187.03	15,008.53	17,774.23
Austria	15,270.15	14,985.18	13,534.08	13,595.24	14,589.40	17,841.93	20,167.10
Azerbaijan	433.00	406.61	390.75	391.23	393.85	424.48	455.27
Belarus	822.57	669.66	568.87	685.41	844.31	1,022.80	1,198.33
Belgium	12,882.37	12,632.98	11,537.96	11,567.65	12,665.56	15,499.44	17,775.11
Bolivia	814.30	793.39	766.45	730.02	686.56	677.41	683.23
Brazil	2,964.41	2,100.54	2,362.60	1,978.54	1,728.32	1,878.46	2,098.89
Bulgaria	1,107.91	1,171.16	1,109.28	1,195.64	1,393.08	1,737.97	2,111.77
Canada	11,369.36	11,904.02	12,501.90	12,376.76	12,671.12	14,795.79	16,347.31
Chile	3,229.45	2,888.15	2,913.95	2,577.77	2,464.34	2,522.12	2,944.85
China	360.06	379.79	411.14	437.31	453.92	489.23	525.32
Colombia	1,600.95	1,349.43	1,283.53	1,260.40	1,228.71	1,151.98	1,352.12
Croatia	2,830.79	2,517.74	2,420.83	2,526.55	2,820.09	3,585.79	4,285.97
Czech Republic	2,875.40	2,843.37	2,683.92	2,936.66	3,543.09	4,164.90	4,815.45
Denmark	16,107.29	15,912.85	13,971.24	13,840.49	14,915.81	18,370.94	20,877.46
Ecuador	1,164.32	739.44	706.67	930.25	1,012.95	1,050.34	1,079.50
Egypt	1,073.39	1,130.96	1,226.95	1,111.87	1,053.07	857.13	866.97
Estonia	2,465.43	2,429.36	2,321.85	2,490.35	2,921.21	3,839.34	4,517.00
Finland	12,098.66	11,963.49	11,027.04	11,270.40	12,397.64	15,141.06	16,781.75
France	13,825.73	13,607.51	12,230.40	12,314.63	13,308.14	16,348.74	18,486.70
Germany	14,369.37	14,171.42	12,629.59	12,654.22	13,338.59	16,125.04	18,291.38
Greece	8,604.88	8,554.14	7,843.31	8,087.87	9,062.31	11,453.93	13,454.24
Hong Kong, China	14,764.27	13,960.18	13,986.23	13,928.89	13,397.73	12,707.05	12,653.77
Hungary	2,537.21	2,649.96	2,538.91	2,863.11	3,392.00	4,288.86	5,212.31
India	278.26	291.51	284.96	294.09	302.70	330.16	358.56
Indonesia	325.93	507.71	498.62	464.80	582.84	672.59	698.55
Ireland	11,258.59	11,899.81	11,562.77	12,068.04	13,490.95	16,892.12	19,063.27
Israel	9,787.69	9,596.28	10,207.46	9,804.70	8,921.65	9,010.38	9,030.35
Italy	12,534.69	12,441.20	11,389.30	11,429.63	12,333.73	15,112.64	17,308.87
Japan	16,871.73	19,219.33	20,266.66	17,954.28	17,586.87	18,990.97	20,726.62
Jordan	1,323.96	1,300.54	1,467.53	1,509.28	1,480.29	1,442.77	1,470.58
Kazakhstan	1,047.30	792.70	751.41	871.37	932.11	1,074.97	1,308.22
Kuwait	5,673.95	5,636.44	5,945.56	6,514.58	7,183.35	7,203.50	7,355.15
Latvia	1,602.17	1,722.17	1,833.33	1,992.70	2,217.50	2,665.72	3,104.96
Lithuania	1,899.55	1,994.97	2,073.93	2,228.03	2,495.62	3,075.97	3,557.93
Malaysia	1,341.14	1,472.59	1,647.54	1,675.59	1,721.58	1,730.48	1,760.69
Mexico	3,027.36	3,373.72	4,004.06	4,387.72	4,426.48	4,015.51	4,051.64
Morocco	921.30	864.87	828.53	825.93	866.71	1,043.95	1,137.76
Netherlands	12,432.89	12,511.95	11,511.82	11,732.81	12,620.82	15,673.76	17,503.16
New Zealand	8,408.58	8,582.02	7,701.17	7,411.29	8,444.14	10,741.68	12,504.16
Nigeria	307.95	202.74	220.05	275.47	331.90	395.36	448.88
Norway	15,714.90	15,931.78	14,991.32	15,218.09	17,768.25	20,676.09	22,163.70
Pakistan	336.55	343.05	324.84	300.60	330.90	364.68	393.45
Peru	1,640.35	1,438.20	1,478.35	1,502.72	1,543.14	1,657.35	1,765.67
Philippines	661.96	739.85	690.81	646.98	690.90	705.67	718.18
Poland	2,582.16	2,545.53	2,622.28	3,028.67	3,129.63	3,351.43	3,811.10
Portugal	7,124.42	7,219.05	6,576.20	6,709.73	7,232.89	8,821.85	9,997.95
Romania	1,393.60	1,127.84	1,136.20	1,224.42	1,351.69	1,830.38	2,150.85
Russia	1,024.02	666.85	760.95	966.26	1,138.88	1,543.24	1,901.50
Saudi Arabia	3,335.15	3,262.01	3,257.80	3,121.71	3,132.87	3,218.53	3,315.39
Singapore	10,607.80	10,998.63	12,021.24	11,223.12	11,143.50	11,562.56	12,148.43
Slovakia	2,242.38	2,128.41	2,099.25	2,220.47	2,555.87	3,376.71	4,262.67
Slovenia	5,735.09	5,841.14	5,262.16	5,337.60	5,981.96	8,138.70	9,334.18
South Africa	2,003.17	1,922.53	1,834.97	1,577.28	1,418.00	2,197.65	2,637.38
South Korea	3,798.43	4,935.64	5,646.84	5,346.08	5,984.35	6,606.36	7,261.51
Spain	9,430.25	9,609.21	8,880.15	9,081.18	9,994.03	12,568.87	14,453.47
Sweden	13,313.37	13,463.37	12,707.27	11,648.75	12,740.50	15,825.06	17,742.87
Switzerland	22,236.91	21,955.91	20,020.49	20,413.20	22,276.19	26,014.37	28,806.09
Taiwan	7,276.61	7,924.49	8,015.73	8,209.79	7,962.42	7,956.14	8,398.20
Thailand	1,123.75	1,260.77	1,258.17	1,192.27	1,284.29	1,376.49	1,487.08
Tunisia	1,264.29	1,303.95	1,211.75	1,235.62	1,321.73	1,601.39	1,716.50
Turkey	2,218.86	2,070.75	2,169.60	1,572.71	1,802.41	2,317.10	2,697.83
Turkmenistan	199.31	259.16	325.87	438.25	518.29	672.32	725.83
Ukraine	461.36	336.65	332.31	409.58	442.67	496.09	568.81
United Arab Emirates	8,741.97	7,861.82	7,163.75	6,901.82	6,629.86	6,688.26	6,780.44
United Kingdom	15,183.84	15,633.36	15,387.55	15,264.64	16,571.55	18,677.97	22,073.15
USA	21,658.75	22,926.19	24,368.96	25,239.78	26,238.81	27,335.06	28,656.41
Venezuela	2,846.55	2,913.54	3,076.81	3,311.76	2,388.67	2,658.84	2,861.46
Vietnam	254.70	257.07	262.99	267.86	280.64	298.38	303.00

Source: National statistical offices/OECD/Eurostat/Euromonitor International

Real growth in total consumer expenditure (national currencies) 1998-2004

Table: 1.20

1990=100

	1998	1999	2000	2001	2002	2003	2004
Algeria	107.6	116.0	118.8	124.1	133.1	139.0	145.7
Argentina	88.8	87.2	87.1	82.5	68.4	56.9	52.7
Australia	128.9	134.3	137.2	140.2	144.7	146.4	150.9
Austria	115.1	118.4	121.1	122.3	122.9	124.1	125.3
Azerbaijan							
Belarus							
Belgium	113.5	116.1	119.8	121.0	124.5	125.6	128.7
Bolivia	133.8	137.5	137.9	140.9	145.3	151.1	154.1
Brazil	158.9	170.1	182.7	186.9	188.9	191.0	192.7
Bulgaria	45.0	48.0	47.2	48.3	50.0	50.6	52.0
Canada	120.0	124.7	128.6	130.9	134.2	137.3	139.7
Chile	168.3	163.1	170.2	173.2	177.5	179.4	184.8
China	199.9	215.7	234.7	250.0	263.4	282.7	293.9
Colombia	120.4	114.7	120.8	123.0	124.9	127.6	131.2
Croatia	74.7	72.7	75.9	75.5	78.3	83.3	87.8
Czech Republic	92.9	96.2	97.5	100.2	102.2	103.3	105.8
Denmark	121.4	122.3	121.2	121.2	121.4	122.7	125.7
Ecuador	16.4	7.0	3.5	3.4	3.3	3.2	3.3
Egypt	138.8	144.9	159.7	165.1	175.3	180.6	176.7
Estonia							
Finland	114.9	118.5	122.5	125.9	130.0	131.5	132.4
France	110.6	114.3	117.4	120.3	121.9	122.9	124.4
Germany	113.6	117.2	119.2	120.7	119.6	119.5	121.3
Greece	121.5	123.9	127.8	131.6	135.6	138.3	143.7
Hong Kong, China	119.6	119.1	125.6	128.4	128.6	126.6	128.1
Hungary	104.8	109.6	115.2	120.5	121.8	127.6	130.7
India	136.2	144.7	144.4	153.4	158.3	161.8	167.2
Indonesia	204.7	210.5	216.6	223.5	230.3	232.7	240.0
Ireland	151.4	167.5	180.3	187.1	192.8	197.0	199.8
Israel	148.3	154.5	164.3	164.9	163.2	161.2	163.4
Italy	118.4	121.8	125.8	126.9	127.4	127.1	129.7
Japan	111.5	111.1	111.8	112.9	115.2	115.5	117.8
Jordan	150.3	151.4	174.9	181.9	180.3	176.4	178.5
Kazakhstan							
Kuwait	116.9	120.3	123.1	133.5	147.6	147.2	150.5
Latvia	191.0	197.2	210.4	229.3	244.6	262.6	270.5
Lithuania							
Malaysia	138.0	146.2	166.7	170.9	176.1	178.9	183.2
Mexico	120.9	122.9	133.8	138.3	139.4	137.2	140.3
Morocco	116.5	112.7	116.7	125.0	126.4	132.9	133.7
Netherlands	120.0	125.2	130.8	132.3	131.7	134.3	135.4
New Zealand	122.7	127.5	130.6	133.1	136.3	136.9	137.8
Nigeria	167.7	116.4	124.8	155.4	183.3	210.5	219.2
Norway	131.1	135.1	140.2	141.9	145.9	148.0	151.2
Pakistan	146.9	162.2	163.8	173.9	183.4	194.7	202.1
Peru	127.6	127.0	131.9	134.3	140.1	147.7	151.1
Philippines	126.6	129.6	134.1	139.4	149.2	158.5	160.5
Poland	133.4	139.9	143.3	147.7	149.3	151.2	156.1
Portugal	126.0	131.9	135.7	137.4	137.0	135.7	137.2
Romania	77.6	74.3	72.6	77.8	79.6	93.6	96.4
Russia	62.4	55.3	59.4	64.1	69.7	80.8	83.9
Saudi Arabia	142.6	144.9	150.0	150.3	155.6	163.6	172.7
Singapore	117.4	125.1	138.9	135.8	137.7	140.4	142.8
Slovakia							
Slovenia							
South Africa	124.2	128.0	134.1	138.3	142.0	151.8	157.1
South Korea	165.2	181.7	194.6	203.2	216.0	220.6	226.3
Spain	122.4	128.7	133.7	137.3	140.3	143.5	146.1
Sweden	113.2	118.5	123.0	124.4	126.0	127.9	130.3
Switzerland	106.8	108.8	110.4	112.0	113.1	113.9	115.9
Taiwan	177.7	187.6	196.4	198.4	203.9	204.7	209.3
Thailand	135.8	140.6	146.7	152.8	159.5	164.1	169.1
Tunisia	137.7	145.8	153.8	163.2	169.7	183.2	185.2
Turkey	121.0	111.9	115.0	107.5	106.2	110.2	114.0
Turkmenistan							
Ukraine							
United Arab Emirates	140.6	132.5	127.5	128.4	129.0	133.3	136.2
United Kingdom	122.8	127.8	131.0	135.1	139.0	140.2	144.0
USA	122.7	128.2	133.0	135.1	139.4	143.2	147.4
Venezuela	104.3	97.6	101.6	105.4	101.6	121.7	128.9
Vietnam	84.9	87.6	93.8	101.0	107.1	113.5	115.4

Source: National statistical offices/OECD/Eurostat/Euromonitor International

World Health Trends

■ **Life Expectancy**

Life expectancy at birth: total population 1998-2004

Table: 2.1

years/% change

	1998	1999	2000	2001	2002	2003	2004	% change 1998-2004
Algeria	68.7	68.9	68.9	69.4	69.3	69.5	69.6	1.35
Argentina	73.4	73.6	73.7	73.9	74.5	74.7	75.1	2.36
Australia	79.7	79.8	79.8	80.0	80.4	80.7	80.9	1.47
Austria	78.4	78.5	78.6	79.0	79.4	79.5	79.8	1.90
Azerbaijan	63.0	63.2	62.3	63.6	65.8	66.7	67.8	7.74
Belarus	68.5	68.5	69.0	68.5	68.3	68.5	68.4	-0.09
Belgium	77.5	77.7	77.8	78.0	78.3	78.5	78.8	1.66
Bolivia	61.6	62.0	62.2	62.7	63.2	63.7	64.1	4.14
Brazil	68.1	68.3	68.4	68.7	68.9	69.2	69.5	1.98
Bulgaria	71.6	71.6	71.6	71.5	71.9	72.2	72.3	1.07
Canada	79.0	79.1	79.1	79.3	79.8	80.0	80.3	1.61
Chile	75.9	76.1	76.1	76.3	76.7	76.8	77.2	1.58
China	70.5	70.8	70.8	71.2	71.1	71.3	71.3	1.18
Colombia	69.9	70.2	70.7	70.7	71.8	72.5	73.1	4.51
Croatia	72.5	72.7	72.9	72.9	74.8	75.5	76.5	5.43
Czech Republic	74.8	75.0	75.1	75.3	75.8	76.0	76.2	1.93
Denmark	76.7	76.9	76.9	77.2	77.2	77.3	77.3	0.69
Ecuador	69.9	70.1	69.7	70.3	70.6	70.9	71.1	1.75
Egypt	65.5	65.9	66.3	66.5	67.1	67.5	68.0	3.94
Estonia	70.5	70.7	71.0	71.2	71.1	71.3	71.3	1.16
Finland	77.4	77.5	77.7	77.8	78.2	78.3	78.5	1.53
France	78.8	78.9	79.1	79.3	79.7	80.2	80.4	2.08
Germany	77.6	77.8	78.0	78.2	78.7	78.9	79.2	2.04
Greece	77.9	78.0	78.0	78.1	78.4	78.7	78.8	1.12
Hong Kong, China	79.4	79.5	79.6	79.8	80.0	80.1	80.3	1.14
Hungary	71.0	71.3	71.5	71.7	72.6	73.0	73.6	3.63
India	59.8	60.2	60.6	60.8	61.0	61.3	61.5	2.95
Indonesia	64.7	65.2	65.4	65.9	66.4	66.8	67.2	3.80
Ireland	76.0	76.2	76.3	76.5	77.1	77.4	77.8	2.24
Israel	78.1	78.2	78.5	78.5	79.3	79.8	80.2	2.73
Italy	78.9	79.0	79.1	79.3	79.7	79.9	80.1	1.48
Japan	80.8	81.0	81.3	81.4	81.8	82.2	82.5	2.16
Jordan	70.3	70.6	70.7	70.8	70.8	71.0	71.1	1.11
Kazakhstan	62.5	62.7	62.5	63.0	63.6	64.2	64.7	3.39
Kuwait	75.0	75.1	75.4	75.3	76.2	76.8	77.3	3.11
Latvia	69.8	70.1	70.5	70.7	70.3	70.2	70.2	0.44
Lithuania	72.1	72.4	72.6	72.9	71.9	71.8	71.3	-1.07
Malaysia	71.3	71.5	71.7	71.7	72.0	72.3	72.6	1.88
Mexico	73.6	73.8	74.2	74.2	74.3	74.5	74.7	1.44
Morocco	68.3	68.7	69.3	69.4	70.8	71.5	72.3	5.90
Netherlands	78.0	78.1	78.1	78.3	78.5	78.7	78.9	1.18
New Zealand	78.1	78.2	78.3	78.5	78.9	79.2	79.4	1.71
Nigeria	51.1	51.3	51.6	51.6	48.8	48.0	46.6	-8.88
Norway	78.3	78.5	78.7	78.8	79.0	79.3	79.5	1.45
Pakistan	60.2	60.6	61.2	61.3	61.4	61.5	61.9	2.79
Peru	67.8	68.1	68.1	68.5	69.7	70.3	71.0	4.74
Philippines	67.1	67.4	67.4	67.7	68.3	68.8	69.1	2.99
Poland	73.4	73.6	73.9	74.0	74.7	75.0	75.4	2.72
Portugal	75.9	76.1	76.4	76.5	77.0	77.3	77.8	2.42
Romania	71.1	71.1	71.1	71.1	71.5	71.7	71.8	1.04
Russia	65.6	65.6	65.2	65.2	64.8			
Saudi Arabia	70.2	70.5	70.3	70.5	70.8	71.0	71.2	1.39
Singapore	78.3	78.5	78.4	78.8	79.5	79.9	80.3	2.67
Slovakia	72.9	73.0	73.3	73.3	74.0	74.4	74.8	2.66
Slovenia	75.2	75.4	75.7	75.9	76.7	77.0	77.5	3.12
South Africa	54.0	52.2	51.2	49.0	50.7	50.3	50.4	-6.79
South Korea	74.4	74.6	74.6	74.9	75.5	75.7	75.9	2.08
Spain	78.6	78.7	78.8	78.9	79.5	79.8	80.2	1.97
Sweden	79.6	79.7	79.8	80.0	80.4	80.5	80.7	1.42
Switzerland	79.8	79.9	79.9	80.2	80.6	80.7	81.0	1.47
Taiwan	72.7	73.0	73.3	73.5	73.8	74.0	74.3	2.24
Thailand	68.3	68.5	68.8	68.9	69.3	69.6	69.9	2.37
Tunisia	70.5	70.8	70.9	71.1	71.6	72.0	72.3	2.52
Turkey	68.3	68.6	68.9	69.0	70.0	70.5	71.1	4.10
Turkmenistan	61.8	62.1	62.4	62.5	62.7	63.1	63.3	2.50
Ukraine	67.7	67.7	67.8	67.7	67.2	67.2	66.9	-1.14
United Arab Emirates	72.3	72.4	71.6	71.7	72.5	72.7	73.0	1.01
United Kingdom	77.0	77.2	77.0	77.5	78.2	78.5	78.9	2.52
USA	76.4	76.6	76.8	77.0	77.3	77.4	77.6	1.62
Venezuela	73.1	73.3	73.4	73.6	73.9	74.1	74.3	1.67
Vietnam	68.3	68.7	69.1	69.3	69.6	70.0	70.3	2.90

Source: Euromonitor International from World Bank

Healthy life expectancy at birth: total population 1998-2002

Table: 2.2

years/% change

	1998	2002	% change 1998-2002
Algeria	62.0	57.8	-6.7
Argentina	67.0	63.1	-5.8
Australia	73.0	71.6	-1.9
Austria	72.0	71.0	-1.4
Azerbaijan	64.0	52.8	-17.5
Belarus	62.0	58.4	-5.8
Belgium	72.0	69.7	-3.1
Bolivia	53.0	50.8	-4.1
Brazil	59.0	56.7	-4.0
Bulgaria	64.0	63.0	-1.5
Canada	72.0	69.9	-3.0
Chile	69.0	66.1	-4.2
China	62.0	63.2	1.9
Colombia	63.0	58.7	-6.8
Croatia	67.0	63.3	-5.5
Czech Republic	68.0	66.6	-2.0
Denmark	69.0	70.1	1.6
Ecuador	61.0	56.7	-7.1
Egypt	58.0	59.5	2.5
Estonia	63.0	62.0	-1.5
Finland	70.0	70.1	0.1
France	73.0	71.3	-2.4
Germany	70.0	70.2	0.4
Greece	73.0	70.4	-3.5
Hong Kong, China			
Hungary	64.0	61.8	-3.5
India	53.0	51.4	-3.0
Indonesia	60.0	56.7	-5.5
Ireland	70.0	69.0	-1.4
Israel	70.0		
Italy	73.0		
Japan	75.0		
Jordan	60.0	73.6	22.6
Kazakhstan	56.0	58.5	4.5
Kuwait	63.0	52.4	-16.8
Latvia	62.0	60.0	-3.2
Lithuania	64.0	61.1	-4.5
Malaysia	61.0	63.8	4.6
Mexico	65.0	60.4	-7.1
Morocco	59.0	55.4	-6.2
Netherlands	72.0	69.9	-2.9
New Zealand	69.0	70.3	1.9
Nigeria	38.0	41.9	10.2
Norway	72.0	70.8	-1.7
Pakistan	56.0	50.9	-9.0
Peru	59.0	57.4	-2.7
Philippines	59.0	55.5	-6.0
Poland	66.0	64.3	-2.5
Portugal	69.0	66.8	-3.1
Romania	62.0	60.9	-1.8
Russia	61.0	56.7	-7.1
Saudi Arabia	65.0	60.0	-7.7
Singapore	69.0	68.7	-0.4
Slovakia	67.0	64.1	-4.3
Slovenia	68.0	67.7	-0.5
South Africa	40.0	41.3	3.3
South Korea	65.0	67.4	3.7
Spain	73.0	70.9	-2.9
Sweden	73.0	71.8	-1.6
Switzerland	72.0	72.8	1.1
Taiwan			
Thailand	60.0	58.6	-2.4
Tunisia	61.0	61.3	0.5
Turkey	63.0	59.8	-5.1
Turkmenistan	54.0	50.3	-6.9
Ukraine	63.0	57.4	-8.9
United Arab Emirates	65.0	62.5	-3.9
United Kingdom	72.0	69.6	-3.3
USA	70.0	67.6	-3.4
Venezuela	65.0	61.1	-6.1
Vietnam	58.0	58.6	1.1

Source: Euromonitor International from World Bank

Life expectancy at birth: males 1998-2001

Table: 2.3

years/% change

	1998	2001	% change 1998-2001
Algeria	67.1	67.7	0.97
Argentina	69.6	70.4	1.20
Australia	77.1	77.4	0.35
Austria	75.4	75.9	0.72
Azerbaijan	59.9	60.7	1.35
Belarus	62.8	62.9	0.13
Belgium	74.3	74.8	0.73
Bolivia	60.0	61.1	1.86
Brazil	64.9	65.5	0.97
Bulgaria	68.4	68.4	0.03
Canada	76.3	76.6	0.35
Chile	72.8	73.2	0.53
China	69.2	69.8	0.94
Colombia	65.7	66.7	1.58
Croatia	68.4	68.9	0.79
Czech Republic	71.3	71.9	0.84
Denmark	74.4	74.8	0.58
Ecuador	67.1	67.6	0.75
Egypt	64.2	65.3	1.68
Estonia	64.9	65.7	1.25
Finland	74.0	74.5	0.73
France	75.1	75.6	0.72
Germany	74.6	75.1	0.72
Greece	75.2	75.5	0.36
Hong Kong, China	76.6	77.1	0.58
Hungary	66.5	67.3	1.22
India	59.1	60.0	1.50
Indonesia	63.3	64.4	1.71
Ireland	73.3	73.8	0.67
Israel	75.7	76.1	0.57
Italy	75.9	76.2	0.36
Japan	77.5	77.9	0.56
Jordan	68.0	68.6	0.95
Kazakhstan	58.3	58.8	0.93
Kuwait	74.5	74.9	0.58
Latvia	64.1	65.2	1.68
Lithuania	66.9	67.7	1.21
Malaysia	68.7	69.2	0.79
Mexico	71.1	71.6	0.71
Morocco	66.4	67.5	1.63
Netherlands	75.5	75.8	0.36
New Zealand	75.7	76.1	0.57
Nigeria	50.1	50.6	1.09
Norway	75.7	76.1	0.57
Pakistan	59.9	61.0	1.80
Peru	65.5	66.3	1.18
Philippines	63.4	64.8	2.22
Poland	69.3	69.9	0.94
Portugal	72.2	72.7	0.75
Romania	67.7	67.8	0.13
Russia	59.0	58.9	-0.16
Saudi Arabia	67.8	68.4	0.96
Singapore	76.0	76.5	0.71
Slovakia	68.8	69.3	0.79
Slovenia	71.5	72.1	0.91
South Africa	51.7	47.7	-7.70
South Korea	70.6	71.2	0.92
Spain	74.9	75.3	0.58
Sweden	77.3	77.7	0.56
Switzerland	77.0	77.3	0.35
Taiwan	73.8	75.4	2.09
Thailand	65.0	65.7	1.04
Tunisia	68.4	69.0	0.95
Turkey	66.2	67.0	1.23
Turkmenistan	57.8	58.9	1.87
Ukraine	62.1	62.2	0.12
United Arab Emirates	70.3	70.7	0.61
United Kingdom	74.6	75.1	0.72
USA	73.8	74.3	0.73
Venezuela	70.2	70.7	0.74
Vietnam	65.8	66.9	1.64

Source: Euromonitor International from World Bank

Healthy life expectancy at birth: males 1998-2001

Table: 2.4

years/% change

	1998	2001	% change 1998-2001
Algeria	64.0	55.8	-12.80
Argentina	71.0	60.6	-14.71
Australia	69.0	70.1	1.58
Austria	61.0	68.9	12.98
Azerbaijan	56.0	50.3	-10.24
Belarus	69.0	53.9	-21.84
Belgium	52.0	67.7	30.16
Bolivia	55.0	48.0	-12.67
Brazil	61.0	52.2	-14.36
Bulgaria	70.0	60.8	-13.08
Canada	66.0	68.2	3.31
Chile	61.0	64.4	5.62
China	60.0	62.0	3.36
Colombia	63.0	55.3	-12.28
Croatia	62.0	59.7	-3.70
Czech Republic	67.0	63.8	-4.82
Denmark	60.0	69.3	15.51
Ecuador	59.0	56.6	-4.13
Egypt	58.0	56.4	-2.84
Estonia	67.0	58.0	-13.48
Finland	69.0	67.7	-1.85
France	67.0	69.0	3.05
Germany	70.0	68.3	-2.49
Greece		69.0	
Hong Kong, China	60.0		
Hungary	53.0	58.0	9.40
India	59.0	51.5	-12.65
Indonesia	68.0	56.1	-17.44
Ireland	69.0	67.6	-1.96
Israel	70.0	68.0	-2.81
Italy	72.0	69.2	-3.84
Japan	61.0	71.4	17.01
Jordan	52.0	57.2	9.95
Kazakhstan	63.0	49.0	-22.26
Kuwait	57.0	64.1	12.51
Latvia	61.0	55.2	-9.57
Lithuania	61.0	56.9	-6.76
Malaysia	62.0	57.6	-7.12
Mexico	59.0	62.6	6.12
Morocco	70.0	54.9	-21.61
Netherlands	67.0	68.7	2.49
New Zealand	38.0	69.1	81.94
Nigeria	69.0	40.0	-42.02
Norway	55.0	69.3	26.04
Pakistan	58.0	50.4	-13.14
Peru	57.0	54.7	-3.96
Philippines	62.0	51.1	-17.51
Poland	66.0	62.1	-5.93
Portugal	59.0	64.3	8.90
Romania	56.0	58.6	4.58
Russia	65.0	51.5	-20.82
Saudi Arabia	67.0	57.4	-14.26
Singapore	64.0	67.9	6.16
Slovakia	65.0	61.6	-5.20
Slovenia	39.0	65.1	67.01
South Africa	62.0	40.0	-35.46
South Korea	70.0	64.5	-7.86
Spain	71.0	68.7	-3.30
Sweden	70.0	70.5	0.71
Switzerland		71.1	
Taiwan	58.0		
Thailand	62.0	56.4	-9.04
Tunisia	64.0	58.9	-8.01
Turkey	52.0	58.5	12.51
Turkmenistan	58.0	46.7	-19.43
Ukraine	65.0	52.9	-18.55
United Arab Emirates	70.0	61.7	-11.87
United Kingdom	68.0	68.4	0.64
USA	63.0	66.4	5.34
Venezuela	59.0	57.1	-3.28
Vietnam		55.9	

Source: *Euromonitor International from World Bank*

Healthy life expectancy at 60: males 1998-2001

Table: 2.5

years/% change

	1998	2001	% change 1998-2001
Algeria	15.0	10.3	-31.3
Argentina	17.0	11.9	-30.0
Australia	15.0	16.4	9.1
Austria	13.0	15.7	21.0
Azerbaijan	10.0	8.5	-15.5
Belarus	16.0	9.5	-40.6
Belgium	12.0	14.8	23.4
Bolivia	12.0	8.4	-30.2
Brazil	12.0	9.4	-21.9
Bulgaria	16.0	11.5	-28.0
Canada	14.0	15.3	9.4
Chile	12.0	13.3	10.4
China	14.0	12.7	-9.3
Colombia	11.0	10.7	-2.8
Croatia	13.0	10.1	-22.5
Czech Republic	14.0	12.8	-8.7
Denmark	13.0	15.5	18.9
Ecuador	12.0	9.4	-22.0
Egypt	11.0	9.4	-14.5
Estonia	14.0	11.1	-20.6
Finland	17.0	15.2	-10.8
France	14.0	16.1	14.8
Germany	17.0	15.0	-12.0
Greece		15.7	
Hong Kong, China	12.0		
Hungary	11.0	10.4	-5.4
India	16.0	9.7	-39.5
Indonesia	14.0	10.6	-24.2
Ireland	16.0	13.9	-13.0
Israel	16.0	15.8	-1.5
Italy	18.0	15.5	-13.8
Japan	10.0	17.1	70.9
Jordan	9.0	9.9	10.0
Kazakhstan	11.0	8.7	-21.1
Kuwait	11.0	12.2	10.7
Latvia	13.0	10.0	-23.3
Lithuania	10.0	11.0	10.0
Malaysia	15.0	9.2	-38.5
Mexico	12.0	14.5	20.8
Morocco	15.0	9.2	-38.6
Netherlands	14.0	15.0	7.4
New Zealand	9.0	15.9	76.3
Nigeria	15.0	7.0	-53.4
Norway	11.0	15.6	42.3
Pakistan	12.0	9.3	-22.2
Peru	10.0	10.7	6.6
Philippines	12.0	8.0	-33.0
Poland	14.0	11.9	-15.0
Portugal	12.0	13.4	11.5
Romania	10.0	11.1	11.3
Russia	13.0	8.5	-34.9
Saudi Arabia	14.0	10.0	-28.2
Singapore	13.0	14.5	11.5
Slovakia	13.0	11.5	-11.6
Slovenia	7.0	13.3	90.7
South Africa	10.0	8.9	-11.3
South Korea	17.0	12.9	-24.3
Spain	17.0	15.2	-10.3
Sweden	16.0	16.5	2.9
Switzerland		16.9	
Taiwan	14.0		
Thailand	11.0	12.0	9.3
Tunisia	16.0	10.8	-32.7
Turkey	9.0	11.2	24.3
Turkmenistan	12.0	6.8	-43.5
Ukraine	12.0	8.8	-27.0
United Arab Emirates	16.0	10.6	-33.8
United Kingdom	15.0	15.0	-0.2
USA	13.0	14.9	14.3
Venezuela	10.0	11.6	15.8
Vietnam		9.9	

Source: Euromonitor International from World Bank

Life expectancy at birth: females 1998-2004

Table: 2.6

years/% change

	1998	1999	2000	2001	2002	2003	2004	% change 1998-2004
Algeria	70.3	70.6	71.2	71.2	71.2	71.4	71.6	1.86
Argentina	77.2	77.4	77.8	77.9	78.1	78.3	78.6	1.86
Australia	82.3	82.4	82.1	82.6	83.0	83.2	83.4	1.30
Austria	81.4	81.5	81.4	81.8	82.2	82.4	82.7	1.64
Azerbaijan	66.1	66.3	68.9	68.7	68.6	69.4	70.5	6.72
Belarus	74.1	74.1	74.0	74.2	74.3	74.4	74.4	0.39
Belgium	80.8	80.9	80.9	81.2	81.5	81.7	81.9	1.40
Bolivia	63.1	63.6	63.6	64.3	64.7	65.1	65.4	3.61
Brazil	71.3	71.6	71.9	72.0	72.3	72.5	72.8	2.06
Bulgaria	74.8	74.8	74.9	74.8	75.3	75.5	75.7	1.23
Canada	81.6	81.7	81.5	81.9	82.3	82.5	82.7	1.31
Chile	79.1	79.2	79.5	79.5	80.0	80.2	80.6	1.92
China	71.9	72.2	73.0	72.7	72.7	72.9	73.0	1.54
Colombia	74.2	74.4	75.1	74.8	76.3	76.9	77.7	4.69
Croatia	76.7	76.8	77.7	77.1	78.6	79.2	80.0	4.35
Czech Republic	78.3	78.5	78.2	78.8	79.0	79.2	79.4	1.40
Denmark	79.1	79.2	78.5	79.5	79.5	79.6	79.6	0.67
Ecuador	72.7	72.9	74.2	73.2	73.5	73.7	73.9	1.71
Egypt	66.7	67.1	69.1	67.8	69.0	69.6	70.4	5.52
Estonia	76.1	76.2	76.5	76.5	77.1	77.4	77.7	2.15
Finland	80.8	80.9	80.9	81.2	81.5	81.7	81.9	1.40
France	82.5	82.6	83.1	82.9	83.5	83.8	84.1	1.98
Germany	80.7	80.8	80.6	81.1	81.6	81.9	82.2	1.90
Greece	80.5	80.6	80.8	80.8	81.1	81.3	81.4	1.08
Hong Kong, China	82.1	82.2	82.4	82.6	82.7	82.9	83.1	1.15
Hungary	75.6	75.8	75.2	76.1	76.8	77.1	77.6	2.70
India	60.5	60.9	62.7	61.7	62.0	62.2	62.6	3.53
Indonesia	66.2	66.6	67.4	67.4	67.9	68.3	68.7	3.84
Ireland	78.8	78.9	79.7	79.2	79.8	80.1	80.4	2.06
Israel	80.5	80.6	80.6	80.9	81.4	81.7	82.0	1.90
Italy	81.9	82.0	82.4	82.2	82.5	82.7	82.8	1.06
Japan	84.0	84.3	84.7	84.7	85.3	85.6	86.0	2.34
Jordan	72.7	73.0	72.5	73.5	73.3	73.4	73.4	0.98
Kazakhstan	66.8	66.9	68.4	67.2	68.9	69.5	70.5	5.55
Kuwait	75.5	75.6	76.8	75.9	76.9	77.3	77.9	3.22
Latvia	75.6	75.7	75.5	76.0	75.8	75.8	75.8	0.31
Lithuania	77.4	77.6	77.2	77.9	77.6	77.6	77.5	0.18
Malaysia	73.9	74.1	74.1	74.4	74.7	74.9	75.1	1.68
Mexico	76.2	76.4	76.2	76.7	77.0	77.2	77.4	1.59
Morocco	70.2	70.6	70.4	71.3	72.8	73.5	74.4	5.95
Netherlands	80.4	80.5	81.0	80.7	81.1	81.3	81.5	1.33
New Zealand	80.5	80.6	80.9	80.9	81.2	81.4	81.6	1.41
Nigeria	52.2	52.4	51.4	52.6	49.6	48.7	47.2	-9.63
Norway	81.0	81.1	81.4	81.4	81.7	81.9	82.1	1.40
Pakistan	60.4	60.8	60.7	61.5	61.6	61.8	62.1	2.78
Peru	70.1	70.4	71.6	71.8	72.0	72.5	73.2	4.49
Philippines	70.8	71.1	71.1	71.5	71.7	71.9	72.1	1.84
Poland	77.6	77.8	77.7	78.1	78.7	79.0	79.4	2.37
Portugal	79.7	79.8	79.3	80.1	80.5	80.7	81.0	1.67
Romania	74.4	74.4	73.5	74.5	75.0	75.2	75.4	1.33
Russia	72.2	72.2	72.0	72.3	72.1	72.1	72.0	-0.29
Saudi Arabia	72.7	73.0	70.3	70.5	70.8	71.0	71.1	-2.19
Singapore	80.6	80.8	80.2	81.1	81.7	82.0	82.4	2.28
Slovakia	77.0	77.1	77.5	77.4	78.3	78.7	79.2	2.90
Slovenia	79.0	79.2	79.4	79.5	80.5	80.9	81.5	3.22
South Africa	56.4	54.1	52.1	50.3	52.6	52.2	52.4	-7.02
South Korea	78.2	78.4	78.3	78.7	79.4	79.7	78.0	-0.20
Spain	82.3	82.4	82.3	82.6	83.0	83.2	83.4	1.30
Sweden	81.9	82.0	82.0	82.3	82.6	82.8	83.0	1.38
Switzerland	82.5	82.6	82.5	82.8	83.3	83.5	83.8	1.54
Taiwan	71.6	71.6	71.7	71.7	71.7	71.8	71.9	0.39
Thailand	71.5	71.8	72.4	72.2	72.7	73.0	73.3	2.47
Tunisia	72.7	73.0	73.4	73.5	73.9	74.2	74.5	2.49
Turkey	70.4	70.7	72.5	72.3	72.2	72.7	73.3	4.10
Turkmenistan	65.7	66.0	64.9	66.5	66.9	67.2	67.5	2.76
Ukraine	73.2	73.2	73.3	73.3	72.9	72.8	72.6	-0.83
United Arab Emirates	74.3	74.4	76.4	74.7	75.1	75.3	75.6	1.79
United Kingdom	79.4	79.6	79.9	79.9	80.5	80.8	81.2	2.32
USA	79.0	79.2	79.5	79.5	79.8	80.0	80.2	1.57
Venezuela	76.0	76.2	76.5	76.5	76.8	77.0	77.2	1.60
Vietnam	70.7	71.1	71.0	71.8	72.2	72.5	72.9	3.08

Source: Euromonitor International from World Bank

Healthy life expectancy at birth: females 1998-2001

Table: 2.7

years/% change

	1998	2001	% change 1998-2001
Algeria	62.0	59.9	-3.41
Argentina	64.0	65.7	2.65
Australia	71.0	73.2	3.06
Austria	69.0	73.0	5.83
Azerbaijan	61.0	55.4	-9.20
Belarus	56.0	62.8	12.18
Belgium	69.0	71.8	4.03
Bolivia	52.0	53.6	3.08
Brazil	55.0	61.1	11.02
Bulgaria	61.0	65.2	6.93
Canada	70.0	71.6	2.22
Chile	66.0	67.8	2.73
China	61.0	64.3	5.43
Colombia	60.0	62.1	3.52
Croatia	63.0	66.9	6.17
Czech Republic	62.0	69.5	12.03
Denmark	67.0	70.8	5.75
Ecuador	60.0	62.4	3.97
Egypt	59.0	57.0	-3.47
Estonia	58.0	66.1	13.95
Finland	67.0	72.5	8.17
France	69.0	73.5	6.47
Germany	67.0	72.2	7.82
Greece	70.0	71.9	2.68
Hong Kong, China			
Hungary	60.0	65.5	9.20
India	53.0	51.3	-3.21
Indonesia	59.0	57.2	-2.99
Ireland	68.0	70.4	3.49
Israel	69.0	70.8	2.66
Italy	70.0	72.9	4.08
Japan	72.0	75.8	5.23
Jordan	61.0	59.9	-1.79
Kazakhstan	52.0	55.8	7.36
Kuwait	63.0	65.8	4.38
Latvia	57.0	64.9	13.87
Lithuania	61.0	65.4	7.15
Malaysia	61.0	63.2	3.53
Mexico	62.0	65.0	4.77
Morocco	59.0	55.9	-5.33
Netherlands	70.0	71.1	1.59
New Zealand	67.0	71.5	6.79
Nigeria	38.0	43.8	15.15
Norway	69.0	72.2	4.61
Pakistan	55.0	51.5	-6.35
Peru	58.0	60.1	3.61
Philippines	57.0	59.8	4.94
Poland	62.0	66.6	7.43
Portugal	66.0	69.4	5.20
Romania	59.0	63.3	7.23
Russia	56.0	61.9	10.52
Saudi Arabia	65.0	62.5	-3.88
Singapore	67.0	69.5	3.66
Slovakia	64.0	66.6	4.11
Slovenia	65.0	70.3	8.08
South Africa	39.0	42.7	9.40
South Korea	62.0	70.3	13.44
Spain	70.0	73.0	4.35
Sweden	71.0	73.2	3.10
Switzerland	70.0	74.4	6.31
Taiwan			
Thailand	58.0	60.8	4.76
Tunisia	62.0	63.7	2.73
Turkey	64.0	61.1	-4.55
Turkmenistan	52.0	53.8	3.49
Ukraine	58.0	61.8	6.63
United Arab Emirates	65.0	63.3	-2.68
United Kingdom	70.0	70.9	1.23
USA	68.0	68.8	1.22
Venezuela	63.0	65.0	3.24
Vietnam	59.0	61.4	4.07

Source: *Euromonitor International from World Bank*

Healthy life expectancy at 60: females 1998-2001

Table: 2.8

years/% change

	1998	2001	% change 1998-2001
Algeria	12.0	12.2	1.67
Argentina	18.0	15.1	-16.11
Australia	20.0	18.8	-6.00
Austria	19.0	18.5	-2.63
Azerbaijan	16.0	11.0	-31.25
Belarus	15.0	13.0	-13.33
Belgium	20.0	17.8	-10.77
Bolivia	11.0	11.0	-0.16
Brazil	15.0	13.0	-13.04
Bulgaria	15.0	13.9	-7.30
Canada	19.0	17.9	-5.58
Chile	18.0	15.5	-13.89
China	14.0	14.2	1.62
Colombia	15.0	12.9	-14.07
Croatia	16.0	14.4	-9.71
Czech Republic	16.0	16.0	-0.25
Denmark	17.0	16.7	-1.51
Ecuador	13.0	14.2	9.56
Egypt	12.0	9.2	-23.41
Estonia	16.0	15.0	-6.05
Finland	18.0	18.1	0.54
France	22.0	19.1	-13.34
Germany	18.0	17.7	-1.53
Greece	19.0	17.1	-9.80
Hong Kong, China			
Hungary	16.0	14.4	-9.92
India	12.0	10.2	-14.69
Indonesia	16.0	11.1	-30.94
Ireland	17.0	16.1	-5.12
Israel	17.0	16.9	-0.86
Italy	20.0	18.2	-9.12
Japan	22.0	20.7	-5.85
Jordan	9.0	11.5	27.96
Kazakhstan	13.0	10.8	-17.14
Kuwait	12.0	13.0	8.02
Latvia	16.0	14.4	-9.83
Lithuania	16.0	14.8	-7.80
Malaysia	10.0	12.0	20.21
Mexico	17.0	14.9	-12.14
Morocco	11.0	10.0	-9.42
Netherlands	20.0	17.3	-13.39
New Zealand	17.0	17.7	4.36
Nigeria	10.0	9.5	-4.67
Norway	20.0	17.9	-10.66
Pakistan	13.0	10.8	-16.57
Peru	13.0	13.2	1.61
Philippines	12.0	11.9	-0.98
Poland	17.0	14.6	-13.93
Portugal	18.0	16.2	-10.05
Romania	15.0	13.5	-10.18
Russia	15.0	12.7	-15.04
Saudi Arabia	13.0	13.0	0.02
Singapore	17.0	15.8	-7.05
Slovakia	16.0	14.6	-9.04
Slovenia	17.0	16.6	-2.60
South Africa	9.0	11.4	27.15
South Korea	15.0	16.6	10.48
Spain	20.0	18.2	-8.89
Sweden	20.0	18.5	-7.39
Switzerland	21.0	19.4	-7.63
Taiwan			
Thailand	14.0	12.6	-10.21
Tunisia	10.0	13.4	34.28
Turkey	15.0	12.4	-17.49
Turkmenistan	11.0	9.7	-11.68
Ukraine	16.0	12.2	-23.64
United Arab Emirates	13.0	12.3	-5.75
United Kingdom	19.0	16.9	-11.30
USA	18.0	16.6	-7.81
Venezuela	16.0	15.0	-6.51
Vietnam	11.0	12.5	13.87

Source: Euromonitor International from World Bank

■ Sanitation

Population with access to improved sanitary facilities 2000

Table: 2.9

As stated

	Total population (% of total population)	Urban population (% of urban population)	Rural population (% of rural population)
Algeria	99.0	99.0	81.0
Argentina	85.0		
Australia	100.0	100.0	100.0
Austria	100.0	100.0	100.0
Azerbaijan	81.0	90.0	70.0
Belarus		100.0	100.0
Belgium			
Bolivia	70.0	86.0	42.0
Brazil	76.0	84.0	43.0
Bulgaria	100.0	100.0	100.0
Canada	100.0	100.0	99.0
Chile	96.0	96.0	97.0
China	40.0	69.0	27.0
Colombia	86.0	96.0	56.0
Croatia			
Czech Republic			
Denmark			
Ecuador	86.0	92.0	74.0
Egypt	98.0	100.0	96.0
Estonia		93.0	
Finland	100.0	100.0	100.0
France			
Germany			
Greece			
Hong Kong, China			
Hungary	99.0	100.0	98.0
India	28.0	61.0	15.0
Indonesia	55.0	69.0	46.0
Ireland			
Israel			
Italy			
Japan			
Jordan	99.0	100.0	98.0
Kazakhstan	99.0	100.0	98.0
Kuwait			
Latvia			
Lithuania			
Malaysia			98.0
Mexico	74.0	88.0	34.0
Morocco	68.0	86.0	44.0
Netherlands	100.0	100.0	100.0
New Zealand			100.0
Nigeria	54.0	66.0	45.0
Norway		100.0	100.0
Pakistan	62.0	95.0	43.0
Peru	71.0	79.0	49.0
Philippines	83.0	93.0	69.0
Poland			
Portugal			
Romania	53.0	86.0	10.0
Russia			96.0
Saudi Arabia	100.0	100.0	100.0
Singapore	100.0	100.0	
Slovakia	100.0	100.0	100.0
Slovenia			100.0
South Africa	87.0	93.0	80.0
South Korea	63.0	76.0	4.0
Spain			
Sweden	100.0	100.0	100.0
Switzerland	100.0	100.0	100.0
Taiwan			
Thailand	96.0	96.0	96.0
Tunisia	84.0	96.0	62.0
Turkey	90.0	97.0	70.0
Turkmenistan	100.0		
Ukraine	99.0	100.0	98.0
United Arab Emirates			
United Kingdom	100.0	100.0	100.0
USA	100.0	100.0	100.0
Venezuela	68.0	71.0	48.0
Vietnam	47.0	82.0	38.0

Source: National statistics/World Bank

Population with access to improved water source 2000

%

	% of total population with access
Algeria	89.0
Argentina	
Australia	100.0
Austria	100.0
Azerbaijan	78.0
Belarus	100.0
Belgium	
Bolivia	83.0
Brazil	87.0
Bulgaria	100.0
Canada	100.0
Chile	93.0
China	75.0
Colombia	91.0
Croatia	
Czech Republic	
Denmark	100.0
Ecuador	85.0
Egypt	97.0
Estonia	
Finland	100.0
France	
Germany	
Greece	
Hong Kong, China	
Hungary	99.0
India	84.0
Indonesia	78.0
Ireland	
Israel	
Italy	
Japan	
Jordan	96.0
Kazakhstan	91.0
Kuwait	
Latvia	
Lithuania	
Malaysia	
Mexico	88.0
Morocco	80.0
Netherlands	100.0
New Zealand	
Nigeria	62.0
Norway	100.0
Pakistan	90.0
Peru	80.0
Philippines	86.0
Poland	
Portugal	
Romania	58.0
Russia	99.0
Saudi Arabia	95.0
Singapore	100.0
Slovakia	100.0
Slovenia	100.0
South Africa	86.0
South Korea	92.0
Spain	
Sweden	100.0
Switzerland	100.0
Taiwan	
Thailand	84.0
Tunisia	80.0
Turkey	82.0
Turkmenistan	
Ukraine	98.0
United Arab Emirates	
United Kingdom	100.0
USA	100.0
Venezuela	83.0
Vietnam	77.0

Source: Euromonitor International from World Bank

■ **Health Expenditure**

Public expenditure on pharmaceuticals and other medical non-durables 1998-2004

Table: 2.11

US$ million/% real change

	1998	1999	2000	2001	2002	2003	2004	% real growth 1998-2004
Algeria								
Argentina								
Australia	1,943.0	2,281.4	2,549.2	2,499.2	2,698.6	3,273.2	3,938.1	28.18
Austria	1,699.4	1,764.3	1,663.0	1,690.4	1,909.6	2,454.8	2,930.9	28.81
Azerbaijan								
Belarus								
Belgium	1,701.7	1,770.7	1,630.7	1,658.2	1,780.6	2,205.3	2,558.2	11.90
Bolivia								
Brazil								
Bulgaria								
Canada	2,713.9	3,081.3	3,592.3	3,949.0	4,347.1	5,389.5	6,590.1	66.14
Chile								
China								
Colombia								
Croatia								
Czech Republic	842.6	700.4	629.9	702.5	899.4	1,132.8	1,393.8	29.79
Denmark	635.0	632.9	567.1	614.0	739.1	992.2	1,237.7	50.72
Ecuador								
Egypt								
Estonia								
Finland	633.4	651.0	624.7	687.2	808.4	1,085.7	1,332.4	61.38
France	15,949.6	16,699.9	16,121.2	17,218.6	19,465.4	25,348.9	31,022.7	45.05
Germany	20,987.4	21,628.4	19,584.5	21,054.0	23,443.6	29,936.8	35,856.5	32.00
Greece	1,077.3	1,169.8	1,177.4	1,218.8	1,387.2	1,818.2	2,242.4	39.71
Hong Kong, China								
Hungary	678.5	634.9	585.6	666.7	870.6	1,160.6	1,592.5	52.04
India								
Indonesia								
Ireland	469.7	515.6	513.2	638.9	816.0	1,188.4	1,647.5	123.71
Israel								
Italy	8,043.2	8,473.0	8,641.1	11,067.5	11,703.9	13,375.3	15,377.4	37.41
Japan	34,015.7	39,343.3	44,174.5	41,865.1	42,489.4	48,402.4	54,599.2	35.28
Jordan								
Kazakhstan								
Kuwait								
Latvia								
Lithuania								
Malaysia								
Mexico		2.7	17.7	32.8	779.5	726.1	765.3	24,712.10
Morocco								
Netherlands	2,369.8	2,174.5	2,259.1	2,244.3	2,773.5	3,302.4	3,777.4	30.03
New Zealand	435.2	477.9	420.2	418.7	487.5	639.9	779.2	15.67
Nigeria								
Norway								
Pakistan								
Peru								
Philippines								
Poland	837.3	890.1	1,037.7	1,266.8	1,339.7	1,556.2	1,896.7	59.17
Portugal								
Romania								
Russia								
Saudi Arabia								
Singapore								
Slovakia		305.5	314.7	327.0	433.9	642.8	938.2	65.09
Slovenia								
South Africa								
South Korea	116.5	171.7	749.7	2,932.5	3,138.4	3,387.3	5,850.0	2,698.71
Spain	6,724.9	7,031.5	6,550.6	6,872.4	7,916.8	10,340.5	12,732.5	32.53
Sweden	1,939.8	2,072.4	1,955.3	1,761.3	2,014.7	2,533.2	2,939.4	16.82
Switzerland	1,622.3	1,679.6	1,670.4	1,815.6	2,117.9	2,662.9	3,153.9	48.46
Taiwan								
Thailand								
Tunisia								
Turkey		1,696.8	2,045.2	1,617.2	1,972.5	2,472.7	3,351.3	42.50
Turkmenistan								
Ukraine								
United Arab Emirates								
United Kingdom	9,764.4	10,190.0	10,461.0	11,011.2	13,202.5	15,855.4	20,111.0	54.53
USA	19,627.0	23,390.0	27,978.0	32,962.0	37,833.0	43,923.0	52,385.9	97.52
Venezuela								
Vietnam								

Source: Euromonitor International from OECD/national statistics

Private expenditure as a proportion of total health expenditure 1998-2004

Table: 2.12

% of total expenditure

	1998	1999	2000	2001	2002	2003	2004	% change 1998-2004
Algeria								
Argentina								
Australia	7.6	6.6	6.9	7.6	6.5	6.1	5.8	-23.82
Austria	7.6	7.3	7.3	7.4	7.4	7.1	7.0	-8.03
Azerbaijan								
Belarus								
Belgium								
Bolivia								
Brazil								
Bulgaria								
Canada	11.2	11.2	11.5	12.4	12.7	13.1	13.7	22.14
Chile								
China								
Colombia								
Croatia								
Czech Republic								
Denmark	1.4	1.7	1.6	1.6	1.6	1.7	1.7	24.49
Ecuador								
Egypt								
Estonia								
Finland	2.6	2.7	2.6	2.5	2.4	2.4	2.4	-8.21
France	12.6	12.6	12.6	12.9	13.2	13.2	13.3	5.93
Germany	8.0	8.2	8.3	8.4	8.6	8.7	8.9	10.75
Greece								
Hong Kong, China								
Hungary		0.1	0.2	0.3	0.4	0.5	0.6	
India								
Indonesia								
Ireland	8.9	8.0	7.6	6.3	5.4	4.2	3.1	-64.79
Israel								
Italy	0.9	0.9	0.9	0.9	0.9	0.9	0.9	0.00
Japan	0.3	0.3	0.3	0.3	0.3	0.3	0.3	0.00
Jordan								
Kazakhstan								
Kuwait								
Latvia								
Lithuania								
Malaysia								
Mexico	2.2	2.2	2.5	2.8	3.0	3.3	3.6	62.27
Morocco								
Netherlands	16.6	16.9	16.1	16.5	17.1	17.6	18.1	8.84
New Zealand	6.4	6.2	6.3	6.3	5.7	5.5	5.2	-18.75
Nigeria								
Norway								
Pakistan								
Peru								
Philippines								
Poland								
Portugal	1.5	1.5	1.6	1.6	1.7	1.7	1.7	16.00
Romania								
Russia								
Saudi Arabia								
Singapore								
Slovakia								
Slovenia								
South Africa								
South Korea	2.6	2.7	2.9	2.1	2.4	2.4	2.3	-10.16
Spain	3.7	3.8	3.9	4.0	4.1	4.2	4.3	16.22
Sweden								
Switzerland	11.4	10.4	10.5	10.2	9.6	9.2	8.8	-23.25
Taiwan								
Thailand								
Tunisia								
Turkey		4.2	4.4	4.3	4.7	4.9	5.1	
Turkmenistan								
Ukraine								
United Arab Emirates								
United Kingdom								
USA	33.9	34.4	35.1	35.7	36.2	36.5	37.0	9.09
Venezuela								
Vietnam								

Source: Euromonitor International from OECD

Share of total health expenditure in GDP 1998-2004

Table: 2.13

% of total GDP

	1998	1999	2000	2001	2002	2003	2004
Algeria	3.6	3.6	3.8	4.1	4.0	3.9	3.7
Argentina	8.2	9.0	8.9	9.5	9.6	9.3	9.1
Australia	8.6	8.7	8.9	9.2	9.5	9.4	9.2
Austria	8.0	8.0	8.0	8.0	8.0	8.2	7.8
Azerbaijan	2.3	2.0	1.7	1.6	1.7	1.7	1.7
Belarus	5.7	5.8	5.4	5.6	5.5	5.6	5.6
Belgium	8.4	8.5	8.6	8.9	8.9	8.9	8.6
Bolivia	5.0	5.2	5.2	5.3	5.2	5.4	5.5
Brazil	7.4	7.8	7.6	7.6	7.3	7.4	7.5
Bulgaria	3.9	5.0	4.8	4.8	4.7	4.8	4.7
Canada	9.1	9.1	9.1	9.5	9.7	9.6	9.4
Chile	6.9	6.8	6.8	7.0	6.9	6.9	6.7
China	4.8	5.1	5.3	5.5	5.5	5.7	5.9
Colombia	5.8	6.4	5.5	5.5	5.3	5.5	5.3
Croatia	8.8	8.9	9.4	9.0	8.8	9.1	8.8
Czech Republic	7.1	7.1	7.1	7.4	7.4	7.5	7.4
Denmark	8.4	8.5	8.2	8.4	8.6	8.7	8.6
Ecuador	4.4	3.7	4.1	4.5	4.5	4.3	4.1
Egypt	3.9	3.9	3.8	3.9	4.0	4.1	4.3
Estonia	6.0	6.5	5.9	5.5	5.4	5.5	5.3
Finland	6.9	6.9	6.6	7.0	7.3	7.0	7.0
France	9.3	9.3	9.4	9.6	9.9	10.1	10.5
Germany	10.6	10.7	10.6	10.8	11.1	11.6	12.2
Greece	9.4	9.6	9.4	9.4	9.1	9.5	9.5
Hong Kong, China	6.2	6.6	7.0	7.4	7.1	6.8	6.6
Hungary	6.9	6.8	6.7	6.8	7.0	6.9	6.6
India	5.0	5.2	5.1	5.1	4.9	5.0	5.1
Indonesia	2.5	2.6	2.7	2.4	2.4	2.5	2.6
Ireland	6.2	6.2	6.4	6.5	6.4	6.7	6.7
Israel	8.1	8.2	8.2	8.7	8.7	8.5	8.6
Italy	7.7	7.8	8.2	8.4	8.0	8.4	8.8
Japan	7.1	7.5	7.7	8.0	8.4	8.7	8.5
Jordan	8.1	8.6	9.2	9.5	9.9	9.5	9.8
Kazakhstan	3.5	3.5	3.3	3.1	3.0	2.9	2.8
Kuwait	4.4	3.9	3.5	3.9	3.9	3.9	3.8
Latvia	6.8	6.9	6.3	6.4	6.5	6.5	6.2
Lithuania	6.4	6.3	6.2	6.0	6.1	5.9	6.0
Malaysia	3.0	3.1	3.3	3.8	3.8	3.7	3.6
Mexico	5.6	5.7	5.7	6.1	5.8	5.9	5.9
Morocco	4.4	4.4	4.7	5.1	4.9	5.0	4.8
Netherlands	8.6	8.7	8.6	8.9	8.8	8.5	8.3
New Zealand	7.9	8.0	8.0	8.3	8.2	8.4	8.8
Nigeria	3.1	3.0	3.0	3.4	3.4	3.5	3.4
Norway	8.5	8.5	7.6	8.0	8.1	7.9	7.9
Pakistan	3.9	4.0	4.1	3.9	4.0	3.9	3.9
Peru	4.6	4.9	4.7	4.7	4.7	4.7	4.7
Philippines	3.5	3.5	3.4	3.3	3.1	3.2	3.1
Poland	6.4	6.2	5.8	6.1	6.2	6.2	5.9
Portugal	8.6	8.7	9.1	9.2	8.7	8.5	8.1
Romania	6.6	6.8	6.6	6.5	6.3	6.4	6.3
Russia	5.8	5.4	5.3	5.4	5.3	5.2	5.1
Saudi Arabia	5.2	4.5	4.4	4.6	4.4	4.5	4.4
Singapore	4.2	4.0	3.6	3.9	4.1	4.1	4.0
Slovakia	5.8	5.8	5.7	5.7	5.4	5.6	5.6
Slovenia	8.3	8.2	8.0	8.4	8.4	8.8	8.5
South Africa	8.7	8.8	8.7	8.6	8.8	8.4	8.3
South Korea	5.1	5.6	5.9	6.0	6.1	5.9	5.7
Spain	7.5	7.5	7.5	7.5	7.7	7.5	7.9
Sweden	8.3	8.4	8.4	8.7	8.5	8.4	8.1
Switzerland	10.6	10.7	10.7	11.0	10.8	10.7	10.5
Taiwan	0.3	0.3	0.4	0.4	0.4	0.4	0.4
Thailand	3.9	3.7	3.6	3.7	3.5	3.6	3.4
Tunisia	6.3	6.3	6.2	6.4	6.6	6.7	6.5
Turkey	4.8	4.9	5.0	5.0	5.1	5.2	5.0
Turkmenistan	5.0	5.0	4.0	4.1	4.3	4.3	4.5
Ukraine	5.0	4.3	4.2	4.3	4.5	4.7	4.7
United Arab Emirates	4.0	3.7	3.5	3.5	3.6	3.7	3.7
United Kingdom	6.9	7.2	7.3	7.6	7.6	7.8	7.6
USA	13.0	13.0	13.1	13.9	13.7	13.9	13.8
Venezuela	5.4	5.6	5.9	6.0	6.2	6.4	6.3
Vietnam	4.9	4.9	5.2	5.1	5.0	4.9	4.8

Source: Euronmonitor from WHO

Per capita trends in health expenditure 1998-2004

Table: 2.14

US$ per capita

	1998	1999	2000	2001	2002	2003	2004	% change 1998-2004
Algeria	62	61	65	70	77	82	88	41.94
Argentina	679	699	680	680	680	682	683	0.59
Australia	1,711	1,871	1,825	1,739	1,995	2,036	2,107	23.14
Austria	2,040	2,047	1,831	1,805	1,969	2,038	2,107	3.28
Azerbaijan	26	26	25	26	27	27	28	7.69
Belarus	90	73	64	82	93	100	108	20.00
Belgium	2,109	2,139	1,952	1,983	2,159	2,263	2,332	10.57
Bolivia	53	63	61	61	63	63	64	20.75
Brazil	348	246	266	227	206	193	180	-48.28
Bulgaria	79	99	101	121	145	153	161	103.80
Canada	1,842	1,916	2,064	2,124	2,222	2,324	2,411	30.89
Chile	325	293	281	253	246	236	225	-30.77
China	36	40	48	52	63	68	73	102.78
Colombia	240	203	158	159	151	142	139	-42.08
Croatia	387	387	374	366	369	363	359	-7.24
Czech Republic	392	380	358	408	504	532	570	45.41
Denmark	2,725	2,767	2,476	2,568	2,831	2,866	2,931	7.56
Ecuador	84	65	53	80	91	97	104	23.81
Egypt	64	67	67	59	59	56	53	-17.19
Estonia	223	244	221	224	263	269	280	25.56
Finland	1,732	1,710	1,543	1,628	1,852	1,899	1,979	14.26
France	2,306	2,282	2,061	2,103	2,348	2,444	2,529	9.67
Germany	2,772	2,727	2,398	2,418	2,631	2,748	2,864	3.32
Greece	1,083	1,146	1,043	1,044	1,198	1,215	1,254	15.79
Hong Kong, China	1,578	1,726	1,874	2,023	2,173	2,327	2,480	57.20
Hungary	335	345	326	375	496	521	554	65.37
India	22	26	29	29	30	31	32	45.45
Indonesia	12	18	20	21	26	27	29	141.67
Ireland	1,454	1,589	1,579	1,839	2,255	2,477	2,677	84.11
Israel	1,511	1,498	1,617	1,754	1,496	1,436	1,375	-9.00
Italy	1,600	1,597	1,506	1,562	1,737	1,784	1,845	15.31
Japan	2,222	2,601	2,827	2,558	2,476	2,434	2,369	6.62
Jordan	144	148	154	163	165	171	176	22.22
Kazakhstan	53	46	48	48	56	59	63	18.87
Kuwait	557	531	516	539	547	552	564	1.26
Latvia	159	179	182	190	203	211	221	38.99
Lithuania	194	194	212	220	241	257	272	40.21
Malaysia	99	109	129	143	149	158	164	65.66
Mexico	232	272	323	369	381	410	433	86.64
Morocco	56	54	54	53	55	55	56	0.00
Netherlands	2,038	2,076	1,894	2,039	2,369	2,467	2,594	27.28
New Zealand	1,125	1,155	1,055	1,056	1,255	1,288	1,351	20.09
Nigeria	17	17	18	20	19	20	20	17.65
Norway	2,865	3,024	2,850	3,031	3,647	3,855	4,078	42.34
Pakistan	16	15	14	12	13	12	12	-25.00
Peru	102	98	96	94	93	91	90	-11.76
Philippines	32	36	34	29	28	27	25	-21.88
Poland	264	249	244	289	301	318	338	28.03
Portugal	932	985	951	994	1,092	1,128	1,175	26.07
Romania	96	91	96	109	128	136	145	51.04
Russia	112	70	102	128	150	166	180	60.71
Saudi Arabia	354	313	336	360	345	356	362	2.26
Singapore	900	849	824	816	898	914	944	4.89
Slovakia	235	218	208	216	256	269	282	20.00
Slovenia	813	829	765	821	922	953	995	22.39
South Africa	261	266	244	224	206	196	188	-27.97
South Korea	328	435	503	528	577	601	617	88.11
Spain	1,112	1,139	1,028	1,063	1,196	1,215	1,246	12.05
Sweden	2,335	2,396	2,280	2,172	2,494	2,527	2,609	11.73
Switzerland	3,908	3,881	3,572	3,774	4,217	4,329	4,497	15.07
Taiwan	744	843	941	990	1,083	1,170	1,251	68.12
Thailand	73	75	72	66	90	93	98	34.25
Tunisia	126	124	115	120	126	127	129	2.38
Turkey	149	179	196	137	172	180	187	25.50
Turkmenistan	27	29	46	58	79	87	94	248.15
Ukraine	41	27	26	34	40	43	47	14.63
United Arab Emirates	724	704	787	824	802	835	851	17.54
United Kingdom	1,688	1,781	1,784	1,837	2,031	2,114	2,224	31.75
USA	4,096	4,298	4,538	4,869	5,267	5,590	5,941	45.04
Venezuela	220	254	300	261	184	176	162	-26.36
Vietnam	18	18	21	21	23	24	25	38.89

Source: *Euromonitor International from OECD/WHO/national statistics*

Per capita trends in consumer expenditure on health goods and medical services 1998-2004

Table: 2.15

US$ per capita

	1998	1999	2000	2001	2002	2003	2004	% change 1998-2004
Algeria	1,018.3	1,146.6	1,041.9	1,108.4	1,221.7	1,428.0	1,693.5	66.30
Argentina	17,431.7	17,477.7	17,298.6	16,211.1	5,441.6	5,347.7	5,022.1	-71.19
Australia	8,712.6	9,875.2	9,775.5	10,422.9	12,481.5	15,354.5	18,691.1	114.53
Austria	3,947.0	3,922.8	3,545.2	3,533.7	3,862.4	4,775.2	5,445.1	37.95
Azerbaijan	132.9	137.6	133.5	135.0	139.0	152.0	163.1	22.71
Belarus	794.0	645.6	546.9	659.6	809.5	938.5	1,089.6	37.23
Belgium	4,935.4	4,922.4	4,539.6	4,678.3	5,211.5	6,524.0	7,631.4	54.62
Bolivia	182.9	185.1	188.4	183.0	173.2	166.1	173.9	-4.96
Brazil	30,445.7	21,437.5	24,138.3	20,178.2	17,540.0	19,680.9	22,206.1	-27.06
Bulgaria	134.5	122.9	115.3	123.4	145.1	179.7	216.3	60.86
Canada	14,569.3	15,464.5	16,388.7	16,718.5	17,420.9	21,125.0	24,009.9	64.80
Chile	4,349.7	4,248.5	4,615.2	4,398.7	4,532.7	4,698.3	5,592.1	28.56
China	21,688.2	20,224.7	25,576.6	28,416.9	30,795.7	33,093.6	35,624.9	64.26
Colombia	2,489.1	2,193.1	2,217.8	2,313.1	2,374.2	2,298.2	2,743.7	10.23
Croatia	216.7	218.7	206.7	214.2	247.2	316.6	378.2	74.53
Czech Republic	322.6	326.6	357.8	444.6	550.4	709.2	814.8	152.60
Denmark	2,131.5	2,124.4	1,901.9	1,972.2	2,184.9	2,765.8	3,228.1	51.45
Ecuador	374.7	246.9	239.7	320.9	356.3	373.8	386.4	3.11
Egypt	1,581.9	1,684.7	1,865.8	1,725.3	1,651.5	1,334.9	1,360.9	-13.97
Estonia	49.1	55.8	55.6	61.4	85.4	112.5	131.1	166.79
Finland	2,238.6	2,243.7	2,169.7	2,273.8	2,538.2	3,110.5	3,456.7	54.41
France	28,723.4	28,315.8	25,469.9	25,744.7	28,709.2	36,108.1	42,154.2	46.76
Germany	47,765.8	46,344.3	41,634.4	42,326.2	45,776.7	56,261.9	63,935.5	33.85
Greece	4,955.9	4,946.6	4,160.7	4,382.1	5,005.9	6,359.8	7,552.7	52.40
Hong Kong, China	3,997.5	3,976.3	3,982.6	3,959.6	3,901.8	3,933.8	4,088.1	2.27
Hungary	767.5	878.2	874.6	1,057.2	1,328.5	1,729.8	2,112.9	175.30
India	10,703.4	14,592.5	18,583.5	20,804.3	23,824.6	26,995.4	30,189.7	182.06
Indonesia	1,230.1	1,978.9	1,973.3	1,867.2	2,386.8	2,862.4	3,034.7	146.70
Ireland	1,156.1	1,212.5	1,202.4	1,322.2	1,660.3	2,103.0	2,396.9	107.33
Israel	1,231.8	1,092.0	1,033.1	780.9	572.5	615.2	633.1	-48.60
Italy	23,603.1	23,038.0	20,604.0	19,398.3	21,721.2	26,725.8	30,429.3	28.92
Japan	69,771.2	83,538.3	92,744.4	85,944.9	88,056.3	96,087.3	104,593.6	49.91
Jordan	157.6	162.0	189.0	200.6	202.4	211.5	221.5	40.52
Kazakhstan	670.9	492.6	463.7	534.2	584.6	621.0	754.1	12.40
Kuwait	155.5	164.5	170.3	190.2	217.3	228.7	243.6	56.70
Latvia	147.8	156.5	190.5	217.3	234.1	283.4	331.8	124.46
Lithuania	247.1	254.5	260.6	267.9	305.3	369.7	419.9	69.90
Malaysia	658.4	741.1	870.0	906.0	952.8	1,016.1	1,069.7	62.46
Mexico	11,689.5	13,447.6	16,455.3	19,391.2	20,026.3	18,581.0	19,165.8	63.96
Morocco	1,470.6	1,419.2	1,382.3	1,404.7	1,501.6	1,782.6	2,054.1	39.68
Netherlands	7,260.7	7,724.0	6,945.8	7,260.8	7,966.7	10,768.6	12,087.2	66.47
New Zealand	919.0	968.5	880.9	890.8	1,091.0	1,415.7	1,698.8	84.84
Nigeria	1,054.7	658.6	801.0	1,152.6	1,397.5	1,777.0	2,036.0	93.05
Norway	1,877.4	1,931.9	1,867.9	1,962.9	2,355.5	2,731.2	2,892.7	54.08
Pakistan	2,354.9	2,447.5	2,336.9	2,174.2	2,381.4	2,620.3	2,850.7	21.05
Peru	2,162.7	1,914.1	2,003.3	2,076.1	2,154.3	2,262.6	2,438.0	12.73
Philippines	913.0	1,041.8	995.6	886.2	897.2	889.8	929.8	1.85
Poland	4,029.5	4,139.0	4,397.8	5,210.4	5,580.6	5,953.3	6,760.0	67.76
Portugal	3,118.6	3,242.0	3,014.6	3,124.8	3,406.9	4,191.7	4,793.7	53.71
Romania	1,176.7	963.9	969.5	961.2	1,088.8	1,092.3	1,249.0	6.14
Russia	2,730.1	2,194.5	2,493.1	3,159.9	3,748.2	5,078.1	6,152.9	125.37
Saudi Arabia	1,648.6	1,837.1	1,882.2	1,867.3	2,008.0	2,097.8	2,237.2	35.70
Singapore	1,874.5	1,988.6	2,083.3	2,157.3	2,287.3	2,414.2	2,619.9	39.76
Slovakia	116.1	131.6	138.0	162.7	186.2	277.6	347.3	199.05
Slovenia	279.3	283.5	263.4	269.8	305.9	409.9	465.4	66.60
South Africa	5,927.9	6,051.1	5,917.7	5,364.6	5,164.6	8,161.4	9,918.2	67.31
South Korea	12,698.7	16,700.5	18,528.4	18,902.8	21,349.9	23,822.1	26,539.9	109.00
Spain	12,064.2	12,446.9	11,609.5	12,255.8	13,788.5	17,433.9	20,178.0	67.25
Sweden	2,811.0	2,840.6	2,785.1	2,698.4	3,002.6	3,754.3	4,214.5	49.93
Switzerland	21,410.1	21,337.5	19,836.2	20,779.7	23,340.7	27,138.1	29,887.6	39.60
Taiwan	13,148.2	14,968.6	15,695.2	16,648.2	16,709.4	17,169.8	18,299.7	39.18
Thailand	5,271.7	5,841.3	5,734.6	5,517.4	5,904.4	6,449.3	7,059.7	33.92
Tunisia	1,025.5	1,080.8	1,017.6	1,051.0	1,148.6	1,390.7	1,531.7	49.37
Turkey	7,776.9	8,081.9	8,626.9	6,367.0	7,614.8	10,402.8	12,441.4	59.98
Turkmenistan	36.4	44.6	57.3	78.4	97.5	130.0	140.8	286.76
Ukraine	192.7	149.9	135.3	163.6	185.3	201.2	228.4	18.56
United Arab Emirates	764.3	763.8	761.1	780.7	812.3	886.1	929.9	21.66
United Kingdom	13,383.0	13,799.7	13,597.5	13,678.7	15,561.5	19,001.7	22,823.2	70.54
USA	997,757.0	1,054,725.0	1,134,365.0	1,233,583.0	1,341,520.0	1,457,272.0	1,558,943.4	56.24
Venezuela	1,981.8	1,788.7	1,743.2	1,847.8	1,383.2	1,546.1	1,683.5	-15.05
Vietnam	1,478.4	1,516.2	1,574.5	1,628.0	1,730.8	1,819.4	1,877.2	26.98

Source: *National statistical offices/OECD/Eurostat/Euromonitor International*

Real growth in consumer expenditure on health goods and medical services (national currencies) 1998-2004

Table: 2.16

1990=100

	1998	1999	2000	2001	2002	2003	2004
Algeria	96.3	119.7	122.6	128.4	144.0	159.3	169.8
Argentina	104.3	105.8	105.7	100.1	81.8	67.1	60.8
Australia	128.6	139.9	147.5	168.9	186.9	187.4	196.6
Austria	139.7	145.3	148.3	148.3	151.4	153.9	156.4
Azerbaijan							
Belarus							
Belgium	137.5	142.7	148.4	153.7	160.1	164.5	171.4
Bolivia	131.1	137.0	141.8	144.8	147.5	146.2	151.9
Brazil	148.8	156.2	165.7	167.0	165.9	170.9	172.0
Bulgaria	117.9	109.6	107.8	110.6	116.9	118.1	121.6
Canada	142.3	148.7	153.3	159.1	164.3	173.1	179.4
Chile	285.3	298.0	330.6	358.0	390.6	395.2	410.3
China	662.0	626.1	789.8	873.3	953.7	1,013.1	1,048.6
Colombia	112.8	110.4	121.5	129.3	135.9	141.1	145.3
Croatia	86.2	94.0	98.2	97.9	104.8	112.4	118.4
Czech Republic	161.8	171.7	202.2	236.4	247.5	274.5	279.4
Denmark	117.2	118.6	119.6	124.7	128.0	132.4	138.9
Ecuador	15.4	6.7	3.3	3.2	3.2	3.1	3.1
Egypt	135.4	140.2	154.7	160.0	168.8	169.8	164.8
Estonia							
Finland	136.0	141.8	153.4	161.4	168.7	170.9	172.3
France	118.2	122.0	124.8	127.8	132.9	136.5	141.8
Germany	151.3	153.6	157.2	161.4	163.7	166.0	168.7
Greece	150.7	154.2	145.4	152.6	159.9	163.6	171.6
Hong Kong, China	128.4	133.2	139.3	140.9	143.2	147.9	154.4
Hungary	150.4	173.0	186.7	209.8	225.5	244.0	252.3
India	154.8	210.4	268.9	304.9	344.5	360.4	377.9
Indonesia	231.0	241.9	249.4	257.8	267.3	277.1	288.2
Ireland	145.9	158.4	172.1	185.7	211.9	216.3	219.2
Israel	196.4	180.3	166.1	128.1	100.1	102.7	104.5
Italy	175.0	176.8	178.3	168.1	174.7	174.6	176.8
Japan	114.4	119.6	126.5	133.2	142.1	143.7	146.0
Jordan	214.9	219.6	254.5	265.3	262.9	268.5	271.9
Kazakhstan							
Kuwait	120.7	123.8	126.9	139.4	155.6	159.1	165.6
Latvia	194.6	199.6	245.3	282.7	294.3	320.0	333.2
Lithuania							
Malaysia	229.2	243.1	281.0	288.6	298.1	314.6	326.4
Mexico	121.6	125.6	138.8	152.0	154.4	153.1	157.8
Morocco	109.7	107.3	111.2	119.5	121.1	123.5	129.2
Netherlands	144.8	158.6	160.8	165.6	167.0	184.3	185.8
New Zealand	116.7	124.6	128.6	136.9	148.5	150.8	155.0
Nigeria	223.4	143.0	167.2	233.0	269.4	322.0	329.9
Norway	144.8	150.5	159.3	166.0	174.7	175.3	175.9
Pakistan	256.2	280.9	278.5	290.0	296.8	306.9	313.6
Peru	125.0	123.5	128.5	131.2	136.2	138.4	141.1
Philippines	127.1	129.9	134.5	130.2	129.5	131.0	133.6
Poland	168.8	184.4	194.9	206.2	216.0	218.1	225.0
Portugal	86.1	92.0	96.2	98.4	98.5	97.8	99.4
Romania	86.9	84.3	82.4	81.3	85.5	74.8	75.1
Russia	89.4	98.1	105.4	114.1	125.6	146.6	150.4
Saudi Arabia	124.8	141.0	146.1	146.5	157.2	163.3	173.5
Singapore	174.8	187.8	197.4	210.4	223.8	228.7	236.8
Slovakia							
Slovenia							
South Africa	190.5	204.3	215.5	229.2	247.5	265.2	271.4
South Korea	172.3	190.7	196.8	220.2	234.7	240.9	249.0
Spain	157.6	167.3	174.4	183.0	189.9	194.4	198.5
Sweden	128.2	134.1	144.5	154.1	158.2	161.2	163.8
Switzerland	135.9	139.2	143.3	148.5	153.1	152.8	154.2
Taiwan	224.9	246.3	265.0	275.7	291.8	299.8	308.1
Thailand	119.1	120.3	123.3	129.3	133.0	137.8	142.3
Tunisia	156.2	167.0	176.5	187.6	197.1	210.4	216.2
Turkey	276.7	280.1	288.1	270.0	273.9	297.4	311.1
Turkmenistan							
Ukraine							
United Arab Emirates	166.2	162.7	159.8	159.5	161.3	170.7	171.2
United Kingdom	141.2	146.7	150.2	156.0	167.7	182.7	190.0
USA	135.2	139.8	145.5	153.8	164.7	174.9	182.3
Venezuela	177.0	143.0	134.6	134.9	132.4	156.2	164.4
Vietnam	82.3	85.1	91.3	98.5	104.5	108.0	110.1

Source: National statistical offices/OECD/Eurostat/Euromonitor International

Consumer expenditure on health goods and medical services as a proportion of the total 1998-2004

Table: 2.17

% of total consumer expenditure

	1998	1999	2000	2001	2002	2003	2004
Algeria	0.1	0.1	0.1	0.1	0.1	0.1	0.1
Argentina	8.3	8.6	8.6	8.6	2.8	2.9	2.8
Australia	2.5	2.7	2.5	2.5	2.8	3.3	3.9
Austria	3.6	3.5	3.0	2.9	3.1	3.7	4.1
Azerbaijan	0.0	0.0	0.0	0.0	0.0	0.0	0.0
Belarus	0.2	0.0	0.0	0.0	0.0	0.0	0.0
Belgium	4.2	4.1	3.5	3.5	3.8	4.6	5.1
Bolivia	0.5	0.5	0.5	0.5	0.4	0.4	0.4
Brazil	5.3	3.3	3.3	2.5	2.0	1.9	2.0
Bulgaria	0.8	0.7	0.6	0.6	0.6	0.8	0.8
Canada	2.9	2.9	2.9	2.8	2.8	3.2	3.5
Chile	0.0	0.0	0.0	0.0	0.0	0.0	0.0
China	0.6	0.5	0.6	0.6	0.6	0.6	0.6
Colombia	0.0	0.0	0.0	0.0	0.0	0.0	0.0
Croatia	0.3	0.3	0.2	0.2	0.3	0.3	0.3
Czech Republic	0.0	0.0	0.0	0.0	0.0	0.1	0.1
Denmark	0.4	0.4	0.3	0.3	0.3	0.4	0.5
Ecuador	2.7	2.8	2.8	2.8	2.8	2.8	2.7
Egypt	0.7	0.7	0.7	0.6	0.5	0.4	0.4
Estonia	0.1	0.1	0.1	0.1	0.1	0.2	0.2
Finland	4.0	3.9	3.5	3.5	3.7	4.5	4.9
France	4.0	3.8	3.3	3.2	3.4	4.2	4.7
Germany	4.5	4.2	3.7	3.6	3.9	4.8	5.3
Greece	6.1	5.9	4.6	4.6	4.9	5.9	6.5
Hong Kong, China	0.5	0.6	0.5	0.5	0.6	0.6	0.6
Hungary	0.0	0.0	0.0	0.0	0.0	0.0	0.0
India	0.1	0.1	0.1	0.1	0.2	0.2	0.2
Indonesia	0.0	0.0	0.0	0.0	0.0	0.0	0.0
Ireland	3.1	2.9	2.5	2.6	3.0	3.6	3.9
Israel	0.6	0.4	0.4	0.3	0.2	0.2	0.2
Italy	3.7	3.4	2.9	2.6	2.9	3.4	3.7
Japan	0.0	0.0	0.0	0.0	0.0	0.0	0.0
Jordan	3.6	3.6	3.7	3.7	3.7	3.8	3.8
Kazakhstan	0.1	0.0	0.0	0.0	0.0	0.0	0.0
Kuwait	4.2	4.2	4.2	4.2	4.3	4.5	4.7
Latvia	6.5	6.5	7.2	7.3	7.3	8.0	8.5
Lithuania	0.9	0.9	0.9	0.9	1.0	1.1	1.2
Malaysia	0.6	0.6	0.6	0.6	0.6	0.6	0.6
Mexico	0.4	0.4	0.4	0.5	0.5	0.4	0.4
Morocco	0.6	0.6	0.5	0.5	0.5	0.6	0.7
Netherlands	4.2	4.2	3.5	3.5	3.7	4.8	5.3
New Zealand	1.5	1.6	1.3	1.3	1.5	1.9	2.2
Nigeria	0.0	0.0	0.0	0.0	0.0	0.0	0.0
Norway	0.4	0.3	0.3	0.3	0.4	0.4	0.4
Pakistan	0.1	0.1	0.1	0.1	0.1	0.1	0.1
Peru	1.8	1.6	1.5	1.5	1.5	1.5	1.5
Philippines	0.0	0.0	0.0	0.0	0.0	0.0	0.0
Poland	1.2	1.1	1.0	1.1	1.1	1.2	1.3
Portugal	4.9	4.7	4.1	4.1	4.3	5.2	5.7
Romania	0.0	0.0	0.0	0.0	0.0	0.0	0.0
Russia	0.2	0.1	0.1	0.1	0.1	0.1	0.1
Saudi Arabia	0.7	0.7	0.7	0.7	0.8	0.8	0.8
Singapore	3.3	3.3	3.1	3.2	3.4	3.5	3.7
Slovakia	0.0	0.0	0.0	0.0	0.0	0.0	0.0
Slovenia	0.0	0.0	0.0	0.0	0.0	0.0	0.0
South Africa	1.3	1.2	1.1	0.9	0.8	1.1	1.2
South Korea	0.0	0.0	0.0	0.0	0.0	0.0	0.0
Spain	3.6	3.5	3.0	3.0	3.2	3.9	4.3
Sweden	0.3	0.3	0.3	0.3	0.3	0.3	0.4
Switzerland	9.4	9.1	8.2	8.4	9.3	10.6	11.4
Taiwan	0.2	0.3	0.3	0.3	0.3	0.3	0.3
Thailand	0.2	0.2	0.2	0.2	0.2	0.2	0.2
Tunisia	7.7	7.5	6.5	6.2	6.3	6.9	7.2
Turkey	0.0	0.0	0.0	0.0	0.0	0.0	0.0
Turkmenistan	0.0	0.0	0.0	0.0	0.0	0.0	0.0
Ukraine	0.3	0.2	0.2	0.2	0.2	0.2	0.2
United Arab Emirates	0.8	0.9	0.9	0.9	0.9	0.9	0.9
United Kingdom	2.5	2.4	2.3	2.2	2.4	2.8	3.2
USA	17.0	16.9	16.9	17.6	18.3	18.9	19.1
Venezuela	0.0	0.0	0.0	0.0	0.0	0.0	0.0
Vietnam	0.0	0.0	0.0	0.0	0.0	0.0	0.0

Source: National statistical offices/OECD/Eurostat/Euromonitor International

Consumer expenditure on health goods and medical services by sector 2004

Table: 2.18

% value

	Pharmaceuticals, medical appliances& equipment	Outpatient services	Hospital services
Algeria	38.3	19.3	42.4
Argentina			
Australia	45.7	48.7	5.7
Austria	22.1	49.6	28.3
Azerbaijan	45.8	50.6	3.7
Belarus	9.6	79.8	10.5
Belgium	34.5	35.2	30.3
Bolivia	71.1	23.1	5.8
Brazil	41.1	50.3	8.6
Bulgaria	16.1	75.2	8.7
Canada	39.8	55.0	5.2
Chile	58.3	30.6	11.1
China	49.9	28.0	22.1
Colombia	71.4	11.0	17.6
Croatia	68.8	26.6	4.5
Czech Republic	78.9	17.9	3.1
Denmark	50.4	39.0	10.7
Ecuador	84.3	12.4	3.3
Egypt	25.1	23.6	51.3
Estonia	65.7	32.2	2.2
Finland	47.2	37.7	15.1
France	42.8	36.2	20.9
Germany	35.2	38.0	26.7
Greece	10.2	89.8	
Hong Kong, China	18.6	50.9	30.5
Hungary	79.6	16.2	4.3
India	43.8	39.3	16.8
Indonesia	57.9	31.0	11.1
Ireland	24.2	24.7	51.1
Israel	74.0	20.7	5.3
Italy	50.5	40.5	9.0
Japan	45.1	34.0	20.9
Jordan	31.0	59.8	9.2
Kazakhstan	41.5	54.1	4.4
Kuwait	53.1	40.4	6.5
Latvia	62.3	26.0	11.8
Lithuania	84.0	10.1	5.9
Malaysia	31.9	41.2	26.9
Mexico	37.1	44.5	18.4
Morocco	30.0	49.7	20.4
Netherlands	35.8	29.2	35.0
New Zealand	27.1	44.3	28.6
Nigeria	31.5	58.9	9.7
Norway	46.0	52.4	1.6
Pakistan	40.1	1.1	58.7
Peru	38.1	49.5	12.3
Philippines	27.2	53.6	19.2
Poland	69.6	28.1	2.2
Portugal	29.5	70.5	
Romania	81.6	16.5	1.9
Russia	8.1	87.9	4.0
Saudi Arabia	65.2	29.7	5.1
Singapore	29.2	42.8	28.1
Slovakia	74.1	24.5	1.4
Slovenia	49.7	31.7	18.7
South Africa	22.6	66.0	11.3
South Korea	24.0	45.4	30.6
Spain	31.6	54.1	14.3
Sweden	46.3	50.4	3.3
Switzerland	16.5	67.9	15.7
Taiwan	68.6	8.6	22.9
Thailand	25.9	43.0	31.1
Tunisia	26.7	3.5	69.8
Turkey	42.2	53.3	4.5
Turkmenistan	49.2	48.1	2.6
Ukraine	37.6	42.3	20.0
United Arab Emirates	32.4	57.4	10.3
United Kingdom	61.2	23.3	15.6
USA	17.6	40.2	42.2
Venezuela	63.6	15.5	20.9
Vietnam	28.6	47.6	23.7

Source: National statistical offices/OECD/Eurostat/Euromonitor International

© **Euromonitor International 2005**

■ **Healthcare Infrastructure and Services**

Hospitals and clinics 1998-2004

number/% change

	1998	1999	2000	2001	2002	2003	2004	% change 1998-2004
Algeria	233	235	236	236	237	238	239	2.58
Argentina	6,723	7,206	7,548	7,883	8,192	8,510	8,700	29.41
Australia	1,236	1,257	1,257	1,260	1,262	1,267	1,270	2.75
Austria	330	325	312	310	278	267	258	-21.82
Azerbaijan	746	739	735	735	731	725	722	-3.22
Belarus	836	833	830	826	824	823	822	-1.67
Belgium	958	958	958	959	961	963	964	0.63
Bolivia	2,435	2,438	2,441	2,439	2,437	2,433	2,431	-0.16
Brazil	6,391	6,582	6,782	6,782	6,845	6,902	6,967	9.01
Bulgaria	276	280	249	244	251	249	248	-10.14
Canada	1,062	1,063	1,063	1,065	1,066	1,067	1,068	0.56
Chile	213	212	211	210	209	208	207	-2.82
China	67,081	66,935	66,509	65,424	64,548	63,319	62,290	-7.14
Colombia								
Croatia	78	78	77	78	79	79	80	2.56
Czech Republic	207	203	211	202	201	200	198	-4.35
Denmark	81	80	64	60	59	58	57	-29.63
Ecuador	3,480	3,492	3,501	3,501	3,496	3,485	3,480	0.00
Egypt	331	321	333	327	326	324	322	-2.72
Estonia	78	78	68	68	51	50	49	-37.18
Finland	343	363	389	390	391	394	398	16.03
France	1,064	1,079	1,054	1,060	1,053	1,048	1,042	-2.07
Germany	2,263	2,242	2,235	3,628	3,781	3,800	3,821	68.85
Greece	492	483	475	467	460	453	446	-9.35
Hong Kong, China	102	105	102	104	107	110	113	10.78
Hungary	167	172	178	184	191	195	199	19.16
India	15,356	15,452	15,549	15,623	15,741	15,828	15,936	3.78
Indonesia	1,112	1,111	1,145	1,164	1,182	1,207	1,228	10.43
Ireland								
Israel	317	327	343	354	363	372	377	18.93
Italy	1,581	1,580	1,580	1,580	1,581	1,582	1,583	0.13
Japan	161,540	163,270	165,451	167,555	169,079	171,061	172,973	7.08
Jordan	83	84	86	91	95	97	99	19.28
Kazakhstan	991	917	938	981	1,005	1,029	1,051	6.05
Kuwait	85	86	90	91	92	94	95	11.76
Latvia	150	151	142	140	129	131	132	-12.00
Lithuania	187	186	187	189	188	191	192	2.67
Malaysia	111	114	115					
Mexico	816	817	819	819	820	821	823	0.86
Morocco	143	144	145	148	152	156	159	11.19
Netherlands	698	693	685	690	690	689	688	-1.43
New Zealand	387	412	433	444	453	462	470	21.45
Nigeria								
Norway								
Pakistan	872	879	876	907	920	933	947	8.60
Peru	472	475	503	483	478	477	476	0.85
Philippines	1,713	1,794	1,712	1,740	1,741	1,745	1,752	2.28
Poland	715	698	716	736	739	747	758	6.01
Portugal	1,115	1,123	1,116	1,122	1,146	1,154	1,166	4.57
Romania	414	425	439	442	449	450	452	9.18
Russia	11,100	10,900	10,700	10,465	10,234	10,063	9,889	-10.91
Saudi Arabia	182	186	55	55	55	56	57	-68.68
Singapore	23	28	28	28	29	29	29	26.09
Slovakia								
Slovenia	26	26	27	27	27	27	27	3.85
South Africa								
South Korea	38,037	40,244	42,082	43,675	47,430	49,412	51,333	34.96
Spain								
Sweden								
Switzerland								
Taiwan	17,731	17,770	18,082	18,265	18,228	18,203	18,180	2.53
Thailand	3,608	3,627	3,682	3,712	3,773	3,821	3,822	5.93
Tunisia	163	164	167	167	168	170	172	5.52
Turkey	19,441	19,474	18,631	18,750	18,668	18,484	18,266	-6.04
Turkmenistan	323	310	296	280	270	265	259	-19.81
Ukraine	3,300	3,200	3,086	2,976	2,860	2,740	2,644	-19.88
United Arab Emirates	59	60	59	62	65	67	69	16.95
United Kingdom								
USA	6,021	5,890	5,810	5,801	5,731	5,764	5,716	-5.07
Venezuela	561	563	567	567	567	566	564	0.53
Vietnam	1,944	1,857						

Source: Euromonitor International from national statistics

In-patient beds 1998-2004

Table: 2.20

'000/% change

	1998	1999	2000	2001	2002	2003	2004	% change 1998-2004
Algeria	58	58	58	57	58	58	58	-0.59
Argentina	77	77	78					
Australia	73	72	73	73	74	74	74	0.89
Austria	51	51	50	50	50	50	50	-2.68
Azerbaijan	72	71	70	69	68	67	66	-7.95
Belarus	127	127	127	127	128	128	128	1.34
Belgium	46	45	45	44	43	43	42	-8.08
Bolivia	11	11	12	12	12	12	12	5.89
Brazil	480	487	493	494	499	503	507	5.47
Bulgaria	81	73	67	63	56	45	44	-45.51
Canada	105	98	98	98	98	98	98	-6.45
Chile	42	42	41	40	40	40	40	-4.45
China	3,141	3,159	3,177	3,201	3,136	3,129	3,113	-0.89
Colombia	48	48	48	48	48	48	49	2.16
Croatia	27	27	27	27	25	25	25	-8.39
Czech Republic	69	67	67	67	67	66	66	-4.82
Denmark	18	18	21	21	21	21	21	18.85
Ecuador	18	18	18	20	20	20	21	16.28
Egypt	33	34	34	35	36	37	38	13.01
Estonia	11	10	10	9	8	8	8	-23.87
Finland	13,433	12,939	12,481	12,208	12,119	11,999	11,888	-11.50
France	410	402	392	393	395	396	397	-3.01
Germany	534	529	523	516	511	506	502	-5.97
Greece	42	42	42	42	42	43	43	2.18
Hong Kong, China	33	34	33	35	36	37	37	13.06
Hungary	66	65	64	61	60	60	59	-9.89
India	922	933	948	969	978	997	1,009	9.43
Indonesia	123	123	126	127	128	130	131	6.36
Ireland	11	11	11	12	12	12	12	7.41
Israel	36	38	39	39	40	40	40	9.59
Italy	285	261	251					
Japan	1,892	1,873	1,864	1,856	1,839	1,828	1,816	-4.02
Jordan	9	9	9	9	9	10	10	5.49
Kazakhstan	124	108	107	110	112	115	117	-5.10
Kuwait	4	4	5	5	5	5	5	16.20
Latvia	23	22	21	19	17	18	19	-20.09
Lithuania	36	35	34	32	31	30	29	-18.57
Malaysia	27	28	29					
Mexico	98	103	105	105	106	107	109	10.25
Morocco	26	25	26	26	28	29	30	16.84
Netherlands	58	57	55	53	52	51	50	-13.53
New Zealand	24	24	24	24	24	24	24	3.02
Nigeria								
Norway	14	14	14	14	14	14	14	-1.53
Pakistan	91	92	94	98	99	99	100	9.86
Peru	42	46	44	42	43	43	43	0.79
Philippines	82	84	81					
Poland	213	205	191	188	188	187	185	-13.16
Portugal	33	34	35	36	36	37	38	15.23
Romania	165	164	167	168	169	170	171	3.93
Russia	1,717	1,672	1,672	1,642	1,615	1,592	1,577	-8.15
Saudi Arabia	27	28	28	28	28	28	28	2.09
Singapore	11	12	12	12	12	12	12	5.36
Slovakia	38	38	56	55	54	54	54	41.28
Slovenia	11	11	11	10	10	10	10	-8.95
South Africa								
South Korea	236	259	287	289	316	322	323	36.74
Spain	128	139	147	151	155	156	157	22.72
Sweden	23	22	22	31	32	33	33	44.61
Switzerland	31	32	30	29	27	26	25	-19.87
Taiwan	125	123	126	128	133	136	139	11.92
Thailand	366	370	410	414	430	442	447	22.00
Tunisia	16	16	17	17	17	17	17	7.70
Turkey	140	143	146	147	150	153	156	11.41
Turkmenistan	36	35	34	33	32	31	30	-16.22
Ukraine	483	469	461	453	449	447	445	-7.87
United Arab Emirates	8	7	7	8	8	8	8	-4.39
United Kingdom	230	230	230	230	230	232	234	1.74
USA	842	831	825	823	817	814	812	-3.59
Venezuela	44	49	49	49	49	49	49	11.46
Vietnam	199	196	198	204	213	217	221	11.00

Source: *Euromonitor International from OECD/national statistics*

Hospital admissions 1998-2004

Table: 2.21

number/% change

	1998	1999	2000	2001	2002	2003	2004	% change 1998-2004
Algeria								
Argentina								
Australia								
Austria	2,246,381	2,329,887	2,370,977	2,416,263	2,512,275	2,537,575	2,596,405	15.58
Azerbaijan	400,220	382,916	385,173	394,417	398,293	406,064	411,629	2.85
Belarus	2,957,838	2,962,015	2,926,973	2,992,786	2,908,655	2,906,940	2,894,920	-2.13
Belgium	2,013,054							
Bolivia								
Brazil								
Bulgaria	1,331,831	1,298,709	1,261,151	1,212,167	1,294,645	1,289,482	1,298,391	-2.51
Canada								
Chile								
China								
Colombia								
Croatia	686,073	682,961	689,190	700,524	696,519	710,943	713,343	3.97
Czech Republic	2,021,010	1,992,302	2,052,772	2,072,932	2,148,276	2,186,831	2,227,879	10.24
Denmark	966,354	989,442	1,004,516	1,015,059	1,028,623	1,040,390	1,054,240	9.09
Ecuador								
Egypt								
Estonia	282,914	282,302	279,470	268,741	259,772	249,630	240,020	-15.16
Finland	1,381,731	1,380,476	1,382,552	1,350,163	1,361,044	1,347,108	1,322,998	-4.25
France	13,497,976	13,509,484	13,541,664	13,568,676	13,595,688	13,568,209	13,758,910	1.93
Germany	18,604,298	18,994,362	19,317,636	19,418,936	19,668,219	19,800,984	20,233,442	8.76
Greece	1,620,768	1,688,596	1,756,424	1,824,252	1,892,080	1,946,189	2,015,570	24.36
Hong Kong, China								
Hungary	2,344,708	2,357,854	2,405,460	2,429,504	2,498,987	2,520,410	2,592,696	10.58
India								
Indonesia								
Ireland	547,389	541,484	561,529	570,653	566,829	582,037	584,796	6.83
Israel	1,135,184	1,152,886	1,158,554	1,206,122	1,215,156	1,231,840	1,261,416	11.12
Italy	10,182,892	9,672,963	9,279,501	9,255,297	8,803,602	8,435,061	8,111,174	-20.35
Japan								
Jordan								
Kazakhstan	2,346,025	2,195,384	2,214,351	2,306,982	2,427,000	2,495,213	2,551,301	8.75
Kuwait								
Latvia	537,843	537,857	525,141	486,886	466,288	441,243	415,922	-22.67
Lithuania	894,866	905,466	862,919	836,691	819,312	778,645	757,968	-15.30
Malaysia								
Mexico								
Morocco								
Netherlands	1,556,788	1,526,068	1,488,812	1,487,033	1,453,045	1,421,251	1,412,163	-9.29
New Zealand								
Nigeria								
Norway	712,883	730,568	749,394	787,584	805,840	830,963	851,008	19.38
Pakistan								
Peru								
Philippines								
Poland	5,339,126	5,685,288	6,007,091	6,336,215	6,670,198	6,994,503	7,296,147	36.65
Portugal	1,196,282	1,221,699	1,144,549	1,169,020	1,143,154	1,126,133	1,110,255	-7.19
Romania	4,577,841	4,653,375	5,024,995	5,458,747	5,449,589	5,712,762	5,912,313	29.15
Russia	30,184,113	30,458,497	31,724,846	32,296,942	32,559,646	33,127,697	33,680,133	11.58
Saudi Arabia								
Singapore								
Slovakia	1,095,175	1,044,213	1,075,208	1,061,996	1,022,339	1,022,981	1,030,511	-5.90
Slovenia	325,742	328,819	332,601	330,302	327,175	326,933	325,885	0.04
South Africa								
South Korea								
Spain	4,592,343	4,721,698	4,824,961	4,928,224	5,031,488	5,124,482	5,279,919	14.97
Sweden	1,464,625	1,437,623	1,407,863	1,391,850	1,386,000	1,347,189	1,345,738	-8.12
Switzerland	1,207,203							
Taiwan								
Thailand								
Tunisia								
Turkey	4,640,357	4,864,134	5,075,170	5,290,024	5,508,263	5,732,650	5,888,445	26.90
Turkmenistan								
Ukraine	9,606,114	9,536,600	9,557,970	9,686,347	9,575,106	9,570,653	9,637,147	0.32
United Arab Emirates								
United Kingdom	8,964,200	9,064,867	9,155,867	9,246,867	9,337,867	9,438,296	9,443,708	5.35
USA								
Venezuela								
Vietnam								

Source: EU/WHO

In-patient surgical procedures 1998-2004

Table: 2.22

'000/% change

	1998	1999	2000	2001	2002	2003	2004	% change 1998-2004
Algeria								
Argentina								
Australia								
Austria	1,037.1	1,050.6	1,055.6	1,066.2	1,084.0	1,079.2	1,099.3	6.00
Azerbaijan		81.3	83.1	87.8	89.5	93.9	96.6	
Belarus		670.0						
Belgium								
Bolivia								
Brazil								
Bulgaria								
Canada								
Chile								
China								
Colombia								
Croatia								
Czech Republic								
Denmark	408.1	406.7	406.4	404.7	403.6	403.4	399.6	-2.06
Ecuador								
Egypt								
Estonia	94.4	94.7	92.3	87.3	87.4	84.5	82.4	-12.76
Finland	457.2	463.4	467.8	451.0	474.1	474.3	475.1	3.92
France								
Germany	5,904.2	6,368.9	6,711.5	7,074.6	7,412.0	7,769.8	8,192.3	38.75
Greece								
Hong Kong, China								
Hungary	1,310.9	1,264.6	1,271.3	1,238.1	1,245.5	1,237.2	1,229.3	-6.23
India								
Indonesia								
Ireland	556.0	682.4	817.4	1,009.7	1,273.4	1,335.8	1,422.2	155.79
Israel	483.5	487.0	501.6	525.2	546.3	560.1	577.8	19.49
Italy	3,160.6	3,222.1	3,203.4	3,258.6	3,266.9	3,324.1	3,351.8	6.05
Japan								
Jordan								
Kazakhstan								
Kuwait								
Latvia	149.3	154.1	153.3	144.2	148.3	145.3	145.3	-2.71
Lithuania	235.3	250.8	254.5	256.8	266.0	271.2	273.5	16.26
Malaysia								
Mexico								
Morocco								
Netherlands								
New Zealand								
Nigeria								
Norway								
Pakistan								
Peru								
Philippines								
Poland								
Portugal	596.4	597.6	580.7	607.2	609.6	616.2	627.2	5.16
Romania	3,219.5	2,998.2	3,608.1	3,040.3	3,612.9	3,548.1	3,623.8	12.56
Russia	8,496.2	8,465.0	8,587.0	8,751.0	8,728.7	8,777.9	8,941.6	5.24
Saudi Arabia								
Singapore								
Slovakia	37.3	34.0	33.4	34.1	33.3	33.4	33.4	-10.32
Slovenia				109.0	114.9	121.3	127.3	
South Africa								
South Korea								
Spain	2,087.5							
Sweden	544.9	556.8	547.8	551.0	565.8	565.7	563.6	3.45
Switzerland								
Taiwan								
Thailand								
Tunisia								
Turkey	1,438.2	1,494.6	1,638.1	1,875.9	2,053.7	2,177.2	2,333.2	62.23
Turkmenistan								
Ukraine			2,445.8	2,439.7	2,478.3	2,467.1	2,515.7	
United Arab Emirates								
United Kingdom								
USA								
Venezuela								
Vietnam								

Source: EU/WHO

Out-patient contacts 1998-2004

Table: 2.23

per capita/% change

	1998	1999	2000	2001	2002	2003	2004	% change 1998-2004
Algeria								
Argentina								
Australia								
Austria	6.5	6.7	6.7	6.7	6.6	6.7	6.9	6.15
Azerbaijan		5.1	5.0	4.9	4.5	4.3	4.4	
Belarus	11.6	11.9	11.7	11.6	11.4	11.9	11.2	-3.45
Belgium	7.7	7.5	7.5	7.4	7.3	7.5	7.2	-6.13
Bolivia								
Brazil								
Bulgaria	5.5	5.4	5.2	5.1	4.7	4.8	4.5	-18.18
Canada								
Chile								
China								
Colombia								
Croatia	6.5	6.6	7.0	7.3	7.5	7.6	8.0	22.89
Czech Republic	14.5	14.5	14.8	14.8	14.8	14.4	14.9	2.76
Denmark	6.0	5.8	6.1	6.2	6.2	6.1	6.1	1.67
Ecuador								
Egypt								
Estonia	6.4	6.3	6.7	6.5	6.4	6.6	6.8	6.25
Finland	4.2	4.3	4.3	4.3	4.2	4.3	4.3	2.38
France	6.7	6.8	6.9	6.9	7.0	6.9	7.2	7.78
Germany	7.0	7.2	7.4	7.6	7.9	8.2	8.4	20.69
Greece								
Hong Kong, China								
Hungary	10.6	10.9	11.1	11.3	11.9	12.0	12.1	14.15
India								
Indonesia								
Ireland								
Israel			7.1					
Italy		6.0						
Japan								
Jordan								
Kazakhstan	5.7	5.4	5.5	5.7	6.2	6.1	6.2	8.77
Kuwait								
Latvia	4.6	4.9	4.8	4.8	4.6	4.4	4.5	-2.17
Lithuania	6.9	6.9	6.3	6.5	6.4	6.4	6.2	-10.14
Malaysia								
Mexico								
Morocco								
Netherlands	5.7	5.8	5.9	5.8	5.6	5.8	5.5	-3.51
New Zealand								
Nigeria								
Norway								
Pakistan								
Peru								
Philippines								
Poland	5.4	5.3	5.4	5.5	5.3	5.6	5.8	7.41
Portugal	3.4	3.4	3.5	3.6	3.6	3.8	3.7	8.82
Romania	6.8	6.4	5.1	5.4	5.7	5.6	5.6	-17.65
Russia	9.1	9.3	9.4	9.5	9.6	10.0	9.7	6.59
Saudi Arabia								
Singapore								
Slovakia	16.4	16.4	16.3	14.6	14.5	13.1	13.7	-16.62
Slovenia	7.1	7.4	6.8	6.7	6.4	6.1	5.8	-18.31
South Africa								
South Korea								
Spain				8.7				
Sweden								
Switzerland								
Taiwan								
Thailand								
Tunisia								
Turkey	2.1	2.1	2.4	2.6	2.9	3.0	3.2	52.38
Turkmenistan								
Ukraine	9.7	9.7	10.0	10.1	10.3	10.5	10.3	6.19
United Arab Emirates								
United Kingdom	5.4	5.3	5.0	4.8	4.8	4.2	3.9	-27.78
USA								
Venezuela								
Vietnam								

Source: EU/WHO

Doctors 1998-2004

number/% change

	1998	1999	2000	2001	2002	2003	2004	% change 1998-2004
Algeria	29,970	31,130	32,337	33,034	34,025	34,873	35,417	18.17
Argentina					107,412	108,568	109,141	
Australia	44,684	45,999	47,372	49,392	47,559	47,017	46,865	4.88
Austria	24,368	24,505	25,332	26,286	26,711	27,233	27,825	14.19
Azerbaijan	28,500	28,500	29,033	29,100	29,226	29,457	29,732	4.32
Belarus	45,200	45,900	45,800	44,900	44,800	44,800	44,600	-1.33
Belgium	38,109	38,769	39,519	40,167	40,763	41,521	42,380	11.21
Bolivia	2,542	2,652	2,907	3,021	3,068	3,121	3,137	23.39
Brazil								
Bulgaria	28,476	27,940	27,304	26,683	25,856	25,316	24,768	-13.02
Canada	62,937	63,651	64,454	65,226	66,289	67,193	68,132	8.25
Chile	8,308	10,552	11,707	12,356	12,835	12,982	13,049	57.07
China	2,000,000	2,045,000	2,076,000	2,100,000	1,844,000	1,726,000	1,692,000	-15.40
Colombia	40,551	40,632	40,618	40,605	40,486	40,334	40,240	-0.77
Croatia	8,600	8,046	7,751	7,779	7,790	7,808	7,824	-9.02
Czech Republic	31,192	31,653	34,604	35,222	35,750	36,752	37,182	19.20
Denmark	16,635	16,917	17,165	17,443	17,802	18,116	18,445	10.88
Ecuador	16,588	17,075	18,335	19,376	20,109	20,360	20,597	24.17
Egypt	49,677	41,021	39,204	40,422	41,783	42,368	42,571	-14.30
Estonia	4,311	4,426	4,414	4,293	4,208	4,138	4,050	-6.05
Finland	15,436	15,794	15,905	16,110	16,272	16,435	16,616	7.64
France	191,700	193,200	194,000	196,000	198,700	201,400	203,929	6.38
Germany	260,461	263,447	267,965	272,296	275,167	279,432	283,942	9.02
Greece	44,753	46,124	47,251	47,944	49,060	50,193	51,217	14.44
Hong Kong, China	9,527	9,818	10,130	10,139	10,052	9,934	9,815	3.02
Hungary	31,638	31,768	30,621	29,448	32,452	33,760	34,558	9.23
India	503,947	493,582	483,117	472,719	462,294	451,879	441,922	-12.31
Indonesia	19,291	25,535	21,467	20,912	20,738	20,632	20,486	6.19
Ireland	8,102	8,469	8,438	9,166	9,444	10,270	10,399	28.35
Israel	22,684							
Italy	234,000	241,000	234,000	249,000	253,000	237,000	234,000	0.00
Japan	246,548	249,852	253,469	259,342	260,500	264,157	267,826	8.63
Jordan	2,447	2,638	2,815	2,967	2,911	2,872	2,859	16.84
Kazakhstan	53,200	50,600	49,000	51,300	53,700	54,600	54,900	3.20
Kuwait	3,117	3,178	3,204	3,270	3,323	3,373	3,431	10.07
Latvia	7,964	8,041	8,134	7,744	7,921	7,883	7,824	-1.76
Lithuania	14,622	14,578	14,034	14,031	13,856	13,682	13,567	-7.22
Malaysia	15,016	15,076	15,619					
Mexico	121,230	133,615	139,958	150,572	155,735	160,297	163,865	35.17
Morocco	10,771	11,907	12,439	12,955	13,955	14,437	14,657	36.08
Netherlands	46,101	48,987	50,856	52,602	49,366	50,854	51,906	12.59
New Zealand	8,491	8,616	8,615	8,491	8,403	8,395	8,383	-1.27
Nigeria	22,481	22,495	22,504	22,534	22,568	22,609	22,653	0.77
Norway	12,110	12,473	12,813	13,388	15,586	16,279	16,882	39.41
Pakistan	82,682	87,105	91,823	96,248	99,378	102,003	104,723	26.66
Peru	27,880	28,775	30,108	31,743	32,395	33,156	33,731	20.99
Philippines	2,848	2,948	2,985	2,999	2,960	2,877	2,826	-0.77
Poland	90,086	87,524	85,031	86,706	88,070	90,512	92,979	3.21
Portugal	31,087	31,758	32,498	33,233	34,015	34,833	35,454	14.05
Romania	41,310	42,975	42,371	42,339	42,678	43,170	43,748	5.90
Russia	680,000	683,000	680,000	698,000	710,000	720,000	728,000	7.06
Saudi Arabia	13,807	14,077	13,975	13,876	13,876	13,918	13,922	0.83
Singapore	5,148	5,325	5,577	5,922	6,029	6,292	6,487	26.01
Slovakia	18,837	19,059	19,303	18,982	18,743	18,784	18,794	-0.23
Slovenia	1,363	1,413	1,417	1,467	1,521	1,564	1,607	17.90
South Africa	29,369	30,521	31,336	31,687	31,614	31,098	31,012	5.59
South Korea	47,387	50,424	49,220	53,189	57,779	60,412	62,861	32.65
Spain	111,000	117,200	127,100	124,900	120,200	118,660	118,178	6.47
Sweden	24,957	25,428	26,979	27,579	28,405	29,368	30,144	20.78
Switzerland	23,679	24,026	25,216	25,395	25,921	26,569	27,269	15.16
Taiwan	30,629	31,757	33,323	34,548	35,633	36,709	37,312	21.82
Thailand	17,955	18,140	18,025	18,779	19,392	19,790	20,297	13.04
Tunisia	6,819	7,149	7,444	7,761	7,964	8,095	8,143	19.42
Turkey	77,344	81,988	85,117	90,757	91,000	91,224	91,278	18.02
Turkmenistan	12,691							
Ukraine	227,000	226,000	226,000	226,000	226,664	227,829	228,863	0.82
United Arab Emirates	5,664	5,235	5,222	6,003	6,328	6,540	6,633	17.11
United Kingdom	112,889	115,089	117,579	120,912	123,236	126,113	129,439	14.66
USA	777,900	797,600	813,800	836,200	858,128	882,246	905,292	16.38
Venezuela	40,355	34,905	35,454	35,424	36,132	36,439	36,760	-8.91
Vietnam	34,200	37,100	39,600	41,200	46,323	48,025	49,072	43.49

Source: Euromonitor International from OECD/national statistics

Nurses 1998-2004

number/% change

	1998	1999	2000	2001	2002	2003	2004	% change 1998-2004
Algeria								
Argentina								
Australia	197,458	200,049	200,910	201,753	202,000	203,349	204,216	3.42
Austria	71,849	73,084	74,601	74,948	74,922	75,621	76,301	6.20
Azerbaijan	60,700	58,100	58,000	57,900	58,896	59,230	59,560	-1.88
Belarus	74,567	75,214	75,643	76,074	76,060	76,220	76,289	2.31
Belgium	52,232	53,819	55,406	56,996	58,306	59,851	61,264	17.29
Bolivia	7,852	7,858	7,860	7,865	7,869	7,873	7,882	0.38
Brazil								
Bulgaria	47,343	44,114	43,435	42,707	41,829	41,325	40,950	-13.50
Canada	307,087	306,967	310,887	310,234	292,212	287,593	284,307	-7.42
Chile	3,479	3,677	3,841	4,001	4,117	4,214	4,283	23.11
China	1,219,000	1,245,000	1,267,000	1,287,000	1,247,000	1,228,000	1,222,000	0.25
Colombia								
Croatia	41,235	40,998	40,661	40,327	39,929	39,486	39,302	-4.69
Czech Republic	88,165	88,564	91,285	93,682	95,498	97,929	100,250	13.71
Denmark	49,474	50,178	50,905	51,529	51,990	52,597	53,173	7.48
Ecuador								
Egypt	107,696	92,489	79,429	83,879	86,650	87,644	87,878	-18.40
Estonia	7,706	7,587	7,456	7,489	8,294	8,556	8,765	13.74
Finland	37,600	39,300	42,700	44,800	46,900	48,254	49,356	31.27
France	373,938	381,047	397,279	412,231	425,981	439,115	454,019	21.42
Germany	769,715	779,005	790,899	801,237	815,639	830,947	846,904	10.03
Greece	40,932	41,151	42,129	42,919	43,663	44,666	45,595	11.39
Hong Kong, China	39,157	38,960	40,388	41,906	42,259	42,541	42,620	8.84
Hungary	82,843	50,415	81,210	84,947	86,853	88,519	90,189	8.87
India	583,531	592,352	595,326	597,663	598,325	605,872	609,438	4.44
Indonesia	162,060	162,014	163,412	164,241	165,772	166,242	166,641	2.83
Ireland	48,579	50,940	53,072	57,059	60,084	61,221	61,324	26.24
Israel	35,700							
Italy	302,662	298,350	299,166	307,302	312,707	317,660	324,079	7.08
Japan	985,821		1,042,468	1,071,438	1,096,967	1,107,428	1,130,002	14.63
Jordan	1,728	1,882	1,999	1,963	2,016	2,064	2,087	20.78
Kazakhstan	120,000	114,100	112,300	109,100	110,900	111,100	111,200	-7.33
Kuwait	7,684	7,338	8,232	8,467	8,704	8,906	9,095	18.36
Latvia	10,576	10,453	10,378	10,129	10,001	9,923	9,872	-6.66
Lithuania	28,813	29,450	28,017	27,787	26,918	26,127	25,527	-11.40
Malaysia	18,134	20,914	23,255					
Mexico	203,007	213,629	208,318	222,389	225,958	228,796	231,243	13.91
Morocco								
Netherlands	197,000	200,500	213,100	205,800	198,274	194,754	192,924	-2.07
New Zealand	36,736	36,770	36,976	37,303	37,097	36,514	36,504	-0.63
Nigeria	99,716	103,322	106,828	110,833	114,342	117,912	120,898	21.24
Norway	43,638	45,133	46,128	46,877	47,991	49,120	50,191	15.02
Pakistan	32,938	35,979	37,528	40,019	41,599	42,277	43,040	30.67
Peru			20,587					
Philippines	4,389	4,945	5,303	5,580	5,643	5,704	5,745	30.90
Poland	213,127	197,153	189,632	186,491	185,892	183,990	182,103	-14.56
Portugal	37,747	37,487	37,477	39,529	40,210	40,892	41,421	9.73
Romania	92,055	92,453	92,762					
Russia	1,621,000	1,612,000	1,564,000	1,618,894	1,674,364	1,732,432	1,780,701	9.85
Saudi Arabia	35,463	36,887	37,614	38,612	39,369	39,965	40,231	13.44
Singapore	11,491	11,765	12,353	12,828	13,308	13,740	14,089	22.61
Slovakia	39,702	40,380	39,428	38,352	38,130	37,935	37,903	-4.53
Slovenia	13,460	13,120	13,120	13,120	13,341	13,452	13,543	0.62
South Africa	174,754	174,895	175,126	175,214	175,314	175,388	175,575	0.47
South Korea	53,954	59,104	59,791	68,013	75,239	76,952	77,399	43.45
Spain	243,100	257,600	258,000	269,500	298,800	315,285	328,634	35.18
Sweden	73,562	74,657	78,380	95,109	102,337	106,693	109,123	48.34
Switzerland			77,120	77,232	77			
Taiwan	71,214	75,598	79,176	82,762	89,564	93,120	95,066	33.49
Thailand	63,708	68,008	70,978	77,008	80,174	81,391	81,820	28.43
Tunisia								
Turkey	110,305	111,541	113,190	117,037	117,838	119,960	122,397	10.96
Turkmenistan	22,879	22,412	22,355	22,025	21,873	21,783	21,680	-5.24
Ukraine	557,000	549,000	548,451	547,902	552,234	558,921	564,798	1.40
United Arab Emirates	12,288	10,390	10,762	12,280	13,211	13,764	13,966	13.66
United Kingdom	490,000	515,000	515,000	530,000	545,000	561,109	576,091	17.57
USA	2,180,040	2,201,810	2,249,440	2,262,020	2,291,851	2,322,901	2,356,334	8.09
Venezuela								
Vietnam	46,500	45,454	45,000	45,400	50,569	51,712	52,351	12.58

Source: Euromonitor International from OECD/national statistics

Midwives 1998-2004

Table: 2.26

number/% change

	1998	1999	2000	2001	2002	2003	2004	% change 1998-2004
Algeria								
Argentina								
Australia	11,756	12,567	12,976	13,865	14,340	14,871	15,061	28.11
Austria			1,093	1,132	1,168	1,212	1,252	
Azerbaijan								
Belarus	6,893	6,713	6,521	6,365	6,282	6,188	6,094	-11.59
Belgium								
Bolivia								
Brazil								
Bulgaria	5,826	5,459	5,292	5,165	5,057	4,992	4,942	-15.17
Canada								
Chile	2,133	2,171	2,213	2,254	2,291	2,331	2,372	11.20
China	49,000	44,000	41,700	40,300	38,823	37,721	36,848	-24.80
Colombia								
Croatia								
Czech Republic								
Denmark								
Ecuador								
Egypt								
Estonia	542	554	507	453	422	410	402	-25.83
Finland	4,025	4,049	3,980	3,952	3,934	3,921	3,910	-2.86
France	10,165	13,921	14,353	14,725	15,153	15,520	15,796	55.40
Germany								
Greece								
Hong Kong, China	12,006	12,072	12,172	12,272	12,395	12,537	12,661	5.46
Hungary	2,277	2,279	2,113	2,059	2,020	1,997	1,975	-13.26
India								
Indonesia								
Ireland								
Israel								
Italy								
Japan	24,202	24,457	24,694	24,972	25,252	25,544	25,734	6.33
Jordan	668	716	845	832	806	801	796	19.16
Kazakhstan								
Kuwait								
Latvia								
Lithuania	1,757	1,820	1,828	1,836	1,857	1,881	1,899	8.07
Malaysia								
Mexico								
Morocco								
Netherlands	1,422	1,507	1,576	1,627	1,725	1,825	1,883	32.42
New Zealand								
Nigeria	71,681	73,240	74,699	76,401	78,122	79,521	80,946	12.93
Norway								
Pakistan	22,103	22,401	22,525	22,711	22,985	23,231	23,523	6.42
Peru								
Philippines	14,962	16,173	17,176	17,522	17,409	16,768	16,698	11.60
Poland	24,434	24,221	21,997	21,843	21,743	21,538	21,406	-12.39
Portugal								
Romania								
Russia	93,800	89,300	85,700	84,200	84,900	85,100	85,600	-8.74
Saudi Arabia								
Singapore	456	449	437	415	393	371	358	-21.49
Slovakia								
Slovenia								
South Africa	229							
South Korea	1,268	1,428	1,080	1,227	1,174	1,162	1,147	-9.54
Spain	6,148	6,102	6,144	6,164	6,236	6,342	6,414	4.33
Sweden								
Switzerland								
Taiwan	845	889	929	969	1,006	1,039	1,071	26.75
Thailand								
Tunisia								
Turkey	41,059	41,271	41,590	42,447	43,032	43,656	44,321	7.94
Turkmenistan	3,611	3,575	3,439	3,370	3,260	3,136	3,044	-15.70
Ukraine								
United Arab Emirates								
United Kingdom								
USA								
Venezuela								
Vietnam	13,100	13,631	13,900	14,300	15,619	16,354	17,033	30.02

Source: Euromonitor International from national statistics

Consultations with general practitioners 1998-2004

Table: 2.27

per capita/% change

	1998	1999	2000	2001	2002	2003	2004	% change 1998-2004
Algeria								
Argentina								
Australia	6.6	6.5	6.4	6.4	6.2	6.0	5.9	-10.61
Austria	6.5	6.7	6.7	6.7	6.7	6.7	6.7	3.08
Azerbaijan								
Belarus								
Belgium	7.9	7.9	7.9	7.8	7.8	7.8	7.7	-2.41
Bolivia								
Brazil								
Bulgaria								
Canada	6.4	6.4	6.4	6.3	6.2	6.2	6.1	-5.00
Chile								
China								
Colombia								
Croatia								
Czech Republic	12.4	12.3	12.6	12.7	12.9	13.1	13.3	7.18
Denmark	6.8	6.6	6.9	7.0	7.1	7.3	7.5	9.71
Ecuador								
Egypt								
Estonia								
Finland	4.2	4.3	4.3	4.3	4.3	4.3	4.3	2.38
France	6.6	6.6	6.9	6.9	6.9	6.9	6.9	4.55
Germany	7.1	7.2	7.3	7.5	7.6	7.7	7.8	10.42
Greece	2.5	2.5	2.5	2.4	2.4	2.4	2.3	-6.40
Hong Kong, China								
Hungary	10.6	10.9	11.1	11.3	11.9	12.1	12.4	17.17
India								
Indonesia								
Ireland								
Israel								
Italy	6.0	6.1	6.0	5.9	5.8	5.7	5.6	-6.83
Japan	14.5	14.5	14.4	14.5	14.5	14.5	14.5	-0.23
Jordan								
Kazakhstan								
Kuwait								
Latvia								
Lithuania								
Malaysia								
Mexico	2.3	2.5	2.5	2.5	2.5	2.5	2.5	8.70
Morocco								
Netherlands	5.6	5.8	5.9	5.8	5.6	5.6	5.5	-1.31
New Zealand				4.4				
Nigeria								
Norway	4.8	4.9	5.3	5.2	5.4	5.5	5.6	17.26
Pakistan								
Peru								
Philippines								
Poland	5.4	5.3	5.4	5.5	5.6	5.7	5.8	8.26
Portugal	3.4	3.5	3.5	3.6	3.6	3.7	3.7	9.80
Romania								
Russia								
Saudi Arabia								
Singapore								
Slovakia	15.0	15.0	15.0	13.0	13.0	13.0	13.0	-13.33
Slovenia								
South Africa								
South Korea		8.8	9.2	9.8	10.6	10.8	11.0	
Spain								
Sweden	2.9	2.8	2.9	2.9	2.9	2.9	3.0	2.07
Switzerland					3.4			
Taiwan								
Thailand								
Tunisia								
Turkey	2.1	2.1	2.5	2.6	3.9	4.0	4.0	90.48
Turkmenistan								
Ukraine								
United Arab Emirates								
United Kingdom	5.4	5.1	4.9	4.5	4.4	4.4	4.3	-20.37
USA	10.1	10.4	8.9	9.0	8.9	8.9	8.9	-11.55
Venezuela								
Vietnam								

Source: Euromonitor International from OECD

Active pharmacists 1998-2004

Table: 2.28

number/% change

	1998	1999	2000	2001	2002	2003	2004	% change 1998-2004
Algeria	4,299	4,600	4,814	5,003	5,122	5,235	5,374	25.01
Argentina								
Australia	11,600	11,829	15,000	12,500	12,900	16,500	17,208	48.34
Austria	4,337	4,439	4,532	4,581	4,704	4,810	4,912	13.26
Azerbaijan	2,607	2,634	2,666	2,685	2,706	2,726	2,754	5.64
Belarus								
Belgium	10,087	10,437	10,724	10,939	11,775	12,079	12,386	22.79
Bolivia								
Brazil								
Bulgaria	1,529	1,452	1,390	1,355	1,330	1,310	1,305	-14.65
Canada	18,037	19,872	19,623	19,588	20,504	20,726	21,112	17.05
Chile	323	321	320	322	324	326	328	1.55
China	424,000	418,000	412,000	406,000	399,071	391,871	385,383	-9.11
Colombia								
Croatia	1,550	1,502	1,493	1,575	1,620	1,662	1,703	9.87
Czech Republic	4,559	4,786	5,059	5,199	5,397	5,518	5,622	23.32
Denmark	2,404	2,643	2,666	2,685	2,638	2,695	2,705	12.52
Ecuador								
Egypt	3,548	3,278	2,842	3,375	4,354	4,654	4,813	35.65
Estonia	1,315	1,367	1,400	1,440	1,484	1,525	1,569	19.32
Finland	7,462	7,569	7,660	7,755	7,838	7,930	8,022	7.50
France	61,712	63,038	64,338	65,526	67,937	69,655	71,525	15.90
Germany	45,465	46,064	46,078	45,869	46,513	46,742	46,981	3.33
Greece	8,767	8,928	8,977	9,057	9,181	9,297	9,424	7.49
Hong Kong, China	1,212	1,273	1,315	1,352	1,372	1,378	1,400	15.51
Hungary	4,789	4,762	4,905	5,024	5,070	5,123	5,141	7.35
India								
Indonesia				3,466	3,469	3,482		
Ireland	2,762	2,886	3,044	3,165	3,144	3,385	3,509	27.05
Israel								
Italy	60,974	61,326	62,862	63,008	64,130	64,576	64,860	6.37
Japan	187,710	192,544	199,797	205,561	212,720	219,906	227,050	20.96
Jordan	173	177	189	213	226	235	244	41.04
Kazakhstan	11,100	11,100	11,200	11,200	11,234	11,267	11,289	1.70
Kuwait	479	447	448	451	454	458	461	-3.76
Latvia								
Lithuania	2,895	2,970	2,995	3,020	3,056	3,098	3,131	8.15
Malaysia	2,129							
Mexico								
Morocco	5,026	4,298	5,197	6,375	8,640	9,037	9,258	84.20
Netherlands	2,922	2,965	3,069	3,148	3,224	3,298	3,372	15.40
New Zealand	2,944	3,405	3,733	3,843	3,927	3,999	4,026	36.75
Nigeria	7,230	7,316	7,330	7,381	7,396	7,405	7,438	2.88
Norway					1,595	1,610	1,622	
Pakistan								
Peru								
Philippines								
Poland	20,572	21,857	22,161	23,774	24,421	24,653	24,855	20.82
Portugal	7,505	7,797	8,056	8,322	8,565	8,789	9,018	20.16
Romania	1,642	1,598	1,588	1,490	1,467	1,426	1,396	-14.98
Russia								
Saudi Arabia	652	642	661	676	680	690	699	7.21
Singapore	998	1,043	1,098	1,141	1,191	1,236	1,271	27.35
Slovakia	2,236	2,253	2,400	2,344	2,420	2,460	2,481	10.96
Slovenia	887	917	1,079	1,122	1,255	1,272	1,284	44.76
South Africa	9,948	9,959	9,971	9,986	10,003	10,021	10,050	1.03
South Korea	3,131	3,120	2,312	2,607	2,704	2,748	2,772	-11.47
Spain	28,100	27,100	32,600	41,000	37,400	37,186	37,013	31.72
Sweden	5,249	5,317						
Switzerland	1,651	1,640	1,658	1,621	1,618	1,618	1,614	-2.24
Taiwan	22,763	23,940	24,407	24,895	25,352	26,134	26,789	17.69
Thailand	5,911	6,062	6,384	6,823	7,080	7,326	7,434	25.77
Tunisia	1,623	1,690	1,951	1,998	2,050	2,101	2,130	31.24
Turkey	21,441	22,065	23,266	22,922	22,500	22,423	22,403	4.49
Turkmenistan								
Ukraine								
United Arab Emirates								
United Kingdom	33,724	31,964	29,751	28,136	27,000	26,348	26,437	-21.61
USA	190,900	193,400	196,100	199,852	203,016	206,198	209,155	9.56
Venezuela								
Vietnam	12,800	12,900	13,700	14,600	15,679	16,533	17,171	34.15

Source: Euromonitor International from OECD/national statistics

Dentists 1998-2004

number/% change

Table: 2.29

	1998	1999	2000	2001	2002	2003	2004	% change 1998-2004
Algeria	7,954	8,086	8,197	8,350	8,579	8,755	8,881	11.65
Argentina								
Australia	8,500	8,750	8,991	9,000	9,150	9,232	9,402	10.61
Austria	3,813	3,721	3,732	3,838	4,109	4,239	4,340	13.82
Azerbaijan	2,279	2,242	2,240	2,238	2,304	2,367	2,402	5.40
Belarus	6,157	6,336	6,415	6,415	6,392	6,334	6,270	1.84
Belgium	8,240	8,326	8,465	8,512	8,553	8,634	8,712	5.73
Bolivia	515	518	519	527	534	543	551	6.99
Brazil	7,524	7,825	8,105	8,105	8,123	8,141	8,153	8.36
Bulgaria	4,838	4,684	4,562	4,511	4,480	4,426	4,382	-9.43
Canada	16,490	16,908	17,314	17,691	17,961	18,326	18,676	13.26
Chile	1,078	1,355	1,367	1,372	1,386	1,396	1,403	30.15
China								
Colombia								
Croatia	1,121	769	664	615	548	523	499	-55.49
Czech Republic	6,386	6,426	6,658	6,698	6,697	6,791	6,836	7.05
Denmark	4,857	4,830	4,817	4,825	4,834	4,808	4,805	-1.07
Ecuador								
Egypt	3,903	4,754	5,459	5,770	6,128	6,274	6,437	64.92
Estonia	985	1,012	1,015	1,095	1,135	1,170	1,201	21.93
Finland	4,833	4,826	4,794	4,731	4,636	4,574	4,503	-6.83
France	39,457	40,088	40,539	40,426	40,481	40,648	40,685	3.11
Germany	62,277	62,564	63,202	63,854	64,484	65,172	66,101	6.14
Greece	11,947	12,152	12,362	12,394	12,585	12,769	12,958	8.46
Hong Kong, China	1,724	1,779	1,826	2,028	2,060	2,076	2,088	21.11
Hungary	4,505	4,618	4,365	3,640	4,843	5,020	5,096	13.12
India								
Indonesia								
Ireland	1,713	1,794	1,899	2,006	2,102	2,171	2,230	30.18
Israel	6,834							
Italy	31,000	35,000	23,000	31,000	31,000	31,000	31,000	0.00
Japan	86,847	87,786	89,668	90,583	91,783	93,156	94,349	8.64
Jordan	307	350	396	431	471	492	503	63.84
Kazakhstan	4,095							
Kuwait	425	492	517	522	534	552	559	31.53
Latvia	1,064	1,026	1,278	1,350	1,392	1,416	1,435	34.87
Lithuania	2,259	2,306	2,446	2,490	2,309	2,372	2,421	7.17
Malaysia	2,058	1,909	2,144					
Mexico	8,807	9,465	9,777	9,669	9,891	10,117	10,326	17.25
Morocco	1,964	2,111	2,299	2,453	2,578	2,665	2,750	40.02
Netherlands	7,215	7,284	7,397	7,509	7,623	7,749	7,887	9.31
New Zealand	1,496	1,558	1,591	1,601	1,645	1,685	1,710	14.30
Nigeria	1,596	1,635	1,696	1,750	1,778	1,802	1,829	14.60
Norway	3,642	3,635	3,608	3,628	3,853	3,984	4,111	12.88
Pakistan	3,444	3,867	4,175	4,622	4,821	4,999	5,108	48.32
Peru								
Philippines	1,713	2,027	2,280	2,465	2,533	2,574	2,598	51.66
Poland	17,323	13,260	11,758	10,124	10,775	10,924	11,084	-36.02
Portugal	3,322	3,769	4,370	4,799	4,841	4,922	5,024	51.23
Romania	5,367	5,261	4,983	5,057	5,019	4,940	4,873	-9.20
Russia	54,400	56,000	56,800	57,200	57,600	57,800	58,100	6.80
Saudi Arabia	201	237	262	278	284	290	293	45.77
Singapore	914	942	1,028	1,087	1,130	1,183	1,224	33.92
Slovakia	2,490	2,253	2,400	2,344	2,556	2,586	2,618	5.14
Slovenia	1,201	1,199	1,188	1,208	1,231	1,242	1,255	4.50
South Africa	4,387	4,412	4,448	4,981	5,100	5,213	5,290	20.58
South Korea	12,070	13,199	13,593	13,814	14,679	15,171	15,430	27.84
Spain	16,133	16,891	17,538	18,507	19,292	20,008	20,536	27.29
Sweden	7,667	7,837	7,722	7,763	7,856	7,919	7,941	3.57
Switzerland	3,470	3,449	3,468	3,432	3,501	3,514	3,533	1.82
Taiwan	7,895	8,244	8,597	8,940	9,211	9,379	9,454	19.75
Thailand	3,917	4,026	4,141	4,299	4,470	4,625	4,769	21.75
Tunisia	1,276	1,301	1,315	1,380	1,394	1,427	1,462	14.58
Turkey	13,421	14,226	16,002	15,866	16,000	16,285	16,556	23.36
Turkmenistan	883	896	904	915	924	931	933	5.66
Ukraine	19,595							
United Arab Emirates	838	880	750	784	1,071	1,127	1,160	38.42
United Kingdom	24,174	24,785	25,234	25,914	26,490	27,179	27,900	15.41
USA	151,300	152,200	155,200	157,571	160,197	162,506	164,778	8.91
Venezuela								
Vietnam								

Source: Euromonitor International from OECD/national statistics

■ **Immunisation**

Vaccination rate against MMR (measles, mumps, rubella) 1998-2004

Table: 2.30

% of target population

	1998	1999	2000	2001	2002	2003	2004
Algeria	75	83	83	83	81	81	80
Argentina	99	99	56	94	97	97	99
Australia	86	89	92	93	94	95	96
Austria				65	79	92	93
Azerbaijan	98	98	99	99	97	98	97
Belarus	98	98	98	99	99	99	99
Belgium				75	82	89	96
Bolivia	77	99	99	99	99	99	99
Brazil	96	99	99	95	93	91	89
Bulgaria	96		89	90	92	94	95
Canada	96						
Chile	94	96	97	99	95	96	96
China	97	85		79	98	99	99
Colombia	73	75	75	90	93	96	99
Croatia	93	92	93	94	95	95	96
Czech Republic	95	97	99	99	99	99	99
Denmark	91	92	93	94	99	99	99
Ecuador	88	99	99	99	80	88	86
Egypt	98	96	98	97	97	98	98
Estonia	89	92	93	95	95	97	99
Finland				96	96	96	96
France					85	88	88
Germany			89	90	92	92	93
Greece		88					
Hong Kong, China							
Hungary	99	99	99	99	99	99	99
India	84	87	89	56	67	57	50
Indonesia	91	88	73	76	44	42	32
Ireland	77	77	77	73	73	71	70
Israel	94	94	94	94	95	95	95
Italy	55	70	72	74	77	79	81
Japan			96	98	99	99	99
Jordan	86	83	94	99	95	97	98
Kazakhstan	99	99	99	95	95	94	93
Kuwait	99	96	99	99	99	99	99
Latvia	97	97	97	98	98	99	99
Lithuania	97	97	97	97	98	98	98
Malaysia	86	87	88	88	92	93	94
Mexico	96	95	96	95	96	97	98
Morocco	91	90	93	96	96	97	98
Netherlands	96	96	96	96	96	96	96
New Zealand	81	83	85	85	87	89	90
Nigeria	26		30				
Norway	93	93	93	93	88	90	89
Pakistan	76	81	75	75	63	68	66
Peru	93	92	93	97	95	97	98
Philippines	87		80	75	73	69	66
Poland		97	97	97	98	98	98
Portugal	96	96	96	96	92	93	92
Romania	97	98	98	98	98	98	99
Russia	94	97	98	98	98	99	99
Saudi Arabia	93	92	92	94	97	97	98
Singapore	96	93	90	89	91	92	90
Slovakia	99	99	99	99	99	98	98
Slovenia	93	98	95	94	95	97	98
South Africa	82	82	95	72	78	76	75
South Korea	85	90	95	66	97	86	86
Spain	93	93	94	95	97	97	97
Sweden			95	94	91	88	86
Switzerland	81	81	80	81	79	79	79
Taiwan							
Thailand		96	94	94	94	93	93
Tunisia	94	99	85	92	94	96	98
Turkey	80	82	86	90	82	88	89
Turkmenistan	99	97	97	98	88	90	92
Ukraine	96	99	99	99	99	99	99
United Arab Emirates	95	96	94	94	94	94	93
United Kingdom	91	90	88	85	83	82	80
USA	92	92	91	91	91	91	91
Venezuela	94	82	84	49	62	70	72
Vietnam	96	93	97	97	96	96	96

Source: WHO

Vaccination rate against DTP (diphtheria, tetanus, pertussis) 2000-2004

Table: 2.31

% of target population

	2000	2001	2002	2003	2004
Algeria		92	93	94	95
Argentina	88	92	95	98	98
Australia					
Austria		64	77	78	87
Azerbaijan		98	97	97	97
Belarus					
Belgium		95	95	95	95
Bolivia	98	97	99	99	99
Brazil	99	90	97	94	93
Bulgaria	95	95	90	89	86
Canada					
Chile	98	99	99	99	99
China		79	98	99	99
Colombia	75	73	71	70	68
Croatia		94	99	99	99
Czech Republic					
Denmark		97	97	96	96
Ecuador	99	99	99	99	99
Egypt	98	98	98	98	98
Estonia	0	89	90	90	91
Finland		99	99	99	99
France					
Germany					
Greece					
Hong Kong, China					
Hungary	99	99	99	99	99
India		71	77	83	89
Indonesia	87	82	81	80	79
Ireland					
Israel	97	97	97	99	99
Italy			98	98	98
Japan	99	99	99	99	99
Jordan	89	99	96	96	95
Kazakhstan	97	95	95	95	95
Kuwait	97	97	97	97	97
Latvia	99	100	99	99	99
Lithuania	99	99	98	98	98
Malaysia	95	95	95	96	96
Mexico	90	91	92	93	94
Morocco	97	98	95	94	93
Netherlands					
New Zealand	89	89	89	89	89
Nigeria	48	52	56	60	64
Norway			92	92	92
Pakistan	88	86	77	73	67
Peru	91	91	91	91	90
Philippines	81	58	75	65	62
Poland					
Portugal					
Romania					
Russia					
Saudi Arabia		99	97	95	94
Singapore					
Slovakia		99	99	99	99
Slovenia		96	97	98	98
South Africa	95	87	88	83	80
South Korea	97	59	97	98	98
Spain					
Sweden					
Switzerland		98	98	98	98
Taiwan					
Thailand	99	99	99	99	99
Tunisia	94	96	96	97	98
Turkey	92	95	82	80	75
Turkmenistan	97	96	99	99	100
Ukraine		96	97	97	98
United Arab Emirates	96	96	96	96	96
United Kingdom					
USA	99	98	97	97	96
Venezuela	92	85	77	70	62
Vietnam	97	99	85	82	76

Source: WHO

Vaccination rate against polio 1998-2004

Table: 2.32

% of target population

	1998	1999	2000	2001	2002	2003	2004
Algeria	80	83	85	89	86	89	90
Argentina	74	91	85	88	91	90	90
Australia	86	88	91	92	93	94	96
Austria					83	85	85
Azerbaijan	98	99	99	99	100	99	100
Belarus	99	99	99	99	99	99	99
Belgium				95	95	95	95
Bolivia	75	89	89	90	99	99	99
Brazil	96	98	95	95	97	95	95
Bulgaria	97		98	94	94	92	90
Canada							
Chile	93	95	98	99	95	97	97
China	98	85	90	79	98	95	98
Colombia	72	75	78	83	83	87	90
Croatia	93	93	94	94	95	95	96
Czech Republic	97	98	97	97	97	97	96
Denmark	99	99	96	97	98	99	99
Ecuador	83	70	83	92	90	89	87
Egypt	95	97	98	99	97	98	98
Estonia	94	95	93	94	98	97	97
Finland				95	95	95	95
France					98	98	98
Germany			95	96	96	97	98
Greece		87					
Hong Kong, China							
Hungary	99	99	99	99	99	99	99
India	90	93	95	70	70	75	76
Indonesia	93	90	74	77	75	76	76
Ireland	85	86	85	84	83	82	80
Israel	96		92	92	93	93	94
Italy	96	97	98	98	99	99	99
Japan			99	81	99	99	99
Jordan	91	85	94	97	95	96	97
Kazakhstan	99	99	97	95	95	93	92
Kuwait	94	94	94	94	94	94	94
Latvia	94	99	96	97	98	98	99
Lithuania	88	88	92	97	97	97	96
Malaysia	93	93	95	95	97	98	99
Mexico	96	96	89	89	92	92	93
Morocco	93	91	95	93	95	94	93
Netherlands	97				98	98	98
New Zealand	82	85	82	82	82	82	82
Nigeria	22		38	40	45	42	38
Norway				95	91	90	90
Pakistan	79	80	74	74	71	72	70
Peru	96	96	95	92	95	92	92
Philippines	87		75	90	70	73	71
Poland		98	98	98	98	98	98
Portugal	96				94	94	94
Romania	98	98	99	99	99	99	99
Russia	94	97	97	97	97	97	97
Saudi Arabia	94	93	94	97	95	97	97
Singapore	96	95	93	91	92	90	90
Slovakia	98	99	99	99	98	98	98
Slovenia	90	93	93	93	92	92	91
South Africa		72	96	80	84	88	90
South Korea	71		99	59	99	99	99
Spain			95	96	96	97	98
Sweden			99	99	99	99	99
Switzerland				92	94	96	98
Taiwan							
Thailand		97	97	97	97	97	97
Tunisia	96	99	96	98	96	96	95
Turkey	76		85	88	78	77	73
Turkmenistan	99	98	98	94	99	99	99
Ukraine	98	98	99	99	99	99	99
United Arab Emirates	94	94	94	94	94	94	94
United Kingdom	93		92	94	91	91	90
USA	91	90	90	89	90	89	89
Venezuela	64	87	86	88	88	89	89
Vietnam	94	93	96	97	92	94	94

Source: WHO

■ Infectious Diseases

Incidence of measles 1998-2002

number

	1998	1999	2000	2001	2002
Algeria	3,301	2,503		2,686	5,862
Argentina	10,229	313	6	0	
Australia	327	235	108	141	32
Austria	0	1		0	
Azerbaijan	2,891	1,081	210	574	4,353
Belarus	517	153	21	45	14
Belgium	0			83	
Bolivia	1,004	1,441	122	0	0
Brazil	2,781	908	36	1	1
Bulgaria	80	24	46	8	0
Canada	12	29	206	34	7
Chile	6	31	0	0	0
China	53,030	61,840	71,093	88,962	58,341
Colombia	61	44	1	3	139
Croatia	648	31	9	8	6
Czech Republic	19	2	9	6	4
Denmark			14	11	32
Ecuador	0	0	0	2	0
Egypt	4,868	1,547	2,633	2,150	653
Estonia	17	12	9	0	0
Finland	1			1	0
France			10,000		5,185
Germany				6,024	4,657
Greece	66	69	56	12	5
Hong Kong, China					
Hungary	23	1	1	20	0
India	33,990	21,013	22,236	37,969	51,780
Indonesia	1,034	4,767	3,344	3,825	14,492
Ireland	204	147		241	243
Israel	8	14	36	19	2
Italy	4,072	2,908	1,457		9,385
Japan	899		22,497	22,552	33,812
Jordan	428	115	32	61	19
Kazakhstan	1,935	1,391	245	94	18
Kuwait	90	13	6		
Latvia	3	0	0	1	
Lithuania	18	23	19	7	103
Malaysia	483	2,576	6,187	2,198	408
Mexico	0	0	30	3	
Morocco	7,863	10,853	7,368	2,724	6,000
Netherlands	9	2,368	1,019		3
New Zealand	164	106	65	65	21
Nigeria	143,098		212,183	168,107	42,007
Norway			0	4	5
Pakistan	2,333	2,940	2,064	3,849	3,903
Peru	10	12	1	0	0
Philippines	1,984	2,981	7,120	7,360	7,003
Poland	2,255	99	77	133	33
Portugal	96	50	45		8
Romania	9,547	240	35	10	14
Russia	6,215	7,428	4,800	2,072	580
Saudi Arabia	5,519	2,815		155	311
Singapore	114	65	141	408	211
Slovakia	530	0	0	0	0
Slovenia	13	1		0	0
South Africa	977	385	1,459	1,166	1,043
South Korea	4		32,088	23,044	41
Spain	446	246	152		67
Sweden			59	5	9
Switzerland	2,000	800		700	
Taiwan					
Thailand	13,734	3,167	4,074	7,319	
Tunisia	123	101	47	231	98
Turkey	27,120	16,329	16,244	30,509	7,823
Turkmenistan	1,035	452	113	9	11
Ukraine	5,107	1,389	817	16,970	7,587
United Arab Emirates	296	117	69	30	53
United Kingdom	74		104	73	314
USA	100	100	85	116	37
Venezuela	4	0	22	115	2,392
Vietnam	11,690	14,134	16,512	12,058	6,755

Source: WHO

Incidence of diphtheria 1998-2002

Table: 2.34

number

	1998	1999	2000	2001	2002
Algeria	57	17		3	0
Argentina	2	0	0	0	
Australia	0	0	0	1	0
Austria	0	0	0	0	0
Azerbaijan	20	19	7	0	0
Belarus	36	38	52	25	7
Belgium	0			0	1
Bolivia	8	2	1	3	5
Brazil	217	53	46	10	64
Bulgaria	0	0	0	0	0
Canada	0	1	0	1	2
Chile	0	0	0	0	
China	40	16	19	12	11
Colombia	2	0	11	0	3
Croatia	0	0	0	0	0
Czech Republic	0	0	0	0	0
Denmark			0	0	0
Ecuador	21	5	1	1	4
Egypt	3	2	0	0	0
Estonia	0	0	2	2	0
Finland	0			2	0
France			0		1
Germany	1	1	0	0	1
Greece	0	0	0	0	0
Hong Kong, China					
Hungary	0	0	0	0	0
India	1,378	1,786	3,094	5,101	5,472
Indonesia	14	114	23	34	51
Ireland	0	0		0	0
Israel	1	3	0	0	1
Italy	0	0	0		0
Japan	1		1	1	0
Jordan	0	0	0	0	0
Kazakhstan	75	17	13	14	14
Kuwait	0	0	0		
Latvia	67	81	264	91	45
Lithuania	2	6	2	0	3
Malaysia	5	6	1	4	2
Mexico	0	0	0	0	
Morocco	0	0	0	0	0
Netherlands	0	1	0		0
New Zealand	1	0	0	0	1
Nigeria	708		3,995	2,468	790
Norway			0	0	0
Pakistan	20	12	13	19	22
Peru	2	8	0	0	0
Philippines	83	64	88	73	62
Poland	0	0	1	0	0
Portugal	0	0	0		0
Romania	0	0	0	0	0
Russia	1,409	838	771	909	778
Saudi Arabia	0	0		0	9
Singapore	0	0	0		0
Slovakia	0	0	0	0	0
Slovenia	0	0		0	0
South Africa	4	0	2	0	1
South Korea	0			0	
Spain	0	0	0		0
Sweden			0	0	0
Switzerland	0	0	0	0	0
Taiwan					
Thailand	43	52	15	11	
Tunisia	0	0	0	0	0
Turkey	6	4	4	5	2
Turkmenistan	18	49	30	2	1
Ukraine	706	375	365	283	285
United Arab Emirates	0	1	0	0	0
United Kingdom	0		2	4	6
USA	1	1	2	2	1
Venezuela	0	0	0	0	0
Vietnam	130	81	113	133	105

Source: WHO

Incidence of polio 1998-2002

number

	1998	1999	2000	2001	2002
Algeria	0	10	0	1	0
Argentina	0	0	0	0	
Australia	0	0	0	0	0
Austria	0	0	0	0	0
Azerbaijan	0	0	0	0	0
Belarus	0	0	0	0	0
Belgium	0	0	0	0	0
Bolivia	0	0	0	0	0
Brazil	0	0	0	0	0
Bulgaria	0	0	0	3	0
Canada	0	0	0		0
Chile	0	0	0	0	
China	0	1	0	0	0
Colombia	0	0	0	0	0
Croatia	0	0	0	0	0
Czech Republic	0	0	0	0	0
Denmark	0	0	0	0	0
Ecuador	0	0	0	0	0
Egypt	35	9	4	5	7
Estonia	0	0	0	0	0
Finland	0	0	0	0	0
France	0	0	0		0
Germany	0	0	0	0	0
Greece	0	0	0	0	0
Hong Kong, China					
Hungary	0	0	0	0	
India	4,322	2,817	265	268	1,600
Indonesia	49	39	35	0	0
Ireland	0	0	0	0	0
Israel	0	0	0	0	0
Italy	0	0	0	0	0
Japan	0	0	0		0
Jordan	0	0	0	0	0
Kazakhstan	0	0	0	0	0
Kuwait	0	0	0	0	
Latvia	0	0	0	0	0
Lithuania	0	0	0	0	0
Malaysia	0	0	0	0	0
Mexico	0	0	0	0	
Morocco	0	0	0	0	0
Netherlands	0	0	0	0	0
New Zealand	0	0	0	0	0
Nigeria	312	981	638	56	202
Norway	0	0	0	0	0
Pakistan	341	558	199	116	90
Peru	0	0	0	0	0
Philippines	0	0	0	3	0
Poland	0	0	0	0	0
Portugal	0	0	0	0	0
Romania	0	0	0	0	0
Russia	0	0	0	0	0
Saudi Arabia	1	0	0	0	0
Singapore	0	0	0	0	0
Slovakia	0	0	0	0	0
Slovenia	0	0	0		0
South Africa	104	4	0	0	0
South Korea	0	0	0	0	0
Spain	0	0	0	0	0
Sweden	0	0	0	0	0
Switzerland	0	0	0	0	0
Taiwan					
Thailand	31	24	20	0	
Tunisia	0	0	0	0	0
Turkey	26	0	0	0	0
Turkmenistan	0	0	0	0	0
Ukraine	0	0	0	0	0
United Arab Emirates	0	0	0	0	0
United Kingdom	0	0	0		0
USA	0	0	0		0
Venezuela	0	0	0	0	0
Vietnam	0	0	0	0	0

Source: WHO

Incidence of AIDS 1998-2004

Table: 2.36

number

	1998	1999	2000	2001	2002	2003	2004
Algeria	49	40	58	17	58	62	65
Argentina	1,899	1,401	528	482	612	541	471
Australia	301	181	212	27	182	189	176
Austria	111	89	84	70	70	17	23
Azerbaijan	3	8	19	17	14	7	8
Belarus	4	5	3	2	21	12	15
Belgium	165	98	105	126	187	76	86
Bolivia	42	34	43	73	79	82	75
Brazil	24,017	20,009	15,013	3,024	3,041	2,988	4,203
Bulgaria	3	11	16	14	13	5	6
Canada	639	527	471	384	357	218	250
Chile	492	553	553	654	536	204	250
China	136	230	233	231	292	302	280
Colombia	1,125	906	867	1,157	1,602	1,406	1,503
Croatia	12	16	19	7	20	1	5
Czech Republic	8	16	13	3	8	4	6
Denmark	71	73	60	19	43	34	25
Ecuador	186	325	313	299	325	326	282
Egypt	23	34	44	35	46	52	63
Estonia	6	12	390	1,474	899	258	240
Finland	20	10	16	10	21	12	15
France	2,098	1,785	1,825	787	2,004	1,091	1,020
Germany	943	578	1,474	484	1,008	837	752
Greece	146	137	143	44	91	35	29
Hong Kong, China	63	61	67	24	35	37	25
Hungary	36	37	27	12	26	13	18
India	1,148	952	2,098	2,399	2,514	2,604	2,361
Indonesia	75	57	166	185	232	239	321
Ireland	41	41	21	4	13	5	6
Israel	36	137	50	39	78	22	32
Italy	2,483	2,201	1,903	989	1,753	894	762
Japan	231	300	327	155	132	138	143
Jordan	11	3	14	7	8	8	9
Kazakhstan	9	5	8	10	29	57	32
Kuwait	19	4	12	5	9	10	7
Latvia	11	17	24	42	55	58	50
Lithuania	8	7	8	7	9	6	7
Malaysia	875	1,200	1,168	1,302	1,193	1,076	1,082
Mexico	4,758	4,372	4,855	4,297	4,854	4,922	3,828
Morocco	93	165	112	129	149	152	138
Netherlands	291	234	192	76	234	61	75
New Zealand	29	33	27	26	22	20	25
Nigeria	18,490	16,188	9,715	3,661	3,989	2,026	1,756
Norway	36	23	38	6	33	3	8
Pakistan	23	17	15	8	10	10	9
Peru	1,031	1,009	615	775	893	902	802
Philippines	45	78	40	56	44	47	45
Poland	132	113	109	56	130	62	75
Portugal	874	1,010	1,123	931	822	289	245
Romania	678	492	490	192	222	72	78
Russia	4,058	19,953	59,257	88,422	50,373	39,505	32,101
Saudi Arabia	39	24	24	39	48	52	43
Singapore	125	140	143	152	146	143	151
Slovakia	3	2	4	5	2	1	2
Slovenia	14	9	7	3	2	2	3
South Africa							
South Korea	35	34	32	42	41	40	39
Spain	4,222	3,427	2,847	2,942	2,356	1,243	1,189
Sweden	63	74	54	21	59	26	32
Switzerland	423	262	257	175	199	282	301
Taiwan	151	175	221	236	267	289	172
Thailand	27,485	27,010	26,114	24,042	21,650	13,585	12,621
Tunisia	44	42	48	43	39	37	41
Turkey	29	28	46	27	44	27	22
Turkmenistan							
Ukraine	287	580	648	361	1,353	1,915	1,528
United Arab Emirates	1	2	3	2	4	1	2
United Kingdom	963	790	737	824	807	810	803
USA	43,894	46,143	42,156	43,265	42,786	42,135	41,895
Venezuela	0						
Vietnam	953	970	1,164	742	783	764	738

Source: UNAIDS/World Health Organisation

■ Causes of Death

Deaths from heart disease 1998-2004

number per 100,000 inhabitants

	1998	1999	2000	2001	2002	2003	2004
Algeria							
Argentina	60.1	62.3	64.4	66.6	68.8	71.1	73.3
Australia	151.1	145.9	141.2	136.4	131.6	126.9	123.3
Austria	216.7	212.0	200.3	193.3	185.3	177.3	169.6
Azerbaijan	209.8	134.6	214.3	190.2	192.4	194.6	187.7
Belarus	447.1	492.6	474.8	499.4	513.5	527.7	547.7
Belgium	122.5	123.2	123.9	124.6	125.3	126.0	126.2
Bolivia	48.7	46.1	47.2	46.0	46.1	45.3	45.0
Brazil	44.9	44.8	44.8	44.7	44.7	44.6	44.2
Bulgaria	270.1	254.3	243.3	229.3	216.3	203.3	191.5
Canada	142.2	139.2	136.2	133.3	130.3	127.5	123.5
Chile	53.8	53.0	53.3	53.3	53.3	53.3	52.8
China	53.9	52.1	54.5	50.5	48.9	45.8	42.8
Colombia	53.7	54.0	53.1	52.3	51.3	50.0	49.2
Croatia	211.4	197.5	213.2	209.1	209.9	210.8	208.8
Czech Republic	233.5	238.5	227.6	227.3	224.4	221.5	218.0
Denmark	189.2	180.8	171.1	161.7	152.4	143.4	134.9
Ecuador	18.6	19.8	18.4	18.7	18.5	18.4	18.5
Egypt							
Estonia	444.4	418.7	433.6	421.5	416.2	410.9	405.6
Finland	248.8	251.3	249.2	250.2	250.4	250.7	252.4
France	78.0	76.9	76.8	76.5	76.2	75.9	75.4
Germany	217.9	213.3	211.9	209.7	207.5	205.3	204.0
Greece	116.7	120.9	117.0	115.2	113.4	111.6	109.1
Hong Kong, China	32.4	34.1	37.9	38.6	39.9	40.8	41.9
Hungary	310.9	312.8	297.2	293.4	286.6	279.9	274.1
India	41.5	44.3	40.4	40.2	40.0	39.8	39.5
Indonesia	36.9	37.4	41.6	42.3	44.1	45.2	46.3
Ireland	195.4	188.5	183.4	177.8	172.4	167.0	161.4
Israel	113.0	116.7	121.2	125.8	130.5	135.3	140.2
Italy	136.1	131.7	133.3	133.3	133.4	133.4	133.8
Japan	57.2	58.9	59.4	60.1	60.9	61.6	62.7
Jordan							
Kazakhstan	250.1	244.1	243.0	240.6	238.2	235.7	233.8
Kuwait	37.4	35.5	29.3	26.0	22.2	18.5	15.7
Latvia	435.4	404.0	406.9	387.2	373.3	359.5	348.1
Lithuania	379.0	360.1	341.3	322.6	304.0	285.6	267.8
Malaysia	32.7	33.4	33.9	34.4	35.5	36.2	37.2
Mexico	44.7	45.3	44.6	44.7	44.6	44.5	44.2
Morocco							
Netherlands	121.7	115.8	112.3	108.4	104.5	100.6	96.3
New Zealand	163.6	175.3	175.4	178.4	181.4	184.4	186.4
Nigeria							
Norway	199.1	196.0	189.9	184.7	179.5	174.3	167.7
Pakistan	32.4	33.3	31.5	31.4	30.5	30.1	29.9
Peru		7.1	13.4	15.1	21.4	27.4	34.7
Philippines	61.5	59.0	64.9	67.2	67.3	68.8	70.9
Poland	137.8	147.6	143.8	142.9	140.1	137.7	136.8
Portugal	94.2	92.1	88.3	85.6	82.6	79.6	76.6
Romania	252.4	256.6	242.6	240.6	235.6	230.5	225.9
Russia	349.0	383.5	452.8	497.0	547.0	596.4	650.5
Saudi Arabia							
Singapore	95.1	96.9	91.3	90.6	88.5	86.4	84.3
Slovakia	266.2	268.8	290.4	299.5	311.9	324.5	336.4
Slovenia	141.1	132.9	132.6	130.2	127.8	125.4	122.1
South Africa	29.9	30.3	30.7	31.1	31.4	31.7	31.7
South Korea	16.2	18.5	21.5	24.3	27.4	30.7	34.5
Spain	84.9	80.4	73.7	67.3	61.2	55.4	50.4
Sweden	245.2	239.1	235.0	230.4	225.8	221.3	218.9
Switzerland	244.2	241.6	256.4	260.4	284.2	271.2	277.4
Taiwan	36.6	35.1	39.8	38.4	38.6	37.7	36.8
Thailand	42.3	44.4	47.9	44.0	45.7	43.7	42.6
Tunisia							
Turkey	82.2	77.9	74.7	78.6	76.6	78.5	79.9
Turkmenistan	146.5	123.3	112.1	98.5	98.6	87.5	80.3
Ukraine	538.7	573.4	607.6	642.6	677.7	713.2	755.4
United Arab Emirates							
United Kingdom	234.2	221.9	215.6	208.0	200.4	193.0	185.8
USA	170.1	194.2	199.7	210.2	220.9	231.9	245.2
Venezuela	64.8	64.0	65.0	64.7	64.8	64.9	65.1
Vietnam	41.3	39.9	39.0	39.8	40.4	41.0	41.8

Source: WHO/Euromonitor International

Deaths from lung cancer 1998-2004

Table: 2.38

number per 100,000 inhabitants

	1998	1999	2000	2001	2002	2003	2004
Algeria							
Argentina	21.7	20.6	19.5	18.4	17.2	16.0	15.0
Australia	36.1	35.7	35.6	35.3	35.0	34.7	34.3
Austria	41.1	40.1	40.3	39.6	39.0	38.4	37.6
Azerbaijan	8.8	9.4	9.1	9.9	10.1	10.3	10.7
Belarus	38.2	37.6	37.1	36.2	35.4	34.4	33.4
Belgium	64.1	63.7	63.3	62.9	62.5	62.1	61.6
Bolivia	21.7	19.4	18.9	19.8	20.0	20.7	21.3
Brazil	8.7	8.9	9.2	9.4	9.7	9.9	10.1
Bulgaria	35.8	37.3	35.6	35.8	35.3	34.6	34.3
Canada	53.8	53.5	53.8	54.2	54.5	54.7	54.6
Chile	12.1	12.3	12.3	12.3	12.4	12.4	12.4
China	45.1	43.1	40.7	40.8	41.5	41.6	42.3
Colombia	7.4	7.1	6.5	6.3	6.1	5.9	5.7
Croatia	57.1	54.8	56.5	55.6	55.4	55.1	54.7
Czech Republic	52.8	54.7	55.7	57.4	58.9	60.3	62.0
Denmark	61.6	60.8	59.2	57.6	55.9	54.1	52.6
Ecuador	3.7	3.5	3.6	3.4	3.3	3.2	3.1
Egypt							
Estonia	48.4	45.2	50.1	49.6	50.4	51.1	50.9
Finland	37.4	35.1	35.7	34.3	33.5	32.6	31.5
France	42.7	43.0	43.8	44.4	45.1	45.8	46.4
Germany	46.3	45.9	46.3	46.5	46.7	46.9	46.9
Greece	51.5	51.9	52.6	53.2	53.8	54.4	54.6
Hong Kong, China	22.9	22.1	20.7	21.8	21.6	22.3	22.9
Hungary	78.1	78.3	78.0	78.1	77.9	77.7	76.8
India	35.7	36.1	36.9	35.8	37.2	36.9	37.3
Indonesia	23.0	20.2	18.8	20.2	20.0	20.9	21.6
Ireland	41.1	38.7	39.9	40.1	40.3	40.4	40.9
Israel	19.7	19.8	19.7	19.6	19.5	19.4	19.5
Italy	54.8	54.9	55.3	55.6	55.9	56.2	56.2
Japan	40.6	41.6	42.9	44.1	45.4	46.7	48.3
Jordan							
Kazakhstan	27.4	25.8	25.9	25.5	25.1	24.8	24.3
Kuwait	3.3	2.6	3.3	3.1	2.9	2.7	2.5
Latvia	43.0	46.3	43.8	44.9	45.0	45.0	45.4
Lithuania	39.3	39.6	37.2	36.4	35.2	33.8	33.0
Malaysia	23.9	25.9	26.4	26.2	25.9	25.6	25.5
Mexico	6.5	6.6	6.3	6.3	6.2	6.2	6.2
Morocco							
Netherlands	55.0	55.2	55.0	54.9	54.7	54.4	54.5
New Zealand	36.4	38.5	38.9	39.8	40.7	41.5	42.4
Nigeria							
Norway	38.0	38.3	37.4	36.8	36.2	35.6	35.3
Pakistan	28.9	24.8	26.6	25.7	25.7	25.1	24.4
Peru		2.0	4.3	4.2	6.2	7.8	9.5
Philippines	29.9	28.8	26.9	28.3	27.5	28.1	28.7
Poland	48.6	49.8	51.8	52.3	53.8	55.0	56.6
Portugal	28.5	27.3	28.1	27.5	27.2	26.8	26.5
Romania	36.0	35.4	37.9	38.3	39.0	39.7	40.7
Russia	41.0	40.8	40.2	37.3	32.8	26.8	23.6
Saudi Arabia							
Singapore	30.1	29.1	27.5	26.4	25.2	23.9	22.9
Slovakia	41.3	40.2	41.6	41.2	41.2	41.0	40.6
Slovenia	46.2	49.0	50.2	51.8	53.5	55.2	56.7
South Africa	9.9	9.7	9.5	9.3	9.0	8.7	8.5
South Korea	20.5	22.1	24.4	26.4	28.6	30.9	33.5
Spain	43.7	44.5	45.0	45.3	45.3	45.0	44.9
Sweden	33.0	33.9	33.8	33.9	34.1	34.2	34.6
Switzerland	37.5	36.8	32.7	27.0	23.6	19.4	16.4
Taiwan	18.1	18.0	17.6	17.1	16.9	16.5	16.3
Thailand	28.9	31.2	29.4	31.0	31.0	31.9	33.0
Tunisia							
Turkey	41.6	40.3	38.5	39.6	39.5	40.2	40.4
Turkmenistan	4.2	3.6	2.9	2.3	2.2	2.5	2.4
Ukraine	38.6	37.9	38.2	37.3	36.4	35.3	34.3
United Arab Emirates							
United Kingdom	59.0	57.5	57.0	56.1	55.2	54.3	53.1
USA	57.2	55.8	55.1	53.9	52.5	50.8	49.0
Venezuela	8.4	8.9	8.7	9.0	9.1	9.3	9.5
Vietnam	20.6	20.5	22.6	20.6	20.3	18.9	17.9

Source: WHO/Euromonitor International

Deaths from chronic liver disease and cirrhosis 1998-2004

Table: 2.39

number per 100,000 inhabitants

	1998	1999	2000	2001	2002	2003	2004
Algeria							
Argentina	9.4	9.8	10.2	10.7	11.1	11.6	12.0
Australia	5.9	5.8	5.9	6.0	6.0	6.1	6.1
Austria	23.6	21.6	22.4	21.3	20.7	20.0	19.3
Azerbaijan							
Belarus							
Belgium	11.9	11.9	11.8	11.7	11.7	11.6	11.5
Bolivia	7.3	7.5	7.8	8.1	8.2	8.4	8.6
Brazil	9.8	9.9	10.1	10.2	10.4	10.5	10.7
Bulgaria	20.7	18.4	19.1	17.7	16.9	16.1	15.3
Canada	7.2	7.0	7.1	7.1	7.1	7.1	7.1
Chile	22.7	20.5	19.3	17.8	16.4	15.0	13.7
China	11.1	10.8	10.5	10.6	10.0	9.9	9.7
Colombia	4.3	4.3	4.3	4.2	4.1	4.1	4.1
Croatia	33.3	34.4	32.9	33.1	32.9	32.7	32.5
Czech Republic	18.5	18.1	18.0	17.7	17.5	17.2	16.8
Denmark	15.5	17.0	17.5	18.0	18.3	18.5	18.9
Ecuador	10.5	10.4	10.2	10.1	9.9	9.8	9.6
Egypt							
Estonia	18.9	16.2	19.9	19.2	19.6	20.1	20.3
Finland	12.7	12.1	13.0	13.0	13.2	13.4	13.4
France	16.3	15.8	15.6	15.3	15.0	14.7	14.5
Germany	21.8	21.5	20.9	20.3	19.8	19.2	18.8
Greece	5.7	6.1	6.3	6.5	6.7	6.9	7.1
Hong Kong, China	7.8	7.7	7.7	8.0	8.1	8.3	8.5
Hungary	71.2	71.0	67.5	66.3	64.5	62.7	61.0
India	10.0	9.8	9.6	9.3	9.5	9.4	9.4
Indonesia	6.9	6.7	6.7	7.1	7.1	7.4	7.6
Ireland	4.3	4.4	4.6	4.7	4.8	5.0	5.2
Israel	4.9	4.3	4.1	3.7	3.4	3.1	2.8
Italy	20.8	19.9	19.1	18.3	17.4	16.6	16.0
Japan	11.2	11.4	11.2	11.1	11.0	10.9	10.7
Jordan							
Kazakhstan	20.7	19.4	19.1	18.6	18.1	17.5	17.0
Kuwait	1.8	1.5	1.6	1.4	1.2	1.0	0.9
Latvia	15.4	13.9	14.5	13.8	13.3	12.9	12.3
Lithuania	16.5	14.6	15.1	14.1	13.4	12.7	12.0
Malaysia	8.9	8.6	8.4	8.6	9.0	9.3	9.6
Mexico	26.0	25.4	25.3	24.8	24.5	24.1	23.7
Morocco							
Netherlands	5.3	5.3	5.3	5.2	5.2	5.1	5.0
New Zealand	2.9	3.8	3.8	4.1	4.3	4.6	4.9
Nigeria							
Norway	5.9	5.2	5.2	5.0	4.8	4.7	4.6
Pakistan	8.3	8.1	7.9	7.6	7.7	7.5	7.4
Peru	12.9	10.3	10.4	10.4	8.8	8.7	8.3
Philippines	12.4	12.3	12.2	12.7	13.2	13.7	14.4
Poland	13.6	15.1	14.3	14.6	14.2	14.0	14.0
Portugal	20.8	19.3	17.8	16.4	15.1	13.8	12.7
Romania	54.8	47.6	46.4	41.5	37.7	34.1	30.5
Russia		17.8	20.2	26.5	31.2	36.5	44.4
Saudi Arabia							
Singapore	4.2	4.3	3.0	2.7	2.6	2.6	2.5
Slovakia	25.3	26.7	25.9	26.6	26.8	26.9	27.2
Slovenia	32.2	34.0	35.5	37.0	38.6	40.2	42.3
South Africa	9.3	10.6	12.0	13.4	14.9	16.4	18.3
South Korea	24.1	22.0	21.3	19.2	17.2	14.9	13.1
Spain	15.9	15.1	14.4	13.7	13.0	12.3	11.8
Sweden	6.5	6.4	7.0	7.4	7.8	8.1	8.5
Switzerland	10.3	10.5	8.7	9.1	9.2	8.9	9.0
Taiwan	6.0	5.7	5.4	5.2	5.0	4.8	4.6
Thailand	9.7	9.6	9.5	9.4	9.1	8.9	8.7
Tunisia							
Turkey	8.5	8.1	7.8	8.5	8.2	8.6	9.0
Turkmenistan							
Ukraine							
United Arab Emirates							
United Kingdom	9.1	9.6	10.2	10.7	11.1	11.6	12.0
USA	9.3	10.7	11.1	11.7	12.4	13.1	13.8
Venezuela	7.5	7.8	8.0	8.2	8.4	8.7	8.9
Vietnam	8.3	8.0	7.8	7.6	7.5	7.3	7.2

Source: WHO/Euromonitor International

Deaths from ulcers of the stomach and duodenum 1998-2004

Table: 2.40

number per 100,000 inhabitants

	1998	1999	2000	2001	2002	2003	2004
Algeria							
Argentina	1.1	1.1	1.0	1.0	1.0	0.9	0.9
Australia	2.4	2.4	2.3	2.2	2.1	2.0	1.9
Austria	3.5	2.9	3.2	2.9	2.8	2.6	2.4
Azerbaijan	3.6	3.4	3.6	3.7	3.7	3.7	3.8
Belarus	3.9	3.7	3.7	3.6	3.5	3.3	3.1
Belgium	3.4	3.3	3.2	3.2	3.1	3.1	3.0
Bolivia	28.4	28.8	29.2	29.7	30.8	31.5	32.5
Brazil	1.6	1.4	1.3	1.2	1.1	1.0	0.9
Bulgaria	3.5	3.0	2.7	2.3	2.0	1.7	1.4
Canada	1.6	1.5	1.5	1.5	1.4	1.4	1.4
Chile	1.5	1.8	1.8	1.8	1.9	2.0	2.1
China	37.4	36.3	34.5	32.1	31.5	29.8	28.3
Colombia	2.5	2.5	2.7	2.8	2.8	2.9	3.0
Croatia	5.1	5.1	5.3	5.4	5.5	5.6	5.7
Czech Republic	5.0	5.1	5.9	6.3	6.7	7.2	7.7
Denmark	10.7	10.6	10.4	10.3	10.1	9.8	9.5
Ecuador	2.5	2.1	2.1	1.8	1.6	1.4	1.2
Egypt							
Estonia	6.3	4.9	6.0	5.4	5.2	5.0	4.7
Finland	4.5	5.0	5.2	5.6	5.9	6.2	6.6
France	2.6	2.5	2.5	2.5	2.5	2.5	2.5
Germany	4.1	4.0	4.0	4.0	3.9	3.9	3.9
Greece	2.7	2.6	2.8	2.9	3.0	3.1	3.2
Hong Kong, China	20.3	19.1	20.6	21.1	20.9	21.1	21.5
Hungary	9.4	9.0	9.4	9.3	9.3	9.3	9.3
India	27.6	25.9	27.7	25.8	25.8	24.6	23.6
Indonesia	30.9	28.9	27.5	29.5	28.8	29.9	30.6
Ireland	4.2	5.1	4.7	4.6	4.5	4.5	4.5
Israel	1.6	1.6	1.5	1.4	1.5	1.3	1.2
Italy	3.5	3.3	3.3	3.2	3.2	3.1	3.1
Japan	3.1	3.2	3.3	3.3	3.4	3.5	3.5
Jordan							
Kazakhstan	3.8	1.0	1.1	1.2	1.0	0.9	0.8
Kuwait	0.2	0.2	0.3	0.3	0.4	0.4	0.4
Latvia	6.0	5.1	6.6	6.4	6.6	6.8	6.9
Lithuania	4.3	4.3	4.5	4.6	4.6	4.6	4.6
Malaysia	18.9	19.2	18.4	18.8	18.6	18.8	19.1
Mexico	3.1	3.0	2.8	2.7	2.5	2.3	2.2
Morocco							
Netherlands	2.3	2.3	2.3	2.2	2.1	2.1	2.0
New Zealand	2.9	2.6	2.1	2.3	2.1	1.9	1.8
Nigeria							
Norway	5.2	6.4	6.8	7.3	7.8	8.3	8.9
Pakistan	26.4	28.9	29.2	28.0	27.5	26.6	25.7
Peru		1.5	1.4	1.3	1.3	1.2	1.1
Philippines	31.9	30.9	29.9	32.4	32.0	33.6	34.9
Poland	3.8	3.8	3.9	4.1	4.2	4.4	4.6
Portugal	3.9	4.1	3.4	3.3	3.0	2.8	2.6
Romania	3.6	3.4	4.1	4.2	4.4	4.6	4.8
Russia	5.7	6.3	6.0	6.0	5.7	5.2	5.0
Saudi Arabia							
Singapore	2.2	2.9	1.6	1.6	1.3	1.2	1.1
Slovakia	4.7	4.8	5.0	5.1	5.2	5.3	5.4
Slovenia	5.0	6.3	6.4	6.9	7.3	7.7	8.1
South Africa	2.9	3.0	3.1	3.2	3.3	3.4	3.5
South Korea	1.5	1.3	1.5	1.5	1.4	1.4	1.4
Spain	2.5	2.3	2.2	2.1	2.0	1.8	1.7
Sweden	5.2	5.3	5.4	5.6	5.7	5.9	6.1
Switzerland	2.7	2.7	1.8	2.1	1.9	2.0	2.1
Taiwan	19.2	18.9	20.7	18.9	18.5	17.2	16.1
Thailand	18.7	17.1	18.9	16.4	15.5	13.7	12.4
Tunisia							
Turkey	36.0	32.4	33.4	35.5	35.6	37.1	38.8
Turkmenistan	2.4	2.3	2.2	2.0	1.8	1.7	1.6
Ukraine	4.3	4.1	4.2	4.1	4.0	3.9	3.8
United Arab Emirates							
United Kingdom	7.3	7.4	7.4	7.4	7.4	7.4	7.3
USA	1.7	1.7	1.5	1.4	1.2	1.0	0.9
Venezuela	2.0	2.1	1.8	1.8	1.7	1.6	1.5
Vietnam	21.8	19.4	20.1	19.2	18.3	17.4	16.5

Source: WHO/Euromonitor International

Deaths from infectious and parasitic diseases 1998-2004

Table: 2.41

number per 100,000 inhabitants

	1998	1999	2000	2001	2002	2003	2004
Algeria							
Argentina							
Australia	6.6	6.9	6.6	6.4	6.5	6.3	6.2
Austria	3.3	3.3	2.9	2.8	2.6	2.7	2.6
Azerbaijan							
Belarus	9.3	9.5	9.7	9.9	10.1	9.8	9.8
Belgium							
Bolivia							
Brazil							
Bulgaria							
Canada							
Chile							
China	30.0	30.0	30.0	30.0	30.0	29.4	29.1
Colombia							
Croatia							
Czech Republic	2.2	2.2	2.1	2.1	2.0	2.2	2.2
Denmark	4.7	4.9	4.6	3.9	3.8	4.0	3.8
Ecuador							
Egypt							
Estonia	12.4	12.6	12.6	12.7	13.0	13.1	13.2
Finland	5.3	5.5	5.4	5.5	5.5	5.4	5.4
France	9.1	8.8	8.1	8.1	7.8	7.3	7.1
Germany	6.5	7.6	7.2	7.7	7.3	7.5	7.6
Greece	5.3	4.1	4.9	4.3	4.7	4.9	4.9
Hong Kong, China	12.0	11.3	11.0	10.9	11.0	10.8	10.7
Hungary	5.9	5.6	4.9	4.8	4.3	4.1	3.9
India							
Indonesia							
Ireland	5.4	5.5	5.7	5.9	6.0	5.5	5.4
Israel							
Italy	5.9	5.6	5.4	5.4	6.1	4.7	4.5
Japan	10.3	10.8	10.8	11.1	11.0	10.9	10.9
Jordan							
Kazakhstan							
Kuwait							
Latvia	19.5	19.8	20.1	20.4	20.7	20.6	20.6
Lithuania							
Malaysia	17.8	17.6	17.5	17.7	17.9	16.9	16.6
Mexico							
Morocco	5.3	5.3	5.3	5.3	5.3	5.1	5.0
Netherlands	7.6	8.1	7.7	8.0	8.0	7.7	7.7
New Zealand	3.9	3.8	3.6	3.4	3.3	2.9	2.7
Nigeria							
Norway	7.1	7.5	7.8	8.1	8.5	7.7	7.7
Pakistan							
Peru							
Philippines							
Poland	6.2	5.7	5.9	5.6	5.5	5.8	5.8
Portugal	19.3	20.8	19.4	19.9	20.0	19.8	19.8
Romania	16.3	14.4	14.1	15.4	15.0	14.1	14.2
Russia	19.0	24.6	25.0	21.0	20.3	20.2	18.7
Saudi Arabia							
Singapore	9.2	7.9	6.9	6.9	6.6	6.6	6.4
Slovakia	2.3	2.7	3.2	3.6	3.8	3.2	3.2
Slovenia			103.0				
South Africa							
South Korea	15.8	15.1	14.4	13.7	13.0	13.4	13.2
Spain	12.3	12.3	11.9	11.7	10.3	10.0	9.3
Sweden	5.9	6.5	6.4	6.8	7.0	6.5	6.5
Switzerland	7.2	6.7	5.4	4.6	4.5	5.1	5.0
Taiwan	27.3	25.1	25.4	24.7	24.0	23.9	23.4
Thailand							
Tunisia							
Turkey							
Turkmenistan							
Ukraine							
United Arab Emirates							
United Kingdom	5.1	5.2	5.0	5.1	4.9	5.0	5.0
USA	15.7	18.0	15.5	16.1	16.0	15.9	16.1
Venezuela							
Vietnam							

Source: Euromonitor International from OECD/WHO/national statistics

Deaths from malignant neoplasms (cancer) 1998-2004

Table: 2.42

number per 100,000 inhabitants

	1998	1999	2000	2001	2002	2003	2004
Algeria							
Argentina							
Australia	167.9	163.4	164.4	163.9	158.5	156.8	155.3
Austria	168.6	167.0	164.8	160.1	161.3	155.8	153.2
Azerbaijan	63.4	66.3	64.1	63.1	61.6	60.9	59.6
Belarus	193.6	195.1	196.6	198.1	198.6	199.6	202.0
Belgium							
Bolivia							
Brazil							
Bulgaria							
Canada							
Chile							
China	225.8	223.2	240.6	234.2	230.3	225.0	220.0
Colombia							
Croatia			267.7				
Czech Republic	225.0	223.5	224.2	224.0	223.2	223.8	224.8
Denmark	211.9	210.6	208.0	209.9	212.1	210.8	213.2
Ecuador							
Egypt							
Estonia	235.0	224.8	216.1	207.7	207.9	208.3	204.3
Finland	150.5	147.4	145.3	143.0	142.6	140.9	138.5
France	179.9	178.2	179.1	178.4	176.5	175.8	173.0
Germany	179.1	175.3	175.1	169.8	168.7	164.9	162.8
Greece	150.4	154.0	151.8	153.4	154.0	152.5	153.0
Hong Kong, China	162.1	165.4	169.2	173.3	172.9	175.7	176.5
Hungary	264.1	245.3	239.8	246.9	245.6	249.9	255.9
India							
Indonesia							
Ireland	196.0	194.8	193.2	191.9	190.4	187.2	184.1
Israel							
Italy	174.6	170.6	169.1	167.8	165.4	162.1	159.5
Japan	155.7	154.6	153.4	154.4	153.4	153.1	154.5
Jordan							
Kazakhstan	133.0	129.6	129.1	128.6	129.7	130.4	130.4
Kuwait							
Latvia	231.8	235.0	238.2	241.4	244.7	244.4	245.8
Lithuania							
Malaysia	19.8	21.3	21.2	20.9	20.8	20.0	19.4
Mexico							
Morocco	10.5	10.0	10.0	9.9	9.9	9.7	9.7
Netherlands	192.4	194.2	191.1	191.3	190.6	188.3	188.7
New Zealand	189.1	184.0	182.0	178.0	174.0	172.0	168.3
Nigeria							
Norway	168.0	168.3	164.2	163.1	161.2	162.2	163.2
Pakistan							
Peru							
Philippines	43.2						
Poland	170.1	198.7	202.5	212.8	208.9	206.7	209.8
Portugal	162.8	161.3	159.9	159.1	158.4	157.0	157.6
Romania	174.4	176.4	184.1	191.4	194.4	190.8	191.5
Russia	201.0	205.0	206.0	209.0	211.0	215.0	218.1
Saudi Arabia							
Singapore	104.3	105.5	106.5	105.8	104.3	102.3	101.9
Slovakia	223.9	215.8	212.6	211.4	206.2	200.5	197.6
Slovenia	241.2	245.7	241.9	241.0	237.6	235.0	230.9
South Africa							
South Korea	171.9	169.5	167.1	164.7	162.3	161.1	159.6
Spain	165.7	164.4	164.1	163.7	163.2	162.4	161.8
Sweden	152.3	151.3	150.8	150.0	149.3	150.6	149.0
Switzerland	153.7	150.6	148.7	147.1	146.0	143.5	142.7
Taiwan	134.0	135.3	135.7	136.1	136.4	135.9	136.6
Thailand							
Tunisia							
Turkey							
Turkmenistan							
Ukraine							
United Arab Emirates							
United Kingdom	188.8	184.7	182.4	181.5	179.1	176.1	174.9
USA	174.8	174.7	171.9	170.9	169.6	168.0	166.6
Venezuela							
Vietnam							

Source: Euromonitor International from OECD/WHO/national statistics

Deaths from diseases of the circulatory system 1998-2004

Table: 2.43

number per 100,000 inhabitants

	1998	1999	2000	2001	2002	2003	2004
Algeria							
Argentina	249.0	235.0	232.0	232.0	230.4	227.0	226.0
Australia	224.0	212.6	209.8	200.1	195.3	188.9	180.8
Austria	328.3	319.2	296.8	279.0	263.0	262.0	252.1
Azerbaijan	250.9	254.8	262.2	261.6	264.3	267.6	267.5
Belarus	700.2	715.9	732.0	748.5	764.4	780.7	798.4
Belgium	234.0	228.0	220.0	216.0	197.0	195.0	187.7
Bolivia							
Brazil							
Bulgaria							
Canada	216.0	211.0	208.0	206.0	198.0	190.0	184.5
Chile							
China	224.2	223.0	225.0	224.0	221.6	219.0	215.1
Colombia							
Croatia							
Czech Republic	476.5	467.1	441.9	434.9	425.1	417.2	408.5
Denmark	251.1	240.0	228.7	225.8	217.4	212.7	208.7
Ecuador							
Egypt							
Estonia	732.6	700.5	679.6	659.3	663.7	671.0	668.2
Finland	292.3	284.2	277.0	269.5	268.8	263.7	261.2
France	168.4	163.6	162.3	160.9	159.3	158.6	156.0
Germany	301.3	291.9	290.6	286.0	279.0	270.0	265.6
Greece	314.2	303.4	300.0	298.2	291.6	284.4	279.7
Hong Kong, China	133.1	136.3	137.2	138.7	140.5	142.9	146.0
Hungary	556.5	470.7	412.9	477.7	472.0	476.0	503.6
India							
Indonesia							
Ireland	324.6	322.9	309.0	298.0	282.0	275.0	262.7
Israel							
Italy	243.2	231.3	230.0	228.0	223.0	219.0	215.7
Japan	151.3	150.6	145.8	145.0	142.8	139.8	137.6
Jordan							
Kazakhstan	498.6	489.4	500.5	499.0	498.0	498.0	492.7
Kuwait							
Latvia	775.6	780.0	784.4	782.1	780.2	779.0	772.5
Lithuania							
Malaysia	60.9	62.6	63.6	64.2	64.7	61.3	60.9
Mexico							
Morocco	37.0	38.0	38.0	38.8	39.3	37.7	37.9
Netherlands	235.2	229.7	221.9	215.7	218.1	209.3	207.3
New Zealand	247.4	240.0	237.0	215.0	200.0	185.0	172.0
Nigeria							
Norway	258.3	252.1	246.6	240.8	235.2	242.5	239.2
Pakistan							
Peru							
Philippines							
Poland	379.8	446.2	421.9	427.9	428.8	417.1	412.2
Portugal	316.6	309.3	289.4	290.0	278.0	264.5	256.2
Romania	737.9	736.0	702.2	712.8	701.9	698.9	697.8
Russia	751.0	818.0	852.0	901.0	948.0	998.0	1,055.2
Saudi Arabia							
Singapore	145.6	147.1	143.1	134.5	137.9	130.9	126.2
Slovakia	548.7	517.7	512.9	510.7	508.9	507.6	501.3
Slovenia	398.1	388.3	236.9	234.5	232.5	214.2	205.9
South Africa							
South Korea	196.7	190.2	183.7	177.2	170.7	173.3	169.6
Spain	215.2	203.7	198.8	189.5	181.3	197.3	197.0
Sweden	259.9	253.4	246.7	246.5	240.1	233.5	228.8
Switzerland	209.5	204.5	199.5	194.5	189.6	197.6	195.6
Taiwan	50.5	51.3	52.2	52.9	52.7	50.1	49.9
Thailand							
Tunisia							
Turkey							
Turkmenistan							
Ukraine							
United Arab Emirates							
United Kingdom	276.2	265.4	256.1	255.0	246.2	236.4	231.8
USA	264.7	261.0	253.5	248.8	243.4	239.0	236.7
Venezuela							
Vietnam							

Source: Euromonitor International from OECD/WHO/national statistics

Deaths from diseases of the respiratory system 1998-2004

number per 100,000 inhabitants

	1998	1999	2000	2001	2002	2003	2004
Algeria							
Argentina							
Australia	42.9	41.6	39.0	38.2	37.5	35.5	34.3
Austria	27.9	31.1	31.1	29.5	32.4	31.0	31.2
Azerbaijan	59.4	55.4	53.1	51.9	51.1	49.8	48.4
Belarus	67.4	66.6	65.8	65.0	64.2	65.5	65.5
Belgium							
Bolivia							
Brazil							
Bulgaria							
Canada							
Chile							
China	140.8	140.7	133.5	141.7	139.6	136.1	137.8
Colombia							
Croatia			46.6				
Czech Republic	33.0	36.7	38.3	38.7	43.2	44.9	47.2
Denmark	66.7	64.2	63.6	63.3	62.8	62.5	62.1
Ecuador							
Egypt							
Estonia	41.6	35.9	34.1	33.5	32.7	29.2	27.9
Finland	54.0	53.9	54.1	54.1	54.0	54.0	54.5
France	42.4	42.1	42.2	42.4	41.0	41.4	41.1
Germany	37.0	38.2	39.6	37.5	38.2	37.1	36.2
Greece	41.1	42.7	42.2	44.1	41.9	40.0	39.6
Hong Kong, China	92.0	83.8	78.7	71.7	70.2	68.4	64.9
Hungary	41.5	39.9	33.2	31.6	26.6	23.8	21.2
India							
Indonesia							
Ireland	114.2	125.4	124.1	120.0	118.0	119.0	117.3
Israel							
Italy	35.8	36.7	36.8	37.2	37.8	37.9	38.3
Japan	61.1	67.8	67.7	72.2	75.6	68.9	68.8
Jordan							
Kazakhstan	74.9	68.3	71.1	67.6	65.7	70.5	70.4
Kuwait							
Latvia	34.6	33.8					
Lithuania							
Malaysia							
Mexico							
Morocco	7.0	7.0	7.0	7.0	7.1	6.8	6.7
Netherlands	63.9	64.1	63.9	65.2	65.7	66.4	67.4
New Zealand	49.2	45.0	38.0	33.0	29.0	25.0	21.6
Nigeria							
Norway	50.4	55.3	54.5	57.4	59.4	54.5	54.7
Pakistan							
Peru							
Philippines							
Poland	29.6	44.4	44.3	44.1	41.4	40.8	39.9
Portugal	70.8	83.2	72.6	77.3	78.2	76.0	76.7
Romania	70.8	74.3	66.1	63.1	62.9	60.8	59.7
Russia		65.0	70.7	73.0	75.0	81.0	85.1
Saudi Arabia							
Singapore	62.9	59.7	62.3	53.4	57.8	56.0	54.5
Slovakia	44.4	47.5	52.5	56.2	60.2	52.1	51.4
Slovenia	77.2	79.1	79.0	70.4	71.1	69.1	65.8
South Africa							
South Korea	41.7	40.3	38.9	37.5	36.1	36.7	36.1
Spain	60.8	69.3	70.4	76.4	77.2	79.5	83.3
Sweden	36.2	38.7	34.5	34.8	33.9	33.6	33.3
Switzerland	37.9	38.6	41.1	42.4	43.9	40.4	40.0
Taiwan	9.1	8.2	8.0	7.8	7.5	7.6	7.5
Thailand							
Tunisia							
Turkey							
Turkmenistan							
Ukraine							
United Arab Emirates							
United Kingdom	100.4	108.5	108.5	114.0	115.1	107.5	107.6
USA	67.5	64.5	65.6	64.0	63.1	63.3	61.9
Venezuela							
Vietnam							

Source: Euromonitor International from OECD/WHO/national statistics

Deaths from diseases of the digestive system 1998-2004

Table: 2.45

number per 100,000 inhabitants

	1998	1999	2000	2001	2002	2003	2004
Algeria							
Argentina	32.7	33.2	33.5	33.7	35.0	35.1	35.6
Australia	17.9	18.2	17.9	18.5	19.6	20.5	21.3
Austria	31.7	29.4	30.5	29.2	27.0	26.5	25.5
Azerbaijan	48.7	47.3	46.5	45.6	45.0	44.2	43.2
Belarus	21.7	22.5	23.1	23.0	24.1	24.4	25.1
Belgium	30.2	30.6	30.9	31.3	31.2	30.9	30.7
Bolivia	28.4	28.8	29.2	29.7	30.8	29.9	30.2
Brazil	39.5	40.0	40.8	40.0	40.4	40.1	39.8
Bulgaria	26.4	25.5	24.0	23.0	22.1	21.7	20.9
Canada	21.2	20.7	20.3	19.8	19.4	19.1	18.8
Chile	24.0	24.4	24.6	25.5	25.4	25.5	25.6
China	37.4	36.3	34.5	32.1	31.5	30.9	29.7
Colombia	28.6	29.3	29.7	29.7	30.3	30.8	30.9
Croatia	38.6	38.1	37.5	37.1	36.1	35.8	35.4
Czech Republic	33.2	33.3	33.0	29.6	28.4	30.7	29.9
Denmark	36.5	38.8	39.9	41.8	42.0	43.3	44.9
Ecuador	32.6	29.7	30.1	34.2	34.0	34.6	36.6
Egypt							
Estonia	31.5	29.8	33.5	32.7	33.6	32.4	32.2
Finland	27.9	27.0	27.9	26.7	26.9	26.2	25.9
France	30.5	29.3	28.4	27.6	27.2	27.0	26.4
Germany	33.4	32.6	32.8	31.9	32.2	31.7	31.0
Greece	15.1	15.3	15.1	14.9	14.5	15.0	14.9
Hong Kong, China	20.3	19.1	20.6	21.1	20.9	20.7	20.8
Hungary	83.9	78.1	75.5	72.3	71.8	70.4	68.2
India	27.6	25.9	27.7	25.8	25.8	24.5	23.4
Indonesia	30.9	28.9	27.5	29.5	28.8	29.8	30.4
Ireland	24.6	25.6	25.0	25.4	25.1	24.5	24.4
Israel	17.4	17.9	16.4	15.2	14.0	14.1	13.5
Italy	28.7	27.2	25.8	25.0	23.1	22.9	22.0
Japan	19.7	20.0	18.4	17.9	16.9	15.6	14.6
Jordan							
Kazakhstan	40.4	38.0	41.4	37.3	36.5	35.3	33.8
Kuwait							
Latvia	29.7	31.1	31.8	28.5	29.2	30.8	30.3
Lithuania	23.9	24.9	25.7	23.8	23.7	24.1	23.7
Malaysia	18.9	19.2	18.4	18.8	18.6	18.2	18.2
Mexico	86.9	87.3	87.8	86.9	89.6	87.9	87.8
Morocco							
Netherlands	23.6	23.3	22.6	22.2	21.8	22.3	22.2
New Zealand	14.3	13.5	12.0	11.0	9.0	7.5	6.4
Nigeria							
Norway	19.5	19.4	18.9	18.9	18.8	18.8	18.8
Pakistan	26.4	28.9	29.2	28.0	27.5	26.9	26.3
Peru	28.1	30.4	31.8	31.4	31.8	31.7	32.0
Philippines	31.9	30.9	29.9	32.4	32.0	31.1	31.8
Poland	31.8	34.9	34.6	38.0	36.6	35.2	35.1
Portugal	35.4	33.4	31.2	31.8	31.6	30.8	30.5
Romania	71.6	65.4	64.0	70.9	69.4	67.2	67.7
Russia		42.0	45.0				
Saudi Arabia							
Singapore	32.4	31.2	29.9	32.5	32.5	30.7	31.0
Slovakia	44.4	47.0	45.9	43.1	43.1	42.6	42.0
Slovenia	39.2	40.8	42.1	41.3	42.3	41.6	41.2
South Africa							
South Korea	12.9	12.3	11.9	13.2	13.1	11.5	11.3
Spain	32.9	32.0	30.3	29.7	29.0	28.0	27.2
Sweden	18.5	18.2	17.1	16.9	15.7	15.3	14.7
Switzerland	20.6	20.9	22.0	21.9	22.9	21.5	21.3
Taiwan	19.2	18.9	20.7	18.9	18.5	19.1	18.7
Thailand	18.7	17.1	18.9	16.4	15.5	14.6	13.3
Tunisia							
Turkey	36.0	32.4	33.4	35.5	35.6	35.2	35.7
Turkmenistan	33.1	29.8	28.2	29.7	30.0	30.9	31.6
Ukraine	30.4	31.2	31.8	30.2	30.2	29.2	28.3
United Arab Emirates							
United Kingdom	27.6	28.4	28.1	28.8	28.4	28.1	27.9
USA	24.0	24.7	24.5	24.9	25.1	24.0	24.0
Venezuela	33.9	32.4	31.6	33.9	33.3	34.1	35.2
Vietnam	21.8	19.4	20.1	19.2	18.3	17.9	17.2

Source: Euromonitor International from OECD/WHO/national statistics

Deaths from all other diseases 1998-2004

Table: 2.46

number per 100,000 inhabitants

	1998	1999	2000	2001	2002	2003	2004
Algeria							
Argentina	337.6	350.8	360.4	355.5	336.2	332.2	322.3
Australia	85.9	84.1	82.7	81.4	82.8	80.6	79.4
Austria	91.0	86.4	82.1	76.9	75.6	73.5	70.7
Azerbaijan							
Belarus	183.5	164.6	147.6	142.4	144.6	140.0	138.9
Belgium							
Bolivia							
Brazil							
Bulgaria							
Canada							
Chile							
China	637.6	482.1	347.2	341.6	338.9	342.3	342.4
Colombia							
Croatia			78.3				
Czech Republic	153.5	154.5	155.5	155.6	157.2	157.9	157.8
Denmark	87.2	86.1	85.7	87.7	88.1	88.8	90.7
Ecuador							
Egypt							
Estonia							
Finland	99.3	98.9	95.1	91.7	89.9	89.1	87.0
France	73.3	73.0	73.0	73.4	71.0	71.6	70.5
Germany	89.1	84.4	80.6	77.2	73.1	69.5	65.8
Greece	127.7	124.7	122.5	119.8	122.1	117.1	114.7
Hong Kong, China	62.5	61.0	59.5	58.0	56.5	54.9	53.1
Hungary	173.1	142.9	138.7	158.0	161.7	155.8	163.6
India							
Indonesia							
Ireland	99.7	105.3	98.6	100.0	99.4	97.4	96.0
Israel							
Italy	93.8	88.9	89.5	86.1	83.7	88.1	88.3
Japan	89.8	88.4	84.2	82.0	79.3	84.7	84.5
Jordan							
Kazakhstan	138.7	125.9	124.1	125.2	124.4	123.4	124.3
Kuwait							
Latvia	184.6	192.0					
Lithuania							
Malaysia							
Mexico							
Morocco	94.0	94.0	94.0	96.5	97.9	93.5	93.8
Netherlands	88.0	91.0	88.7	89.9	90.2	87.9	87.0
New Zealand	79.2	76.0	70.0	63.0	58.0	52.0	47.0
Nigeria							
Norway	92.7	89.2	87.2	84.3	81.6	85.5	85.2
Pakistan							
Peru							
Philippines							
Poland		126.5	121.7	204.3	265.0	143.6	151.7
Portugal	187.7	186.8	174.5	175.5	169.8	163.3	158.8
Romania							
Russia							
Saudi Arabia							
Singapore							
Slovakia	120.5	110.1	106.7	105.3	98.7	91.8	86.6
Slovenia							
South Africa							
South Korea							
Spain	94.7	95.5	94.4	94.5	95.1	94.5	95.1
Sweden	82.7	83.3	84.0	84.7	85.3	83.9	83.8
Switzerland	70.1	69.0	67.3	67.9	66.9	65.8	64.9
Taiwan							
Thailand							
Tunisia							
Turkey							
Turkmenistan							
Ukraine							
United Arab Emirates							
United Kingdom	94.6	93.1	91.4	91.1	90.0	88.4	87.6
USA	79.3	88.1	87.4	92.8	96.7	86.7	86.6
Venezuela							
Vietnam							

Source: Euromonitor International from OECD/WHO/national statistics

Deaths from motor traffic accidents 1998-2004

Table: 2.47

number per 100,000 inhabitants

	1998	1999	2000	2001	2002	2003	2004
Algeria							
Argentina	31.5	32.4	33.6	33.7	31.9	30.9	30.0
Australia	10.1	10.1	10.7	11.2	11.9	11.0	11.2
Austria	10.7	12.3	11.2	10.8	11.4	10.4	10.1
Azerbaijan							
Belarus	22.7	23.8	25.0	25.3	26.5	26.7	27.2
Belgium							
Bolivia							
Brazil							
Bulgaria							
Canada	9.4						
Chile							
China	7.8	8.4	9.0	9.7	10.4	9.2	9.3
Colombia							
Croatia	14.9	15.0	16.4	17.9	18.7	18.9	20.0
Czech Republic	8.1	14.1	14.1	15.1	20.2	20.6	23.2
Denmark	9.4	8.9	8.9	9.1	9.2	9.4	9.7
Ecuador							
Egypt							
Estonia							
Finland	8.6	8.5	7.5	7.3	7.2	7.1	7.0
France	13.8	13.5	13.6	13.7	13.3	13.4	13.4
Germany	9.5	9.8	9.1	9.6	10.3	9.9	10.3
Greece	20.3	19.7	18.7	18.8	18.0	17.2	16.7
Hong Kong, China	222.0	217.0	171.0	152.3	144.4	135.2	125.5
Hungary	15.4	14.1	13.3	13.6	13.2	13.2	13.1
India							
Indonesia							
Ireland	11.5	10.4	10.2	9.4	8.8	9.7	9.5
Israel							
Italy	13.0	12.6	13.0	12.9	12.8	12.4	12.1
Japan	9.2	8.8	8.4	8.0	7.6	8.4	8.4
Jordan							
Kazakhstan							
Kuwait							
Latvia	26.0	25.0	25.0	25.0	24.5	25.8	26.2
Lithuania							
Malaysia	14.9	15.2	15.4	15.5	15.6	14.8	14.5
Mexico							
Morocco							
Netherlands	6.8	7.2	6.7	6.7	6.7	6.7	6.8
New Zealand	14.5	14.4	14.3	14.1	14.0	13.8	13.6
Nigeria							
Norway	8.7	7.8	8.8	8.5	8.5	8.3	8.2
Pakistan							
Peru							
Philippines							
Poland	16.9	17.5	16.5	16.6	16.4	16.8	16.8
Portugal	18.7	15.6	13.0	12.8	10.1	7.3	6.1
Romania							
Russia							
Saudi Arabia							
Singapore	5.9	5.4	5.5	4.5	4.6	4.3	4.0
Slovakia	19.1	15.2	14.4	13.9	11.5	9.2	7.8
Slovenia	17.2	17.9	16.8	16.9	15.8	15.6	15.1
South Africa							
South Korea	34.1	33.0	32.6	32.9	33.2	32.2	31.9
Spain	14.8	14.7	15.3	15.4	15.7	15.2	15.2
Sweden	5.6	5.6	5.6	5.7	5.7	5.6	5.6
Switzerland							
Taiwan	11.6	11.0	10.4	9.7	9.7	9.6	9.4
Thailand							
Tunisia							
Turkey							
Turkmenistan							
Ukraine							
United Arab Emirates							
United Kingdom	5.8	5.8	5.6	5.5	5.4	5.3	5.2
USA	15.5	16.2	15.9	16.3	16.5	15.7	15.6
Venezuela							
Vietnam							

Source: Euromonitor International from OECD/WHO/national statistics

Deaths from injury and poisoning 1998-2004

Table: 2.48

number per 100,000 inhabitants

	1998	1999	2000	2001	2002	2003	2004
Algeria							
Argentina							
Australia	41.0	40.9	42.5	40.6	41.3	40.1	39.5
Austria	43.9	45.8	46.0	42.9	42.6	40.8	39.5
Azerbaijan							
Belarus	108.2	117.0	126.5	126.8	136.7	131.9	132.7
Belgium							
Bolivia							
Brazil							
Bulgaria							
Canada							
Chile							
China	62.1	62.3	58.3	63.3	62.3	60.3	60.7
Colombia							
Croatia			66.3				
Czech Republic	59.5	58.6	59.2	59.0	58.7	58.5	58.9
Denmark	48.2	47.9	46.2	46.6	50.2	51.7	53.4
Ecuador							
Egypt							
Estonia	162.2	156.1	150.0	144.2	144.8	145.4	144.6
Finland	68.6	67.0	65.4	63.9	63.7	62.7	62.4
France	57.6	56.7	56.8	56.8	55.0	55.4	54.6
Germany	34.0	33.9	31.6	30.1	28.8	27.4	26.1
Greece	38.6	38.2	38.2	38.0	37.8	38.1	38.4
Hong Kong, China	28.7	30.5	30.4	31.3	31.3	31.5	31.9
Hungary	86.3	77.5	70.4	74.9	71.7	73.6	75.1
India							
Indonesia							
Ireland	41.3	40.1	41.3	40.9	40.9	39.6	39.2
Israel							
Italy	35.6	34.3	34.0	32.9	32.0	33.6	33.5
Japan	46.6	46.2	48.6	49.2	50.2	48.1	47.5
Jordan							
Kazakhstan	138.7	126.0	140.7	137.1	138.1	138.0	138.3
Kuwait							
Latvia	73.9	71.0					
Lithuania							
Malaysia							
Mexico							
Morocco	12.2	11.4	11.4	11.2	11.2	11.0	10.9
Netherlands	26.5	27.6	26.2	26.5	26.3	26.1	26.1
New Zealand	43.5	42.3	41.9	40.5	39.2	38.6	37.9
Nigeria							
Norway	40.8	42.4	43.1	44.3	45.4	42.5	42.0
Pakistan							
Peru							
Philippines							
Poland	68.0	65.8	61.3	61.7	58.3	55.0	52.5
Portugal	47.0	44.3	40.7	40.6	37.7	34.6	32.5
Romania	72.1	64.3	64.3	63.9	63.1	62.5	61.5
Russia							
Saudi Arabia							
Singapore							
Slovakia	59.5	54.5	54.3	53.4	50.9	48.3	46.2
Slovenia			16.0	16.0	16.0	16.1	16.2
South Africa							
South Korea	76.4	73.7	71.0	68.3	65.6	66.8	65.9
Spain	36.6	35.1	35.3	34.4	33.7	35.0	34.9
Sweden	36.8	35.5	35.7	35.0	34.4	35.5	35.3
Switzerland	40.0	38.7	37.8	36.7	35.6	37.4	37.2
Taiwan							
Thailand							
Tunisia							
Turkey							
Turkmenistan							
Ukraine							
United Arab Emirates							
United Kingdom	27.4	27.7	27.5	27.7	27.7	27.2	27.1
USA	51.0	51.4	50.7	50.7	50.5	49.6	48.8
Venezuela							
Vietnam							

Source: Euromonitor International from OECD/WHO/national statistics

Deaths from suicide and self-inflicted injury 1998-2004

Table: 2.49

number per 100,000 inhabitants

	1998	1999	2000	2001	2002	2003	2004
Algeria							
Argentina							
Australia	13.4	12.5	13.1	13.1	13.0	12.7	12.6
Austria	16.5	16.3	16.5	15.4	16.2	15.9	15.7
Azerbaijan	31.9	27.9	26.4	24.3	23.3	21.5	19.9
Belarus	35.0	35.3	35.6	35.9	36.2	35.8	35.7
Belgium							
Bolivia	6.6	6.6	6.7	6.9	6.7	6.9	6.9
Brazil							
Bulgaria							
Canada							
Chile	6.2	6.4	6.6	6.7	6.7	6.8	6.8
China	14.1	14.3	11.3	15.3	14.6	13.6	14.6
Colombia							
Croatia	22.9	21.7	21.1	20.7	20.6	19.7	19.4
Czech Republic	13.7	13.6	13.8	13.8	13.7	13.8	13.8
Denmark	12.1	11.9	10.9	10.1	9.9	9.6	9.1
Ecuador							
Egypt							
Estonia							
Finland	21.5	21.2	20.4	19.3	19.5	18.8	18.4
France	15.4	15.0	14.9	14.7	14.3	14.3	14.0
Germany	11.7	11.2	10.9	10.3	9.8	9.1	8.6
Greece	3.2	3.1	3.3	3.2	3.3	3.2	3.2
Hong Kong, China							
Hungary	27.3	27.7	26.5	24.3	23.8	22.8	21.8
India	10.2	10.7	10.9	11.3	11.6	11.9	12.4
Indonesia							
Ireland	13.2	11.1	12.1	11.0	10.5	11.2	11.0
Israel							
Italy	6.3	5.7	5.5	5.4	5.0	4.6	4.3
Japan	20.4	20.0	22.9	23.6	24.9	22.4	22.1
Jordan	0.1	0.1	0.1	0.1	0.1	0.1	0.1
Kazakhstan	28.7	26.8	29.9	29.7	30.3	29.5	29.6
Kuwait							
Latvia	34.3	34.8	35.3	35.8	36.3	36.2	36.9
Lithuania							
Malaysia	1.6	2.1	2.3	2.4	2.4	2.3	2.3
Mexico							
Morocco							
Netherlands	8.5	8.5	8.2	8.2	8.0	8.1	8.1
New Zealand	15.2	15.5	15.8	16.1	16.5	17.0	17.5
Nigeria							
Norway	11.8	12.7	13.0	13.7	14.3	12.9	12.8
Pakistan							
Peru							
Philippines							
Poland	13.1	13.7	13.8	14.6	14.2	13.6	13.6
Portugal	4.7	4.5	4.2	4.2	4.0	3.9	3.8
Romania							
Russia							
Saudi Arabia							
Singapore	9.5	7.8	8.7	7.5	7.7	7.1	6.6
Slovakia	11.5	11.9	12.4	12.7	13.1	12.8	13.0
Slovenia	30.8	29.8	29.8	30.3	29.8	29.3	29.3
South Africa							
South Korea	14.5	14.9	15.3	15.7	16.1	15.4	15.6
Spain	6.9	6.7	6.6	6.4	6.2	6.5	6.4
Sweden	11.9	12.0	11.8	11.8	11.7	11.8	11.9
Switzerland	16.5	15.4	14.9	14.0	13.2	14.7	14.6
Taiwan	10.0	10.4	10.4	10.5	10.6	10.4	10.4
Thailand							
Tunisia							
Turkey							
Turkmenistan							
Ukraine							
United Arab Emirates							
United Kingdom	6.9	6.9	7.1	7.2	7.3	7.0	7.0
USA	10.7	10.1	9.9	9.5	9.1	9.6	9.5
Venezuela	0.2	0.3	0.2	0.2	0.2	0.2	0.2
Vietnam							

Source: Euromonitor International from OECD/WHO/national statistics

■ Smoking

Smoking prevalence in population aged 15+ 1998-2004

Table: 2.50

% of population aged 15+

	1998	1999	2000	2001	2002	2003	2004
Algeria	33.5	34.2	35.1	35.9	36.7	38.2	39.3
Argentina	37.1	38.6	40.4	42.1	43.7	44.3	45.0
Australia	23.1	22.8	22.5	21.8	21.9	21.1	21.3
Austria	29.3	28.9	29.0	28.7	28.7	28.4	28.3
Azerbaijan	22.9	22.8	22.6	22.5	22.4	22.3	22.2
Belarus	26.6	26.3	26.9	26.3	26.6	28.6	28.2
Belgium	27.0	29.0	30.0	28.0	28.0	28.7	28.4
Bolivia	33.6	33.4	33.1	32.7	32.4	32.2	32.2
Brazil	33.7	33.5	33.3	33.5	33.2	33.1	32.9
Bulgaria	36.5	37.1	37.4	37.5	38.2	38.5	38.9
Canada	23.2	23.8	20.9	21.3	20.8	20.5	20.5
Chile	25.6	26.1	26.6	26.3	26.8	26.4	25.9
China	41.0	41.1	41.6	42.1	42.5	42.7	43.0
Colombia	22.3	22.8	23.2	23.2	23.2	22.8	23.3
Croatia	30.9	30.8	30.3	30.1	30.2	30.4	30.1
Czech Republic	25.1	23.5	29.1	23.3	24.1	22.6	22.1
Denmark	33.0	31.0	30.5	29.5	28.0	30.4	30.2
Ecuador	31.6	31.5	31.5	31.4	31.4	31.1	31.1
Egypt	36.5	36.6	37.0	37.2	37.2	37.6	37.7
Estonia	29.4	29.4	29.4	29.0	28.9	28.7	28.3
Finland	25.0	23.0	23.0	24.0	23.4	23.4	23.6
France	26.7	26.4	27.0	25.8	25.4	25.7	25.4
Germany	31.4	23.5	34.5	32.4	34.6	34.8	32.5
Greece	38.2	37.9	37.6	37.4	37.1	36.8	36.6
Hong Kong, China	19.1	18.6	17.9	18.1	17.6	17.8	18.2
Hungary	32.5	32.5	30.6	32.1	32.6	32.6	32.3
India	35.9	36.0	36.2	36.1	37.2	37.3	38.0
Indonesia	39.0	38.9	38.2	38.4	37.9	38.0	37.7
Ireland	31.0	31.5	31.8	32.4	33.1	33.4	33.6
Israel	28.0	27.6	27.0	36.3	36.4	36.9	37.2
Italy	24.7	24.7	24.4	24.1	23.5	22.4	22.6
Japan	35.3	34.3	34.3	33.6	33.4	33.0	32.7
Jordan	30.1	30.3	30.5	30.8	31.4	31.9	32.4
Kazakhstan	31.1	31.7	28.0	23.9	21.7	20.6	20.4
Kuwait	30.9	30.6	30.1	29.7	29.2	29.2	28.8
Latvia	37.3	29.2	36.9	36.2	35.4	34.7	33.9
Lithuania	28.3	32.5	32.0	33.5	33.5	33.1	33.0
Malaysia	34.9	34.6	33.8	34.2	34.4	34.8	34.7
Mexico	27.1	28.6	29.1	29.5	29.7	30.0	30.2
Morocco	28.1	28.2	28.6	28.8	28.8	29.1	29.2
Netherlands	34.6	33.8	32.4	34.5	33.5	32.9	32.8
New Zealand	26.0	25.0	26.0	25.0	23.9	23.7	22.9
Nigeria	15.2	15.5	14.8	14.9	14.6	14.9	14.4
Norway	32.9	32.3	31.2	29.6	29.6	31.9	31.9
Pakistan	24.4	24.8	25.0	25.7	26.2	27.0	27.6
Peru	33.7	31.5	31.7	32.2	33.1	33.3	33.3
Philippines	35.2	35.2	35.7	35.4	35.7	35.8	35.9
Poland	29.8	29.5	32.0	32.0	32.0	28.7	28.4
Portugal	20.7	20.5	21.1	20.9	21.1	22.2	22.7
Romania			20.8				
Russia	36.0	42.5	42.1	41.7	41.5	41.2	41.5
Saudi Arabia	26.4	25.7	27.3	27.3	27.7	28.0	28.4
Singapore	25.8	25.8	26.0	26.0	26.1	26.3	25.9
Slovakia	29.0	41.3	42.8	45.8	47.4	48.3	49.6
Slovenia	25.3	24.5	23.9	23.7	23.4	23.2	23.1
South Africa	34.6	34.8	34.9	35.5	35.8	36.2	36.5
South Korea	35.2	35.7	35.3	35.4	35.1	34.9	34.7
Spain	33.4	33.7	34.2	34.4	34.4	34.6	34.5
Sweden	19.1	19.3	18.9	18.9	17.8	18.4	18.0
Switzerland	30.2	30.8	30.5	30.2	29.0	29.8	29.6
Taiwan	35.2	35.1	34.8	34.7	34.4	34.1	33.7
Thailand	31.3	31.1	31.1	31.2	31.4	30.8	30.8
Tunisia	37.4	36.9	36.9	36.7	36.4	36.2	36.0
Turkey	48.8	49.3	50.1	50.4	51.1	51.8	52.5
Turkmenistan	25.7	26.3	26.1	26.5	27.6	27.0	27.5
Ukraine	37.5	37.1	34.0	33.8	33.6	33.5	33.4
United Arab Emirates	26.2	26.0	25.7	25.9	25.1	25.4	25.6
United Kingdom	27.0	27.0	27.0	27.0	26.6	25.4	24.8
USA	20.3	19.9	19.1	19.0	18.6	18.1	17.7
Venezuela	35.1	36.6	37.6	37.9	38.9	39.7	40.6
Vietnam	38.8	39.0	39.7	39.9	40.1	40.5	41.5

Source: WHO/OECD/Euromonitor International

Smoking prevalence in male population aged 15+ 1998-2004

Table: 2.51

% of male population aged 15+

	1998	1999	2000	2001	2002	2003	2004
Algeria	43.8	44.5	44.7	45.1	45.8	45.7	45.6
Argentina	45.7	46.8	47.9	48.1	48.2	48.4	48.5
Australia	25.4	24.9	24.0	24.0	23.7	22.8	22.4
Austria	34.9	34.3	34.1	33.8	33.0	32.5	32.0
Azerbaijan	30.5	30.2	29.9	29.6	29.6	29.5	29.3
Belarus	54.9	53.7	54.0	53.3	53.0	52.1	51.2
Belgium	30.0	31.0	36.0	34.0	32.9	32.8	32.3
Bolivia	42.7	42.3	41.6	41.2	40.8	40.5	40.0
Brazil	37.9	37.7	37.9	37.6	37.4	37.1	36.8
Bulgaria	49.9	50.4	50.5	51.4	51.7	52.5	52.9
Canada	25.4	22.5	21.2	22.0	20.9	21.0	20.9
Chile	26.0	24.2	24.7	23.9	23.3	23.5	22.9
China	64.2	65.3	66.1	66.9	66.8	67.3	67.3
Colombia	24.1	24.5	25.2	25.6	26.3	26.8	27.4
Croatia	29.6	28.4	34.1	27.2	26.7	26.8	26.9
Czech Republic	31.1	30.1	36.2	26.4	30.9	29.2	28.9
Denmark	34.0	35.0	32.0	33.5	30.5	29.7	28.8
Ecuador	45.5	45.4	45.2	45.3	44.8	44.6	44.5
Egypt	56.5	56.9	56.9	56.4	56.8	56.5	56.6
Estonia	42.3	43.4	44.1	44.8	45.0	45.8	46.3
Finland	30.0	27.0	27.0	29.0	27.5	26.5	26.2
France	31.9	31.4	33.0	33.0	31.7	33.1	33.6
Germany	38.6	30.9	28.2	27.6	27.9	27.6	27.5
Greece	47.9	47.5	46.8	45.5	45.0	44.7	44.7
Hong Kong, China	27.1	26.6	25.6	25.9	25.4	25.4	25.4
Hungary	40.2	44.0	38.2	38.3	37.3	37.7	36.8
India	57.2	57.0	56.3	57.7	57.4	58.1	58.8
Indonesia	63.0	61.4	60.0	58.3	57.8	57.8	57.5
Ireland	32.0	32.2	32.5	33.2	33.6	33.8	34.3
Israel	33.0	31.0	30.0	40.5	40.6	40.6	40.5
Italy	32.6	32.8	31.9	31.6	29.8	29.4	29.5
Japan	55.2	54.0	53.5	52.0	52.0	51.0	50.4
Jordan	44.6	44.8	45.4	46.4	47.3	48.2	49.1
Kazakhstan	56.8	57.9	58.9	46.5	44.3	42.7	41.2
Kuwait	38.2	38.6	37.8	36.8	36.7	35.9	35.5
Latvia	58.0	49.1	57.5	56.8	56.1	56.4	55.7
Lithuania	48.5	52.0	51.5	50.6	50.0	49.5	49.1
Malaysia	44.2	42.7	43.4	45.7	46.3	48.0	49.5
Mexico	41.5	42.0	42.4	42.4	42.7	42.7	43.0
Morocco	34.7	35.5	35.9	35.9	36.4	36.5	36.8
Netherlands	38.5	36.0	35.9	38.9	37.9	34.9	34.0
New Zealand	26.0	26.0	25.0	25.1	24.8	24.8	24.7
Nigeria	15.4	15.5	15.2	15.4	16.0	17.0	16.9
Norway	33.5	32.4	31.3	29.5	29.5	30.9	30.6
Pakistan	34.6	34.7	36.0	36.6	38.0	38.8	39.0
Peru	47.3	48.9	48.3	50.6	50.0	49.9	49.8
Philippines	57.6	58.3	57.2	57.4	57.3	57.3	57.4
Poland	39.0	39.5	40.0	40.0	40.0	36.9	36.8
Portugal	32.9	32.8	32.5	32.5	32.2	31.8	31.6
Romania			32.3				
Russia	63.2	62.1	61.5	61.3	60.9	60.8	60.3
Saudi Arabia	34.8	35.7	35.6	36.3	36.6	37.2	37.7
Singapore	28.9	28.9	26.9	28.5	28.4	29.5	30.1
Slovakia	44.1	53.0	53.0	52.7	53.6	53.8	54.0
Slovenia	31.9	30.0	29.0	28.0	27.5	27.3	27.0
South Africa	53.9	54.6	55.5	56.1	56.2	57.0	56.7
South Korea	64.1	65.1	64.5	64.9	64.4	64.1	64.0
Spain	42.1	42.1	42.1	42.1	42.1	42.0	42.0
Sweden	17.0	19.2	16.8	17.9	16.3	14.9	14.4
Switzerland	35.6	35.3	34.7	34.4	34.0	33.6	33.3
Taiwan	55.8	55.0	54.5	53.9	53.6	53.1	52.7
Thailand	48.3	48.1	47.9	48.1	46.8	46.5	46.0
Tunisia	61.6	62.1	62.3	62.4	61.8	61.9	61.7
Turkey	67.9	67.9	68.2	68.7	68.4	68.4	68.3
Turkmenistan	37.5	40.0	39.8	40.0	40.0	40.5	40.6
Ukraine	55.2	57.7	58.0	61.5	61.9	61.2	61.4
United Arab Emirates	25.0	25.5	26.2	26.3	25.9	26.1	26.5
United Kingdom	28.0	28.5	29.0	28.0	25.4	25.1	24.6
USA	21.6	20.6	21.0	20.5	20.2	19.7	19.4
Venezuela	45.2	45.9	46.5	47.2	48.3	49.0	49.3
Vietnam	69.9	69.5	69.7	69.6	69.2	69.2	68.4

Source: WHO/OECD/Euromonitor International

Smoking prevalence in female population aged 15+ 1998-2004

Table: 2.52

% of female population aged 15+

	1998	1999	2000	2001	2002	2003	2004
Algeria	23.1	23.8	25.5	26.5	27.5	30.6	32.9
Argentina	29.1	31.2	33.5	36.7	39.5	40.6	41.8
Australia	20.8	20.8	21.1	19.6	20.2	19.4	20.2
Austria	24.2	23.9	23.8	24.1	24.8	24.6	24.9
Azerbaijan	15.9	16.1	16.1	16.0	15.8	15.8	15.7
Belarus	4.6	4.8	6.7	6.3	6.3	8.6	8.6
Belgium	23.0	26.0	26.0	22.0	23.4	24.9	24.7
Bolivia	24.8	24.9	24.9	24.6	24.4	24.2	24.7
Brazil	29.8	29.4	28.9	29.6	29.3	29.3	29.2
Bulgaria	23.9	24.6	25.2	24.6	25.7	25.4	25.9
Canada	21.2	25.1	20.6	20.6	20.8	19.9	20.1
Chile	25.3	28.0	28.3	28.6	30.1	29.1	28.8
China	17.6	16.6	16.6	16.8	18.0	17.8	18.3
Colombia	20.6	21.2	21.3	20.9	20.3	19.1	19.4
Croatia	32.0	33.0	26.6	32.7	33.3	33.7	32.9
Czech Republic	19.6	17.3	22.0	20.4	18.1	16.5	15.8
Denmark	31.0	27.0	29.0	25.5	26.0	31.1	31.5
Ecuador	17.8	17.7	17.9	17.5	18.1	17.6	17.8
Egypt	16.1	15.7	16.3	17.3	16.8	17.8	17.7
Estonia	19.6	19.7	19.9	19.1	17.9	22.9	22.1
Finland	20.0	20.0	20.0	20.0	19.9	20.6	21.2
France	21.9	21.9	21.0	19.2	19.6	18.8	17.8
Germany	22.1	16.5	19.5	18.0	16.8	17.2	16.6
Greece	27.6	28.4	29.0	29.0	28.5	28.3	28.1
Hong Kong, China	11.4	10.9	10.7	10.7	10.5	10.9	11.7
Hungary	25.7	21.0	21.0	23.0	28.4	28.0	28.3
India	13.2	13.8	14.9	13.3	15.8	15.3	15.9
Indonesia	15.2	16.7	16.7	18.7	18.3	18.5	18.2
Ireland	31.0	31.4	31.7	31.9	32.5	327.0	33.6
Israel	25.0	24.4	24.0	32.3	32.3	33.5	34.1
Italy	17.5	17.3	17.4	17.1	17.6	16.0	16.2
Japan	16.5	15.7	16.2	16.3	15.8	16.1	16.1
Jordan	13.9	14.2	13.8	13.4	13.7	13.7	13.9
Kazakhstan	8.0	8.3	8.6	7.6	6.8	6.4	5.7
Kuwait	18.0	16.0	16.3	17.3	16.3	17.8	17.5
Latvia	20.4	13.0	20.0	19.3	18.4	16.9	16.0
Lithuania	12.5	16.1	15.8	19.1	19.5	19.3	19.5
Malaysia	25.3	26.2	24.0	22.4	22.2	21.2	19.5
Mexico	13.8	16.2	16.8	17.5	17.6	18.1	18.3
Morocco	21.6	21.0	21.4	21.9	21.4	21.8	21.7
Netherlands	30.7	31.7	29.2	30.2	29.2	31.0	31.6
New Zealand	26.0	24.1	26.9	24.9	23.2	22.6	21.2
Nigeria	15.0	15.5	14.4	14.4	13.2	12.8	11.9
Norway	32.3	32.2	31.1	29.7	29.7	32.8	33.2
Pakistan	13.7	14.5	13.5	14.4	13.9	14.7	15.8
Peru	20.2	14.1	15.1	13.8	16.2	16.8	16.8
Philippines	12.9	12.2	14.3	13.5	14.1	14.2	14.4
Poland	21.3	20.3	25.0	25.0	25.0	21.1	20.7
Portugal	9.6	9.5	10.8	10.4	11.1	13.5	14.5
Romania			10.1				
Russia	9.7	25.8	25.7	25.1	25.2	24.6	25.6
Saudi Arabia	15.4	12.6	16.4	15.6	16.2	16.2	16.5
Singapore	22.8	22.8	25.1	23.6	24.0	23.1	21.8
Slovakia	14.7	30.5	33.4	39.5	41.6	43.3	45.5
Slovenia	20.3	20.3	20.2	20.1	20.1	20.0	19.9
South Africa	17.2	17.0	16.5	17.3	17.8	18.0	18.9
South Korea	6.9	6.9	6.7	6.5	6.5	6.2	5.9
Spain	25.6	26.4	26.8	27.2	27.4	27.7	27.9
Sweden	21.1	19.4	21.0	19.9	19.3	21.7	21.5
Switzerland	25.1	26.6	26.6	26.3	25.0	26.3	26.1
Taiwan	13.8	14.4	14.4	15.0	14.5	14.6	14.2
Thailand	14.9	14.9	15.1	15.0	16.7	15.9	16.3
Tunisia	13.2	11.8	11.5	11.1	11.0	10.5	10.3
Turkey	29.5	30.4	31.8	31.9	33.6	35.0	36.5
Turkmenistan	14.4	13.3	13.0	13.6	15.8	14.1	15.0
Ukraine	22.8	19.9	14.0	14.0	13.8	13.7	13.8
United Arab Emirates	29.5	27.2	24.3	24.7	22.8	23.7	23.4
United Kingdom	26.0	25.6	25.0	26.0	27.7	25.7	25.0
USA	19.1	19.2	17.3	17.6	17.2	16.7	16.1
Venezuela	25.0	27.3	28.7	28.6	29.5	30.4	31.9
Vietnam	8.5	9.4	10.5	10.8	11.7	12.5	15.2

Source: WHO/OECD/Euromonitor International

■ **Nutrition and Obesity**

Obese population (BMI 30kg/sq m or more) 1998-2004

Table: 2.53

% of population aged 15+

	1998	1999	2000	2001	2002	2003	2004
Algeria	4.1	4.0	4.0	4.0	4.2	4.3	4.3
Argentina	10.7	11.2	11.2	11.3	11.5	11.6	11.7
Australia	20.4	20.8	21.5	21.6	22.0	22.9	23.1
Austria	9.1	9.1	10.1	12.6	14.5	16.3	17.8
Azerbaijan	7.6	7.5	7.6	7.7	7.7	7.7	7.7
Belarus	6.8	6.7	6.7	6.7	6.7	6.5	6.5
Belgium	11.3	11.6	11.7	12.6	13.5	13.9	14.5
Bolivia	8.3	8.4	8.6	8.6	8.6	8.7	8.7
Brazil	10.7	11.0	11.1	11.2	11.3	11.4	11.5
Bulgaria	13.3	13.6	13.9	13.9	14.1	14.1	14.1
Canada	14.6	14.6	14.8	14.9	15.2	15.7	16.0
Chile	16.1	17.8	18.1	18.4	18.9	19.1	19.5
China	4.0	4.0	4.1	4.2	4.3	4.4	4.5
Colombia	19.7	21.0	21.0	21.0	21.0	21.3	21.4
Croatia	7.8	8.0	8.3	9.0	9.2	9.6	10.0
Czech Republic	13.3	14.2	14.4	14.6	14.8	15.0	15.2
Denmark	9.2	9.8	9.5	10.6	12.0	12.4	13.0
Ecuador	13.2	13.6	13.6	13.8	14.0	14.2	14.4
Egypt	5.6	5.6	5.6	5.7	5.7	5.8	5.9
Estonia	15.0	15.5	15.9	16.3	16.8	17.2	17.6
Finland	9.5	10.1	11.2	11.4	12.8	13.5	13.9
France	8.6	9.0	9.0	10.0	12.6	14.5	15.2
Germany	14.8	15.6	16.8	17.9	19.0	20.1	20.5
Greece	8.0	8.5	9.2	10.1	10.3	11.0	11.4
Hong Kong, China	5.2	5.2	5.2	5.2	5.2	5.2	5.2
Hungary	19.0	19.1	19.3	19.4	19.5	19.6	19.7
India	5.1	5.2	5.3	5.4	5.3	5.4	5.4
Indonesia	5.7	5.8	5.8	5.8	5.7	5.7	5.7
Ireland	9.6	10.0	10.2	10.3	10.4	10.6	10.7
Israel	17.8	17.9	17.8	17.8	17.8	18.0	18.1
Italy	8.4	8.5	8.6	9.0	9.2	9.3	9.6
Japan	2.1	2.2	2.1	2.4	2.4	2.6	2.7
Jordan	14.5	14.4	14.6	14.6	14.7	14.7	14.7
Kazakhstan	5.6	5.8	5.3	5.4	5.5	5.6	5.7
Kuwait	33.8	35.3	35.5	36.2	36.5	37.1	37.6
Latvia	9.0	9.3	10.0	11.5	13.0	13.5	13.8
Lithuania	8.8	9.6	10.8	12.9	14.0	14.5	14.9
Malaysia	6.2	6.5	6.5	6.5	6.5	6.7	6.7
Mexico	22.6	20.1	20.2	20.5	20.0	20.0	19.8
Morocco	4.1	4.0	4.0	4.0	4.1	4.1	4.1
Netherlands	8.4	9.0	9.1	10.8	11.0	11.3	12.5
New Zealand	16.1	16.3	16.3	16.4	16.5	16.6	16.7
Nigeria	18.7	18.5	18.8	19.7	19.9	20.6	21.1
Norway	8.0	8.7	9.2	10.3	11.5	11.9	12.2
Pakistan	5.6	5.6	5.7	5.8	5.7	5.8	5.8
Peru	10.1	8.1	8.1	8.2	9.3	9.7	10.2
Philippines	5.1	4.0	3.9	4.3	5.5	5.7	5.8
Poland	11.5	12.0	12.2	12.5	12.7	13.0	13.3
Portugal	14.0	14.2	14.4	14.8	15.4	15.9	16.2
Romania	22.3	21.7	21.0	20.4	20.0	20.0	19.7
Russia	18.1	18.2	18.0	18.0	17.5	17.5	17.5
Saudi Arabia	26.3	26.4	26.7	27.0	27.4	27.7	28.0
Singapore	6.3	6.5	6.5	6.6	6.7	6.7	6.7
Slovakia	15.8	16.8	16.5	16.8	17.0	17.0	17.2
Slovenia	10.8	10.8	10.9	11.0	11.1	11.1	11.2
South Africa	19.3	20.1	20.8	21.5	22.1	23.0	25.4
South Korea	2.2	2.5	2.4	2.5	2.5	2.5	2.5
Spain	11.7	11.9	12.0	12.0	12.0	12.2	12.4
Sweden	9.8	10.0	10.8	10.9	11.0	11.1	11.1
Switzerland	6.1	5.4	5.4	5.5	5.5	5.6	5.6
Taiwan	6.1	6.1	6.2	6.0	5.9	5.8	5.7
Thailand	3.6	3.7	3.8	3.8	3.6	3.6	3.7
Tunisia	5.5	5.0	5.1	5.2	5.0	5.0	4.9
Turkey	13.1	12.9	12.9	12.9	13.0	13.0	13.1
Turkmenistan	4.3	4.2	4.2	4.3	4.2	4.3	4.3
Ukraine	12.2	12.3	12.3	12.4	12.5	12.7	12.7
United Arab Emirates	26.3	26.4	26.7	26.7	26.8	26.8	26.8
United Kingdom	19.3	19.9	20.3	22.3	23.0	24.5	25.9
USA	26.2	27.1	27.6	28.3	30.9	32.3	33.7
Venezuela	13.3	13.0	12.9	12.7	12.5	12.3	12.1
Vietnam	4.1	4.2	4.2	4.2	4.3	4.2	4.3

Source: *OECD/International Obesity Taskforce/Euromonitor International*

Average supply of calories per day 1998-2004

Table: 2.54

calories per capita/% change

	1998	1999	2000	2001	2002	2003	2004	% change 1998-2004
Algeria	2,933.8	2,976.5	2,943.7	3,006.1	3,021.5	3,035.5	3,057.4	4.21
Argentina	3,178.0	3,177.7	3,179.9	3,052.6	2,992.1	2,934.2	3,066.2	-3.52
Australia	3,052.3	3,063.6	3,087.5	3,129.3	3,053.6	3,013.9	3,181.8	4.24
Austria	3,671.3	3,732.9	3,760.6	3,779.5	3,673.3	3,612.3	3,557.7	-3.09
Azerbaijan	2,159.5	2,277.6	2,392.7	2,476.3	2,574.8	2,678.5	2,784.4	28.94
Belarus	3,248.8	3,086.6	2,988.1	3,031.1	3,000.3	2,972.3	2,955.5	-9.03
Belgium	3,629.0	3,643.0	3,589.1	3,576.9	3,583.8	3,577.7	3,571.1	-1.60
Bolivia	2,171.3	2,209.4	2,236.8	2,277.1	2,235.2	2,218.7	2,208.4	1.71
Brazil	2,953.3	2,992.8	2,981.2	2,999.9	3,049.5	3,085.1	3,062.3	3.69
Bulgaria	2,787.4	2,823.3	2,802.7	2,751.0	2,847.9	2,852.6	2,875.6	3.16
Canada	3,454.4	3,513.0	3,546.9	3,545.2	3,589.3	3,625.2	3,656.6	5.85
Chile	2,796.5	2,800.1	2,824.8	2,847.5	2,863.2	2,880.4	2,898.6	3.65
China	2,977.4	2,960.9	2,969.1	2,953.3	2,951.0	2,947.6	2,941.5	-1.21
Colombia	2,533.9	2,556.8	2,574.8	2,576.6	2,584.6	2,593.7	2,600.6	2.63
Croatia	2,610.7	2,688.3	2,705.8	2,807.0	2,799.0	2,813.6	2,839.4	8.76
Czech Republic	3,254.1	3,118.3	3,064.8	3,119.1	3,171.3	3,207.4	3,249.7	-0.14
Denmark	3,383.8	3,387.2	3,389.8	3,397.2	3,439.3	3,469.6	3,500.0	3.43
Ecuador	2,687.1	2,704.4	2,702.1	2,755.2	2,754.0	2,762.9	2,777.0	3.35
Egypt	3,336.0	3,348.6	3,336.0	3,349.0	3,338.0	3,331.9	3,328.8	-0.22
Estonia	2,917.2	3,060.6	2,985.3	2,992.9	3,002.2	3,096.1	3,105.1	6.44
Finland	3,143.4	3,125.2	3,111.5	3,153.9	3,100.4	3,171.0	3,129.6	-0.44
France	3,591.3	3,588.8	3,600.9	3,646.4	3,653.9	3,669.0	3,689.4	2.73
Germany	3,398.1	3,391.2	3,433.0	3,492.7	3,495.6	3,515.5	3,538.7	4.14
Greece	3,626.4	3,666.6	3,647.6	3,694.5	3,721.1	3,743.6	3,735.6	3.01
Hong Kong, China	3,331.6	3,367.8	3,388.3	3,441.1	3,476.3	3,511.9	3,551.6	6.60
Hungary	3,348.5	3,344.8	3,487.2	3,441.6	3,483.2	3,528.2	3,557.2	6.23
India	2,329.2	2,438.7	2,414.8	2,385.8	2,459.0	2,499.9	2,535.5	8.86
Indonesia	2,864.1	2,895.7	2,919.7	2,911.4	2,903.9	2,902.9	2,898.5	1.20
Ireland	3,653.3	3,685.0	3,692.9	3,642.0	3,656.4	3,658.4	3,653.6	0.01
Israel	3,552.4	3,532.3	3,605.2	3,661.0	3,666.0	3,689.7	3,716.3	4.61
Italy	3,628.1	3,685.4	3,701.0	3,696.7	3,670.6	3,656.5	3,642.8	0.41
Japan	2,754.4	2,771.4	2,799.7	2,788.6	2,760.9	2,746.2	2,731.2	-0.84
Jordan	2,612.6	2,624.8	2,641.7	2,688.1	2,673.5	2,674.2	2,681.1	2.62
Kazakhstan	2,531.9	2,222.8	2,389.6	2,570.8	2,676.6	2,718.7	2,773.8	9.55
Kuwait	3,102.2	3,054.3	3,084.0	3,062.9	3,010.0	2,978.0	2,945.0	-5.07
Latvia	2,872.2	2,882.7	2,920.1	3,016.8	2,938.0	2,909.4	2,893.3	0.73
Lithuania	3,260.8	3,192.0	3,353.6	3,400.3	3,324.5	3,310.7	3,397.2	4.18
Malaysia	2,846.1	2,856.8	2,899.9	2,892.1	2,881.1	2,880.9	2,877.0	1.09
Mexico	3,119.2	3,125.8	3,160.8	3,160.1	3,144.7	3,138.8	3,130.7	0.37
Morocco	3,138.4	3,060.5	3,026.1	3,046.5	3,051.8	3,053.5	3,060.4	-2.49
Netherlands	3,207.1	3,252.9	3,374.1	3,326.1	3,362.3	3,400.0	3,424.6	6.78
New Zealand	3,172.2	3,197.3	3,228.1	3,213.8	3,219.2	3,226.0	3,229.9	1.82
Nigeria	2,773.5	2,765.3	2,704.0	2,684.4	2,725.5	2,739.0	2,751.1	-0.81
Norway	3,352.4	3,393.5	3,363.6	3,425.5	3,484.2	3,528.0	3,579.3	6.77
Pakistan	2,445.8	2,455.5	2,447.1	2,425.7	2,418.8	2,410.1	2,399.9	-1.88
Peru	2,512.7	2,510.1	2,529.1	2,550.2	2,570.9	2,591.5	2,612.6	3.98
Philippines	2,330.8	2,374.4	2,375.5	2,371.3	2,379.3	2,383.4	2,387.1	2.42
Poland	3,355.9	3,353.7	3,382.4	3,369.8	3,374.5	3,380.2	3,383.6	0.83
Portugal	3,604.9	3,735.7	3,750.9	3,754.7	3,740.9	3,733.5	3,727.4	3.40
Romania	3,291.8	3,315.2	3,361.8	3,424.4	3,454.6	3,494.3	3,538.4	7.49
Russia	2,869.7	2,898.2	2,915.9	3,011.7	3,071.8	3,131.4	3,201.0	11.54
Saudi Arabia	2,808.6	2,831.0	2,837.9	2,850.4	2,844.5	2,843.6	2,844.0	1.26
Singapore	3,101.7	3,087.5	3,161.2	3,022.0	3,008.2	2,988.7	2,951.9	-4.83
Slovakia	3,129.2	3,023.8	2,869.3	2,873.9	2,888.9	2,874.7	2,868.3	-8.34
Slovenia	2,997.4	3,135.3	3,111.1	2,932.5	3,001.4	3,015.9	3,007.3	0.33
South Africa	2,820.4	2,843.8	2,886.4	2,909.1	2,956.1	2,999.4	3,039.2	7.76
South Korea	2,935.7	3,056.7	3,063.1	3,054.5	3,058.0	3,060.5	3,060.2	4.24
Spain	3,297.7	3,337.8	3,369.9	3,349.2	3,370.6	3,385.7	3,396.8	3.01
Sweden	3,084.7	3,166.1	3,089.2	3,131.1	3,185.4	3,217.5	3,255.1	5.52
Switzerland	3,296.6	3,256.2	3,441.0	3,448.9	3,526.2	3,612.0	3,683.8	11.75
Taiwan	3,170.6	3,151.2	3,197.1	3,255.6	3,274.7	3,306.8	3,342.4	5.42
Thailand	2,453.8	2,442.8	2,435.3	2,455.8	2,467.3	2,476.1	2,488.0	1.39
Tunisia	3,333.1	3,397.9	3,303.9	3,272.2	3,237.8	3,218.8	3,185.9	-4.42
Turkey	3,375.3	3,336.7	3,371.8	3,346.5	3,357.0	3,364.3	3,368.4	-0.20
Turkmenistan	2,770.5	2,728.3	2,711.5	2,702.8	2,741.6	2,762.7	2,781.5	0.40
Ukraine	2,824.3	2,781.5	2,897.9	3,003.2	3,053.6	3,128.1	3,205.4	13.49
United Arab Emirates	3,150.3	3,173.8	3,166.9	3,205.2	3,224.7	3,241.6	3,262.2	3.55
United Kingdom	3,344.9	3,395.6	3,357.6	3,420.7	3,412.2	3,411.5	3,418.7	2.21
USA	3,664.3	3,705.3	3,813.7	3,795.6	3,774.1	3,774.0	3,768.0	2.83
Venezuela	2,312.8	2,281.9	2,348.2	2,370.4	2,336.3	2,327.8	2,320.7	0.34
Vietnam	2,472.8	2,499.8	2,534.5	2,566.2	2,566.2	2,577.5	2,589.9	4.74

Source: *UN Food and Agriculture Organisation, FAOSTAT*

Average supply of protein per day 1998-2004

Table: 2.55

grams per capita/% change

	1998	1999	2000	2001	2002	2003	2004	% change 1998-2004
Algeria	82.6	82.8	79.4	80.2	80.7	80.6	80.8	-2.18
Argentina	101.5	104.7	104.8	99.6	96.0	97.8	99.6	-1.87
Australia	100.6	102.9	103.6	104.1	103.5	103.3	103.1	2.49
Austria	108.6	110.4	109.7	111.0	109.6	108.8	108.3	-0.28
Azerbaijan	65.8	67.6	71.3	73.1	74.5	76.4	78.3	19.00
Belarus	95.5	91.9	85.5	89.1	86.1	83.8	82.5	-13.61
Belgium	102.7	104.8	88.8	89.8	88.6	85.8	84.0	-18.21
Bolivia	54.7	58.8	59.0	59.4	59.3	59.3	59.4	8.59
Brazil	78.0	80.3	80.4	80.8	82.8	83.2	82.6	5.90
Bulgaria	88.4	89.0	85.9	84.3	88.4	89.6	90.1	1.92
Canada	102.8	106.2	107.0	106.3	105.0	104.1	103.2	0.39
Chile	76.5	75.9	77.4	78.1	78.4	78.9	79.4	3.79
China	81.0	80.9	82.7	82.3	81.5	81.2	80.8	-0.25
Colombia	60.2	59.9	60.2	60.7	60.6	60.7	60.9	1.16
Croatia	65.7	69.7	70.4	74.4	74.6	75.6	77.0	17.20
Czech Republic	96.4	90.6	89.0	91.0	94.1	96.3	98.7	2.39
Denmark	105.8	107.9	107.1	110.7	109.7	109.5	109.8	3.78
Ecuador	56.4	55.9	55.8	56.4	57.9	58.0	58.2	3.19
Egypt	93.5	94.1	94.7	94.9	95.4	95.9	96.3	2.99
Estonia	91.4	94.7	90.6	93.0	93.0	93.4	94.1	2.95
Finland	102.5	100.9	100.4	102.3	101.0	100.4	100.1	-2.34
France	117.2	116.8	117.5	118.9	119.2	119.8	120.5	2.82
Germany	96.0	95.8	96.0	99.6	100.1	101.1	100.4	4.58
Greece	115.9	118.1	117.0	115.9	115.7	115.2	114.7	-1.04
Hong Kong, China	105.7	108.2	112.1	110.7	114.1	116.8	119.0	12.58
Hungary	86.0	88.2	94.0	94.8	96.8	99.4	101.7	18.26
India	55.4	57.3	56.1	55.9	57.3	58.0	58.7	5.96
Indonesia	62.0	66.2	65.9	64.2	64.2	63.9	63.4	2.26
Ireland	113.6	116.3	115.3	115.0	114.2	113.5	112.9	-0.62
Israel	116.5	115.4	122.4	126.8	128.6	131.8	129.4	11.12
Italy	111.3	114.3	115.0	113.9	113.1	112.5	112.8	1.35
Japan	91.4	91.6	92.8	91.7	91.8	91.9	91.2	-0.19
Jordan	67.9	68.4	71.3	70.1	67.4	66.0	67.2	-0.99
Kazakhstan	81.8	72.4	76.2	81.6	84.7	88.6	93.0	13.69
Kuwait	92.9	88.9	86.6	84.0	79.8	76.4	73.2	-21.21
Latvia	79.2	79.3	79.4	79.9	80.2	80.5	80.8	2.02
Lithuania	98.5	99.5	104.7	107.7	111.0	109.3	106.4	8.02
Malaysia	74.6	76.2	76.6	75.7	76.3	76.6	76.7	2.82
Mexico	86.1	87.4	89.8	91.5	90.8	91.1	91.5	6.27
Morocco	83.5	82.7	80.9	84.1	84.8	85.5	84.5	1.20
Netherlands	104.8	103.4	109.3	110.7	107.5	109.8	113.0	7.82
New Zealand	95.0	98.1	95.0	97.7	99.9	101.3	103.2	8.63
Nigeria	62.9	62.6	62.1	60.3	61.1	61.2	61.1	-2.86
Norway	104.2	104.8	104.3	106.6	107.6	108.6	109.8	5.37
Pakistan	63.2	62.6	62.4	61.8	61.9	61.8	61.7	-2.37
Peru	63.4	63.6	65.6	66.6	67.1	68.0	68.9	8.68
Philippines	54.8	54.7	55.2	56.2	56.1	56.3	56.6	3.28
Poland	99.7	99.5	99.5	98.7	99.4	99.7	99.8	0.10
Portugal	115.2	118.9	118.4	120.2	118.4	117.4	116.7	1.30
Romania	104.5	102.6	101.4	104.5	107.4	109.7	112.3	7.46
Russia	88.8	87.1	86.0	88.5	91.4	93.6	96.1	8.22
Saudi Arabia	76.0	78.2	75.6	74.6	73.8	72.7	73.7	-3.03
Singapore	107.5	106.8	106.2	103.2	102.4	101.2	99.8	-7.16
Slovakia	85.6	82.9	77.5	77.0	77.6	77.1	76.8	-10.28
Slovenia	99.1	107.4	104.7	102.5	102.6	101.9	101.1	2.02
South Africa	71.7	73.2	76.4	75.7	76.2	77.0	76.5	6.69
South Korea	80.4	88.3	86.4	88.7	89.6	90.2	91.1	13.31
Spain	111.0	109.9	110.7	110.9	111.7	112.4	113.0	1.80
Sweden	100.4	103.1	101.7	104.0	106.6	108.6	107.8	7.37
Switzerland	92.4	90.2	94.0	94.6	96.0	97.7	96.8	4.76
Taiwan	102.0	105.0	102.2	104.9	105.2	105.3	105.9	3.82
Thailand	56.9	56.4	56.1	56.7	57.0	57.3	57.7	1.41
Tunisia	90.6	91.8	90.9	90.9	87.0	88.6	90.2	-0.44
Turkey	97.2	97.0	96.4	95.3	95.4	95.7	95.8	-1.44
Turkmenistan	79.4	78.5	77.6	79.2	79.4	79.6	80.0	0.76
Ukraine	81.3	78.9	80.2	82.9	84.1	85.6	87.3	7.38
United Arab Emirates	98.4	101.7	99.6	100.2	101.0	101.3	101.7	3.35
United Kingdom	98.9	99.6	99.4	102.1	102.4	103.0	104.0	5.16
USA	112.3	114.7	114.4	114.1	114.0	113.9	113.8	1.34
Venezuela	62.6	60.8	62.1	64.5	63.8	64.0	64.4	2.88
Vietnam	58.8	59.4	60.4	61.7	62.3	63.1	64.0	8.84

Source: UN Food and Agriculture Organisation, FAOSTAT

Average supply of fat per day 1998-2004

Table: 2.56

grams per capita/% change

	1998	1999	2000	2001	2002	2003	2004	% change 1998-2004
Algeria	67.6	69.4	67.9	72.8	72.3	72.6	72.9	7.84
Argentina	119.5	111.6	108.3	102.9	106.1	106.9	107.1	-10.38
Australia	128.2	132.2	137.1	139.3	131.2	130.3	130.9	2.11
Austria	161.9	163.4	162.4	164.3	158.2	154.5	151.4	-6.49
Azerbaijan	34.8	39.0	37.0	39.2	42.0	44.1	46.5	33.62
Belarus	101.4	101.4	94.6	102.5	97.8	95.1	94.0	-7.30
Belgium	158.7	158.3	158.8	159.7	159.6	159.7	159.9	0.76
Bolivia	58.5	48.2	49.5	48.4	51.9	54.4	56.6	-3.25
Brazil	88.1	90.0	91.6	91.5	93.7	91.4	91.8	4.20
Bulgaria	93.8	93.6	92.5	92.2	96.0	98.4	100.7	7.36
Canada	148.8	147.1	147.1	145.8	146.2	146.3	146.3	-1.68
Chile	82.5	81.4	83.1	84.6	84.0	84.1	84.3	2.18
China	79.0	80.6	84.4	86.0	90.3	94.4	98.3	24.43
Colombia	64.9	65.4	65.7	65.4	65.3	65.3	65.2	0.46
Croatia	70.1	89.6	92.0	92.7	81.3	83.3	84.6	20.68
Czech Republic	115.8	112.9	111.1	115.0	118.0	120.4	123.3	6.48
Denmark	133.6	136.6	138.8	140.4	139.5	139.5	139.6	4.49
Ecuador	91.6	88.6	89.8	96.9	100.9	98.6	97.2	6.11
Egypt	56.6	57.7	58.8	59.3	59.8	60.4	61.0	7.77
Estonia	100.6	103.3	88.6	90.9	91.0	93.5	95.7	-4.87
Finland	130.3	125.3	119.6	123.5	123.0	122.3	122.5	-5.99
France	165.6	164.6	167.3	170.0	170.8	172.3	173.8	4.95
Germany	147.1	144.0	145.5	141.8	146.4	149.1	151.2	2.79
Greece	151.5	151.3	147.0	148.5	152.7	155.1	157.7	4.09
Hong Kong, China	138.3	136.9	138.1	142.4	143.4	145.1	147.2	6.44
Hungary	135.4	133.8	146.5	143.7	147.2	151.4	154.5	14.11
India	44.6	51.2	52.1	50.0	49.6	49.2	48.6	8.97
Indonesia	56.4	58.2	58.8	60.1	59.4	59.3	59.3	5.14
Ireland	138.2	137.7	137.7	130.9	132.3	132.1	131.1	-5.14
Israel	126.0	123.6	135.0	141.4	139.0	140.6	142.4	13.02
Italy	154.8	157.6	157.2	157.7	158.1	158.3	158.6	2.45
Japan	80.7	81.9	86.6	86.8	84.6	84.0	83.3	3.22
Jordan	80.1	75.6	77.6	84.2	81.5	81.3	81.9	2.25
Kazakhstan	62.3	63.6	71.6	74.1	76.0	79.3	80.4	29.05
Kuwait	104.3	108.6	111.4	112.1	109.1	107.7	106.4	2.01
Latvia	87.3	89.4	98.2	107.2	109.6	114.7	112.4	28.75
Lithuania	80.7	85.7	96.7	97.3	97.9	100.5	102.5	27.01
Malaysia	84.9	85.0	84.8	83.3	81.8	80.5	79.2	-6.71
Mexico	87.1	86.9	86.8	86.0	87.5	88.3	88.9	2.07
Morocco	61.6	61.5	60.0	59.7	58.2	56.9	55.8	-9.42
Netherlands	141.7	141.5	145.7	145.1	144.3	144.3	144.1	1.69
New Zealand	113.3	114.9	112.6	112.4	115.3	116.9	118.4	4.50
Nigeria	64.8	64.8	62.6	61.7	62.0	61.7	61.4	-5.25
Norway	137.1	137.9	137.2	141.2	145.4	148.8	145.6	6.20
Pakistan	65.2	67.8	65.0	65.4	65.1	64.5	64.1	-1.69
Peru	44.2	45.4	47.7	47.3	48.0	48.8	49.4	11.76
Philippines	43.6	49.4	48.9	46.1	48.4	49.5	50.2	15.14
Poland	112.0	112.6	111.7	111.4	112.8	113.5	114.1	1.87
Portugal	130.8	138.3	139.6	139.2	139.8	140.4	140.9	7.72
Romania	88.7	91.0	93.9	96.7	96.1	96.7	97.5	9.92
Russia	77.5	75.8	77.4	80.9	83.0	85.4	84.6	9.16
Saudi Arabia	77.0	79.5	85.0	85.4	86.7	88.6	90.2	17.14
Singapore	103.5	103.4	108.6	100.6	103.3	104.8	105.0	1.45
Slovakia	121.2	116.8	101.9	111.2	111.5	111.1	112.5	-7.18
Slovenia	113.2	112.7	107.0	110.7	106.3	103.2	101.1	-10.69
South Africa	72.3	70.9	72.5	75.6	77.5	79.7	82.1	13.55
South Korea	71.3	72.3	74.9	75.2	77.1	78.9	80.5	12.90
Spain	149.9	149.0	150.6	149.8	150.9	151.8	152.5	1.73
Sweden	125.5	130.0	122.3	123.6	125.6	126.0	127.4	1.51
Switzerland	148.4	143.6	149.2	153.0	156.2	160.1	158.4	6.74
Taiwan	151.9	159.5	148.7	147.1	142.9	138.4	134.6	-11.39
Thailand	51.4	50.8	50.3	50.4	51.1	51.5	51.9	0.97
Tunisia	94.6	103.6	98.8	96.6	95.0	96.4	97.2	2.75
Turkey	87.5	86.2	91.9	87.6	91.6	90.6	90.2	3.09
Turkmenistan	73.5	74.2	72.4	64.9	62.9	60.3	57.3	-22.04
Ukraine	73.2	73.6	74.3	76.2	81.7	83.4	80.2	9.56
United Arab Emirates	103.1	102.2	94.4	95.4	97.8	98.3	99.2	-3.78
United Kingdom	142.0	143.3	142.2	142.5	138.9	137.4	136.2	-4.08
USA	143.6	147.5	155.8	157.8	156.5	157.4	158.0	10.03
Venezuela	59.7	59.1	60.7	63.7	63.6	64.3	65.3	9.38
Vietnam	37.6	40.0	40.2	42.7	45.5	48.0	50.8	35.11

Source: UN Food and Agriculture Organisation, FAOSTAT

■ **Over-the-Counter Healthcare**

Trends in OTC healthcare retail sales 1998-2004

Table: 2.57

US$ million/% real growth (national currencies)

	1998	1999	2000	2001	2002	2003	2004	% real growth 1998-2004
Algeria	20.6	21.5	21.6	22.4	25.0	29.8	31.8	
Argentina	551.6	581.1	594.6	587.7	200.3	298.2	371.4	28.59
Australia	943.8	1,035.3	985.6	934.3	1,042.0	1,300.3	1,535.0	10.68
Austria	376.4	374.3	331.1	330.7	360.3	456.8	514.9	7.78
Azerbaijan								
Belarus								
Belgium	649.6	635.9	566.6	564.1	599.4	730.6	819.1	0.82
Bolivia								
Brazil	3,686.4	2,680.6	2,694.8	2,169.3	1,892.5	1,795.5	2,082.2	-16.55
Bulgaria	31.7	35.9	37.3	42.8	48.9	65.2	78.2	38.91
Canada	1,529.6	1,614.6	1,703.2	1,701.9	1,762.5	2,024.3	2,201.8	7.37
Chile	177.8	170.2	168.7	151.8	146.8	152.2	179.9	13.80
China	5,329.2	4,425.7	3,703.3	3,355.3	3,523.9	4,026.4	4,637.4	-0.24
Colombia	234.2	251.0	271.1	291.4	310.4	288.8	317.0	37.58
Croatia								
Czech Republic	136.0	140.5	135.2	147.8	179.1	216.2	242.8	14.34
Denmark	288.5	286.3	257.7	259.1	280.1	343.9	379.5	3.29
Ecuador								
Egypt	336.4	355.5	368.9	345.2	326.2	273.9	276.4	14.03
Estonia								
Finland	320.4	316.8	281.8	285.4	307.4	380.3	431.4	8.47
France	2,547.4	2,476.1	2,202.3	2,186.2	2,314.1	2,840.9	3,147.3	0.29
Germany	4,609.3	4,571.5	4,146.6	4,052.3	4,244.6	5,149.4	5,794.0	1.97
Greece	123.7	123.5	113.4	117.9	134.5	172.3	196.2	16.96
Hong Kong, China	216.4	222.5	232.0	237.6	244.0	253.9	257.6	30.58
Hungary	121.0	128.5	122.3	134.7	160.8	196.3	227.7	9.46
India	708.5	755.3	806.5	853.0	910.0	1,033.1	1,144.4	31.91
Indonesia	240.7	391.8	482.1	470.4	619.6	799.4	911.5	79.39
Ireland	126.5	128.0	120.0	125.6	142.4	186.8	221.1	22.19
Israel	133.3	129.5	137.3	142.5	154.0	176.2	190.5	47.96
Italy	2,801.6	2,807.2	2,466.6	2,436.0	2,685.8	3,449.6	3,871.0	5.50
Japan	15,508.6	18,600.9	19,900.8	17,923.6	17,512.7	19,319.9	20,652.4	9.19
Jordan	2.8	3.3	3.2	3.3	3.0	3.2	3.5	
Kazakhstan								
Kuwait	8.1	8.1	8.8	9.5	10.4	11.8	12.5	
Latvia								
Lithuania								
Malaysia	183.7	210.1	233.1	254.0	271.2	287.0	299.3	32.64
Mexico	1,251.2	1,326.5	1,436.2	1,539.2	1,581.2	1,519.3	1,616.0	7.45
Morocco	164.8	174.6	174.9	178.8	199.2	242.9	272.6	32.77
Netherlands	431.3	436.0	403.6	419.9	476.7	607.6	689.6	19.62
New Zealand	87.9	93.4	86.2	83.1	94.8	123.0	144.0	9.98
Nigeria								
Norway	327.6	333.1	312.8	321.2	379.5	450.7	490.1	16.90
Pakistan								
Peru								
Philippines	287.8	367.1	407.1	413.7	462.0	510.2	559.3	75.53
Poland	434.6	454.9	505.1	615.6	680.1	778.5	874.3	47.09
Portugal	196.2	193.2	171.1	175.7	201.4	257.8	291.1	11.14
Romania	106.6	87.7	87.9	88.1	97.9	118.1	135.9	11.12
Russia	749.2	583.3	654.3	771.8	925.5	1,087.6	1,213.9	
Saudi Arabia	286.8	295.7	306.0	321.7	338.5	355.0	372.7	27.58
Singapore	136.0	140.8	146.8	149.4	156.0	169.8	176.5	20.48
Slovakia	72.0	65.0	61.7	62.3	70.3	91.8	108.9	-8.43
Slovenia								
South Africa	570.3	540.6	494.8	420.3	360.9	528.5	646.0	-0.91
South Korea	1,443.2	1,840.8	2,143.5	1,855.6	2,127.4	1,974.1	2,001.3	-9.14
Spain	1,031.0	1,036.5	949.8	954.6	1,051.2	1,325.4	1,481.0	5.66
Sweden	574.1	564.6	526.5	479.2	536.7	668.6	754.7	11.63
Switzerland	676.1	672.9	613.4	623.0	678.2	794.6	855.0	1.71
Taiwan	890.7	976.4	994.7	1,075.8	1,073.9	1,126.9	1,212.1	27.02
Thailand	278.8	311.6	305.1	288.1	314.8	345.4	375.9	18.30
Tunisia	10.8	11.1	10.8	11.1	12.3	14.7	15.6	
Turkey	786.0	832.1	894.3	807.4	956.4	1,181.6	1,335.2	
Turkmenistan								
Ukraine	199.1	137.1	138.5	170.1	201.4	231.3	252.9	47.18
United Arab Emirates	5.1	5.5	6.3	6.9	7.1	7.1	7.7	
United Kingdom	3,161.9	3,330.2	3,305.0	3,271.0	3,484.9	3,926.9	4,509.7	6.48
USA	26,718.9	27,637.9	27,929.3	28,037.6	28,714.8	31,030.7	32,216.7	2.80
Venezuela	271.7	337.9	385.6	466.2	327.1	373.1	393.0	41.86
Vietnam	91.8	95.7	109.4	118.8	120.2	125.8	128.8	40.63

Source: *Euromonitor International from trade sources*

Per capita trends in OTC healthcare retail sales 1998-2004

Table: 2.58

US$ per capita

	1998	1999	2000	2001	2002	2003	2004
Algeria	20.6	21.5	21.6	22.4	25.0	29.8	31.8
Argentina	551.6	581.1	594.6	587.7	200.3	298.2	371.4
Australia	943.8	1,035.3	985.6	934.3	1,042.0	1,300.3	1,535.0
Austria	376.4	374.3	331.1	330.7	360.3	456.8	514.9
Azerbaijan							
Belarus							
Belgium	649.6	635.9	566.6	564.1	599.4	730.6	819.1
Bolivia							
Brazil	3,686.4	2,680.6	2,694.8	2,169.3	1,892.5	1,795.5	2,082.2
Bulgaria	31.7	35.9	37.3	42.8	48.9	65.2	78.2
Canada	1,529.6	1,614.6	1,703.2	1,701.9	1,762.5	2,024.3	2,201.8
Chile	177.8	170.2	168.7	151.8	146.8	152.2	179.9
China	5,329.2	4,425.7	3,703.3	3,355.3	3,523.9	4,026.4	4,637.4
Colombia	234.2	251.0	271.1	291.4	310.4	288.8	317.0
Croatia							
Czech Republic	136.0	140.5	135.2	147.8	179.1	216.2	242.8
Denmark	288.5	286.3	257.7	259.1	280.1	343.9	379.5
Ecuador							
Egypt	336.4	355.5	368.9	345.2	326.2	273.9	276.4
Estonia							
Finland	320.4	316.8	281.8	285.4	307.4	380.3	431.4
France	2,547.4	2,476.1	2,202.3	2,186.2	2,314.1	2,840.9	3,147.3
Germany	4,609.3	4,571.5	4,146.6	4,052.3	4,244.6	5,149.4	5,794.0
Greece	123.7	123.5	113.4	117.9	134.5	172.3	196.2
Hong Kong, China	216.4	222.5	232.0	237.6	244.0	253.9	257.6
Hungary	121.0	128.5	122.3	134.7	160.8	196.3	227.7
India	708.5	755.3	806.5	853.0	910.0	1,033.1	1,144.4
Indonesia	240.7	391.8	482.1	470.4	619.6	799.4	911.5
Ireland	126.5	128.0	120.0	125.6	142.4	186.8	221.1
Israel	133.3	129.5	137.3	142.5	154.0	176.2	190.5
Italy	2,801.6	2,807.2	2,466.6	2,436.0	2,685.8	3,449.6	3,871.0
Japan	15,508.6	18,600.9	19,900.8	17,923.6	17,512.7	19,319.9	20,652.4
Jordan	2.8	3.3	3.2	3.3	3.0	3.2	3.5
Kazakhstan							
Kuwait	8.1	8.1	8.8	9.5	10.4	11.8	12.5
Latvia							
Lithuania							
Malaysia	183.7	210.1	233.1	254.0	271.2	287.0	299.3
Mexico	1,251.2	1,326.5	1,436.2	1,539.2	1,581.2	1,519.3	1,616.0
Morocco	164.8	174.6	174.9	178.8	199.2	242.9	272.6
Netherlands	431.3	436.0	403.6	419.9	476.7	607.6	689.6
New Zealand	87.9	93.4	86.2	83.1	94.8	123.0	144.0
Nigeria							
Norway	327.6	333.1	312.8	321.2	379.5	450.7	490.1
Pakistan							
Peru							
Philippines	287.8	367.1	407.1	413.7	462.0	510.2	559.3
Poland	434.6	454.9	505.1	615.6	680.1	778.5	874.3
Portugal	196.2	193.2	171.1	175.7	201.4	257.8	291.1
Romania	106.6	87.7	87.9	88.1	97.9	118.1	135.9
Russia	749.2	583.3	654.3	771.8	925.5	1,087.6	1,213.9
Saudi Arabia	286.8	295.7	306.0	321.7	338.5	355.0	372.7
Singapore	136.0	140.8	146.8	149.4	156.0	169.8	176.5
Slovakia	72.0	65.0	61.7	62.3	70.3	91.8	108.9
Slovenia							
South Africa	570.3	540.6	494.8	420.3	360.9	528.5	646.0
South Korea	1,443.2	1,840.8	2,143.5	1,855.6	2,127.4	1,974.1	2,001.3
Spain	1,031.0	1,036.5	949.8	954.6	1,051.2	1,325.4	1,481.0
Sweden	574.1	564.6	526.5	479.2	536.7	668.6	754.7
Switzerland	676.1	672.9	613.4	623.0	678.2	794.6	855.0
Taiwan	890.7	976.4	994.7	1,075.8	1,073.9	1,126.9	1,212.1
Thailand	278.8	311.6	305.1	288.1	314.8	345.4	375.9
Tunisia	10.8	11.1	10.8	11.1	12.3	14.7	15.6
Turkey	786.0	832.1	894.3	807.4	956.4	1,181.6	1,335.2
Turkmenistan							
Ukraine	199.1	137.1	138.5	170.1	201.4	231.3	252.9
United Arab Emirates	5.1	5.5	6.3	6.9	7.1	7.1	7.7
United Kingdom	3,161.9	3,330.2	3,305.0	3,271.0	3,484.9	3,926.9	4,509.7
USA	26,718.9	27,637.9	27,929.3	28,037.6	28,714.8	31,030.7	32,216.7
Venezuela	271.7	337.9	385.6	466.2	327.1	373.1	393.0
Vietnam	91.8	95.7	109.4	118.8	120.2	125.8	128.8

Source: Euromonitor International from trade sources

OTC healthcare retail sales by sector 2004

Table: 2.59

% of total OTC sales

	Analgesics	Cough, cold and allergy remedies	Digestive remedies	Medicated skin care	Vitamins and dietary supplements	Smoking cessation aids	Eye care	Ear care
Algeria	13.0	20.6	11.9	18.9	29.5			
Argentina	36.5	20.4	16.0	13.0	11.1	0.2	0.9	0.1
Australia	13.3	18.0	6.0	9.9	38.8	6.6	2.6	0.4
Austria	10.6	31.4	7.2	11.7	29.6	1.5	0.6	0.2
Azerbaijan								
Belarus								
Belgium	17.0	22.3	10.8	7.1	31.5	2.6	1.1	0.2
Bolivia								
Brazil	22.4	27.2	14.7	12.9	17.6	0.3	1.4	0.1
Bulgaria	31.6	22.3	6.2	8.0	25.4			
Canada	18.8	24.5	8.9	13.5	25.2	4.6	1.4	0.3
Chile	26.3	23.3	11.5	15.8	16.7	0.1	2.9	0.3
China	3.1	14.2	3.0	3.6	72.8		1.8	
Colombia	28.3	22.9	15.8	9.3	18.5	0.2	0.0	0.0
Croatia								
Czech Republic	26.9	20.8	10.3	9.0	26.0			
Denmark	18.9	14.4	10.7	9.4	29.7	9.2	2.2	0.6
Ecuador								
Egypt	19.3	23.2	17.4	11.7	24.1		1.5	0.3
Estonia								
Finland	17.4	17.0	13.8	10.8	27.0	7.8	1.5	0.1
France	16.7	20.1	11.8	12.1	22.2	5.2	2.6	0.4
Germany	16.1	22.8	10.7	16.9	24.2	0.9	1.8	0.1
Greece	15.4	23.2	6.3	18.5	25.5	1.2	3.8	0.0
Hong Kong, China	12.4	21.9	9.6	4.3	48.7	0.5	0.6	0.1
Hungary	22.6	24.7	13.9	9.4	23.5			
India	22.4	22.3	10.7	8.7	31.8		0.5	0.3
Indonesia	16.8	21.5	6.9	12.4	35.4		1.2	
Ireland	26.4	20.0	7.4	13.0	18.7	9.2	1.0	0.7
Israel	16.0	12.4	10.7	13.1	39.9	0.2	3.3	1.0
Italy	14.7	17.4	11.9	11.7	33.9	0.2	3.1	0.3
Japan	6.7	14.5	8.7	8.3	55.6	0.4	2.6	0.0
Jordan	24.8	37.9	14.8	16.7	3.9			
Kazakhstan								
Kuwait	5.1	5.5	3.6	4.8	78.4			
Latvia								
Lithuania								
Malaysia	12.5	18.4	4.7	7.7	52.0	0.2	2.2	0.4
Mexico	16.0	33.3	13.1	12.9	19.2	0.3	2.4	0.2
Morocco	20.5	22.4	17.3	18.9	12.8	1.2	1.6	0.9
Netherlands	14.1	27.9	7.1	6.7	34.4	1.1	0.2	0.1
New Zealand	10.8	24.3	2.6	12.6	34.0	5.7	5.3	0.8
Nigeria								
Norway	14.7	15.2	6.8	7.0	46.6	5.1	1.5	0.1
Pakistan								
Peru								
Philippines	26.7	24.5	6.3	8.5	32.2		0.7	0.0
Poland	24.2	21.3	11.4	7.7	23.4			
Portugal	26.3	17.7	17.7	15.2	11.7	0.2	3.9	0.0
Romania	25.2	12.2	15.9	7.8	31.1			
Russia	13.9	18.5	12.2	9.2	35.4			
Saudi Arabia	20.2	27.7	15.5	16.8	15.1	0.3	1.3	0.6
Singapore	8.7	25.6	4.7	7.4	50.5	0.2	1.0	0.2
Slovakia	24.1	17.1	9.6	11.6	31.0			
Slovenia								
South Africa	29.9	29.8	7.5	15.3	11.5	0.5	1.8	0.5
South Korea	7.4	5.8	7.8	5.2	71.8	0.6	0.3	
Spain	19.0	27.8	15.3	11.5	17.4	1.3	2.2	0.1
Sweden	16.3	27.3	6.3	7.8	28.2	7.7	0.8	0.4
Switzerland	13.5	26.6	10.9	16.6	16.3	1.2	1.9	1.1
Taiwan	4.1	8.4	3.7	5.7	77.2	0.1	0.5	
Thailand	14.6	23.6	5.6	9.8	42.8		1.8	0.1
Tunisia	13.0	20.6	11.9	18.9	29.5			
Turkey	28.3	28.4	10.4	7.1	9.3	0.0	4.2	2.6
Turkmenistan								
Ukraine	10.1	34.3	12.6	7.7	26.1			
United Arab Emirates	14.5	21.8	5.8	13.1	40.7			
United Kingdom	20.2	23.1	11.6	16.0	17.9	3.4	2.4	0.4
USA	11.8	15.8	10.8	9.7	45.3	2.0	1.6	0.2
Venezuela	8.3	22.6	9.5	9.9	46.5	0.0	1.1	0.7
Vietnam	14.5	19.3	18.5	8.8	28.0		3.2	0.6

Source: Euromonitor International from trade sources

OTC healthcare retail sales by sector (continued) 2004

Table: 2.60

% of total OTC sales

	Adult mouthcare	Calming and sleeping products	Wound treatments	Other	Total
Algeria					
Argentina	0.7	0.3	0.8	0.0	100.0
Australia	1.4	0.5	2.2	0.3	100.0
Austria	0.8	2.9	3.5	0.0	100.0
Azerbaijan					
Belarus					
Belgium	1.4	0.9	5.1	0.2	100.0
Bolivia					
Brazil	0.0	1.4	2.0	0.0	100.0
Bulgaria					
Canada	0.1	0.6	2.1	0.0	100.0
Chile	0.7	0.7	1.8	0.0	100.0
China	0.3	0.1	0.3		
Colombia	0.2	0.3	4.4	0.0	100.0
Croatia					
Czech Republic					
Denmark	0.2	1.9	2.5	0.4	100.0
Ecuador					
Egypt	0.5	1.0	1.2		
Estonia					
Finland	0.4	1.2	2.9	0.1	100.0
France	1.5	3.0	4.1	0.2	100.0
Germany	0.6	4.7	1.1	0.0	100.0
Greece	1.8	1.0	3.1	0.0	100.0
Hong Kong, China	0.7	0.4	0.7	0.0	100.0
Hungary					
India	0.5		2.8		
Indonesia	1.7	0.0	4.1		
Ireland	1.6	0.7	1.4	0.0	100.0
Israel	1.9	0.5	0.8	0.2	100.0
Italy	2.5	0.3	4.1	0.0	100.0
Japan	1.1	1.1	0.9	0.0	100.0
Jordan					
Kazakhstan					
Kuwait					
Latvia					
Lithuania					
Malaysia	0.5		1.4		
Mexico	0.9	0.4	1.3	0.0	100.0
Morocco	1.1	1.4	1.9	0.0	100.0
Netherlands	0.5	2.4	5.5	0.0	100.0
New Zealand	0.8	0.1	2.8	0.1	100.0
Nigeria					
Norway	0.7	0.2	1.6	0.5	100.0
Pakistan					
Peru					
Philippines	0.6		0.4		
Poland					
Portugal	3.8	2.0	0.2	1.3	100.0
Romania					
Russia					
Saudi Arabia	1.3	0.0	1.2	0.0	100.0
Singapore	0.4	0.3	1.1	0.0	100.0
Slovakia					
Slovenia					
South Africa	1.1	0.2	1.6	0.4	100.0
South Korea	0.4	0.1	0.5		
Spain	2.7	1.0	1.7	0.0	100.0
Sweden	2.1	0.7	1.8	0.6	100.0
Switzerland	1.7	3.6	6.4	0.1	100.0
Taiwan	0.0		0.3		
Thailand	0.5	0.2	0.8		
Tunisia					
Turkey	0.6	8.4	0.8	0.0	100.0
Turkmenistan					
Ukraine					
United Arab Emirates					
United Kingdom	1.4	1.0	1.4	1.4	100.0
USA	0.5	0.5	1.9	0.0	100.0
Venezuela	0.1	0.9	0.3	0.0	100.0
Vietnam	0.7	3.7	2.6		

Source: Euromonitor International from trade sources

■ **Health and Wellness**

Trends in retail sales of organic packaged foods 2002-2004

US$ million/US$ per capita/% real growth (national currencies)

	2002	2003	2004	US$ per capita 2004	% real growth 2002-2004
Algeria					
Argentina					
Australia	116.2	165.7	229.7	11.51	31.57
Austria					
Azerbaijan					
Belarus					
Belgium	126.9	158.2	184.1	17.84	3.25
Bolivia					
Brazil					
Bulgaria					
Canada	296.2	376.6	456.5	14.44	19.78
Chile					
China	13.4	16.4	21.0	0.02	48.78
Colombia					
Croatia					
Czech Republic					
Denmark	183.0	252.1	318.1	58.85	24.57
Ecuador					
Egypt					
Estonia					
Finland	36.7	48.6	60.3	11.55	20.01
France	376.0	494.6	611.9	10.26	15.24
Germany	1,172.3	1,444.4	1,668.6	20.38	2.32
Greece	7.0	10.2	16.0	1.52	58.27
Hong Kong, China	3.8	4.5	5.2	0.68	41.24
Hungary	21.7	30.7	40.7	4.07	37.80
India					
Indonesia					
Ireland	34.6	49.5	66.5	16.84	34.18
Israel					
Italy	755.0	1,018.8	1,302.3	22.43	21.39
Japan	340.0	385.9	438.5	3.45	10.06
Jordan					
Kazakhstan					
Kuwait					
Latvia					
Lithuania					
Malaysia					
Mexico	2.0	2.0	2.3	0.02	21.24
Morocco					
Netherlands	228.3	300.7	375.9	23.05	17.65
New Zealand					
Nigeria					
Norway	35.5	45.2	53.0	11.57	22.87
Pakistan					
Peru					
Philippines					
Poland	8.2	11.1	13.8	0.36	46.34
Portugal					
Romania					
Russia	16.2	16.4	17.6	0.12	
Saudi Arabia					
Singapore					
Slovakia					
Slovenia					
South Africa					
South Korea	46.2	81.8	113.5	2.30	118.02
Spain	38.8	52.7	67.1	1.69	20.20
Sweden	244.5	339.5	433.7	48.79	27.48
Switzerland	347.5	451.5	540.9	74.57	20.92
Taiwan	1.0	1.1	6.6	0.29	546.28
Thailand	23.0	26.5	33.1	0.52	24.47
Tunisia					
Turkey					
Turkmenistan					
Ukraine					
United Arab Emirates					
United Kingdom	960.5	1,140.4	1,404.8	23.48	12.04
USA	4,314.8	5,013.3	5,646.6	19.88	24.63
Venezuela					
Vietnam					

Source: *Euromonitor International from trade sources*

Trends in retail sales of fortified/functional foods 2002-2004

Table: 2.62

US$ million/US$ per capita/% real growth (national currencies)

	2002	2003	2004	US$ per capita 2004	% real growth 2002-2004
Algeria					
Argentina					
Australia	298.9	411.6	540.8	27.09	20.38
Austria					
Azerbaijan					
Belarus					
Belgium	144.1	188.7	234.9	22.77	16.06
Bolivia					
Brazil	1,214.0	1,273.8	1,480.6	8.36	-4.66
Bulgaria					
Canada	189.4	224.7	276.8	8.76	13.59
Chile					
China	403.8	485.0	573.7	0.44	35.21
Colombia					
Croatia					
Czech Republic					
Denmark	71.1	89.7	105.6	19.53	6.43
Ecuador					
Egypt					
Estonia					
Finland	142.2	189.7	233.2	44.70	19.88
France	633.6	873.6	1,090.1	18.28	21.85
Germany	1,277.5	1,643.3	1,948.8	23.80	9.66
Greece	162.5	229.9	293.4	27.74	25.13
Hong Kong, China	120.0	125.7	131.6	17.28	12.53
Hungary	28.7	40.1	49.3	4.93	26.36
India					
Indonesia					
Ireland	84.3	118.7	158.2	40.07	31.06
Israel					
Italy	679.3	958.9	1,257.7	21.66	30.29
Japan	6,637.3	7,545.5	8,519.8	67.00	9.54
Jordan					
Kazakhstan					
Kuwait					
Latvia					
Lithuania					
Malaysia					
Mexico	85.1	100.8	124.6	1.19	50.33
Morocco					
Netherlands	219.3	301.0	396.5	24.31	29.17
New Zealand					
Nigeria					
Norway	107.4	130.3	143.1	31.22	9.52
Pakistan					
Peru					
Philippines					
Poland	57.4	71.5	87.0	2.25	31.02
Portugal					
Romania					
Russia	51.5	62.9	75.2	0.53	
Saudi Arabia					
Singapore					
Slovakia					
Slovenia					
South Africa					
South Korea	1,529.3	1,692.2	1,693.3	34.33	-1.67
Spain	973.8	1,355.4	1,708.6	43.13	22.06
Sweden	121.8	170.4	209.1	23.53	23.38
Switzerland	181.5	220.4	257.6	35.51	10.28
Taiwan	209.5	215.5	238.4	10.38	10.27
Thailand	276.7	306.9	355.1	5.61	11.20
Tunisia					
Turkey					
Turkmenistan					
Ukraine					
United Arab Emirates					
United Kingdom	1,008.3	1,189.2	1,441.1	24.08	9.48
USA	4,455.6	4,828.2	5,215.8	18.36	11.48
Venezuela					
Vietnam					

Source: Euromonitor International from trade sources

Trends in retail sales of packaged foods for food intolerances 1998-2004

Table: 2.63

US$ million/US$ per capita/% real growth (national currencies)

	2002	2003	2004	US$ per capita 2004	% real growth 2002-2004
Algeria					
Argentina					
Australia	31.3	40.0	53.3	2.67	13.38
Austria					
Azerbaijan					
Belarus					
Belgium	15.6	19.6	22.9	2.22	4.48
Bolivia					
Brazil	8.9	10.2	12.8	0.07	12.39
Bulgaria					
Canada	179.3	211.9	239.0	7.56	3.61
Chile					
China	6.4	7.7	10.0	0.01	48.62
Colombia					
Croatia					
Czech Republic					
Denmark	6.3	8.7	10.9	2.02	25.37
Ecuador					
Egypt					
Estonia					
Finland	37.2	57.8	71.7	13.74	40.65
France	93.7	126.1	159.6	2.68	20.67
Germany	483.5	610.8	709.9	8.67	5.55
Greece	0.2	0.2	0.3	0.03	47.50
Hong Kong, China					
Hungary	19.6	26.6	30.9	3.09	15.82
India					
Indonesia					
Ireland	6.5	8.7	10.8	2.73	15.27
Israel					
Italy	67.9	108.4	176.3	3.04	82.89
Japan	80.8	90.1	100.6	0.79	6.19
Jordan					
Kazakhstan					
Kuwait					
Latvia					
Lithuania					
Malaysia					
Mexico	81.9	81.9	90.8	0.87	13.80
Morocco					
Netherlands	49.9	61.8	71.9	4.41	2.96
New Zealand					
Nigeria					
Norway	18.2	24.8	29.4	6.42	32.99
Pakistan					
Peru					
Philippines					
Poland	3.6	4.4	5.3	0.14	27.58
Portugal					
Romania					
Russia	35.1	38.7	42.7	0.30	
Saudi Arabia					
Singapore					
Slovakia					
Slovenia					
South Africa					
South Korea	0.2	0.2	0.6	0.01	238.98
Spain	38.4	49.0	62.4	1.57	13.05
Sweden	112.5	159.6	203.4	22.89	29.98
Switzerland	44.9	53.9	62.1	8.55	7.49
Taiwan	4.1	4.1	4.8	0.21	11.43
Thailand	6.5	7.4	8.8	0.14	16.89
Tunisia					
Turkey					
Turkmenistan					
Ukraine					
United Arab Emirates					
United Kingdom	93.2	124.8	158.0	2.64	29.90
USA	1,543.6	1,680.7	1,922.5	6.77	18.61
Venezuela					
Vietnam					

Source: *Euromonitor International from trade sources*

Retail sales of packaged foods for food intolerance by sector 2004

Table: 2.64

% value

	Diabetic	Gluten free	Lactose free
Algeria			
Argentina			
Australia		12.4	87.6
Austria			
Azerbaijan			
Belarus			
Belgium	18.4	13.9	67.7
Bolivia			
Brazil			100.0
Bulgaria			
Canada	4.1	0.4	95.5
Chile			
China	99.9		0.1
Colombia			
Croatia			
Czech Republic			
Denmark		100.0	
Ecuador			
Egypt			
Estonia			
Finland	20.0	37.0	42.9
France	2.0	88.2	9.8
Germany	11.1	4.5	84.3
Greece	100.0		
Hong Kong, China			
Hungary	51.1	44.5	4.3
India			
Indonesia			
Ireland	15.3	51.3	33.5
Israel			
Italy	5.3	41.9	52.8
Japan	55.8	7.3	36.8
Jordan			
Kazakhstan			
Kuwait			
Latvia			
Lithuania			
Malaysia			
Mexico	0.9		99.1
Morocco			
Netherlands	67.7	10.6	21.8
New Zealand			
Nigeria			
Norway		57.1	42.9
Pakistan			
Peru			
Philippines			
Poland	27.0	73.0	
Portugal			
Romania			
Russia	88.8		11.2
Saudi Arabia			
Singapore			
Slovakia			
Slovenia			
South Africa			
South Korea			100.0
Spain	56.1	40.2	3.7
Sweden	8.3	37.7	54.0
Switzerland	73.4	21.2	5.4
Taiwan			100.0
Thailand			100.0
Tunisia			
Turkey			
Turkmenistan			
Ukraine			
United Arab Emirates			
United Kingdom	14.6	60.6	24.8
USA	9.5	9.3	81.2
Venezuela			
Vietnam			

Source: Euromonitor International from trade sources

World Health Rankings

■ **Rankings**

Life expectancy at birth: total population 2004

Table 3.1

years

Rank	Country	2004
I	Japan	83
2	Switzerland	81
3	Australia	81
4	Sweden	81
5	France	80
6	Canada	80
6	Hong Kong, China	80
6	Singapore	80
9	Israel	80
9	Spain	80
II	Italy	80
12	Austria	80
13	Norway	80
14	New Zealand	79
15	Germany	79
16	Netherlands	79
16	United Kingdom	79
18	Belgium	79
18	Greece	79
20	Finland	79
21	Ireland	78
21	Portugal	78
23	USA	78
24	Slovenia	78
25	Denmark	77
25	Kuwait	77
27	Chile	77
28	Croatia	77
29	Czech Republic	76
30	South Korea	76
31	Poland	75
32	Argentina	75
33	Slovakia	75
34	Mexico	75
35	Taiwan	74
35	Venezuela	74
37	Hungary	74
38	Colombia	73
39	United Arab Emirates	73
40	Malaysia	73
41	Bulgaria	72
41	Morocco	72
41	Tunisia	72
44	Romania	72
45	China	71
45	Estonia	71
45	Lithuania	71
48	Saudi Arabia	71
49	Ecuador	71
49	Jordan	71
49	Turkey	71
52	Peru	71
53	Vietnam	70
54	Latvia	70
55	Thailand	70
56	Algeria	70
57	Brazil	70
58	Philippines	69
59	Belarus	68
60	Egypt	68
61	Azerbaijan	68
62	Indonesia	67
63	Ukraine	67
64	Kazakhstan	65
65	Bolivia	64
66	Turkmenistan	63
67	Pakistan	62
68	India	62
69	South Africa	50
70	Nigeria	47

Source:*Euromonitor International from World Bank*

Healthy life expectancy at birth: total population 2002

Table 3.2

years

Rank	Country	2002
I	Jordan	74
2	Switzerland	73
3	Australia	72
3	Sweden	72
5	Austria	71
5	France	71
5	Norway	71
5	Spain	71
9	Belgium	70
9	Canada	70
9	Denmark	70
9	Finland	70
9	Germany	70
9	Greece	70
9	Netherlands	70
9	New Zealand	70
9	United Kingdom	70
18	Ireland	69
18	Singapore	69
20	Slovenia	68
20	USA	68
22	Czech Republic	67
22	Portugal	67
22	South Korea	67
25	Chile	66
26	Malaysia	64
26	Poland	64
26	Slovakia	64
29	Argentina	63
29	Bulgaria	63
29	China	63
29	Croatia	63
33	Estonia	62
33	Hungary	62
33	United Arab Emirates	62
36	Lithuania	61
36	Romania	61
36	Tunisia	61
36	Venezuela	61
40	Latvia	60
40	Mexico	60
40	Saudi Arabia	60
40	Turkey	60
44	Colombia	59
44	Egypt	59
44	Kazakhstan	59
44	Thailand	59
44	Vietnam	59
49	Algeria	58
49	Belarus	58
51	Brazil	57
51	Ecuador	57
51	Indonesia	57
51	Peru	57
51	Russia	57
51	Ukraine	57
57	Morocco	55
57	Philippines	55
59	Azerbaijan	53
60	Kuwait	52
61	Bolivia	51
61	India	51
61	Pakistan	51
64	Turkmenistan	50
65	Nigeria	42
66	South Africa	41

Source:*Euromonitor International from World Bank*

Healthy life expectancy at 60: males 2001   Table 3.3

years

Rank	Country	2001
1	Japan	17
1	Switzerland	17
3	Australia	16
3	Austria	16
3	France	16
3	Greece	16
3	Israel	16
3	Italy	16
3	New Zealand	16
3	Norway	16
3	Sweden	16
12	Belgium	15
12	Canada	15
12	Denmark	15
12	Finland	15
12	Germany	15
12	Netherlands	15
12	Spain	15
12	United Kingdom	15
12	USA	15
21	Ireland	14
21	Mexico	14
21	Singapore	14
24	Chile	13
24	China	13
24	Czech Republic	13
24	Portugal	13
24	Slovenia	13
24	South Korea	13
30	Argentina	12
30	Bulgaria	12
30	Kuwait	12
30	Poland	12
30	Thailand	12
30	Venezuela	12
36	Colombia	11
36	Estonia	11
36	Indonesia	11
36	Lithuania	11
36	Peru	11
36	Romania	11
36	Slovakia	11
36	Tunisia	11
36	Turkey	11
36	United Arab Emirates	11
46	Algeria	10
46	Belarus	10
46	Croatia	10
46	Hungary	10
46	India	10
46	Jordan	10
46	Latvia	10
46	Saudi Arabia	10
46	Vietnam	10
55	Brazil	9
55	Ecuador	9
55	Egypt	9
55	Kazakhstan	9
55	Malaysia	9
55	Morocco	9
55	Pakistan	9
55	South Africa	9
55	Ukraine	9
64	Azerbaijan	8
64	Bolivia	8
64	Philippines	8
64	Russia	8
68	Nigeria	7
68	Turkmenistan	7

Source:Euromonitor International from World Bank

Healthy life expectancy at 60: females 2001   Table 3.4

years

Rank	Country	2001
1	Japan	21
2	Australia	19
2	Austria	19
2	France	19
2	Sweden	19
2	Switzerland	19
7	Belgium	18
7	Canada	18
7	Finland	18
7	Germany	18
7	Italy	18
7	New Zealand	18
7	Norway	18
7	Spain	18
15	Denmark	17
15	Greece	17
15	Israel	17
15	Netherlands	17
15	Slovenia	17
15	South Korea	17
15	United Kingdom	17
15	USA	17
23	Chile	16
23	Czech Republic	16
23	Ireland	16
23	Portugal	16
23	Singapore	16
28	Argentina	15
28	Estonia	15
28	Lithuania	15
28	Mexico	15
28	Poland	15
28	Slovakia	15
28	Venezuela	15
35	Bulgaria	14
35	China	14
35	Croatia	14
35	Ecuador	14
35	Hungary	14
35	Latvia	14
41	Belarus	13
41	Brazil	13
41	Colombia	13
41	Kuwait	13
41	Peru	13
41	Romania	13
41	Russia	13
41	Saudi Arabia	13
41	Thailand	13
41	Tunisia	13
41	Vietnam	13
52	Algeria	12
52	Jordan	12
52	Malaysia	12
52	Philippines	12
52	Turkey	12
52	Ukraine	12
52	United Arab Emirates	12
59	Azerbaijan	11
59	Bolivia	11
59	Indonesia	11
59	Kazakhstan	11
59	Pakistan	11
59	South Africa	11
65	India	10
65	Morocco	10
65	Nigeria	10
65	Turkmenistan	10
69	Egypt	9

Source:Euromonitor International from World Bank

© **Euromonitor International 2005**

Private health expenditure as a proportion of total health expenditure 2004

Table 3.5

% of total expenditure

Rank	Country	2004
I	USA	37.0
2	Netherlands	18.1
3	Canada	13.7
4	France	13.3
5	Germany	8.9
6	Switzerland	8.8
7	Austria	7.0
8	Australia	5.8
9	New Zealand	5.2
10	Turkey	5.1
11	Spain	4.3
12	Mexico	3.6
13	Ireland	3.1
14	Finland	2.4
15	South Korea	2.3
16	Denmark	1.7
16	Portugal	1.7
18	Italy	0.9
19	Hungary	0.6
20	Japan	0.3

Source:Euromonitor International from OECD

Share of total health expenditure in GDP 2004

Table 3.6

% of total GDP

Rank	Country	2004
I	USA	13.8
2	Germany	12.2
3	France	10.5
3	Switzerland	10.5
5	Jordan	9.8
6	Greece	9.5
7	Canada	9.4
8	Australia	9.2
9	Argentina	9.1
10	Croatia	8.8
10	Italy	8.8
10	New Zealand	8.8
13	Belgium	8.6
13	Denmark	8.6
13	Israel	8.6
16	Japan	8.5
16	Slovenia	8.5
18	Netherlands	8.3
18	South Africa	8.3
20	Portugal	8.1
20	Sweden	8.1
22	Norway	7.9
22	Spain	7.9
24	Austria	7.8
25	United Kingdom	7.6
26	Brazil	7.5
27	Czech Republic	7.4
28	Finland	7.0
29	Chile	6.7
29	Ireland	6.7
31	Hong Kong, China	6.6
31	Hungary	6.6
33	Tunisia	6.5
34	Romania	6.3
34	Venezuela	6.3
36	Latvia	6.2
37	Lithuania	6.0
38	China	5.9
38	Mexico	5.9
38	Poland	5.9
41	South Korea	5.7
42	Belarus	5.6
42	Slovakia	5.6
44	Bolivia	5.5
45	Colombia	5.3
45	Estonia	5.3
47	India	5.1
47	Russia	5.1
49	Turkey	5.0
50	Morocco	4.8
50	Vietnam	4.8
52	Bulgaria	4.7
52	Peru	4.7
52	Ukraine	4.7
55	Turkmenistan	4.5
56	Saudi Arabia	4.4
57	Egypt	4.3
58	Ecuador	4.1
59	Singapore	4.0
60	Pakistan	3.9
61	Kuwait	3.8
62	Algeria	3.7
62	United Arab Emirates	3.7
64	Malaysia	3.6
65	Nigeria	3.4
65	Thailand	3.4
67	Philippines	3.1
68	Kazakhstan	2.8
69	Indonesia	2.6
70	Azerbaijan	1.7
71	Taiwan	0.4

Source:Euromonitor International from WHO

Consumer expenditure on health goods and medical services as a proportion of the total 2004

Table 3.7

% of total consumer expenditure

Rank	Country	2004
1	USA	19.13
2	Switzerland	14.18
3	Chile	11.90
4	Taiwan	9.58
5	Belarus	9.22
6	Tunisia	9.03
7	Argentina	8.18
8	South Africa	7.91
9	India	7.84
10	South Korea	7.76
11	Thailand	7.75
12	Vietnam	7.56
13	Turkey	6.42
14	Singapore	6.20
15	Brazil	5.91
16	Morocco	5.86
17	Greece	5.27
18	Australia	5.25
19	China	5.20
20	Peru	5.05
21	Algeria	4.77
22	Pakistan	4.66
23	Hong Kong, China	4.64
24	Latvia	4.61
25	Canada	4.60
25	Poland	4.60
27	Portugal	4.59
28	Colombia	4.55
29	Mexico	4.54
30	Azerbaijan	4.26
31	Netherlands	4.24
32	Germany	4.23
33	Belgium	4.13
34	Hungary	4.01
35	Turkmenistan	3.96
36	Finland	3.95
36	Japan	3.95
38	France	3.80
39	Kazakhstan	3.74
40	Nigeria	3.61
41	Lithuania	3.44
42	Spain	3.43
43	New Zealand	3.39
44	Austria	3.33
45	United Arab Emirates	3.28
46	Ireland	3.16
47	Italy	3.02
48	Bolivia	2.86
48	Denmark	2.86
48	Saudi Arabia	2.86
51	Norway	2.85
52	Ecuador	2.73
53	Jordan	2.72
54	Sweden	2.65
55	Romania	2.61
56	Slovenia	2.49
57	Malaysia	2.38
58	Egypt	2.32
59	Russia	2.27
59	Venezuela	2.27
61	Estonia	2.15
62	Croatia	1.99
63	Indonesia	1.96
64	United Kingdom	1.73
65	Czech Republic	1.66
66	Philippines	1.57
67	Slovakia	1.52
68	Kuwait	1.37
69	Bulgaria	1.32
70	Israel	1.02
71	Ukraine	0.85

Source: National statistical offices/OECD/Eurostat/Euromonitor International

Concentration of hospitals and clinics 2004

Table 3.8

number per 100,000 inhabitants

Rank	Country	2004
1	Japan	135.4
2	South Korea	109.0
3	Taiwan	80.0
4	Bolivia	27.3
5	Ecuador	26.6
6	Turkey	25.4
7	Argentina	23.3
8	New Zealand	11.7
9	Portugal	11.2
10	Belgium	9.3
11	Azerbaijan	8.6
12	Belarus	8.3
13	Finland	7.6
14	Russia	6.9
15	Kazakhstan	6.8
16	Australia	6.3
17	Thailand	6.2
18	Latvia	5.7
19	Lithuania	5.6
20	Ukraine	5.6
21	Israel	5.5
22	Turkmenistan	5.3
23	China	4.8
24	Germany	4.6
25	Netherlands	4.2
26	Greece	4.2
27	Kuwait	3.9
28	Brazil	3.9
29	Estonia	3.6
30	Canada	3.3
31	Bulgaria	3.2
32	Austria	3.2
33	Italy	2.7
34	Venezuela	2.2
35	Philippines	2.1
36	Romania	2.0
37	USA	2.0
38	Hungary	2.0
39	Poland	2.0
40	Czech Republic	1.9
41	Croatia	1.8
42	Jordan	1.8
43	Tunisia	1.7
44	Peru	1.7
45	France	1.7
46	United Arab Emirates	1.7
47	Hong Kong, China	1.6
48	India	1.5
49	Slovenia	1.4
50	Chile	1.3
51	Denmark	1.1
52	Singapore	0.8
53	Mexico	0.8
54	Algeria	0.7
55	Pakistan	0.6
56	Indonesia	0.6
57	Morocco	0.5
58	Egypt	0.5
59	Saudi Arabia	0.2

Source: Euromonitor International from national statistics

Concentration of doctors 2004   Table 3.9

number per 100,000 inhabitants

Rank	Country	2004
1	Russia	511.2
2	Ukraine	483.5
3	Greece	481.1
4	Belarus	452.4
5	Belgium	407.8
6	Italy	401.7
7	Lithuania	396.0
8	Switzerland	372.7
9	Norway	368.5
10	Czech Republic	364.6
11	Kazakhstan	356.1
12	Azerbaijan	353.6
13	Slovakia	349.9
14	Germany	343.6
15	Austria	343.3
16	Hungary	342.3
17	Denmark	341.3
18	France	340.0
19	Portugal	339.4
20	Latvia	337.4
21	Sweden	336.0
22	Netherlands	318.9
23	Bulgaria	318.9
24	Finland	318.7
25	USA	318.4
26	Estonia	299.9
27	Argentina	292.1
28	Spain	290.0
29	Ireland	261.8
30	Poland	241.0
31	Australia	234.2
32	United Kingdom	217.1
33	Canada	213.4
34	Japan	209.7
35	New Zealand	209.0
36	Romania	196.6
37	Singapore	186.5
38	Croatia	176.1
39	Taiwan	164.1
40	United Arab Emirates	158.7
41	Ecuador	157.3
41	Mexico	157.3
43	Kuwait	142.1
44	Venezuela	141.8
45	Hong Kong, China	141.1
46	South Korea	133.5
47	China	129.7
48	Turkey	127.2
49	Peru	123.3
50	Algeria	110.4
51	Colombia	90.3
52	Tunisia	82.4
53	Chile	81.8
54	Slovenia	80.4
55	Pakistan	67.4
56	South Africa	65.2
57	Egypt	62.8
58	Vietnam	59.9
59	Saudi Arabia	59.0
60	Jordan	51.6
61	Morocco	47.6
62	India	41.2
63	Bolivia	35.3
64	Thailand	33.1
65	Nigeria	18.0
66	Indonesia	9.3
67	Philippines	3.4

Source:Euromonitor International from OECD/national statistics

Concentration of nurses 2004   Table 3.10

number per 100,000 inhabitants

Rank	Country	2004
1	Ireland	1,543.6
2	Russia	1,250.4
3	Sweden	1,216.4
4	Ukraine	1,193.1
5	Netherlands	1,185.4
6	Norway	1,095.5
7	Germany	1,024.9
8	Australia	1,020.3
9	Denmark	983.9
10	Czech Republic	982.9
11	United Kingdom	966.4
12	Finland	946.8
13	Austria	941.4
14	New Zealand	909.9
15	Hungary	893.2
16	Canada	890.4
17	Croatia	884.8
18	Japan	884.6
19	USA	828.8
20	Spain	806.5
21	Belarus	773.9
22	France	757.0
23	Lithuania	745.0
24	Kazakhstan	721.3
25	Azerbaijan	708.4
26	Slovakia	705.7
27	Slovenia	677.7
28	Estonia	649.0
29	Hong Kong, China	612.5
30	Belgium	589.5
31	Italy	556.4
32	Bulgaria	527.2
33	Poland	471.9
34	Turkmenistan	442.2
35	Greece	428.3
36	Latvia	425.7
37	Taiwan	418.2
38	Singapore	405.1
39	Portugal	396.6
40	Kuwait	376.8
41	South Africa	369.2
42	United Arab Emirates	334.1
43	Mexico	221.9
44	Saudi Arabia	170.5
44	Turkey	170.5
46	South Korea	164.4
47	Thailand	133.6
48	Egypt	129.6
49	Nigeria	96.3
50	China	93.7
51	Bolivia	88.7
52	Indonesia	75.3
53	Vietnam	63.9
54	India	56.8
55	Jordan	37.7
56	Pakistan	27.7
57	Chile	26.8
58	Philippines	7.0

Source:Euromonitor International from OECD/national statistics

Concentration of active pharmacists 2004

Table 3.11

number per 100,000 inhabitants

Rank	Country	2004
1	Japan	177.8
2	Finland	153.9
3	France	119.3
4	Belgium	119.2
5	Taiwan	117.8
6	Estonia	116.2
7	Italy	111.4
8	New Zealand	100.4
9	Lithuania	91.4
10	Spain	90.8
11	Greece	88.5
12	Ireland	88.3
13	Portugal	86.3
14	Australia	86.0
15	USA	73.6
16	Kazakhstan	73.2
17	Canada	66.1
18	Poland	64.4
19	Slovenia	64.3
20	Austria	60.6
21	Germany	56.9
22	Czech Republic	55.1
23	Hungary	50.9
24	Denmark	50.1
25	Slovakia	46.2
26	United Kingdom	44.4
27	Croatia	38.3
28	Singapore	36.5
29	Norway	35.4
30	Azerbaijan	32.8
31	Turkey	31.2
32	Morocco	30.0
33	China	29.6
34	Switzerland	22.1
35	Tunisia	21.6
36	South Africa	21.1
37	Vietnam	21.0
38	Netherlands	20.7
39	Hong Kong, China	20.1
40	Kuwait	19.1
41	Bulgaria	16.8
42	Algeria	16.8
43	Thailand	12.1
44	Egypt	7.1
45	Romania	6.3
46	Nigeria	5.9
47	South Korea	5.9
48	Jordan	4.4
49	Saudi Arabia	3.0
50	Chile	2.1

Source: Euromonitor International from OECD/national statistics

Concentration of dentists 2004

Table 3.12

number per 100,000 inhabitants

Rank	Country	2004
1	Greece	121.7
2	Norway	89.7
3	Estonia	88.9
4	Denmark	88.9
5	Sweden	88.5
6	Finland	86.4
7	Belgium	83.8
8	Germany	80.0
9	Japan	73.9
10	Lithuania	70.7
11	France	67.8
12	Czech Republic	67.0
13	Belarus	63.6
14	Slovenia	62.8
15	Latvia	61.9
16	Canada	58.5
17	USA	58.0
18	Bulgaria	56.4
19	Ireland	56.1
20	Austria	53.5
21	Italy	53.2
22	Hungary	50.5
23	Spain	50.4
24	Slovakia	48.7
25	Netherlands	48.5
26	Switzerland	48.3
27	Portugal	48.1
28	Australia	47.0
29	United Kingdom	46.8
30	New Zealand	42.6
31	Taiwan	41.6
32	Russia	40.8
33	Singapore	35.2
34	South Korea	32.8
35	Hong Kong, China	30.0
36	Poland	28.7
37	Azerbaijan	28.6
38	United Arab Emirates	27.8
39	Algeria	27.7
40	Kuwait	23.2
41	Turkey	23.1
42	Romania	21.9
43	Turkmenistan	19.0
44	Tunisia	14.8
45	Croatia	11.2
46	South Africa	11.1
47	Mexico	9.9
48	Egypt	9.5
49	Jordan	9.1
50	Morocco	8.9
51	Chile	8.8
52	Thailand	7.8
53	Bolivia	6.2
54	Brazil	4.6
55	Pakistan	3.3
56	Philippines	3.1
57	Nigeria	1.5
58	Saudi Arabia	1.2

Source: Euromonitor International from OECD/national statistics

Concentration of incidence of measles 2002

Table 3.13

number per 100,000 inhabitants

Rank	Country	2002
1	Azerbaijan	52.7
2	Nigeria	35.2
3	Japan	26.5
4	Morocco	20.1
5	Algeria	18.9
6	Italy	16.2
7	Ukraine	15.7
8	Turkey	11.2
9	Venezuela	9.6
10	Philippines	8.8
11	France	8.7
12	Vietnam	8.5
13	Indonesia	6.7
14	Ireland	6.3
15	Singapore	6.2
16	Germany	5.6
17	India	5.0
18	China	4.5
19	Lithuania	3.0
20	Pakistan	2.6
21	South Africa	2.3
22	Malaysia	1.7
23	Saudi Arabia	1.4
23	United Arab Emirates	1.4
25	Egypt	1.0
25	Tunisia	1.0
27	Denmark	0.6
28	New Zealand	0.5
28	United Kingdom	0.5
30	Jordan	0.4
30	Russia	0.4
32	Colombia	0.3
33	Australia	0.2
33	Spain	0.2
33	Turkmenistan	0.2
36	Belarus	0.1
36	Croatia	0.1
36	Kazakhstan	0.1
36	Norway	0.1
36	Poland	0.1
36	Portugal	0.1
36	Romania	0.1
36	South Korea	0.1
36	Sweden	0.1
45	Bolivia	0.0
45	Brazil	0.0
45	Bulgaria	0.0
45	Canada	0.0
45	Chile	0.0
45	Czech Republic	0.0
45	Ecuador	0.0
45	Estonia	0.0
45	Finland	0.0
45	Greece	0.0
45	Hungary	0.0
45	Israel	0.0
45	Netherlands	0.0
45	Peru	0.0
45	Slovakia	0.0
45	Slovenia	0.0
45	USA	0.0

Source: WHO

Concentration of incidence of AIDS 2004

Table 3.14

number per 100,000 inhabitants

Rank	Country	2004
1	Russia	22.54
2	Thailand	20.61
3	Estonia	17.77
4	USA	14.73
5	Singapore	4.34
6	Malaysia	4.23
7	Switzerland	4.11
8	Mexico	3.67
9	Colombia	3.37
10	Ukraine	3.23
11	Peru	2.93
12	Spain	2.92
13	Brazil	2.35
14	Portugal	2.35
15	Latvia	2.16
16	Ecuador	2.15
17	France	1.70
18	Chile	1.57
19	Nigeria	1.40
20	United Kingdom	1.35
21	Italy	1.31
22	Argentina	1.26
23	Germany	0.91
24	Vietnam	0.90
25	Australia	0.88
26	Bolivia	0.84
27	Belgium	0.83
28	Canada	0.78
29	Taiwan	0.76
30	New Zealand	0.62
31	Israel	0.46
32	Denmark	0.46
33	Netherlands	0.46
34	Morocco	0.45
35	Tunisia	0.42
36	Hong Kong, China	0.36
37	Sweden	0.36
38	Romania	0.35
39	Kuwait	0.29
40	Finland	0.29
41	Austria	0.28
42	Greece	0.27
43	India	0.22
44	Kazakhstan	0.21
45	Lithuania	0.20
46	Algeria	0.20
47	Poland	0.19
48	Saudi Arabia	0.18
49	Hungary	0.18
50	Norway	0.18
51	Jordan	0.16
52	Belarus	0.15
53	Ireland	0.15
54	Slovenia	0.15
55	Indonesia	0.14
56	Croatia	0.11
57	Japan	0.11
58	Azerbaijan	0.10
59	Egypt	0.09
60	South Korea	0.08
61	Bulgaria	0.08
62	Czech Republic	0.06
63	Philippines	0.05
64	United Arab Emirates	0.05
65	Slovakia	0.04
66	Turkey	0.03
67	China	0.02
68	Pakistan	0.01

Source: UNAIDS/World Health Organisation

Concentration of deaths from heart disease 2004

Table 3.15

number per 100,000 inhabitants

Rank	Country	2004
1	Ukraine	755.4
2	Russia	650.5
3	Belarus	547.7
4	Estonia	405.6
5	Latvia	348.1
6	Slovakia	336.4
7	Switzerland	277.4
8	Hungary	274.1
9	Lithuania	267.8
10	Finland	252.4
11	USA	245.2
12	Kazakhstan	233.8
13	Romania	225.9
14	Sweden	218.9
15	Czech Republic	218.0
16	Croatia	208.8
17	Germany	204.0
18	Bulgaria	191.5
19	Azerbaijan	187.7
20	New Zealand	186.4
21	United Kingdom	185.8
22	Austria	169.6
23	Norway	167.7
24	Ireland	161.4
25	Israel	140.2
26	Poland	136.8
27	Denmark	134.9
28	Italy	133.8
29	Belgium	126.2
30	Canada	123.5
31	Australia	123.3
32	Slovenia	122.1
33	Greece	109.1
34	Netherlands	96.3
35	Singapore	84.3
36	Turkmenistan	80.3
37	Turkey	79.9
38	Portugal	76.6
39	France	75.4
40	Argentina	73.3
41	Philippines	70.9
42	Venezuela	65.1
43	Japan	62.7
44	Chile	52.8
45	Spain	50.4
46	Colombia	49.2
47	Indonesia	46.3
48	Bolivia	45.0
49	Brazil	44.2
49	Mexico	44.2
51	China	42.8
52	Thailand	42.6
53	Hong Kong, China	41.9
54	Vietnam	41.8
55	India	39.5
56	Malaysia	37.2
57	Taiwan	36.8
58	Peru	34.7
59	South Korea	34.5
60	South Africa	31.7
61	Pakistan	29.9
62	Ecuador	18.5
63	Kuwait	15.7

Source: WHO/Euromonitor International

Concentration of deaths from lung cancer 2004

Table 3.16

number per 100,000 inhabitants

Rank	Country	2004
1	Hungary	76.8
2	Czech Republic	62.0
3	Belgium	61.6
4	Slovenia	56.7
5	Poland	56.6
6	Italy	56.2
7	Croatia	54.7
8	Canada	54.6
8	Greece	54.6
10	Netherlands	54.5
11	United Kingdom	53.1
12	Denmark	52.6
13	Estonia	50.9
14	USA	49.0
15	Japan	48.3
16	Germany	46.9
17	France	46.4
18	Latvia	45.4
19	Spain	44.9
20	New Zealand	42.4
21	China	42.3
22	Ireland	40.9
23	Romania	40.7
24	Slovakia	40.6
25	Turkey	40.4
26	Austria	37.6
27	India	37.3
28	Norway	35.3
29	Sweden	34.6
30	Australia	34.3
30	Bulgaria	34.3
30	Ukraine	34.3
33	South Korea	33.5
34	Belarus	33.4
35	Lithuania	33.0
35	Thailand	33.0
37	Finland	31.5
38	Philippines	28.7
39	Portugal	26.5
40	Malaysia	25.5
41	Pakistan	24.4
42	Kazakhstan	24.3
43	Russia	23.6
44	Hong Kong, China	22.9
44	Singapore	22.9
46	Indonesia	21.6
47	Bolivia	21.3
48	Israel	19.5
49	Vietnam	17.9
50	Switzerland	16.4
51	Taiwan	16.3
52	Argentina	15.0
53	Chile	12.4
54	Azerbaijan	10.7
55	Brazil	10.1
56	Peru	9.5
56	Venezuela	9.5
58	South Africa	8.5
59	Mexico	6.2
60	Colombia	5.7
61	Ecuador	3.1
62	Kuwait	2.5
63	Turkmenistan	2.4

Source: WHO/Euromonitor International

Concentration of deaths from chronic liver disease and cirrhosis 2004

Table 3.17

number per 100,000 inhabitants

Rank	Country	2004
1	Hungary	61.0
2	Russia	44.4
3	Slovenia	42.3
4	Croatia	32.5
5	Romania	30.5
6	Slovakia	27.2
7	Mexico	23.7
8	Estonia	20.3
9	Austria	19.3
10	Denmark	18.9
11	Germany	18.8
12	South Africa	18.3
13	Kazakhstan	17.0
14	Czech Republic	16.8
15	Italy	16.0
16	Bulgaria	15.3
17	France	14.5
18	Philippines	14.4
19	Poland	14.0
20	USA	13.8
21	Chile	13.7
22	Finland	13.4
23	South Korea	13.1
24	Portugal	12.7
25	Latvia	12.3
26	Argentina	12.0
26	Lithuania	12.0
26	United Kingdom	12.0
29	Spain	11.8
30	Belgium	11.5
31	Brazil	10.7
31	Japan	10.7
33	China	9.7
34	Ecuador	9.6
34	Malaysia	9.6
36	India	9.4
37	Switzerland	9.0
37	Turkey	9.0
39	Venezuela	8.9
40	Thailand	8.7
41	Bolivia	8.6
42	Hong Kong, China	8.5
42	Sweden	8.5
44	Peru	8.3
45	Indonesia	7.6
46	Pakistan	7.4
47	Vietnam	7.2
48	Canada	7.1
48	Greece	7.1
50	Australia	6.1
51	Ireland	5.2
52	Netherlands	5.0
53	New Zealand	4.9
54	Norway	4.6
54	Taiwan	4.6
56	Colombia	4.1
57	Israel	2.8
58	Singapore	2.5
59	Kuwait	0.9

Source: WHO/Euromonitor International

Concentration of deaths from ulcers of the stomach and duodenum 2004

Table 3.18

number per 100,000 inhabitants

Rank	Country	2004
1	Turkey	38.8
2	Philippines	34.9
3	Bolivia	32.5
4	Indonesia	30.6
5	China	28.3
6	Pakistan	25.7
7	India	23.6
8	Hong Kong, China	21.5
9	Malaysia	19.1
10	Vietnam	16.4
11	Taiwan	16.1
12	Thailand	12.4
13	Denmark	9.5
14	Hungary	9.3
15	Norway	8.8
16	Slovenia	8.2
17	Czech Republic	7.7
18	United Kingdom	7.3
19	Latvia	6.9
20	Finland	6.6
21	Sweden	6.0
22	Croatia	5.7
23	Slovakia	5.4
24	Russia	5.0
25	Romania	4.8
26	Estonia	4.7
27	Lithuania	4.6
28	Poland	4.6
29	Ireland	4.5
30	Germany	3.9
31	Ukraine	3.8
32	Azerbaijan	3.8
33	Japan	3.5
34	South Africa	3.5
35	Greece	3.2
36	Belarus	3.1
37	Italy	3.1
38	Belgium	3.0
39	Colombia	3.0
40	Portugal	2.6
41	France	2.5
42	Austria	2.4
43	Mexico	2.2
44	Chile	2.1
45	Switzerland	2.1
46	Netherlands	2.0
47	Australia	1.9
48	New Zealand	1.8
49	Spain	1.7
50	Turkmenistan	1.6
51	Venezuela	1.5
52	Bulgaria	1.5
53	Canada	1.4
54	South Korea	1.4
55	Israel	1.2
56	Ecuador	1.2
57	Peru	1.1
58	Singapore	1.1
59	Brazil	0.9
60	USA	0.9
61	Argentina	0.9
62	Kazakhstan	0.8
63	Kuwait	0.4

Source: WHO/Euromonitor International

Concentration of deaths from diseases of the circulatory system 2004

Table 3.19

number per 100,000 inhabitants

Rank	Country	2004
1	Russia	1,055.2
2	Belarus	798.4
3	Latvia	772.5
4	Romania	697.8
5	Estonia	668.2
6	Hungary	503.6
7	Slovakia	501.3
8	Kazakhstan	492.7
9	Poland	412.2
10	Czech Republic	408.5
11	Greece	279.7
12	Azerbaijan	267.5
13	Germany	265.6
14	Ireland	262.7
15	Finland	261.2
16	Portugal	256.2
17	Austria	252.1
18	Norway	239.2
19	USA	236.7
20	United Kingdom	231.8
21	Sweden	228.8
22	Argentina	226.0
23	Italy	215.7
24	China	215.1
25	Denmark	208.7
26	Netherlands	207.3
27	Slovenia	205.9
28	Spain	197.0
29	Switzerland	195.6
30	Belgium	187.7
31	Canada	184.5
32	Australia	180.8
33	New Zealand	172.0
34	South Korea	169.6
35	France	156.0
36	Hong Kong, China	146.0
37	Japan	137.6
38	Singapore	126.2
39	Malaysia	60.9
40	Taiwan	49.9
41	Morocco	37.9

Source: Euromonitor International from OECD/WHO/national statistics

Concentration of deaths from diseases of the respiratory system 2004

Table 3.20

number per 100,000 inhabitants

Rank	Country	2004
1	China	137.8
2	Ireland	117.3
3	United Kingdom	107.6
4	Russia	85.1
5	Spain	83.3
6	Portugal	76.7
7	Kazakhstan	70.4
8	Japan	68.8
9	Netherlands	67.4
10	Slovenia	65.8
11	Belarus	65.5
12	Hong Kong, China	64.9
13	Denmark	62.1
14	USA	61.9
15	Romania	59.7
16	Norway	54.7
17	Finland	54.5
17	Singapore	54.5
19	Slovakia	51.4
20	Azerbaijan	48.4
21	Czech Republic	47.2
22	France	41.1
23	Switzerland	40.0
24	Poland	39.9
25	Greece	39.6
26	Italy	38.3
27	Germany	36.2
28	South Korea	36.1
29	Australia	34.3
30	Sweden	33.3
31	Austria	31.2
32	Estonia	27.9
33	New Zealand	21.6
34	Hungary	21.2
35	Taiwan	7.5
36	Morocco	6.7

Source: Euromonitor International from OECD/WHO/national statistics

Concentration of deaths from diseases of the digestive system 2004

Table 3.21

number per 100,000 inhabitants

Rank	Country	2004
1	Mexico	87.8
2	Hungary	68.2
3	Romania	67.7
4	Denmark	44.9
5	Azerbaijan	43.2
6	Slovakia	42.0
7	Slovenia	41.2
8	Brazil	39.8
9	Ecuador	36.6
10	Turkey	35.7
11	Argentina	35.6
12	Croatia	35.4
13	Venezuela	35.2
14	Poland	35.1
15	Kazakhstan	33.8
16	Estonia	32.2
17	Peru	32.0
18	Philippines	31.8
19	Turkmenistan	31.6
20	Germany	31.0
20	Singapore	31.0
22	Colombia	30.9
23	Belgium	30.7
24	Portugal	30.5
25	Indonesia	30.4
26	Latvia	30.3
27	Bolivia	30.2
28	Czech Republic	29.9
29	China	29.7
30	Ukraine	28.3
31	United Kingdom	27.9
32	Spain	27.2
33	France	26.4
34	Pakistan	26.3
35	Finland	25.9
36	Chile	25.6
37	Austria	25.5
38	Belarus	25.1
39	Ireland	24.4
40	USA	24.0
41	Lithuania	23.7
42	India	23.4
43	Netherlands	22.2
44	Italy	22.0
45	Australia	21.3
45	Switzerland	21.3
47	Bulgaria	20.9
48	Hong Kong, China	20.8
49	Canada	18.8
49	Norway	18.8
51	Taiwan	18.7
52	Malaysia	18.2
53	Vietnam	17.2
54	Greece	14.9
55	Sweden	14.7
56	Japan	14.6
57	Israel	13.5
58	Thailand	13.3
59	South Korea	11.3
60	New Zealand	6.4

Source:*Euromonitor International from OECD/WHO/national statistics*

Concentration of deaths from motor traffic accidents 2004

Table 3.22

number per 100,000 inhabitants

Rank	Country	2004
1	Hong Kong, China	125.5
2	South Korea	31.9
3	Argentina	30.0
4	Belarus	27.2
5	Latvia	26.2
6	Czech Republic	23.2
7	Croatia	20.0
8	Poland	16.8
9	Greece	16.7
10	USA	15.6
11	Spain	15.2
12	Slovenia	15.1
13	Malaysia	14.5
14	New Zealand	13.6
15	France	13.4
16	Hungary	13.1
17	Italy	12.1
18	Australia	11.2
19	Germany	10.3
20	Austria	10.1
21	Denmark	9.7
22	Ireland	9.5
23	Taiwan	9.4
24	China	9.3
25	Japan	8.4
26	Norway	8.2
27	Slovakia	7.8
28	Finland	7.0
29	Netherlands	6.8
30	Portugal	6.1
31	Sweden	5.6
32	United Kingdom	5.2
33	Singapore	4.0

Source:*Euromonitor International from OECD/WHO/national statistics*

Concentration of deaths from injury and poisoning 2004

Table 3.23

number per 100,000 inhabitants

Rank	Country	2004
1	Estonia	144.6
2	Kazakhstan	138.3
3	Belarus	132.7
4	Hungary	75.1
5	South Korea	65.9
6	Finland	62.4
7	Romania	61.5
8	China	60.7
9	Czech Republic	58.9
10	France	54.6
11	Denmark	53.4
12	Poland	52.5
13	USA	48.8
14	Japan	47.5
15	Slovakia	46.2
16	Norway	42.0
17	Australia	39.5
17	Austria	39.5
19	Ireland	39.2
20	Greece	38.4
21	New Zealand	37.9
22	Switzerland	37.2
23	Sweden	35.3
24	Spain	34.9
25	Italy	33.5
26	Portugal	32.5
27	Hong Kong, China	31.9
28	United Kingdom	27.1
29	Germany	26.1
29	Netherlands	26.1
31	Slovenia	16.2
32	Morocco	10.9

Source: Euromonitor International from OECD/WHO/national statistics

Concentration of deaths from suicide and self-inflicted injury 2004

Table 3.24

number per 100,000 inhabitants

Rank	Country	2004
1	Latvia	36.9
2	Belarus	35.7
3	Kazakhstan	29.6
4	Slovenia	29.3
5	Japan	22.1
6	Hungary	21.8
7	Azerbaijan	19.9
8	Croatia	19.4
9	Finland	18.4
10	New Zealand	17.5
11	Austria	15.7
12	South Korea	15.6
13	China	14.6
13	Switzerland	14.6
15	France	14.0
16	Czech Republic	13.8
17	Poland	13.6
18	Slovakia	13.0
19	Norway	12.8
20	Australia	12.6
21	India	12.4
22	Sweden	11.9
23	Ireland	11.0
24	Taiwan	10.4
25	USA	9.5
26	Denmark	9.1
27	Germany	8.6
28	Netherlands	8.1
29	United Kingdom	7.0
30	Bolivia	6.9
31	Chile	6.8
32	Singapore	6.6
33	Spain	6.4
34	Italy	4.3
35	Portugal	3.8
36	Greece	3.2
37	Malaysia	2.3
38	Venezuela	0.2
39	Jordan	0.1

Source: Euromonitor International from OECD/WHO/national statistics

Smoking prevalence in population aged 15+ 2004   Table 3.25

% of population aged 15+

Rank	Country	2004
I	Turkey	52.5
2	Slovakia	49.6
3	Argentina	45.0
4	China	43.0
5	Russia	41.5
5	Vietnam	41.5
7	Venezuela	40.6
8	Algeria	39.3
9	Bulgaria	38.9
10	India	38.0
II	Egypt	37.7
II	Indonesia	37.7
13	Israel	37.2
14	Greece	36.6
15	South Africa	36.5
16	Tunisia	36.0
17	Philippines	35.9
18	Malaysia	34.7
18	South Korea	34.7
20	Spain	34.5
21	Latvia	33.9
22	Taiwan	33.7
23	Ireland	33.6
24	Ukraine	33.4
25	Peru	33.3
26	Lithuania	33.0
27	Brazil	32.9
28	Netherlands	32.8
29	Japan	32.7
30	Germany	32.5
31	Jordan	32.4
32	Hungary	32.3
33	Bolivia	32.2
34	Norway	31.9
35	Ecuador	31.1
36	Thailand	30.8
37	Denmark	30.2
37	Mexico	30.2
39	Croatia	30.1
40	Switzerland	29.6
41	Morocco	29.2
42	Kuwait	28.8
43	Belgium	28.4
43	Poland	28.4
43	Saudi Arabia	28.4
46	Austria	28.3
46	Estonia	28.3
48	Belarus	28.2
49	Pakistan	27.6
50	Turkmenistan	27.5
51	Chile	25.9
51	Singapore	25.9
53	United Arab Emirates	25.6
54	France	25.4
55	United Kingdom	24.8
56	Finland	23.6
57	Colombia	23.3
58	Slovenia	23.1
59	New Zealand	22.9
60	Portugal	22.7
61	Italy	22.6
62	Azerbaijan	22.2
63	Czech Republic	22.1
64	Australia	21.3
65	Canada	20.5
66	Kazakhstan	20.4
67	Hong Kong, China	18.2
68	Sweden	18.0
69	USA	17.7
70	Nigeria	14.4

Source:WHO/OECD/Euromonitor International

Obese population (BMI 30 kg/sq m or more) 2004   Table 3.26

% of population aged 15+

Rank	Country	2004
I	Kuwait	37.6
2	USA	33.7
3	Saudi Arabia	28.0
4	United Arab Emirates	26.8
5	United Kingdom	25.9
6	South Africa	25.4
7	Australia	23.1
8	Colombia	21.4
9	Nigeria	21.1
10	Germany	20.5
II	Mexico	19.8
12	Hungary	19.7
12	Romania	19.7
14	Chile	19.5
15	Israel	18.1
16	Austria	17.8
17	Estonia	17.6
18	Russia	17.5
19	Slovakia	17.2
20	New Zealand	16.7
21	Portugal	16.2
22	Canada	16.0
23	Czech Republic	15.2
23	France	15.2
25	Lithuania	14.9
26	Jordan	14.8
27	Belgium	14.5
28	Ecuador	14.4
29	Bulgaria	14.1
30	Finland	13.9
31	Latvia	13.8
32	Poland	13.3
33	Turkey	13.1
34	Denmark	13.0
35	Ukraine	12.7
36	Netherlands	12.5
37	Spain	12.4
38	Norway	12.2
39	Venezuela	12.1
40	Argentina	11.7
41	Brazil	11.5
42	Greece	11.4
43	Slovenia	11.2
44	Sweden	11.1
45	Ireland	10.7
46	Peru	10.2
47	Croatia	10.0
48	Italy	9.6
49	Bolivia	8.7
50	Azerbaijan	7.7
51	Singapore	6.8
52	Malaysia	6.7
53	Belarus	6.5
54	Egypt	5.9
55	Pakistan	5.8
56	Philippines	5.8
57	Kazakhstan	5.8
58	Indonesia	5.7
58	Taiwan	5.7
60	Switzerland	5.6
61	India	5.4
62	Hong Kong, China	5.2
63	Tunisia	4.9
64	China	4.5
65	Algeria	4.3
65	Turkmenistan	4.3
65	Vietnam	4.3
68	Morocco	4.2
69	Thailand	3.7
70	Japan	2.7
71	South Korea	2.5

Source:OECD/International Obesity Taskforce/Euromonitor International

Average supply of calories per day 2004   Table 3.27

calories per capita

Rank	Country	2004
1	USA	3,768
2	Greece	3,736
3	Portugal	3,727
4	Israel	3,716
5	France	3,689
6	Switzerland	3,684
7	Canada	3,657
8	Ireland	3,654
9	Italy	3,643
10	Norway	3,579
11	Belgium	3,571
12	Austria	3,558
13	Hungary	3,557
14	Hong Kong, China	3,552
15	Germany	3,539
16	Romania	3,538
17	Denmark	3,500
18	Netherlands	3,425
19	United Kingdom	3,419
20	Lithuania	3,397
20	Spain	3,397
22	Poland	3,384
23	Turkey	3,368
24	Taiwan	3,342
25	Egypt	3,329
26	United Arab Emirates	3,262
27	Sweden	3,255
28	Czech Republic	3,250
29	New Zealand	3,230
30	Ukraine	3,205
31	Russia	3,201
32	Tunisia	3,186
33	Australia	3,182
34	Mexico	3,131
35	Finland	3,130
36	Estonia	3,105
37	Argentina	3,066
38	Brazil	3,062
39	Morocco	3,060
39	South Korea	3,060
41	Algeria	3,057
42	South Africa	3,039
43	Slovenia	3,007
44	Belarus	2,956
45	Singapore	2,952
46	Kuwait	2,945
47	China	2,942
48	Chile	2,899
48	Indonesia	2,899
50	Latvia	2,893
51	Malaysia	2,877
52	Bulgaria	2,876
53	Slovakia	2,868
54	Saudi Arabia	2,844
55	Croatia	2,839
56	Azerbaijan	2,784
57	Turkmenistan	2,782
58	Ecuador	2,777
59	Kazakhstan	2,774
60	Nigeria	2,751
61	Japan	2,731
62	Jordan	2,681
63	Peru	2,613
64	Colombia	2,601
65	Vietnam	2,590
66	India	2,536
67	Thailand	2,488
68	Pakistan	2,400
69	Philippines	2,387
70	Venezuela	2,321
71	Bolivia	2,208

*Source:*UN Food and Agriculture Organisation, FAOSTAT

Average supply of protein per day 2004   Table 3.28

grams per capita

Rank	Country	2004
1	Israel	129.4
2	France	120.5
3	Hong Kong, China	119.0
4	Portugal	116.7
5	Greece	114.7
6	USA	113.8
7	Netherlands	113.0
7	Spain	113.0
9	Ireland	112.9
10	Italy	112.8
11	Romania	112.3
12	Denmark	109.8
12	Norway	109.8
14	Austria	108.3
15	Sweden	107.8
16	Lithuania	106.4
17	Taiwan	105.9
18	United Kingdom	104.0
19	Canada	103.2
19	New Zealand	103.2
21	Australia	103.1
22	Hungary	101.7
22	United Arab Emirates	101.7
24	Slovenia	101.1
25	Germany	100.4
26	Finland	100.1
27	Poland	99.8
27	Singapore	99.8
29	Argentina	99.6
30	Czech Republic	98.7
31	Switzerland	96.8
32	Egypt	96.3
33	Russia	96.1
34	Turkey	95.8
35	Estonia	94.1
36	Kazakhstan	93.0
37	Mexico	91.5
38	Japan	91.2
39	South Korea	91.1
40	Tunisia	90.2
41	Bulgaria	90.1
42	Ukraine	87.3
43	Morocco	84.5
44	Belgium	84.0
45	Brazil	82.6
46	Belarus	82.5
47	Algeria	80.8
47	China	80.8
47	Latvia	80.8
50	Turkmenistan	80.0
51	Chile	79.4
52	Azerbaijan	78.3
53	Croatia	77.0
54	Slovakia	76.8
55	Malaysia	76.7
56	South Africa	76.5
57	Saudi Arabia	73.7
58	Kuwait	73.2
59	Peru	68.9
60	Jordan	67.2
61	Venezuela	64.4
62	Vietnam	64.0
63	Indonesia	63.4
64	Pakistan	61.7
65	Nigeria	61.1
66	Colombia	60.9
67	Bolivia	59.4
68	India	58.7
69	Ecuador	58.2
70	Thailand	57.7
71	Philippines	56.6

*Source:*UN Food and Agriculture Organisation, FAOSTAT

Average supply of fat per day 2004

Table 3.29

grams per capita

Rank	Country	2004
1	France	173.8
2	Belgium	159.9
3	Italy	158.6
4	Switzerland	158.4
5	USA	158.0
6	Greece	157.7
7	Hungary	154.5
8	Spain	152.5
9	Austria	151.4
10	Germany	151.2
11	Hong Kong, China	147.2
12	Canada	146.3
13	Norway	145.6
14	Netherlands	144.1
15	Israel	142.4
16	Portugal	140.9
17	Denmark	139.6
18	United Kingdom	136.2
19	Taiwan	134.6
20	Ireland	131.1
21	Australia	130.9
22	Sweden	127.4
23	Czech Republic	123.3
24	Finland	122.5
25	New Zealand	118.4
26	Poland	114.1
27	Slovakia	112.5
28	Latvia	112.4
29	Argentina	107.1
30	Kuwait	106.4
31	Singapore	105.0
32	Lithuania	102.5
33	Slovenia	101.1
34	Bulgaria	100.7
35	United Arab Emirates	99.2
36	China	98.3
37	Romania	97.5
38	Ecuador	97.2
38	Tunisia	97.2
40	Estonia	95.7
41	Belarus	94.0
42	Brazil	91.8
43	Saudi Arabia	90.2
43	Turkey	90.2
45	Mexico	88.9
46	Croatia	84.6
46	Russia	84.6
48	Chile	84.3
49	Japan	83.3
50	South Africa	82.1
51	Jordan	81.9
52	South Korea	80.5
53	Kazakhstan	80.4
54	Ukraine	80.2
55	Malaysia	79.2
56	Algeria	72.9
57	Venezuela	65.3
58	Colombia	65.2
59	Pakistan	64.1
60	Nigeria	61.4
61	Egypt	61.0
62	Indonesia	59.3
63	Turkmenistan	57.3
64	Bolivia	56.6
65	Morocco	55.8
66	Thailand	51.9
67	Vietnam	50.8
68	Philippines	50.2
69	Peru	49.4
70	India	48.6
71	Azerbaijan	46.5

Source: UN Food and Agriculture Organisation, FAOSTAT

Section 4

Country Snapshots

■ Algeria

Socio-economic Parameters

Algeria: Socio-economic parameters 1998-2004

Table: 4.1

As stated

	1998	1999	2000	2001	2002	2003	2004
Population: national estimates at January 1st ('000)	29,074.5	29,534.1	30,004.6	30,494.7	31,005.2	31,531.9	32,068.4
% aged 0-14 yrs	37.2	36.4	35.5	34.7	33.9	33.1	32.3
% aged 15-64 yrs	58.8	59.6	60.4	61.2	61.9	62.7	63.4
% aged 65 + yrs	4.0	4.0	4.1	4.1	4.2	4.2	4.3
% Male	50.5	50.5	50.5	50.5	50.5	50.5	50.5
% Female	49.5	49.5	49.5	49.5	49.5	49.5	49.5
% Urban	58.8	59.6	59.3	60.0	60.7	61.3	62.1
Occupants per household at January 1st (Number)	6.6	6.5	6.4	6.3	6.2	6.1	6.1
Households ('000)	4,426.5	4,560.6	4,696.8	4,840.6	4,982.1	5,132.6	5,285.6
Annual rates of inflation (% growth)	5.0	2.6	0.3	4.2	1.4	2.6	3.6
GDP (DZD million)	2,830,490.0	3,238,200.0	4,098,820.0	4,241,800.0	4,454,800.0	5,124,000.0	5,870,295.0
GDP (US$ million)	48,187.6	48,640.7	54,462.3	54,934.9	55,907.3	66,205.8	81,463.3
GDP (US$ per capita)	1,657.4	1,646.9	1,815.1	1,801.5	1,803.2	2,099.6	2,540.3

Source: Euromonitor International from International Monetary Fund (IMF), International Financial Statistics and World Economic Outlook/UN/national statistics

Life Expectancy

Algeria: Life expectancy 1998-2004

Table: 4.2

As stated

	1998	1999	2000	2001	2002	2003	2004	% change 1998-2004
Life expectancy at birth: total population (years)	68.7	68.9	68.9	69.4	69.3	69.5	69.6	1.35
Life expectancy at birth: total population: year on year growth	0.4	0.4	-0.1	0.7	-0.1	0.2	0.1	
Healthy life expectancy at birth (years)	62.0			57.5	57.8			
Healthy life expectancy at birth: year on year growth					0.6			

Source: Euromonitor International from World Bank

Sanitation

Algeria: Improved sanitary facilities and water source 2000

Table: 4.3

As stated

	2000
Population with access to improved sanitary facilities (% of population)	99.0
Population with access to improved water source (% of population)	89.0
Population with improved access to sanitation facilities, rural (% of rural population with access)	81.0
Population with improved access to sanitation facilities, urban (% of urban population with access)	99.0

Source: National statistics/World Bank

Health Expenditure

Algeria: Public health expenditure 1998-2004

Table: 4.4

As stated

	1998	1999	2000	2001	2002	2003	2004
Share of total health expenditure in GDP (% of total GDP)	3.6	3.6	3.8	4.1	4.0	3.9	3.7
Health expenditure (US$ per capita)	62.0	61.0	65.0	70.0	77.0	82.0	88.0

Source: Euromonitor International from OECD/national statistics

Algeria: Private health expenditure 1998-2004

Table: 4.5

As stated

	1998	1999	2000	2001	2002	2003	2004
Consumer expenditure on health goods and medical services (DZD million)	59,815.6	76,336.0	78,411.0	85,588.0	97,347.8	110,522.1	122,032.9
Consumer expenditure on health goods and medical services: real growth in national currency: 1990 = 100	96.3	119.7	122.6	128.4	144.0	159.3	169.8
Consumer expenditure on health goods and medical services as a percentage of total consumer expenditure	3.7	4.2	4.2	4.2	4.4	4.7	4.8

Source: National statistical offices/OECD/Eurostat/Euromonitor International

Algeria: Consumer expenditure on health goods and medical services by sector 1998-2004

Table: 4.6

% of total consumer expenditure on health goods and medical services

	1998	1999	2000	2001	2002	2003	2004
Pharmaceuticals, medical appliances/ equipment	38.2	37.5	38.0	39.2	39.3	38.9	38.3
Outpatient services	17.1	18.6	18.1	19.0	18.7	19.0	19.3
Hospital services	44.7	43.9	43.9	41.8	42.0	42.2	42.4
Total	100.0	100.0	100.0	100.0	100.0	100.0	100.0

Source: National statistical offices/OECD/Eurostat/Euromonitor International

Healthcare Infrastructure and Services

Algeria: Healthcare infrastructure and services by sector 1998-2004

Table: 4.7

As stated

	1998	1999	2000	2001	2002	2003	2004
Active pharmacists (number)	4,299	4,600	4,814	5,003	5,122	5,235	5,374
Dentists (number)	7,954	8,086	8,197	8,350	8,579	8,755	8,881
Doctors (number)	29,970	31,130	32,337	33,034	34,025	34,873	35,417
Hospitals and clinics (number)	233	235	236	236	237	238	239
In-patient beds ('000)	58	58	58	57	58	58	58

Source: Euromonitor International from national statistics

Algeria: Healthcare infrastructure and services by sector: growth 1998-2004

Table: 4.8

Year on year growth: % change in stated unit

	1998	1999	2000	2001	2002	2003	2004
Active pharmacists (number)	6.9	7.0	4.7	3.9	2.4	2.2	2.7
Dentists (number)	-0.2	1.7	1.4	1.9	2.7	2.1	1.4
Doctors (number)	5.7	3.9	3.9	2.2	3.0	2.5	1.6
Hospitals and clinics (number)	-0.4	0.9	0.4	0.0	0.4	0.4	0.4
In-patient beds (number)	2.3	-0.8	-0.4	-0.5	0.3	0.3	0.3

Source: Euromonitor International from national statistics

Immunisation

Algeria: Vaccination rates by disease type 1998-2004

Table: 4.9

%

	1998	1999	2000	2001	2002	2003	2004
Vaccination rate against DTP (diphtheria, tetanus, pertussis) 1 & 2 (%)				92.0	93.0	94.0	95.0
Vaccination rate against MMR (measles, mumps, rubella) (%)	75.0	83.0	83.0	83.0	81.0	81.0	80.0
Vaccination rate against polio (%)	80.0	83.0	85.0	89.0	86.0	89.0	90.0

Source: WHO

Infectious Diseases

Algeria: Incidence of disease by type 1998-2004

Table: 4.10

Number

	1998	1999	2000	2001	2002	2003	2004
Incidence of AIDS	49	40	58	17	58	62	65
Incidence of diphtheria	57	17		3	0		
Incidence of measles	3,301	2,503		2,686	5,862		
Incidence of polio	0	10	0	1	0		

Source: WHO

Algeria: Incidence of disease by type: growth 1998-2004

Table: 4.11

Year on year growth: %

	1998	1999	2000	2001	2002	2003	2004
Incidence of AIDS	25.6	-18.4	45.0	-70.7	241.2	6.9	4.8
Incidence of diphtheria	90.0	-70.2			-100.0		
Incidence of measles	-83.1	-24.2			118.2		
Incidence of polio			-100.0		-100.0		

Source: WHO

Smoking

Algeria: Smoking prevalence in population aged 15+ 1998-2004

Table: 4.12

% of population aged 15+

	1998	1999	2000	2001	2002	2003	2004
Smoking prevalence in population aged 15+ (% of population aged 15+)	33.5	34.2	35.1	35.9	36.7	38.2	39.3
Smoking prevalence in male population aged 15+ (% of male population)	43.8	44.5	44.7	45.1	45.8	45.7	45.6
Smoking prevalence in female population aged 15+ (% of female population)	23.1	23.8	25.5	26.5	27.5	30.6	32.9

Source: WHO/OECD/Euromonitor International

Nutrition and Obesity

Algeria: Nutrition and obesity 1998-2004

Table: 4.13

As stated

	1998	1999	2000	2001	2002	2003	2004
Average supply of calories per day (calories per capita)	2,933.8	2,976.5	2,943.7	3,006.1	3,021.5	3,035.5	3,057.4
Average supply of fat per day (grams per capita)	67.6	69.4	67.9	72.8	72.3	72.6	72.9
Average supply of protein per day (grams per capita)	82.6	82.8	79.4	80.2	80.7	80.6	80.8
Obese population (BMI 30kg/sq m or more) (% of population aged 15+)	4.1	4.0	4.0	4.0	4.2	4.3	4.3

Source: WHO/OECD/Euromonitor International

Over-the-Counter Healthcare

Algeria: Trends in OTC healthcare retail sales 1998-2004

Table: 4.14

As stated

	1998	1999	2000	2001	2002	2003	2004
OTC Healthcare (US$ million)	20.6	21.5	21.6	22.4	25.0	29.8	31.8
OTC Healthcare (US$ per capita)	0.7	0.7	0.7	0.7	0.8	0.9	1.0

Source: Euromonitor International from industry sources/national statistics

Algeria: OTC healthcare retail sales by sector 1998-2004

Table: 4.15

% of OTC retail value sales

	1998	1999	2000	2001	2002	2003	2004
Analgesics	15.1	14.7	14.3	13.9	13.5	13.2	13.0
Cough, cold and allergy (hay fever) remedies	21.8	21.6	21.4	21.1	21.0	20.9	20.6
Digestive remedies	10.8	11.0	11.2	11.4	11.5	11.6	11.9
Medicated skin care	17.2	17.6	18.1	18.5	18.8	18.9	18.9
Vitamins and dietary supplements	28.7	28.8	28.9	29.0	29.1	29.3	29.5

Source: Euromonitor International from industry sources/national statistics
Notes: Only selected sectors are shown, so values are not expected to sum to 100

■ **Argentina**

Socio-economic Parameters

Argentina: Socio-economic parameters 1998-2004

Table: 4.16

As stated

	1998	1999	2000	2001	2002	2003	2004
Population: national estimates at January 1st ('000)	35,156.3	35,518.8	35,881.4	36,260.1	36,631.6	37,001.3	37,367.8
% aged 0-14 yrs	28.9	28.8	28.6	28.3	28.0	27.8	27.6
% aged 15-64 yrs	61.5	61.5	61.6	61.8	62.1	62.2	62.5
% aged 65+ yrs	9.6	9.7	9.8	9.9	9.9	10.0	10.0
% Male	48.7	48.7	48.7	48.7	48.7	48.7	48.7
% Female	51.3	51.3	51.3	51.3	51.3	51.3	51.3
% Urban	89.3	89.6	89.3	89.6	89.9	90.0	90.2
Occupants per household at January 1st (Number)	3.6	3.6	3.6	3.6	3.6	3.6	3.6
Households ('000)	9,698.1	9,819.1	9,933.7	10,075.8	10,171.4	10,268.8	10,362.2
Annual rates of inflation (% growth)	0.9	-1.2	-0.9	-1.1	25.9	13.4	4.4
GDP (Peso million)	298,948.0	283,523.0	284,204.0	268,697.0	312,580.0	376,232.0	178,923.0
GDP (US$ million)	299,097.5	283,664.8	284,346.2	268,831.4	102,041.6	129,707.0	61,205.8
GDP (US$ per capita)	8,507.6	7,986.3	7,924.6	7,414.0	2,785.6	3,505.5	1,637.9

Source: Euromonitor International from International Monetary Fund (IMF), International Financial Statistics and World Economic Outlook/UN/national statistics

Life Expectancy

Argentina: Life expectancy 1998-2004

Table: 4.17

As stated

	1998	1999	2000	2001	2002	2003	2004	% change 1998-2004
Life expectancy at birth: total population (years)	73.4	73.6	73.7	73.9	74.5	74.7	75.1	2.36
Life expectancy at birth: total population: year on year growth	0.3	0.3	0.2	0.2	0.7	0.3	0.5	
Healthy life expectancy at birth (years)	67.0			62.9	63.1			
Healthy life expectancy at birth: year on year growth					0.3			

Source: Euromonitor International from World Bank

Sanitation

Argentina: Improved sanitary facilities and water source 2000

Table: 4.18

As stated

	2000
Population with access to improved sanitary facilities (% of population)	85.0

Source: National statistics/World Bank

Health Expenditure

Argentina: Public health expenditure 1998-2004

Table: 4.19

As stated

	1998	1999	2000	2001	2002	2003	2004
Share of total health expenditure in GDP (% of total GDP)	8.2	9.0	8.9	9.5	9.6	9.3	9.1
Health expenditure (US$ per capita)	679.0	699.0	680.0	680.0	680.0	682.0	683.0

Source: Euromonitor International from OECD/national statistics

Argentina: Private health expenditure 1998-2004

Table: 4.20

As stated

	1998	1999	2000	2001	2002	2003	2004
Consumer expenditure on health goods and medical services (Peso million)	17,423.0	17,469.0	17,290.0	16,203.0	16,669.0	15,511.6	14,681.1
Consumer expenditure on health goods and medical services: real growth in national currency: 1990 = 100	104.3	105.8	105.7	100.1	81.8	67.1	60.8
Consumer expenditure on health goods and medical services as a percentage of total consumer expenditure	8.3	8.6	8.6	8.6	8.5	8.4	8.2

Source: National statistical offices/OECD/Eurostat/Euromonitor International

Argentina: Consumer expenditure on health goods and medical services by sector 1998-2004

Table: 4.21

% of total consumer expenditure on health goods and medical services

	1998	1999	2000	2001	2002	2003	2004
Pharmaceuticals, medical appliances/ equipment	52.5	51.8	51.3	50.8	50.4		
Outpatient services	38.0	38.7	39.1	39.6	39.9		
Hospital services	9.5	9.6	9.6	9.6	9.7		
Total	100.0	100.0	100.0	100.0	100.0	100.0	100.0

Source: National statistical offices/OECD/Eurostat/Euromonitor International

Healthcare Infrastructure and Services

Argentina: Healthcare infrastructure and services by sector 1998-2004

Table: 4.22

As stated

	1998	1999	2000	2001	2002	2003	2004
Doctors (number)					107,412	108,568	109,141
Hospitals and clinics (number)	6,723	7,206	7,548	7,883	8,192	8,510	8,700
In-patient beds ('000)	77	77	78				

Source: Euromonitor International from national statistics

Argentina: Healthcare infrastructure and services by sector: growth 1998-2004

Table: 4.23

Year on year growth: % change in stated unit

	1998	1999	2000	2001	2002	2003	2004
Doctors (number)						1.1	0.5
Hospitals and clinics (number)	3.9	7.2	4.7	4.4	3.9	3.9	2.2
In-patient beds (number)	0.4	0.5	0.6				

Source: Euromonitor International from national statistics

Immunisation

Argentina: Vaccination rates by disease type 1998-2004

Table: 4.24

%

	1998	1999	2000	2001	2002	2003	2004
Vaccination rate against DTP (diphtheria, tetanus, pertussis) 1 & 2 (%)			88.5	91.5	94.5	98.0	98.0
Vaccination rate against MMR (measles, mumps, rubella) (%)	99.0	99.0	55.6	93.5	97.0	97.0	99.0
Vaccination rate against polio (%)	74.0	91.0	85.0	88.0	91.0	90.0	90.0

Source: WHO

Infectious Diseases

Argentina: Incidence of disease by type 1998-2004

Table: 4.25

Number

	1998	1999	2000	2001	2002	2003	2004
Incidence of AIDS	1,899	1,401	528	482	612	541	471
Incidence of diphtheria	2	0	0	0			
Incidence of measles	10,229	313	6	0			
Incidence of polio	0	0	0	0			

Source: WHO

Argentina: Incidence of disease by type: growth 1998-2004

Table: 4.26

Year on year growth: %

	1998	1999	2000	2001	2002	2003	2004
Incidence of AIDS	-17.3	-26.2	-62.3	-8.7	27.0	-11.6	-12.9
Incidence of diphtheria		-100.0					
Incidence of measles	8,083.2	-96.9	-98.1	-100.0			

Source: WHO

Causes of Death

Argentina: Deaths by disease 1998-2004

Table: 4.27

Number per 100,000 inhabitants

	1998	1999	2000	2001	2002	2003	2004
Death by diseases of the circulatory system	249.0	235.0	232.0	232.0	230.4	227.0	226.0
Deaths from heart disease	60.1	62.3	64.4	66.6	68.8	71.1	73.3
Death by diseases of the digestive system	32.7	33.2	33.5	33.7	35.0	35.1	35.6
Deaths from lung cancer	21.7	20.6	19.5	18.4	17.2	16.0	15.0
Deaths from chronic liver disease and cirrhosis	9.4	9.8	10.2	10.7	11.1	11.6	12.0
Deaths from ulcers of the stomach and duodenum	1.1	1.1	1.0	1.0	1.0	0.9	0.9

Source: WHO/Euromonitor International
Notes: Data is ranked in descending order by year 2004

Argentina: Deaths by disease: growth 1998-2004

Table: 4.28

% year on year growth

	1998	1999	2000	2001	2002	2003	2004
Deaths from chronic liver disease and cirrhosis	4.0	4.3	4.1	4.9	3.7	4.5	3.3
Deaths from heart disease	5.4	3.7	3.4	3.4	3.3	3.3	3.1
Death by diseases of the digestive system	1.2	1.5	0.9	0.6	3.9	0.3	1.5
Death by diseases of the circulatory system	-5.0	-5.6	-1.3	0.0	-0.7	-1.5	-0.4
Deaths from ulcers of the stomach and duodenum	3.0	0.0	-9.1	0.0	0.0	-10.0	-4.0
Deaths from lung cancer	-5.2	-5.1	-5.3	-5.6	-6.5	-7.0	-6.5

Source: WHO/Euromonitor International
Notes: Data is ranked in descending order by year 2004

Argentina: Other selected causes of death: 1998-2004

Table: 4.29

Number per 100,000 inhabitants

	1998	1999	2000	2001	2002	2003	2004
Death by motor traffic accidents	31.5	32.4	33.6	33.7	31.9	30.9	30.0

Source: Euromonitor International from national statistics

Argentina: Other selected causes of death: growth 1998-2004

Table: 4.30

% year on year growth

	1998	1999	2000	2001	2002	2003	2004
Death by motor traffic accidents	2.9	2.9	3.7	0.3	-5.3	-3.1	-3.0

Source: Euromonitor International from national statistics

Smoking

Argentina: Smoking prevalence in population aged 15+ 1998-2004

Table: 4.31

% of population aged 15+

	1998	1999	2000	2001	2002	2003	2004
Smoking prevalence in population aged 15+ (% of population aged 15+)	37.1	38.6	40.4	42.1	43.7	44.3	45.0
Smoking prevalence in male population aged 15+ (% of male population)	45.7	46.8	47.9	48.1	48.2	48.4	48.5
Smoking prevalence in female population aged 15+ (% of female population)	29.1	31.2	33.5	36.7	39.5	40.6	41.8

Source: WHO/OECD/Euromonitor International

Nutrition and Obesity

Argentina: Nutrition and obesity 1998-2004

Table: 4.32

As stated

	1998	1999	2000	2001	2002	2003	2004
Average supply of calories per day (calories per capita)	3,178.0	3,177.7	3,179.9	3,052.6	2,992.1	2,934.2	3,066.2
Average supply of fat per day (grams per capita)	119.5	111.6	108.3	102.9	106.1	106.9	107.1
Average supply of protein per day (grams per capita)	101.5	104.7	104.8	99.6	96.0	97.8	99.6
Obese population (BMI 30kg/sq m or more) (% of population aged 15+)	10.7	11.2	11.2	11.3	11.5	11.6	11.7

Source: WHO/OECD/Euromonitor International

Over-the-Counter Healthcare

Argentina: Trends in OTC healthcare retail sales 1998-2004

Table: 4.33

As stated

	1998	1999	2000	2001	2002	2003	2004
OTC Healthcare (Peso million)	551.4	580.8	594.3	587.4	613.7	865.0	1,091.3
OTC Healthcare: real growth in national currency: 1998 = 100	100.0	106.6	110.1	110.0	91.3	113.4	136.5
OTC Healthcare: year on year (% real growth)	4.0	6.6	3.3	-0.1	-17.0	24.3	20.4
OTC Healthcare (Peso per capita)	15.7	16.4	16.6	16.2	16.8	23.4	29.2

Source: Euromonitor International from industry sources/national statistics

Argentina: OTC healthcare retail sales by sector 1998-2004

Table: 4.34

% of OTC retail value sales

	1998	1999	2000	2001	2002	2003	2004
Analgesics	29.0	29.2	29.5	31.0	33.2	33.5	36.5
Cough, cold and allergy (hay fever) remedies	22.3	23.1	22.5	23.3	23.4	21.7	20.4
Digestive remedies	21.6	21.3	21.5	20.1	19.7	18.9	16.0
Medicated skin care	15.5	15.3	15.2	14.5	12.5	13.3	13.0
Vitamins and dietary supplements	9.6	8.8	8.8	8.5	8.7	9.7	11.1

Source: Euromonitor International from industry sources/national statistics
Notes: Only selected sectors are shown, so values are not expected to sum to 100

■ **Australia**

Socio-economic Parameters

Australia: Socio-economic parameters 1998-2004

Table: 4.35

As stated

	1998	1999	2000	2001	2002	2003	2004
Population: national estimates at January 1st ('000)	18,711.3	18,925.9	19,153.4	19,413.2	19,662.8	19,819.9	20,014.6
% aged 0-14 yrs	21.0	20.9	20.7	20.5	20.3	19.8	19.5
% aged 15-64 yrs	66.7	66.8	66.9	66.9	67.1	67.6	67.7
% aged 65+ yrs	12.2	12.3	12.4	12.5	12.7	12.6	12.7
% Male	49.7	49.6	49.6	49.6	49.6	49.8	49.8
% Female	50.3	50.4	50.4	50.4	50.4	50.2	50.2
% Urban	84.7	84.7	84.7	84.7	84.7	84.8	84.8
Occupants per household at January 1st (Number)	2.8	2.8	2.8	2.7	2.7	2.7	2.7
Households ('000)	6,719.3	6,835.9	6,956.5	7,072.2	7,184.1	7,304.5	7,420.7
Annual rates of inflation (% growth)	0.9	1.5	4.5	4.4	3.0	2.8	2.3
GDP (A$ million)	577,561.0	605,841.0	650,324.0	689,959.0	736,775.0	785,343.0	838,481.0
GDP (US$ million)	362,828.3	390,877.8	377,036.6	356,855.7	400,299.4	509,331.3	616,643.5
GDP (US$ per capita)	19,390.9	20,653.1	19,685.1	18,382.1	20,358.2	25,698.0	30,809.7

Source: Euromonitor International from International Monetary Fund (IMF), International Financial Statistics and World Economic Outlook/UN/national statistics

Life Expectancy

Australia: Life expectancy 1998-2004

Table: 4.36

As stated

	1998	1999	2000	2001	2002	2003	2004	% change 1998-2004
Life expectancy at birth: total population (years)	79.7	79.8	79.8	80.0	80.4	80.7	80.9	1.47
Life expectancy at birth: total population: year on year growth	0.1	0.1	0.0	0.3	0.5	0.3	0.3	
Healthy life expectancy at birth (years)	73.0			71.4	71.6			
Healthy life expectancy at birth: year on year growth					0.3			

Source: Euromonitor International from World Bank

Sanitation

Australia: Improved sanitary facilities and water source 2000

Table: 4.37

As stated

	2000
Population with access to improved sanitary facilities (% of population)	100.0
Population with access to improved water source (% of population)	100.0
Population with improved access to sanitation facilities, rural (% of rural population with access)	100.0
Population with improved access to sanitation facilities, urban (% of urban population with access)	100.0

Source: National statistics/World Bank

Health Expenditure

Australia: Public health expenditure 1998-2004

Table: 4.38

As stated

	1998	1999	2000	2001	2002	2003	2004
Public expenditure on pharmaceuticals and other medical non-durables (A$ million)	3,093.0	3,536.0	4,397.0	4,832.0	4,967.0	5,047.0	5,354.9
Private insurance expenditure (% of total expenditure on health)	7.6	6.6	6.9	7.6	6.5	6.1	5.8
Share of total health expenditure in GDP (% of total GDP)	8.6	8.7	8.9	9.2	9.5	9.4	9.2
Health expenditure (US$ per capita)	1,711.0	1,871.0	1,825.0	1,739.0	1,995.0	2,036.0	2,107.0

Source: Euromonitor International from OECD/national statistics

Australia: Private health expenditure 1998-2004

Table: 4.39

As stated

	1998	1999	2000	2001	2002	2003	2004
Consumer expenditure on health goods and medical services (A$ million)	13,869.0	15,306.0	16,861.0	20,152.0	22,973.0	23,675.2	25,415.3
Consumer expenditure on health goods and medical services: real growth in national currency: 1990 = 100	128.6	139.9	147.5	168.9	186.9	187.4	196.6
Consumer expenditure on health goods and medical services as a percentage of total consumer expenditure	4.0	4.2	4.3	4.9	5.2	5.2	5.3

Source: National statistical offices/OECD/Eurostat/Euromonitor International

Australia: Consumer expenditure on health goods and medical services by sector 1998-2004

Table: 4.40

% of total consumer expenditure on health goods and medical services

	1998	1999	2000	2001	2002	2003	2004
Pharmaceuticals, medical appliances/equipment	41.9	43.3	45.5	45.5	45.6	45.6	45.7
Outpatient services	51.6	50.2	48.6	48.6	48.9	48.8	48.7
Hospital services	6.4	6.5	6.0	5.9	5.6	5.6	5.7
Total	100.0	100.0	100.0	100.0	100.0	100.0	100.0

Source: National statistical offices/OECD/Eurostat/Euromonitor International

Healthcare Infrastructure and Services

Australia: Healthcare infrastructure and services by sector 1998-2004

Table: 4.41

As stated

	1998	1999	2000	2001	2002	2003	2004
Active pharmacists (number)	11,600	11,829	15,000	12,500	12,900	16,500	17,208
Consultations with GPs (general practitioners) (per capita)	7	7	6	6	6	6	6
Dentists (number)	8,500	8,750	8,991	9,000	9,150	9,232	9,402
Doctors (number)	44,684	45,999	47,372	49,392	47,559	47,017	46,865
Hospitals and clinics (number)	1,236	1,257	1,257	1,260	1,262	1,267	1,270
In-patient beds ('000)	73	72	73	73	74	74	74
Midwives (number)	11,756	12,567	12,976	13,865	14,340	14,871	15,061
Nurses (number)	197,458	200,049	200,910	201,753	202,000	203,349	204,216

Source: Euromonitor International from national statistics

Australia: Healthcare infrastructure and services by sector: growth 1998-2004

Table: 4.42

Year on year growth: % change in stated unit

	1998	1999	2000	2001	2002	2003	2004
Active pharmacists (number)	2.1	2.0	26.8	-16.7	3.2	27.9	4.3
Consultations with GPs (general practitioners) (per capita)	-1.5	-1.5	-1.5	0.0	-3.1	-3.2	-1.7
Dentists (number)	3.0	2.9	2.8	0.1	1.7	0.9	1.8
Doctors (number)	1.1	2.9	3.0	4.3	-3.7	-1.1	-0.3
Hospitals and clinics (number)	0.9	1.7	0.0	0.2	0.2	0.4	0.2
In-patient beds (number)	-1.6	-1.0	1.0	0.3	0.3	0.1	0.2
Midwives (number)	4.6	6.9	3.3	6.9	3.4	3.7	1.3
Nurses (number)	0.9	1.3	0.4	0.4	0.1	0.7	0.4

Source: Euromonitor International from national statistics

Immunisation

Australia: Vaccination rates by disease type 1998-2004

Table: 4.43

%

	1998	1999	2000	2001	2002	2003	2004
Vaccination rate against MMR (measles, mumps, rubella) (%)	86.0	89.0	92.4	93.4	94.1	95.0	96.0
Vaccination rate against polio (%)	86.0	88.3	91.4	91.9	92.6	94.0	96.0

Source: WHO

Infectious Diseases

Australia: Incidence of disease by type 1998-2004

Table: 4.44

Number

	1998	1999	2000	2001	2002	2003	2004
Incidence of AIDS	301	181	212	27	182	189	176
Incidence of diphtheria	0	0	0	1	0		
Incidence of measles	327	235	108	141	32		
Incidence of polio	0	0	0	0	0		

Source: WHO

Australia: Incidence of disease by type: growth 1998-2004

Table: 4.45

Year on year growth: %

	1998	1999	2000	2001	2002	2003	2004
Incidence of AIDS	-18.9	-39.9	17.1	-87.3	574.1	3.8	-6.9
Incidence of diphtheria					-100.0		
Incidence of measles	-61.7	-28.1	-54.0	30.6	-77.3		

Source: WHO

Causes of Death

Australia: Deaths by disease 1998-2004

Table: 4.46

Number per 100,000 inhabitants

	1998	1999	2000	2001	2002	2003	2004
Death by diseases of the circulatory system	224.0	212.6	209.8	200.1	195.3	188.9	180.8
Death by malignant neoplasms (cancers)	167.9	163.4	164.4	163.9	158.5	156.8	155.3
Deaths from heart disease	151.1	145.9	141.2	136.4	131.6	126.9	123.3
Death by diseases of the respiratory system	42.9	41.6	39.0	38.2	37.5	35.5	34.3
Deaths from lung cancer	36.1	35.7	35.6	35.3	35.0	34.7	34.3
Death by diseases of the digestive system	17.9	18.2	17.9	18.5	19.6	20.5	21.3
Deaths from chronic liver disease and cirrhosis	5.9	5.8	5.9	6.0	6.0	6.1	6.1
Deaths from ulcers of the stomach and duodenum	2.4	2.4	2.3	2.2	2.1	2.0	1.9

Source: WHO/Euromonitor International
Notes: Data is ranked in descending order by year 2004

Australia: Deaths by disease: growth 1998-2004

Table: 4.47

% year on year growth

	1998	1999	2000	2001	2002	2003	2004
Death by diseases of the digestive system	-2.2	1.7	-1.6	3.4	5.9	4.6	4.1
Deaths from chronic liver disease and cirrhosis	5.0	-1.5	1.8	1.7	0.0	1.7	0.5
Death by malignant neoplasms (cancers)	-0.8	-2.7	0.6	-0.3	-3.3	-1.1	-1.0
Deaths from lung cancer	0.1	-1.0	-0.4	-0.8	-0.8	-0.9	-1.2
Deaths from heart disease	-3.0	-3.4	-3.2	-3.4	-3.5	-3.6	-2.8
Death by diseases of the respiratory system	-27.8	-3.0	-6.3	-2.1	-1.8	-5.3	-3.4
Death by diseases of the circulatory system	-4.4	-5.1	-1.3	-4.6	-2.4	-3.3	-4.3
Deaths from ulcers of the stomach and duodenum	-5.1	-2.0	-3.0	-4.3	-4.5	-4.8	-5.1

Source: WHO/Euromonitor International
Notes: Data is ranked in descending order by year 2004

Australia: Other selected causes of death: 1998-2004

Table: 4.48

Number per 100,000 inhabitants

	1998	1999	2000	2001	2002	2003	2004
Death by injury and poisoning	41.0	40.9	42.5	40.6	41.3	40.1	39.5
Death by suicide and self-inflicted injury	13.4	12.5	13.1	13.1	13.0	12.7	12.6
Death by motor traffic accidents	10.1	10.1	10.7	11.2	11.9	11.0	11.2

Source: Euromonitor International from national statistics
Notes: Data is ranked in descending order by year 2004

Australia: Other selected causes of death: growth 1998-2004

Table: 4.49

% year on year growth

	1998	1999	2000	2001	2002	2003	2004
Death by motor traffic accidents	3.1	0.0	5.9	4.7	6.3	-7.6	1.6
Death by suicide and self-inflicted injury	-2.2	-6.7	4.8	0.0	-0.8	-2.3	-0.9
Death by injury and poisoning	6.5	-0.2	3.9	-4.5	1.7	-2.9	-1.4

Source: Euromonitor International from national statistics
Notes: Data is ranked in descending order by year 2004

Smoking

Australia: Smoking prevalence in population aged 15+ 1998-2004

Table: 4.50

% of population aged 15+

	1998	1999	2000	2001	2002	2003	2004
Smoking prevalence in population aged 15+ (% of population aged 15+)	23.1	22.8	22.5	21.8	21.9	21.1	21.3
Smoking prevalence in male population aged 15+ (% of male population)	25.4	24.9	24.0	24.0	23.7	22.8	22.4
Smoking prevalence in female population aged 15+ (% of female population)	20.8	20.8	21.1	19.6	20.2	19.4	20.2

Source: WHO/OECD/Euromonitor International

Nutrition and Obesity

Australia: Nutrition and obesity 1998-2004

Table: 4.51

As stated

	1998	1999	2000	2001	2002	2003	2004
Average supply of calories per day (calories per capita)	3,052.3	3,063.6	3,087.5	3,129.3	3,053.6	3,013.9	3,181.8
Average supply of fat per day (grams per capita)	128.2	132.2	137.1	139.3	131.2	130.3	130.9
Average supply of protein per day (grams per capita)	100.6	102.9	103.6	104.1	103.5	103.3	103.1
Obese population (BMI 30kg/sq m or more) (% of population aged 15+)	20.4	20.8	21.5	21.6	22.0	22.9	23.1

Source: WHO/OECD/Euromonitor International

Over-the-Counter Healthcare

Australia: Trends in OTC healthcare retail sales 1998-2004

Table: 4.52

As stated

	1998	1999	2000	2001	2002	2003	2004
OTC Healthcare (A$ million)	1,502.4	1,604.6	1,700.0	1,806.4	1,917.9	2,005.0	2,098.2
OTC Healthcare: real growth in national currency: 1998 = 100	100.0	105.3	106.7	108.7	112.0	113.9	116.0
OTC Healthcare: year on year (% real growth)	4.5	5.3	1.4	1.8	3.1	1.7	1.8
OTC Healthcare (A$ per capita)	80.3	84.8	88.8	93.0	97.5	101.2	104.8

Source: Euromonitor International from industry sources/national statistics

Australia: OTC healthcare retail sales by sector 1998-2004

Table: 4.53

% of OTC retail value sales

	1998	1999	2000	2001	2002	2003	2004
Analgesics	14.2	13.7	13.0	12.8	13.1	13.1	13.3
Cough, cold and allergy (hay fever) remedies	19.0	18.9	18.9	18.7	18.6	18.3	18.0
Digestive remedies	6.8	6.6	6.5	6.3	6.1	6.1	6.0
Medicated skin care	11.5	11.4	11.1	10.9	10.5	10.3	9.9
Vitamins and dietary supplements	38.5	38.5	38.6	38.9	38.7	38.9	38.8

Source: Euromonitor International from industry sources/national statistics
Notes: Only selected sectors are shown, so values are not expected to sum to 100

Health and Wellness

Australia: Retail sales of packaged foods by health and wellness category 2002-2004

Table: 4.54

A$ million

	2002	2003	2004
Packaged food: Total	24,195.1	25,319.2	26,243.8
Better for you	2,240.7	2,468.5	2,680.1
For food intolerance	57.6	61.7	68.7
Fortified/functional	550.2	634.7	696.7
Organic	213.9	255.5	295.9

Source: Euromonitor International from industry sources/national statistics

Australia: Per capita sales of packaged foods by health and wellness category 2002-2004

Table: 4.55

A$ per capita

	2002	2003	2004
Better for you	115.2	125.3	134.3
For food intolerance	3.0	3.1	3.4
Fortified/functional	28.3	32.2	34.9
Organic	11.0	13.0	14.8

Source: Euromonitor International from industry sources/national statistics

Australia: Retail sales of packaged food by health and wellness category: % share of total packaged food market 2002-2004

Table: 4.56

% value

	2002	2003	2004
Better for you	9.3	9.7	10.2
For food intolerance	0.2	0.2	0.3
Fortified/functional	2.3	2.5	2.7
Organic	0.9	1.0	1.1

Source: Euromonitor International from industry sources/national statistics

Australia: Retail sales of packaged food by health and wellness category: real growth index 2002-2004

Table: 4.57

2002 =100

	2002	2003	2004
Better for you	100.00	107.07	113.63
For food intolerance	100.00	104.12	113.29
Fortified/functional	100.00	112.10	120.28
Organic	100.00	116.12	131.46

Source: Euromonitor International from industry sources/national statistics

Australia: Retail sales of better-for-you packaged foods by sector 2002-2004

Table: 4.58

% of total packaged food / as stated

	2002	2003	2004	% real change in value 2002-2004
Combination	0.36	0.40	0.44	24.17
Reduced carb	0.18	0.22	0.26	49.24
Reduced fat	7.70	7.97	8.23	10.23
Reduced salt	0.23	0.26	0.29	32.32

Source: Euromonitor International from industry sources/national statistics

Australia: Retail sales of packaged foods for food intolerances by sector 2002-2004

Table: 4.59

% of total packaged food / as stated

	2002	2003	2004	% real change in value 2002-2004
Gluten-free	0.02	0.02	0.03	67.66
Lactose-free	0.22	0.22	0.23	8.31

Source: *Euromonitor International from industry sources/national statistics*

Australia: Retail sales of naturally healthy packaged foods by sector 2002-2004

Table: 4.60

% of total packaged food / as stated

	2002	2003	2004	% real change in value 2002-2004
High fibre	2.06	2.10	2.13	6.71
Other naturally healthy food	0.86	0.87	0.88	4.93
Soy-based dairy alternatives	0.92	0.97	1.01	13.92

Source: *Euromonitor International from industry sources/national statistics*

■ **Austria**

Socio-economic Parameters

Austria: Socio-economic parameters 1998-2004

Table: 4.61

As stated

	1998	1999	2000	2001	2002	2003	2004
Population: national estimates at January 1st ('000)	7,976.8	7,992.3	8,011.6	8,031.6	8,053.1	8,078.5	8,104.9
% aged 0-14 yrs	17.4	17.2	17.0	16.8	16.6	16.5	16.3
% aged 15-64 yrs	67.2	67.4	67.5	67.7	67.9	68.1	68.1
% aged 65 + yrs	15.4	15.4	15.4	15.5	15.5	15.4	15.6
% Male	48.3	48.3	48.4	48.4	48.4	48.5	48.5
% Female	51.7	51.7	51.6	51.6	51.6	51.5	51.5
% Urban	64.5	64.6	64.7	64.8	65.0	65.1	65.3
Occupants per household at January 1st (Number)	2.5	2.4	2.4	2.4	2.4	2.4	2.4
Households ('000)	3,228.0	3,269.3	3,302.5	3,339.7	3,373.3	3,407.0	3,440.8
Annual rates of inflation (% growth)	0.9	0.6	2.4	2.7	1.8	1.4	2.1
GDP (EUR million)	190,018.9	197,068.3	206,675.9	212,515.3	218,337.9	224,135.2	235,107.6
GDP (US$ million)	213,011.2	209,953.8	190,414.5	190,168.6	205,484.9	252,964.5	291,926.7
GDP (US$ per capita)	26,703.9	26,269.4	23,767.4	23,677.7	25,516.2	31,313.2	36,018.6

Source: *Euromonitor International from International Monetary Fund (IMF), International Financial Statistics and World Economic Outlook/UN/national statistics*

Life Expectancy

Austria: Life expectancy 1998-2004

Table: 4.62

As stated

	1998	1999	2000	2001	2002	2003	2004	% change 1998-2004
Life expectancy at birth: total population (years)	78.4	78.5	78.6	79.0	79.4	79.5	79.8	1.90
Life expectancy at birth: total population: year on year growth	0.3	0.2	0.1	0.5	0.5	0.2	0.4	
Healthy life expectancy at birth (years)	72.0			70.7	71.0			
Healthy life expectancy at birth: year on year growth					0.4			

Source: *Euromonitor International from World Bank*

Sanitation

Austria: Improved sanitary facilities and water source 2000

Table: 4.63

As stated

	2000
Population with access to improved sanitary facilities (% of population)	100.0
Population with access to improved water source (% of population)	100.0
Population with improved access to sanitation facilities, rural (% of rural population with access)	100.0
Population with improved access to sanitation facilities, urban (% of urban population with access)	100.0

Source: National statistics/World Bank

Health Expenditure

Austria: Public health expenditure 1998-2004

Table: 4.64

As stated

	1998	1999	2000	2001	2002	2003	2004
Public expenditure on pharmaceuticals and other medical non-durables (EUR million)	1,516.0	1,656.0	1,805.0	1,889.0	2,029.0	2,175.0	2,360.5
Private insurance expenditure (% of total expenditure on health)	7.6	7.3	7.3	7.4	7.4	7.1	7.0
Share of total health expenditure in GDP (% of total GDP)	8.0	8.0	8.0	8.0	8.0	8.2	7.8
Health expenditure (US$ per capita)	2,040.0	2,047.0	1,831.0	1,805.0	1,969.0	2,038.0	2,107.0

Source: Euromonitor International from OECD/national statistics

Austria: Private health expenditure 1998-2004

Table: 4.65

As stated

	1998	1999	2000	2001	2002	2003	2004
Consumer expenditure on health goods and medical services (EUR million)	3,521.0	3,682.0	3,848.0	3,949.0	4,104.0	4,231.0	4,385.3
Consumer expenditure on health goods and medical services: real growth in national currency: 1990 = 100	139.7	145.3	148.3	148.3	151.4	153.9	156.4
Consumer expenditure on health goods and medical services as a percentage of total consumer expenditure	3.2	3.3	3.3	3.2	3.3	3.3	3.3

Source: National statistical offices/OECD/Eurostat/Euromonitor International

Austria: Consumer expenditure on health goods and medical services by sector 1998-2004

Table: 4.66

% of total consumer expenditure on health goods and medical services

	1998	1999	2000	2001	2002	2003	2004
Pharmaceuticals, medical appliances/ equipment	22.3	22.3	22.3	22.1	22.1	21.9	22.1
Outpatient services	48.5	48.5	48.5	48.8	49.2	49.5	49.6
Hospital services	29.2	29.2	29.2	29.1	28.8	28.6	28.3
Total	100.0	100.0	100.0	100.0	100.0	100.0	100.0

Source: National statistical offices/OECD/Eurostat/Euromonitor International

Healthcare Infrastructure and Services

Austria: Healthcare infrastructure and services by sector 1998-2004

Table: 4.67

As stated

	1998	1999	2000	2001	2002	2003	2004
Active pharmacists (number)	4,337	4,439	4,532	4,581	4,704	4,810	4,912
Consultations with GPs (general practitioners) (per capita)	7	7	7	7	7	7	7
Dentists (number)	3,813	3,721	3,732	3,838	4,109	4,239	4,340
Doctors (number)	24,368	24,505	25,332	26,286	26,711	27,233	27,825
Hospital admissions (number)	2,246,381	2,329,887	2,370,977	2,416,263	2,512,275	2,537,575	2,596,405
Hospitals and clinics (number)	330	325	312	310	278	267	258
In-patient beds ('000)	51	51	50	50	50	50	50
In-patient surgical procedures (number)	1,037,131	1,050,562	1,055,642	1,066,157	1,084,016	1,079,205	1,099,313
Midwives (number)		1,093	1,132	1,168	1,212	1,252
Nurses (number)	71,849	73,084	74,601	74,948	74,922	75,621	76,301
Out-patient contacts (per capita)	7	7	7	7	7	7	7

Source: Euromonitor International from national statistics

Austria: Healthcare infrastructure and services by sector: growth 1998-2004

Table: 4.68

Year on year growth: % change in stated unit

	1998	1999	2000	2001	2002	2003	2004
Active pharmacists (number)	1.7	2.4	2.1	1.1	2.7	2.3	2.1
Consultations with GPs (general practitioners) (per capita)	4.8	3.1	0.0	0.0	0.0	0.0	0.0
Dentists (number)	-0.9	-2.4	0.3	2.8	7.1	3.2	2.4
Doctors (number)	4.5	0.6	3.4	3.8	1.6	2.0	2.2
Hospital admissions (number)	4.4	3.7	1.8	1.9	4.0	1.0	2.3
Hospitals and clinics (number)	0.3	-1.5	-4.0	-0.6	-10.3	-4.0	-3.4
In-patient beds (number)	-1.4	-1.0	-1.0	0.2	-0.5	-0.2	-0.2
In-patient surgical procedures (number)	8.3	1.3	0.5	1.0	1.7	-0.4	1.9
Midwives (number)				3.6	3.2	3.8	3.3
Nurses (number)	1.2	1.7	2.1	0.5	0.0	0.9	0.9
Out-patient contacts (per capita)	4.8	3.1	0.0	0.0	-1.5	1.5	3.0

Source: Euromonitor International from national statistics

Immunisation

Austria: Vaccination rates by disease type 1998-2004

Table: 4.69

%

	1998	1999	2000	2001	2002	2003	2004
Vaccination rate against DTP (diphtheria, tetanus, pertussis) 1 & 2 (%)				63.8	76.8	78.0	87.0
Vaccination rate against MMR (measles, mumps, rubella) (%)				65.3	78.5	92.0	93.0
Vaccination rate against polio (%)					82.5	85.0	85.0

Source: WHO

Infectious Diseases

Austria: Incidence of disease by type 1998-2004

Table: 4.70

Number

	1998	1999	2000	2001	2002	2003	2004
Incidence of AIDS	111	89	84	70	70	17	23
Incidence of diphtheria	0	0	0	0	0		
Incidence of measles	0	1		0			
Incidence of polio	0	0	0	0	0		

Source: WHO

Austria: Incidence of disease by type: growth 1998-2004

Table: 4.71

Year on year growth: %

	1998	1999	2000	2001	2002	2003	2004
Incidence of AIDS	-14.6	-19.8	-5.6	-16.7	0.0	-75.7	35.3

Source: WHO

Causes of Death

Austria: Deaths by disease 1998-2004

Table: 4.72

Number per 100,000 inhabitants

	1998	1999	2000	2001	2002	2003	2004
Death by diseases of the circulatory system	328.3	319.2	296.8	279.0	263.0	262.0	252.1
Deaths from heart disease	216.7	212.0	200.3	193.3	185.3	177.3	169.6
Death by malignant neoplasms (cancers)	168.6	167.0	164.8	160.1	161.3	155.8	153.2
Deaths from lung cancer	41.1	40.1	40.3	39.6	39.0	38.4	37.6
Death by diseases of the respiratory system	27.9	31.1	31.1	29.5	32.4	31.0	31.2
Death by diseases of the digestive system	31.7	29.4	30.5	29.2	27.0	26.5	25.5
Deaths from chronic liver disease and cirrhosis	23.6	21.6	22.4	21.3	20.7	20.0	19.3
Deaths from ulcers of the stomach and duodenum	3.5	2.9	3.2	2.9	2.8	2.6	2.4

Source: WHO/Euromonitor International
Notes: Data is ranked in descending order by year 2004

Austria: Deaths by disease: growth 1998-2004

Table: 4.73

% year on year growth

	1998	1999	2000	2001	2002	2003	2004
Death by diseases of the respiratory system	-1.1	11.5	0.0	-5.1	9.8	-4.3	0.8
Death by malignant neoplasms (cancers)	-2.3	-0.9	-1.3	-2.9	0.7	-3.4	-1.7
Deaths from lung cancer	1.7	-2.5	0.5	-1.8	-1.5	-1.5	-2.0
Death by diseases of the digestive system	-1.9	-7.3	3.7	-4.3	-7.5	-1.9	-3.7
Deaths from chronic liver disease and cirrhosis	-2.7	-8.6	3.6	-4.7	-2.8	-3.4	-3.7
Death by diseases of the circulatory system	-2.6	-2.8	-7.0	-6.0	-5.7	-0.4	-3.8
Deaths from heart disease	2.4	-2.2	-5.5	-3.5	-4.1	-4.3	-4.4
Deaths from ulcers of the stomach and duodenum	-11.9	-18.2	11.8	-9.5	-3.4	-7.1	-6.6

Source: WHO/Euromonitor International
Notes: Data is ranked in descending order by year 2004

Austria: Other selected causes of death: 1998-2004

Table: 4.74

Number per 100,000 inhabitants

	1998	1999	2000	2001	2002	2003	2004
Death by injury and poisoning	43.9	45.8	46.0	42.9	42.6	40.8	39.5
Death by suicide and self-inflicted injury	16.5	16.3	16.5	15.4	16.2	15.9	15.7
Death by motor traffic accidents	10.7	12.3	11.2	10.8	11.4	10.4	10.1

Source: Euromonitor International from national statistics
Notes: Data is ranked in descending order by year 2004

Austria: Other selected causes of death: growth 1998-2004

Table: 4.75

% year on year growth

	1998	1999	2000	2001	2002	2003	2004
Death by suicide and self-inflicted injury	-2.4	-1.2	1.2	-6.7	5.2	-1.9	-1.4
Death by motor traffic accidents	-18.3	15.0	-8.9	-3.6	5.6	-8.8	-2.9
Death by injury and poisoning	-6.6	4.3	0.4	-6.7	-0.7	-4.2	-3.2

Source: Euromonitor International from national statistics
Notes: Data is ranked in descending order by year 2004

Smoking

Austria: Smoking prevalence in population aged 15+ 1998-2004

Table: 4.76

% of population aged 15+

	1998	1999	2000	2001	2002	2003	2004
Smoking prevalence in population aged 15+ (% of population aged 15+)	29.3	28.9	29.0	28.7	28.7	28.4	28.3
Smoking prevalence in male population aged 15+ (% of male population)	34.9	34.3	34.1	33.8	33.0	32.5	32.0
Smoking prevalence in female population aged 15+ (% of female population)	24.2	23.9	23.8	24.1	24.8	24.6	24.9

Source: WHO/OECD/Euromonitor International

Nutrition and Obesity

Austria: Nutrition and obesity 1998-2004

Table: 4.77

As stated

	1998	1999	2000	2001	2002	2003	2004
Availability of fruit and vegetables (kg/capita/year)	178.0	212.3	218.0	223.5	245.0	258.8	271.7
Average supply of calories per day (calories per capita)	3,671.3	3,732.9	3,760.6	3,779.5	3,673.3	3,612.3	3,557.7
Average supply of fat per day (grams per capita)	161.9	163.4	162.4	164.3	158.2	154.5	151.4
Average supply of protein per day (grams per capita)	108.6	110.4	109.7	111.0	109.6	108.8	108.3
Obese population (BMI 30kg/sq m or more) (% of population aged 15+)	9.1	9.1	10.1	12.6	14.5	16.3	17.8

Source: WHO/OECD/Euromonitor International

Over-the-Counter Healthcare

Austria: Trends in OTC healthcare retail sales 1998-2004

Table: 4.78

As stated

	1998	1999	2000	2001	2002	2003	2004
OTC Healthcare (EUR million)	335.8	351.3	359.4	369.5	382.8	404.8	419.0
OTC Healthcare: real growth in national currency: 1998 = 100	100.0	104.0	104.0	104.2	106.0	110.5	112.5
OTC Healthcare: year on year (% real growth)	2.0	4.0	-0.1	0.2	1.7	4.3	1.8

Source: Euromonitor International from industry sources/national statistics

Austria: OTC healthcare retail sales by sector 1998-2004

Table: 4.79

% of OTC retail value sales

	1998	1999	2000	2001	2002	2003	2004
Analgesics	11.2	11.0	10.6	10.4	10.8	10.9	10.6
Cough, cold and allergy (hay fever) remedies	29.8	30.4	30.2	30.7	30.4	31.2	31.4
Digestive remedies	58,102.5	55,640.2	53,158.0	50,909.9	49,255.9	47,315.9	46,518.0
Digestive remedies	7.8	7.5	7.4	7.4	7.3	7.2	7.2
Medicated skin care	12.8	12.5	12.3	12.1	12.0	11.7	11.7
Vitamins and dietary supplements	29.2	29.5	30.2	30.1	30.1	29.7	29.6

Source: Euromonitor International from industry sources/national statistics
Notes: Only selected sectors are shown, so values are not expected to sum to 100

■ **Azerbaijan**

Socio-economic Parameters

Azerbaijan: Socio-economic parameters 1998-2004

Table: 4.80

As stated

	1998	1999	2000	2001	2002	2003	2004
Population: national estimates at January 1st ('000)	7,990.5	8,057.0	8,122.9	8,190.6	8,260.5	8,332.6	8,407.6
% aged 0-14 yrs	33.0	32.5	31.9	31.2	30.5	29.6	28.8
% aged 15-64 yrs	61.7	62.1	62.6	63.1	63.6	64.1	64.7
% aged 65+ yrs	5.3	5.4	5.5	5.7	5.9	6.2	6.5
% Male	48.8	48.8	48.8	48.8	48.8	48.7	48.7
% Female	51.2	51.2	51.2	51.2	51.2	51.3	51.3
% Urban	56.7	57.0	57.1	57.4	57.8	58.3	58.7
Occupants per household at January 1st (Number)	2.6	2.6	2.6	2.5	2.5	2.5	2.5
Households ('000)	3,045.9	3,103.1	3,174.3	3,218.9	3,277.6	3,332.0	3,385.2
Annual rates of inflation (% growth)	-0.7	-8.6	1.8	1.5	2.8	2.2	8.1
GDP (AZM million)	17,172,175.0	18,875,300.0	23,590,500.0	26,578,000.0	30,312,300.0	35,053,600.0	41,872,700.0
GDP (US$ million)	4,438.4	4,581.2	5,272.6	5,707.6	6,236.0	7,138.2	8,522.0
GDP (US$ per capita)	555.5	568.6	649.1	696.9	754.9	856.7	1,013.6

Source: Euromonitor International from International Monetary Fund (IMF), International Financial Statistics and World Economic Outlook/UN/national statistics

Life Expectancy

Azerbaijan: Life expectancy 1998-2004

Table: 4.81

As stated

	1998	1999	2000	2001	2002	2003	2004	% change 1998-2004
Life expectancy at birth: total population (years)	63.0	63.2	62.3	63.6	65.8	66.7	67.8	7.74
Life expectancy at birth: total population: year on year growth	0.4	0.4	-1.5	2.1	3.5	1.3	1.8	
Healthy life expectancy at birth (years)	64.0			51.7	52.8			
Healthy life expectancy at birth: year on year growth					2.2			

Source: Euromonitor International from World Bank

Sanitation

Azerbaijan: Improved sanitary facilities and water source 2000

Table: 4.82

As stated

	2000
Population with access to improved sanitary facilities (% of population)	81.0
Population with access to improved water source (% of population)	78.0
Population with improved access to sanitation facilities, rural (% of rural population with access)	70.0
Population with improved access to sanitation facilities, urban (% of urban population with access)	90.0

Source: National statistics/World Bank

Health Expenditure

Azerbaijan: Public health expenditure 1998-2004

Table: 4.83

As stated

	1998	1999	2000	2001	2002	2003	2004
Share of total health expenditure in GDP (% of total GDP)	2.3	2.0	1.7	1.6	1.7	1.7	1.7
Health expenditure (US$ per capita)	26.0	26.0	25.0	26.0	27.0	27.0	28.0

Source: Euromonitor International from OECD/national statistics

Azerbaijan: Private health expenditure 1998-2004

Table: 4.84

As stated

	1998	1999	2000	2001	2002	2003	2004
Consumer expenditure on health goods and medical services (AZM million)	514,244.0	566,788.7	597,331.3	628,699.0	675,483.0	746,268.5	801,390.2
Consumer expenditure on health goods and medical services as a percentage of total consumer expenditure	3.8	4.2	4.2	4.2	4.3	4.3	4.3

Source: National statistical offices/OECD/Eurostat/Euromonitor International

Azerbaijan: Consumer expenditure on health goods and medical services by sector 1998-2004

Table: 4.85

% of total consumer expenditure on health goods and medical services

	1998	1999	2000	2001	2002	2003	2004
Pharmaceuticals, medical appliances/ equipment	43.7	44.7	44.7	45.5	45.2	45.4	45.8
Outpatient services	49.0	51.0	51.5	50.8	51.2	51.0	50.6
Hospital services	7.3	4.3	3.8	3.7	3.6	3.6	3.7
Total	100.0	100.0	100.0	100.0	100.0	100.0	100.0

Source: National statistical offices/OECD/Eurostat/Euromonitor International

Healthcare Infrastructure and Services

Azerbaijan: Healthcare infrastructure and services by sector 1998-2004

Table: 4.86

As stated

	1998	1999	2000	2001	2002	2003	2004
Active pharmacists (number)	2,607	2,634	2,666	2,685	2,706	2,726	2,754
Dentists (number)	2,279	2,242	2,240	2,238	2,304	2,367	2,402
Doctors (number)	28,500	28,500	29,033	29,100	29,226	29,457	29,732
Hospital admissions (number)	400,220	382,916	385,173	394,417	398,293	406,064	411,629
Hospitals and clinics (number)	746	739	735	735	731	725	722
In-patient beds ('000)	72	71	70	69	68	67	66
In-patient surgical procedures (number)		81,263	83,062	87,803	89,505	93,886	96,647
Nurses (number)	60,700	58,100	58,000	57,900	58,896	59,230	59,560
Out-patient contacts (per capita)		5	5	5	5	4	4

Source: Euromonitor International from national statistics

Azerbaijan: Healthcare infrastructure and services by sector: growth 1998-2004

Table: 4.87

Year on year growth: % change in stated unit

	1998	1999	2000	2001	2002	2003	2004
Active pharmacists (number)	1.0	1.0	1.2	0.7	0.8	0.7	1.0
Dentists (number)	-6.1	-1.6	-0.1	-0.1	2.9	2.7	1.5
Doctors (number)	-1.4	0.0	1.9	0.2	0.4	0.8	0.9
Hospital admissions (number)	-8.1	-4.3	0.6	2.4	1.0	2.0	1.4
Hospitals and clinics (number)	-1.7	-0.9	-0.5	0.0	-0.5	-0.8	-0.4
In-patient beds (number)	-1.0	-1.0	-1.5	-1.3	-1.4	-1.5	-1.5
In-patient surgical procedures (number)			2.2	5.7	1.9	4.9	2.9
Nurses (number)	-4.0	-4.3	-0.2	-0.2	1.7	0.6	0.6
Out-patient contacts (per capita)			-2.0	-1.6	-8.5	-4.4	2.3

Source: Euromonitor International from national statistics

Immunisation

Azerbaijan: Vaccination rates by disease type 1998-2004

Table: 4.88

%

	1998	1999	2000	2001	2002	2003	2004
Vaccination rate against DTP (diphtheria, tetanus, pertussis) 1 & 2 (%)				97.7	97.3	97.0	97.0
Vaccination rate against MMR (measles, mumps, rubella) (%)	97.7	98.4	98.5	98.9	97.5	98.0	97.0
Vaccination rate against polio (%)	98.1	98.9	98.9	98.6	99.5	99.0	100.0

Source: WHO

Infectious Diseases

Azerbaijan: Incidence of disease by type 1998-2004

Table: 4.89

Number

	1998	1999	2000	2001	2002	2003	2004
Incidence of AIDS	3	8	19	17	14	7	8
Incidence of diphtheria	20	19	7	0	0		
Incidence of measles	2,891	1,081	210	574	4,353		
Incidence of polio	0	0	0	0	0		

Source: WHO

Azerbaijan: Incidence of disease by type: growth 1998-2004

Table: 4.90

Year on year growth: %

	1998	1999	2000	2001	2002	2003	2004
Incidence of AIDS	-40.0	166.7	137.5	-10.5	-17.6	-50.0	14.3
Incidence of diphtheria	-47.4	-5.0	-63.2	-100.0			
Incidence of measles	326.4	-62.6	-80.6	173.3	658.4		

Source: WHO

Causes of Death

Azerbaijan: Deaths by disease 1998-2004

Table: 4.91

Number per 100,000 inhabitants

	1998	1999	2000	2001	2002	2003	2004
Death by diseases of the circulatory system	250.9	254.8	262.2	261.6	264.3	267.6	267.5
Deaths from heart disease	209.8	134.6	214.3	190.2	192.4	194.6	187.7
Death by malignant neoplasms (cancers)	63.4	66.3	64.1	63.1	61.6	60.9	59.6
Death by diseases of the respiratory system	59.4	55.4	53.1	51.9	51.1	49.8	48.4
Death by diseases of the digestive system	48.7	47.3	46.5	45.6	45.0	44.2	43.2
Deaths from lung cancer	8.8	9.4	9.1	9.9	10.1	10.3	10.7
Deaths from ulcers of the stomach and duodenum	3.6	3.4	3.6	3.7	3.7	3.7	3.8

Source: WHO/Euromonitor International
Notes: Data is ranked in descending order by year 2004

Azerbaijan: Deaths by disease: growth 1998-2004

Table: 4.92

% year on year growth

	1998	1999	2000	2001	2002	2003	2004
Deaths from lung cancer	-10.3	7.4	-2.9	8.4	2.0	2.0	3.6
Deaths from ulcers of the stomach and duodenum	-13.6	-5.4	6.2	3.4	0.0	0.0	2.0
Death by diseases of the circulatory system	-19.9	1.6	2.9	-0.2	1.0	1.2	0.0
Death by diseases of the digestive system	-0.8	-2.9	-1.7	-1.9	-1.3	-1.8	-2.2
Death by malignant neoplasms (cancers)	1.8	4.6	-3.3	-1.6	-2.4	-1.1	-2.2
Death by diseases of the respiratory system	-13.9	-6.7	-4.2	-2.3	-1.5	-2.5	-2.9
Deaths from heart disease	-3.2	-35.8	59.2	-11.2	1.2	1.1	-3.6

Source: WHO/Euromonitor International
Notes: Data is ranked in descending order by year 2004

Azerbaijan: Other selected causes of death: 1998-2004

Table: 4.93

Number per 100,000 inhabitants

	1998	1999	2000	2001	2002	2003	2004
Death by suicide and self-inflicted injury	31.9	27.9	26.4	24.3	23.3	21.5	19.9

Source: Euromonitor International from national statistics

Azerbaijan: Other selected causes of death: growth 1998-2004

Table: 4.94

% year on year growth

	1998	1999	2000	2001	2002	2003	2004
Death by suicide and self-inflicted injury	-7.3	-12.5	-5.4	-8.0	-4.1	-7.7	-7.5

Source: Euromonitor International from national statistics

Smoking

Azerbaijan: Smoking prevalence in population aged 15+ 1998-2004

Table: 4.95

% of population aged 15+

	1998	1999	2000	2001	2002	2003	2004
Smoking prevalence in population aged 15+ (% of population aged 15+)	22.9	22.8	22.6	22.5	22.4	22.3	22.2
Smoking prevalence in male population aged 15+ (% of male population)	30.5	30.2	29.9	29.6	29.6	29.5	29.3
Smoking prevalence in female population aged 15+ (% of female population)	15.9	16.1	16.1	16.0	15.8	15.8	15.7

Source: WHO/OECD/Euromonitor International

Nutrition and Obesity

Azerbaijan: Nutrition and obesity 1998-2004

Table: 4.96

As stated

	1998	1999	2000	2001	2002	2003	2004
Availability of fruit and vegetables (kg/capita/year)	133.0	149.3	152.1	178.4	189.5	204.0	216.0
Average supply of calories per day (calories per capita)	2,159.5	2,277.6	2,392.7	2,476.3	2,574.8	2,678.5	2,784.4
Average supply of fat per day (grams per capita)	34.8	39.0	37.0	39.2	42.0	44.1	46.5
Average supply of protein per day (grams per capita)	65.8	67.6	71.3	73.1	74.5	76.4	78.3
Microbiological food-borne diseases (per 100000 population)	0.0	4.0	2.0	0.0	0.0	0.0	0.0
Obese population (BMI 30kg/sq m or more) (% of population aged 15+)	7.6	7.5	7.6	7.7	7.7	7.7	7.7

Source: WHO/OECD/Euromonitor International

■ Belarus

Socio-economic Parameters

Belarus: Socio-economic parameters 1998-2004

Table: 4.97

As stated

	1998	1999	2000	2001	2002	2003	2004
Population: national estimates at January 1st ('000)	10,093.0	10,050.9	10,019.5	9,990.4	9,950.9	9,898.6	9,858.3
% aged 0-14 yrs	20.4	19.6	18.9	18.3	17.5	16.9	16.2
% aged 15-64 yrs	66.4	67.1	67.8	68.2	68.7	69.1	69.5
% aged 65+ yrs	13.2	13.3	13.3	13.5	13.8	14.0	14.3
% Male	46.9	47.0	46.9	46.9	46.9	46.9	46.8
% Female	53.1	53.0	53.1	53.1	53.1	53.1	53.2
% Urban	70.2	70.7	71.2	71.1	71.0	72.2	72.6
Occupants per household at January 1st (Number)	2.6	2.6	2.6	2.6	2.5	2.5	2.5
Households ('000)	3,830.1	3,855.0	3,898.7	3,909.4	3,931.2	3,940.1	3,950.9
Annual rates of inflation (% growth)	72.9	293.7	168.6	61.1	42.5	28.4	18.1
GDP (BRb million)	702,161.0	3,026,060.0	9,133,800.0	17,173,200.0	26,138,300.0	36,564,800.0	49,445,200.0
GDP (US$ million)	15,222.1	12,138.5	10,417.8	12,354.8	14,594.9	17,825.4	22,888.5
GDP (US$ per capita)	1,508.2	1,207.7	1,039.8	1,236.7	1,466.7	1,800.8	2,321.7

Source: Euromonitor International from International Monetary Fund (IMF), International Financial Statistics and World Economic Outlook/UN/national statistics

Life Expectancy

Belarus: Life expectancy 1998-2004

Table: 4.98

As stated

	1998	1999	2000	2001	2002	2003	2004	% change 1998-2004
Life expectancy at birth: total population (years)	68.5	68.5	69.0	68.5	68.3	68.5	68.4	-0.09
Life expectancy at birth: total population: year on year growth	0.1	0.0	0.7	-0.7	-0.3	0.2	-0.1	
Healthy life expectancy at birth (years)	62.0			58.8	58.4			
Healthy life expectancy at birth: year on year growth					-0.6			

Source: *Euromonitor International from World Bank*

Sanitation

Belarus: Improved sanitary facilities and water source 2000

Table: 4.99

As stated

	2000
Population with access to improved water source (% of population)	100.0
Population with improved access to sanitation facilities, rural (% of rural population with access)	100.0
Population with improved access to sanitation facilities, urban (% of urban population with access)	100.0

Source: *National statistics/World Bank*

Health Expenditure

Belarus: Public health expenditure 1998-2004

Table: 4.100

As stated

	1998	1999	2000	2001	2002	2003	2004
Share of total health expenditure in GDP (% of total GDP)	5.7	5.8	5.4	5.6	5.5	5.6	5.6
Health expenditure (US$ per capita)	90.0	73.0	64.0	82.0	93.0	100.0	108.0

Source: *Euromonitor International from OECD/national statistics*

Belarus: Private health expenditure 1998-2004

Table: 4.101

As stated

	1998	1999	2000	2001	2002	2003	2004
Consumer expenditure on health goods and medical services (BRb million)	36,624.1	160,946.0	479,512.5	916,836.8	1,449,674.2	1,925,072.6	2,353,838.7
Consumer expenditure on health goods and medical services as a percentage of total consumer expenditure	9.6	9.6	9.6	9.6	9.6	9.3	9.2

Source: *National statistical offices/OECD/Eurostat/Euromonitor International*

Belarus: Consumer expenditure on health goods and medical services by sector 1998-2004

Table: 4.102

% of total consumer expenditure on health goods and medical services

	1998	1999	2000	2001	2002	2003	2004
Pharmaceuticals, medical appliances/ equipment	11.1	10.4	9.7	9.7	9.2	9.4	9.6
Outpatient services	77.4	77.3	78.1	79.4	80.1	80.0	79.8
Hospital services	11.5	12.3	12.3	10.9	10.7	10.7	10.5
Total	100.0	100.0	100.0	100.0	100.0	100.0	100.0

Source: *National statistical offices/OECD/Eurostat/Euromonitor International*

Healthcare Infrastructure and Services

Belarus: Healthcare infrastructure and services by sector 1998-2004

Table: 4.103

As stated

	1998	1999	2000	2001	2002	2003	2004
Dentists (number)	6,157	6,336	6,415	6,415	6,392	6,334	6,270
Doctors (number)	45,200	45,900	45,800	44,900	44,800	44,800	44,600
Hospital admissions (number)	2,957,838	2,962,015	2,926,973	2,992,786	2,908,655	2,906,940	2,894,920
Hospitals and clinics (number)	836	833	830	826	824	823	822
In-patient beds ('000)	127	127	127	127	128	128	128
In-patient surgical procedures (number)		670,016					
Midwives (number)	6,893	6,713	6,521	6,365	6,282	6,188	6,094
Nurses (number)	74,567	75,214	75,643	76,074	76,060	76,220	76,289
Out-patient contacts (per capita)	12	12	12	12	11	12	11

Source: Euromonitor International from national statistics

Belarus: Healthcare infrastructure and services by sector: growth 1998-2004

Table: 4.104

Year on year growth: % change in stated unit

	1998	1999	2000	2001	2002	2003	2004
Dentists (number)	4.5	2.9	1.2	0.0	-0.4	-0.9	-1.0
Doctors (number)	1.3	1.5	-0.2	-2.0	-0.2	0.0	-0.4
Hospital admissions (number)	10.9	0.1	-1.2	2.2	-2.8	-0.1	-0.4
Hospitals and clinics (number)	-0.4	-0.4	-0.4	-0.5	-0.2	-0.1	-0.1
In-patient beds (number)	0.4	0.3	0.2	0.2	0.2	0.2	0.3
Midwives (number)	-3.3	-2.6	-2.9	-2.4	-1.3	-1.5	-1.5
Nurses (number)	1.7	0.9	0.6	0.6	0.0	0.2	0.1
Out-patient contacts (per capita)	3.6	2.6	-1.7	-0.9	-1.7	4.4	-5.9

Source: Euromonitor International from national statistics

Immunisation

Belarus: Vaccination rates by disease type 1998-2004

Table: 4.105

%

	1998	1999	2000	2001	2002	2003	2004
Vaccination rate against MMR (measles, mumps, rubella) (%)	98.0	98.0	98.2	98.9	99.0	99.0	99.0
Vaccination rate against polio (%)	99.0	99.0	99.2	99.3	99.0	99.0	99.0

Source: WHO

Infectious Diseases

Belarus: Incidence of disease by type 1998-2004

Table: 4.106

Number

	1998	1999	2000	2001	2002	2003	2004
Incidence of AIDS	4	5	3	2	21	12	15
Incidence of diphtheria	36	38	52	25	7		
Incidence of measles	517	153	21	45	14		
Incidence of polio	0	0	0	0	0		

Source: WHO

Belarus: Incidence of disease by type: growth 1998-2004

Table: 4.107

Year on year growth: %

	1998	1999	2000	2001	2002	2003	2004
Incidence of AIDS	100.0	25.0	-40.0	-33.3	950.0	-42.9	25.0
Incidence of diphtheria	-62.5	5.6	36.8	-51.9	-72.0		
Incidence of measles	283.0	-70.4	-86.3	114.3	-68.9		

Source: WHO

Causes of Death

Belarus: Deaths by disease 1998-2004

Table: 4.108

Number per 100,000 inhabitants

	1998	1999	2000	2001	2002	2003	2004
Death by diseases of the circulatory system	700.2	715.9	732.0	748.5	764.4	780.7	798.4
Deaths from heart disease	447.1	492.6	474.8	499.4	513.5	527.7	547.7
Death by malignant neoplasms (cancers)	193.6	195.1	196.6	198.1	198.6	199.6	202.0
Death by diseases of the respiratory system	67.4	66.6	65.8	65.0	64.2	65.5	65.5
Deaths from lung cancer	38.2	37.6	37.1	36.2	35.4	34.4	33.4
Death by diseases of the digestive system	21.7	22.5	23.1	23.0	24.1	24.4	25.1
Deaths from ulcers of the stomach and duodenum	3.9	3.7	3.7	3.6	3.5	3.3	3.1

Source: WHO/Euromonitor International
Notes: Data is ranked in descending order by year 2004

Belarus: Deaths by disease: growth 1998-2004

Table: 4.109

% year on year growth

	1998	1999	2000	2001	2002	2003	2004
Deaths from heart disease	4.2	10.2	-3.6	5.2	2.8	2.8	3.8
Death by diseases of the digestive system	-0.9	3.7	2.7	-0.4	4.8	1.2	2.8
Death by diseases of the circulatory system	3.9	2.2	2.2	2.3	2.1	2.1	2.3
Death by malignant neoplasms (cancers)	0.9	0.8	0.8	0.8	0.3	0.5	1.2
Death by diseases of the respiratory system	-1.9	-1.2	-1.2	-1.2	-1.2	2.0	-0.1
Deaths from lung cancer	-2.9	-1.7	-1.4	-2.3	-2.2	-2.8	-3.0
Deaths from ulcers of the stomach and duodenum	-1.2	-5.6	1.7	-3.2	-2.8	-5.7	-4.8

Source: WHO/Euromonitor International
Notes: Data is ranked in descending order by year 2004

Belarus: Other selected causes of death: 1998-2004

Table: 4.110

Number per 100,000 inhabitants

	1998	1999	2000	2001	2002	2003	2004
Death by injury and poisoning	108.2	117.0	126.5	126.8	136.7	131.9	132.7
Death by suicide and self-inflicted injury	35.0	35.3	35.6	35.9	36.2	35.8	35.7
Death by motor traffic accidents	22.7	23.8	25.0	25.3	26.5	26.7	27.2

Source: Euromonitor International from national statistics
Notes: Data is ranked in descending order by year 2004

Belarus: Other selected causes of death: growth 1998-2004

% year on year growth

	1998	1999	2000	2001	2002	2003	2004
Death by motor traffic accidents	9.1	4.8	5.0	1.2	4.7	0.8	2.0
Death by injury and poisoning	9.3	8.1	8.1	0.2	7.8	-3.5	0.6
Death by suicide and self-inflicted injury	0.9	0.9	0.8	0.8	0.8	-1.1	-0.2

Source: Euromonitor International from national statistics
Notes: Data is ranked in descending order by year 2004

Smoking

Belarus: Smoking prevalence in population aged 15+ 1998-2004

% of population aged 15+

	1998	1999	2000	2001	2002	2003	2004
Smoking prevalence in population aged 15+ (% of population aged 15+)	26.6	26.3	26.9	26.3	26.6	28.6	28.2
Smoking prevalence in male population aged 15+ (% of male population)	54.9	53.7	54.0	53.3	53.0	52.1	51.2
Smoking prevalence in female population aged 15+ (% of female population)	4.6	4.8	6.7	6.3	6.3	8.6	8.6

Source: WHO/OECD/Euromonitor International

Nutrition and Obesity

Belarus: Nutrition and obesity 1998-2004

As stated

	1998	1999	2000	2001	2002	2003	2004
Availability of fruit and vegetables (kg/capita/year)	111.6	113.4	119.1	122.0	126.0	129.4	134.2
Average supply of calories per day (calories per capita)	3,248.8	3,086.6	2,988.1	3,031.1	3,000.3	2,972.3	2,955.5
Average supply of fat per day (grams per capita)	101.4	101.4	94.6	102.5	97.8	95.1	94.0
Average supply of protein per day (grams per capita)	95.5	91.9	85.5	89.1	86.1	83.8	82.5
Microbiological food-borne diseases (per 100000 population)	24.0	45.0	16.0	8.0	9.0	10.0	10.0
Obese population (BMI 30kg/sq m or more) (% of population aged 15+)	6.8	6.7	6.7	6.7	6.7	6.5	6.5

Source: WHO/OECD/Euromonitor International

■ **Belgium**

Socio-economic Parameters

Belgium: Socio-economic parameters 1998-2004

Table: 4.114

As stated

	1998	1999	2000	2001	2002	2003	2004
Population: national estimates at January 1st ('000)	10,192.3	10,213.8	10,239.1	10,263.4	10,309.7	10,355.0	10,393.1
% aged 0-14 yrs	17.7	17.7	17.6	17.6	17.5	17.4	17.3
% aged 15-64 yrs	65.8	65.7	65.6	65.6	65.6	65.7	65.8
% aged 65 + yrs	16.5	16.6	16.8	16.9	16.9	16.9	16.9
% Male	48.9	48.9	48.9	48.9	48.9	48.9	48.9
% Female	51.1	51.1	51.1	51.1	51.1	51.1	51.1
% Urban	97.2	97.2	97.3	97.3	97.4	97.5	97.5
Occupants per household at January 1st (Number)	2.4	2.4	2.4	2.4	2.4	2.4	2.4
Households ('000)	4,178.7	4,209.1	4,237.8	4,277.7	4,319.0	4,361.9	4,397.6
Annual rates of inflation (% growth)	1.0	1.1	2.5	2.5	1.6	1.6	2.1
GDP (EUR million)	225,409.1	235,710.1	247,791.9	253,800.8	259,948.6	267,353.2	283,117.0
GDP (US$ million)	252,683.6	251,122.2	228,295.5	227,112.8	244,646.0	301,741.4	351,538.7
GDP (US$ per capita)	24,791.7	24,586.7	22,296.5	22,128.4	23,729.6	29,139.6	33,824.3

Source: Euromonitor International from International Monetary Fund (IMF), International Financial Statistics and World Economic Outlook/UN/national statistics

Life Expectancy

Belgium: Life expectancy 1998-2004

Table: 4.115

As stated

	1998	1999	2000	2001	2002	2003	2004	% change 1998-2004
Life expectancy at birth: total population (years)	77.5	77.7	77.8	78.0	78.3	78.5	78.8	1.66
Life expectancy at birth: total population: year on year growth	0.3	0.2	0.1	0.3	0.4	0.3	0.3	
Healthy life expectancy at birth (years)	72.0			69.6	69.7			
Healthy life expectancy at birth: year on year growth					0.2			

Source: Euromonitor International from World Bank

Health Expenditure

Belgium: Public health expenditure 1998-2004

Table: 4.116

As stated

	1998	1999	2000	2001	2002	2003	2004
Public expenditure on pharmaceuticals and other medical non-durables (EUR million)	1,518.0	1,662.0	1,770.0	1,853.0	1,892.0	1,954.0	2,060.3
Share of total health expenditure in GDP (% of total GDP)	8.4	8.5	8.6	8.9	8.9	8.9	8.6
Health expenditure (US$ per capita)	2,109.0	2,139.0	1,952.0	1,983.0	2,159.0	2,263.0	2,332.0

Source: Euromonitor International from OECD/national statistics

Belgium: Private health expenditure 1998-2004

Table: 4.117

As stated

	1998	1999	2000	2001	2002	2003	2004
Consumer expenditure on health goods and medical services (EUR million)	4,402.7	4,620.3	4,927.3	5,228.1	5,537.5	5,780.5	6,146.1
Consumer expenditure on health goods and medical services: real growth in national currency: 1990 = 100	137.5	142.7	148.4	153.7	160.1	164.5	171.4
Consumer expenditure on health goods and medical services as a percentage of total consumer expenditure	3.8	3.8	3.8	3.9	4.0	4.1	4.1

Source: National statistical offices/OECD/Eurostat/Euromonitor International

Belgium: Consumer expenditure on health goods and medical services by sector 1998-2004

Table: 4.118

% of total consumer expenditure on health goods and medical services

	1998	1999	2000	2001	2002	2003	2004
Pharmaceuticals, medical appliances/ equipment	36.0	35.6	35.5	34.9	34.6	34.7	34.5
Outpatient services	34.6	35.0	35.0	34.9	35.0	35.1	35.2
Hospital services	29.5	29.4	29.5	30.2	30.4	30.2	30.3
Total	100.0	100.0	100.0	100.0	100.0	100.0	100.0

Source: National statistical offices/OECD/Eurostat/Euromonitor International

Healthcare Infrastructure and Services

Belgium: Healthcare infrastructure and services by sector 1998-2004

Table: 4.119

As stated

	1998	1999	2000	2001	2002	2003	2004
Active pharmacists (number)	10,087	10,437	10,724	10,939	11,775	12,079	12,386
Consultations with GPs (general practitioners) (per capita)	8	8	8	8	8	8	8
Dentists (number)	8,240	8,326	8,465	8,512	8,553	8,634	8,712
Doctors (number)	38,109	38,769	39,519	40,167	40,763	41,521	42,380
Hospital admissions (number)	2,013,054						
Hospitals and clinics (number)	958	958	958	959	961	963	964
In-patient beds ('000)	46	45	45	44	43	43	42
Nurses (number)	52,232	53,819	55,406	56,996	58,306	59,851	61,264
Out-patient contacts (per capita)	8	8	7	7	7	8	7

Source: Euromonitor International from national statistics

Belgium: Healthcare infrastructure and services by sector: growth 1998-2004

Table: 4.120

Year on year growth: % change in stated unit

	1998	1999	2000	2001	2002	2003	2004
Active pharmacists (number)	2.1	3.5	2.7	2.0	7.6	2.6	2.5
Consultations with GPs (general practitioners) (per capita)	0.0	0.0	0.0	-1.3	0.0	-0.6	-0.5
Dentists (number)	1.8	1.0	1.7	0.6	0.5	0.9	0.9
Doctors (number)	1.8	1.7	1.9	1.6	1.5	1.9	2.1
Hospitals and clinics (number)	-0.1	0.0	0.0	0.1	0.2	0.2	0.1
In-patient beds (number)	-1.5	-1.5	-1.1	-2.0	-1.1	-1.4	-1.2
Nurses (number)	0.5	3.0	2.9	2.9	2.3	2.6	2.4
Out-patient contacts (per capita)	1.3	-2.1	-0.8	-0.7	-1.2	2.6	-4.0

Source: Euromonitor International from national statistics

Immunisation

Belgium: Vaccination rates by disease type 1998-2004

%

	1998	1999	2000	2001	2002	2003	2004
Vaccination rate against DTP (diphtheria, tetanus, pertussis) 1 & 2 (%)				95.0	95.0	95.0	95.0
Vaccination rate against MMR (measles, mumps, rubella) (%)				75.0	82.0	89.0	96.0
Vaccination rate against polio (%)				95.0	95.0	95.0	95.0

Source: WHO

Infectious Diseases

Belgium: Incidence of disease by type 1998-2004

Number

	1998	1999	2000	2001	2002	2003	2004
Incidence of AIDS	165	98	105	126	187	76	86
Incidence of diphtheria	0			0	1		
Incidence of measles	0			83			
Incidence of polio	0	0	0	0	0		

Source: WHO

Belgium: Incidence of disease by type: growth 1998-2004

Year on year growth: %

	1998	1999	2000	2001	2002	2003	2004
Incidence of AIDS	21.3	-40.6	7.1	20.0	48.4	-59.4	13.2
Incidence of measles	-100.0						

Source: WHO

Causes of Death

Belgium: Deaths by disease 1998-2004

Number per 100,000 inhabitants

	1998	1999	2000	2001	2002	2003	2004
Death by diseases of the circulatory system	234.0	228.0	220.0	216.0	197.0	195.0	187.7
Deaths from heart disease	122.5	123.2	123.9	124.6	125.3	126.0	126.2
Deaths from lung cancer	64.1	63.7	63.3	62.9	62.5	62.1	61.6
Death by diseases of the digestive system	30.2	30.6	30.9	31.3	31.2	30.9	30.7
Deaths from chronic liver disease and cirrhosis	11.9	11.9	11.8	11.7	11.7	11.6	11.5
Deaths from ulcers of the stomach and duodenum	3.4	3.3	3.2	3.2	3.1	3.1	3.0

Source: WHO/Euromonitor International
Notes: Data is ranked in descending order by year 2004

Belgium: Deaths by disease: growth 1998-2004

Table: 4.125

% year on year growth

	1998	1999	2000	2001	2002	2003	2004
Deaths from heart disease	0.6	0.6	0.6	0.6	0.6	0.6	0.2
Deaths from chronic liver disease and cirrhosis	-0.8	0.0	-0.8	-0.8	0.0	-0.9	-0.6
Death by diseases of the digestive system	1.0	1.3	1.0	1.3	-0.3	-1.0	-0.6
Deaths from lung cancer	-0.6	-0.6	-0.6	-0.6	-0.6	-0.6	-0.7
Deaths from ulcers of the stomach and duodenum	-2.9	-2.9	-3.0	0.0	-3.1	0.0	-1.9
Death by diseases of the circulatory system	-1.7	-2.6	-3.5	-1.8	-8.8	-1.0	-3.7

Source: WHO/Euromonitor International
Notes: Data is ranked in descending order by year 2004

Smoking

Belgium: Smoking prevalence in population aged 15+ 1998-2004

Table: 4.126

% of population aged 15+

	1998	1999	2000	2001	2002	2003	2004
Smoking prevalence in population aged 15+ (% of population aged 15+)	27.0	29.0	30.0	28.0	28.0	28.7	28.4
Smoking prevalence in male population aged 15+ (% of male population)	30.0	31.0	36.0	34.0	32.9	32.8	32.3
Smoking prevalence in female population aged 15+ (% of female population)	23.0	26.0	26.0	22.0	23.4	24.9	24.7

Source: WHO/OECD/Euromonitor International

Nutrition and Obesity

Belgium: Nutrition and obesity 1998-2004

Table: 4.127

As stated

	1998	1999	2000	2001	2002	2003	2004
Availability of fruit and vegetables (kg/capita/year)	248.6	261.2	246.9	224.8	224.8	215.8	205.2
Average supply of calories per day (calories per capita)	3,629.0	3,643.0	3,589.1	3,576.9	3,583.8	3,577.7	3,571.1
Average supply of fat per day (grams per capita)	158.7	158.3	158.8	159.7	159.6	159.7	159.9
Average supply of protein per day (grams per capita)	102.7	104.8	88.8	89.8	88.6	85.8	84.0
Microbiological food-borne diseases (per 100000 population)	73.0	98.0	63.0	56.0	60.0	56.0	55.0
Obese population (BMI 30kg/sq m or more) (% of population aged 15+)	11.3	11.6	11.7	12.6	13.5	13.9	14.5

Source: WHO/OECD/Euromonitor International

Over-the-Counter Healthcare

Belgium: Trends in OTC healthcare retail sales 1998-2004

Table: 4.128

As stated

	1998	1999	2000	2001	2002	2003	2004
OTC Healthcare (EUR million)	579.5	596.9	615.0	630.4	636.9	647.4	666.6
OTC Healthcare: real growth in national currency: 1998 = 100	100.0	101.9	102.3	102.4	101.8	101.8	103.0
OTC Healthcare: year on year (% real growth)	1.2	1.9	0.5	0.0	-0.6	0.1	1.1

Source: Euromonitor International from industry sources/national statistics

Belgium: OTC healthcare retail sales by sector 1998-2004

Table: 4.129

% of OTC retail value sales

	1998	1999	2000	2001	2002	2003	2004
Analgesics	18.8	18.9	19.0	19.3	18.0	16.9	17.0
Cough, cold and allergy (hay fever) remedies	23.0	22.6	22.3	22.0	22.6	22.6	22.3
Digestive remedies	14.3	13.6	13.1	12.3	11.6	11.2	10.8
Medicated skin care	7.7	7.5	7.4	7.3	7.3	7.3	7.1
Vitamins and dietary supplements	25.9	27.2	28.2	29.2	30.2	31.0	31.5

Source: *Euromonitor International from industry sources/national statistics*
Notes: *Only selected sectors are shown, so values are not expected to sum to 100*

Health and Wellness

Belgium: Retail sales of packaged foods by health and wellness category 2002-2004

Table: 4.130

EUR million

	2002	2003	2004
Packaged food: Total	10,199.8	10,537.7	10,831.9
Better for you	1,099.6	1,180.2	1,244.2
For food intolerance	16.6	17.4	18.0
Fortified/functional	153.2	167.2	184.4
Organic	134.9	140.2	144.4

Source: *Euromonitor International from industry sources/national statistics*

Belgium: Per capita sales of packaged foods by health and wellness category 2002-2004

Table: 4.131

EUR per capita

	2002	2003	2004
Better for you	107.0	114.6	120.6
For food intolerance	1.6	1.7	1.7
Fortified/functional	14.9	16.2	17.9
Organic	13.1	13.6	14.0

Source: *Euromonitor International from industry sources/national statistics*

Belgium: Retail sales of packaged food by health and wellness category: % share of total packaged food market 2002-2004

Table: 4.132

% value

	2002	2003	2004
Better for you	10.8	11.2	11.5
For food intolerance	0.2	0.2	0.2
Fortified/functional	1.5	1.6	1.7
Organic	1.3	1.3	1.3

Source: *Euromonitor International from industry sources/national statistics*

Belgium: Retail sales of packaged food by health and wellness category: real growth index 2002-2004

Table: 4.133

2002 =100

	2002	2003	2004
Better for you	100.00	105.85	110.04
For food intolerance	100.00	103.08	105.39
Fortified/functional	100.00	107.67	117.07
Organic	100.00	102.51	104.15

Source: *Euromonitor International from industry sources/national statistics*

Belgium: Retail sales of better-for-you packaged foods by sector 2002-2004

Table: 4.134

% of total packaged food / as stated

	2002	2003	2004	% real change in value 2002-2004
Combination	0.34	0.39	0.42	26.32
Reduced fat	9.45	9.83	10.08	10.14
Reduced salt	0.21	0.21	0.22	5.98

Source: *Euromonitor International from industry sources/national statistics*

Belgium: Retail sales of packaged foods for food intolerances by sector 2002-2004

Table: 4.135

% of total packaged food / as stated

	2002	2003	2004	% real change in value 2002-2004
Diabetic	0.03	0.03	0.03	2.33
Gluten-free	0.02	0.02	0.02	6.05
Lactose-free	0.11	0.11	0.11	6.12

Source: *Euromonitor International from industry sources/national statistics*

Belgium: Retail sales of naturally healthy packaged foods by sector 2002-2004

Table: 4.136

% of total packaged food / as stated

	2002	2003	2004	% real change in value 2002-2004
High fibre	5.48	5.40	5.38	1.43
Other naturally healthy food	0.81	0.82	0.83	5.91
Soy-based dairy alternatives	0.13	0.14	0.14	8.72

Source: *Euromonitor International from industry sources/national statistics*

■ **Bolivia**

Socio-economic Parameters

Bolivia: Socio-economic parameters 1998-2004

Table: 4.137

As stated

	1998	1999	2000	2001	2002	2003	2004
Population: national estimates at January 1st ('000)	7,899.1	8,066.2	8,232.6	8,398.1	8,562.3	8,725.9	8,889.7
% aged 0-14 yrs	40.2	40.0	39.7	39.4	39.1	38.8	38.4
% aged 15-64 yrs	55.7	55.8	56.0	56.2	56.5	56.8	57.1
% aged 65+ yrs	4.2	4.2	4.3	4.3	4.4	4.4	4.5
% Male	49.7	49.7	49.8	49.8	49.8	49.8	49.8
% Female	50.3	50.3	50.2	50.2	50.2	50.2	50.2
% Urban	61.3	61.9	62.6	62.8	63.0	64.3	64.9
Occupants per household at January 1st (Number)	4.4	4.4	4.3	4.2	4.2	4.2	4.1
Households ('000)	1,790.5	1,851.5	1,916.1	1,977.7	2,036.4	2,094.3	2,152.7
Annual rates of inflation (% growth)	7.7	2.2	4.6	1.6	0.9	3.3	4.4
GDP (Bvs million)	46,822.0	48,156.0	51,928.0	53,790.0	56,818.0	61,959.0	69,626.0
GDP (US$ million)	8,497.4	8,285.0	8,397.8	8,141.5	7,924.4	8,089.5	8,773.1
GDP (US$ per capita)	1,075.7	1,027.1	1,020.1	969.4	925.5	927.1	986.9

Source: *Euromonitor International from International Monetary Fund (IMF), International Financial Statistics and World Economic Outlook/UN/national statistics*

Life Expectancy

Bolivia: Life expectancy 1998-2004

Table: 4.138

As stated

	1998	1999	2000	2001	2002	2003	2004	% change 1998-2004
Life expectancy at birth: total population (years)	61.6	62.0	62.2	62.7	63.2	63.7	64.1	4.14
Life expectancy at birth: total population: year on year growth	0.8	0.7	0.4	0.8	0.8	0.8	0.6	
Healthy life expectancy at birth (years)	53.0			50.4	50.8			
Healthy life expectancy at birth: year on year growth					0.8			

Source: Euromonitor International from World Bank

Sanitation

Bolivia: Improved sanitary facilities and water source 2000

Table: 4.139

As stated

	2000
Population with access to improved sanitary facilities (% of population)	70.0
Population with access to improved water source (% of population)	83.0
Population with improved access to sanitation facilities, rural (% of rural population with access)	42.0
Population with improved access to sanitation facilities, urban (% of urban population with access)	86.0

Source: National statistics/World Bank

Health Expenditure

Bolivia: Public health expenditure 1998-2004

Table: 4.140

As stated

	1998	1999	2000	2001	2002	2003	2004
Share of total health expenditure in GDP (% of total GDP)	5.0	5.2	5.2	5.3	5.2	5.4	5.5
Health expenditure (US$ per capita)	53.0	63.0	61.0	61.0	63.0	63.0	64.0

Source: Euromonitor International from OECD/national statistics

Bolivia: Private health expenditure 1998-2004

Table: 4.141

As stated

	1998	1999	2000	2001	2002	2003	2004
Consumer expenditure on health goods and medical services (Bvs million)	1,008.0	1,076.0	1,165.0	1,209.0	1,241.9	1,272.0	1,379.8
Consumer expenditure on health goods and medical services: real growth in national currency: 1990 = 100	131.1	137.0	141.8	144.8	147.5	146.2	151.9
Consumer expenditure on health goods and medical services as a percentage of total consumer expenditure	2.8	2.9	3.0	3.0	2.9	2.8	2.9

Source: National statistical offices/OECD/Eurostat/Euromonitor International

Bolivia: Consumer expenditure on health goods and medical services by sector 1998-2004

Table: 4.142

% of total consumer expenditure on health goods and medical services

	1998	1999	2000	2001	2002	2003	2004
Pharmaceuticals, medical appliances/ equipment	71.5	70.8	72.3	72.0	71.6	71.4	71.1
Outpatient services	22.7	23.4	22.3	22.5	22.8	22.9	23.1
Hospital services	5.7	5.8	5.5	5.4	5.6	5.6	5.8
Total	100.0	100.0	100.0	100.0	100.0	100.0	100.0

Source: National statistical offices/OECD/Eurostat/Euromonitor International

Healthcare Infrastructure and Services

Bolivia: Healthcare infrastructure and services by sector 1998-2004

Table: 4.143

As stated

	1998	1999	2000	2001	2002	2003	2004
Dentists (number)	515	518	519	527	534	543	551
Doctors (number)	2,542	2,652	2,907	3,021	3,068	3,121	3,137
Hospitals and clinics (number)	2,435	2,438	2,441	2,439	2,437	2,433	2,431
In-patient beds ('000)	11	11	12	12	12	12	12
Nurses (number)	7,852	7,858	7,860	7,865	7,869	7,873	7,882

Source: Euromonitor International from national statistics

Bolivia: Healthcare infrastructure and services by sector: growth 1998-2004

Table: 4.144

Year on year growth: % change in stated unit

	1998	1999	2000	2001	2002	2003	2004
Dentists (number)	0.6	0.6	0.2	1.5	1.3	1.7	1.5
Doctors (number)	5.1	4.3	9.6	3.9	1.6	1.7	0.5
Hospitals and clinics (number)	0.1	0.1	0.1	-0.1	-0.1	-0.2	-0.1
In-patient beds (number)	-10.6	2.1	2.1	0.7	0.3	0.3	0.3
Nurses (number)	0.1	0.1	0.0	0.1	0.1	0.1	0.1

Source: Euromonitor International from national statistics

Immunisation

Bolivia: Vaccination rates by disease type 1998-2004

Table: 4.145

%

	1998	1999	2000	2001	2002	2003	2004
Vaccination rate against DTP (diphtheria, tetanus, pertussis) 1 & 2 (%)			98.0	97.4	99.0	99.0	99.0
Vaccination rate against MMR (measles, mumps, rubella) (%)	77.0	99.0	99.0	99.0	99.0	99.0	99.0
Vaccination rate against polio (%)	75.0	89.0	89.0	89.7	99.0	99.0	99.0

Source: WHO

Infectious Diseases

Bolivia: Incidence of disease by type 1998-2004

Number

	1998	1999	2000	2001	2002	2003	2004
Incidence of AIDS	42	34	43	73	79	82	75
Incidence of diphtheria	8	2	1	3	5		
Incidence of measles	1,004	1,441	122	0	0		
Incidence of polio	0	0	0	0	0		

Source: WHO

Bolivia: Incidence of disease by type: growth 1998-2004

Year on year growth: %

	1998	1999	2000	2001	2002	2003	2004
Incidence of AIDS	162.5	-19.0	26.5	69.8	8.2	3.8	-8.5
Incidence of diphtheria	166.7	-75.0	-50.0	200.0	66.7		
Incidence of measles	14,242.9	43.5	-91.5	-100.0			

Source: WHO

Causes of Death

Bolivia: Deaths by disease 1998-2004

Number per 100,000 inhabitants

	1998	1999	2000	2001	2002	2003	2004
Deaths from heart disease	48.7	46.1	47.2	46.0	46.1	45.3	45.0
Deaths from ulcers of the stomach and duodenum	28.4	28.8	29.2	29.7	30.8	31.5	32.5
Death by diseases of the digestive system	28.4	28.8	29.2	29.7	30.8	29.9	30.2
Deaths from lung cancer	21.7	19.4	18.9	19.8	20.0	20.7	21.3
Deaths from chronic liver disease and cirrhosis	7.3	7.5	7.8	8.1	8.2	8.4	8.6

Source: WHO/Euromonitor International
Notes: Data is ranked in descending order by year 2004

Bolivia: Deaths by disease: growth 1998-2004

% year on year growth

	1998	1999	2000	2001	2002	2003	2004
Deaths from ulcers of the stomach and duodenum	1.8	1.4	1.4	1.7	3.7	2.3	3.2
Deaths from lung cancer	6.4	-10.6	-2.6	4.8	1.0	3.5	2.9
Deaths from chronic liver disease and cirrhosis	5.8	2.7	4.0	3.8	1.2	2.4	1.9
Death by diseases of the digestive system	1.8	1.4	1.4	1.7	3.7	-2.9	1.0
Deaths from heart disease	3.0	-5.3	2.4	-2.5	0.2	-1.7	-0.8

Source: WHO/Euromonitor International
Notes: Data is ranked in descending order by year 2004

Bolivia: Other selected causes of death: 1998-2004

Number per 100,000 inhabitants

	1998	1999	2000	2001	2002	2003	2004
Death by suicide and self-inflicted injury	6.6	6.6	6.7	6.9	6.7	6.9	6.9

Source: Euromonitor International from national statistics

Bolivia: Other selected causes of death: growth 1998-2004

Table: 4.151

% year on year growth

	1998	1999	2000	2001	2002	2003	2004
Death by suicide and self-inflicted injury	11.9	0.0	1.5	3.0	-2.9	3.0	0.5

Source: Euromonitor International from national statistics

Smoking

Bolivia: Smoking prevalence in population aged 15+ 1998-2004

Table: 4.152

% of population aged 15+

	1998	1999	2000	2001	2002	2003	2004
Smoking prevalence in population aged 15+ (% of population aged 15+)	33.6	33.4	33.1	32.7	32.4	32.2	32.2
Smoking prevalence in male population aged 15+ (% of male population)	42.7	42.3	41.6	41.2	40.8	40.5	40.0
Smoking prevalence in female population aged 15+ (% of female population)	24.8	24.9	24.9	24.6	24.4	24.2	24.7

Source: WHO/OECD/Euromonitor International

Nutrition and Obesity

Bolivia: Nutrition and obesity 1998-2004

Table: 4.153

As stated

	1998	1999	2000	2001	2002	2003	2004
Average supply of calories per day (calories per capita)	2,171.3	2,209.4	2,236.8	2,277.1	2,235.2	2,218.7	2,208.4
Average supply of fat per day (grams per capita)	58.5	48.2	49.5	48.4	51.9	54.4	56.6
Average supply of protein per day (grams per capita)	54.7	58.8	59.0	59.4	59.3	59.3	59.4
Obese population (BMI 30kg/sq m or more) (% of population aged 15+)	8.3	8.4	8.6	8.6	8.6	8.7	8.7

Source: WHO/OECD/Euromonitor International

■ Brazil

Socio-economic Parameters

Brazil: Socio-economic parameters 1998-2004

Table: 4.154

As stated

	1998	1999	2000	2001	2002	2003	2004
Population: national estimates at January 1st ('000)	165,687.5	167,909.7	170,143.1	172,385.8	174,633.0	176,876.4	179,113.5
% aged 0-14 yrs	30.0	29.4	28.9	28.5	28.0	27.6	27.3
% aged 15-64 yrs	65.2	65.7	66.1	66.4	66.8	67.0	67.2
% aged 65+ yrs	4.8	4.9	5.0	5.1	5.2	5.3	5.5
% Male	49.4	49.3	49.3	49.3	49.3	49.2	49.2
% Female	50.6	50.7	50.7	50.7	50.7	50.8	50.8
% Urban	80.1	80.7	80.9	81.3	81.8	82.3	82.8
Occupants per household at January 1st (Number)	3.7	3.6	3.6	3.6	3.5	3.5	3.5
Households ('000)	45,187.2	46,306.3	47,376.7	48,473.1	49,510.1	50,558.0	51,604.6
Annual rates of inflation (% growth)	3.2	4.9	7.0	6.8	8.4	14.7	6.6
GDP (R$ million)	914,188.0	973,846.0	1,101,250.0	1,198,740.0	1,346,030.0	1,556,180.0	1,769,200.0
GDP (US$ million)	787,740.0	536,634.1	601,729.9	508,434.0	460,838.2	505,731.1	604,829.9
GDP (US$ per capita)	4,754.4	3,196.0	3,536.6	2,949.4	2,638.9	2,859.2	3,376.8

Source: Euromonitor International from International Monetary Fund (IMF), International Financial Statistics and World Economic Outlook/UN/national statistics

Life Expectancy

Brazil: Life expectancy 1998-2004

Table: 4.155

As stated

	1998	1999	2000	2001	2002	2003	2004	% change 1998-2004
Life expectancy at birth: total population (years)	68.1	68.3	68.4	68.7	68.9	69.2	69.5	1.98
Life expectancy at birth: total population: year on year growth	0.4	0.4	0.1	0.4	0.3	0.4	0.4	
Healthy life expectancy at birth (years)	59.0			56.3	56.7			
Healthy life expectancy at birth: year on year growth					0.7			

Source: Euromonitor International from World Bank

Sanitation

Brazil: Improved sanitary facilities and water source 2000

Table: 4.156

As stated

	2000
Population with access to improved sanitary facilities (% of population)	76.0
Population with access to improved water source (% of population)	87.0
Population with improved access to sanitation facilities, rural (% of rural population with access)	43.0
Population with improved access to sanitation facilities, urban (% of urban population with access)	84.0

Source: National statistics/World Bank

Health Expenditure

Brazil: Public health expenditure 1998-2004

Table: 4.157

As stated

	1998	1999	2000	2001	2002	2003	2004
Share of total health expenditure in GDP (% of total GDP)	7.4	7.8	7.6	7.6	7.3	7.4	7.5
Health expenditure (US$ per capita)	348.0	246.0	266.0	227.0	206.0	193.0	180.0

Source: Euromonitor International from OECD/national statistics

Brazil: Private health expenditure 1998-2004

Table: 4.158

As stated

	1998	1999	2000	2001	2002	2003	2004
Consumer expenditure on health goods and medical services (R$ million)	35,332.9	38,903.3	44,176.5	47,574.3	51,231.5	60,559.9	64,955.6
Consumer expenditure on health goods and medical services: real growth in national currency: 1990 = 100	148.8	156.2	165.7	167.0	165.9	170.9	172.0
Consumer expenditure on health goods and medical services as a percentage of total consumer expenditure	6.2	6.1	6.0	5.9	5.8	5.9	5.9

Source: National statistical offices/OECD/Eurostat/Euromonitor International

Brazil: Consumer expenditure on health goods and medical services by sector 1998-2004

Table: 4.159

% of total consumer expenditure on health goods and medical services

	1998	1999	2000	2001	2002	2003	2004
Pharmaceuticals, medical appliances/ equipment	39.1	39.6	40.1	40.6	41.0	41.1	41.1
Outpatient services	52.2	51.7	51.2	50.7	50.1	50.2	50.3
Hospital services	8.7	8.7	8.7	8.7	8.9	8.7	8.6
Total	100.0	100.0	100.0	100.0	100.0	100.0	100.0

Source: National statistical offices/OECD/Eurostat/Euromonitor International

Healthcare Infrastructure and Services

Brazil: Healthcare infrastructure and services by sector 1998-2004

Table: 4.160

As stated

	1998	1999	2000	2001	2002	2003	2004
Dentists (number)	7,524	7,825	8,105	8,105	8,123	8,141	8,153
Hospitals and clinics (number)	6,391	6,582	6,782	6,782	6,845	6,902	6,967
In-patient beds ('000)	480	487	493	494	499	503	507

Source: Euromonitor International from national statistics

Brazil: Healthcare infrastructure and services by sector: growth 1998-2004

Table: 4.161

Year on year growth: % change in stated unit

	1998	1999	2000	2001	2002	2003	2004
Dentists (number)	3.2	4.0	3.6	0.0	0.2	0.2	0.1
Hospitals and clinics (number)	-0.3	3.0	3.0	0.0	0.9	0.8	0.9
In-patient beds (number)	-2.0	1.3	1.3	0.2	1.0	0.8	0.7

Source: Euromonitor International from national statistics

Immunisation

Brazil: Vaccination rates by disease type 1998-2004

Table: 4.162

%

	1998	1999	2000	2001	2002	2003	2004
Vaccination rate against DTP (diphtheria, tetanus, pertussis) 1 & 2 (%)			99.0	90.0	97.5	94.0	93.0
Vaccination rate against MMR (measles, mumps, rubella) (%)	96.0	99.0	99.0	95.0	93.3	91.0	89.0
Vaccination rate against polio (%)	96.0	98.0	95.0	95.0	97.0	95.0	95.0

Source: WHO

Infectious Diseases

Brazil: Incidence of disease by type 1998-2004

Table: 4.163

Number

	1998	1999	2000	2001	2002	2003	2004
Incidence of AIDS	24,017	20,009	15,013	3,024	3,041	2,988	4,203
Incidence of diphtheria	217	53	46	10	64		
Incidence of measles	2,781	908	36	1	1		
Incidence of polio	0	0	0	0	0		

Source: WHO

Brazil: Incidence of disease by type: growth 1998-2004

Table: 4.164

Year on year growth: %

	1998	1999	2000	2001	2002	2003	2004
Incidence of AIDS	2.0	-16.7	-25.0	-79.9	0.6	-1.7	40.7
Incidence of diphtheria	578.1	-75.6	-13.2	-78.3	540.0		
Incidence of measles	-94.7	-67.3	-96.0	-97.2	0.0		

Source: WHO

Causes of Death

Brazil: Deaths by disease 1998-2004

Table: 4.165

Number per 100,000 inhabitants

	1998	1999	2000	2001	2002	2003	2004
Deaths from heart disease	44.9	44.8	44.8	44.7	44.7	44.6	44.2
Death by diseases of the digestive system	39.5	40.0	40.8	40.0	40.4	40.1	39.8
Deaths from chronic liver disease and cirrhosis	9.8	9.9	10.1	10.2	10.4	10.5	10.7
Deaths from lung cancer	8.7	8.9	9.2	9.4	9.7	9.9	10.1
Deaths from ulcers of the stomach and duodenum	1.6	1.4	1.3	1.2	1.1	1.0	0.9

Source: WHO/Euromonitor International
Notes: Data is ranked in descending order by year 2004

Brazil: Deaths by disease: growth 1998-2004

Table: 4.166

% year on year growth

	1998	1999	2000	2001	2002	2003	2004
Deaths from lung cancer	3.6	2.3	3.4	2.2	3.2	2.1	2.3
Deaths from chronic liver disease and cirrhosis	2.1	1.0	2.0	1.0	2.0	1.0	1.6
Death by diseases of the digestive system	3.1	1.3	2.0	-2.0	1.0	-0.7	-0.8
Deaths from heart disease	-0.2	-0.2	0.0	-0.2	0.0	-0.2	-0.9
Deaths from ulcers of the stomach and duodenum	-5.9	-12.5	-7.1	-7.7	-8.3	-9.1	-9.1

Source: WHO/Euromonitor International
Notes: Data is ranked in descending order by year 2004

Smoking

Brazil: Smoking prevalence in population aged 15+ 1998-2004

Table: 4.167

% of population aged 15+

	1998	1999	2000	2001	2002	2003	2004
Smoking prevalence in population aged 15+ (% of population aged 15+)	33.7	33.5	33.3	33.5	33.2	33.1	32.9
Smoking prevalence in male population aged 15+ (% of male population)	37.9	37.7	37.9	37.6	37.4	37.1	36.8
Smoking prevalence in female population aged 15+ (% of female population)	29.8	29.4	28.9	29.6	29.3	29.3	29.2

Source: WHO/OECD/Euromonitor International

Nutrition and Obesity

Brazil: Nutrition and obesity 1998-2004

Table: 4.168

As stated

	1998	1999	2000	2001	2002	2003	2004
Average supply of calories per day (calories per capita)	2,953.3	2,992.8	2,981.2	2,999.9	3,049.5	3,085.1	3,062.3
Average supply of fat per day (grams per capita)	88.1	90.0	91.6	91.5	93.7	91.4	91.8
Average supply of protein per day (grams per capita)	78.0	80.3	80.4	80.8	82.8	83.2	82.6
Obese population (BMI 30kg/sq m or more) (% of population aged 15+)	10.7	11.0	11.1	11.2	11.3	11.4	11.5

Source: WHO/OECD/Euromonitor International

Over-the-Counter Healthcare

Brazil: Trends in OTC healthcare retail sales 1998-2004

Table: 4.169

As stated

	1998	1999	2000	2001	2002	2003	2004
OTC Healthcare (R$ million)	4,278.2	4,864.6	4,931.8	5,114.6	5,527.7	5,525.0	6,156.8
OTC Healthcare: real growth in national currency: 1998 = 100	100.0	108.4	102.7	99.7	99.3	86.6	90.5
OTC Healthcare: year on year (% real growth)	0.1	8.4	-5.3	-2.9	-0.3	-12.9	4.5
OTC Healthcare (R$ per capita)	25.8	29.0	29.0	29.7	31.7	31.2	34.4

Source: Euromonitor International from industry sources/national statistics

Brazil: OTC healthcare retail sales by sector 1998-2004

Table: 4.170

% of OTC retail value sales

	1998	1999	2000	2001	2002	2003	2004
Analgesics	18.7	19.7	19.6	19.1	18.8	19.3	22.4
Cough, cold and allergy (hay fever) remedies	30.9	30.2	29.9	29.4	30.3	29.3	27.2
Digestive remedies	16.5	15.4	14.6	15.0	14.5	15.0	14.7
Medicated skin care	12.2	12.8	13.4	13.5	13.2	13.2	12.9
Vitamins and dietary supplements	17.4	17.3	17.7	18.1	18.2	17.8	17.6

Source: Euromonitor International from industry sources/national statistics
Notes: Only selected sectors are shown, so values are not expected to sum to 100

Health and Wellness

Brazil: Retail sales of packaged foods by health and wellness category 2002-2004

Table: 4.171

R$ million

	2002	2003	2004
Packaged food: Total	96,336.2	111,940.7	119,258.3
Better for you	2,837.1	3,359.9	3,659.1
For food intolerance	25.9	31.4	35.6
Fortified/functional	3,545.8	3,919.5	4,134.0

Source: Euromonitor International from industry sources/national statistics

Brazil: Per capita sales of packaged foods by health and wellness category 2002-2004

Table: 4.172

R$ per capita

	2002	2003	2004
Better for you	16.4	19.2	20.7
For food intolerance	0.2	0.2	0.2
Fortified/functional	20.5	22.4	23.4

Source: *Euromonitor International from industry sources/national statistics*

Brazil: Retail sales of packaged food by health and wellness category: % share of total packaged food market 2002-2004

Table: 4.173

% value

	2002	2003	2004
Better for you	2.9	3.0	3.1
For food intolerance	0.0	0.0	0.0
Fortified/functional	3.7	3.5	3.5

Source: *Euromonitor International from industry sources/national statistics*

Brazil: Retail sales of packaged food by health and wellness category: real growth index 2002-2004

Table: 4.174

2002 =100

	2002	2003	2004
Better for you	100.00	102.98	105.60
For food intolerance	100.00	105.51	112.53
Fortified/functional	100.00	96.12	95.46

Source: *Euromonitor International from industry sources/national statistics*

Brazil: Retail sales of better-for-you packaged foods by sector 2002-2004

Table: 4.175

% of total packaged food / as stated

	2002	2003	2004	% real change in value 2002-2004
Combination	0.14	0.15	0.15	4.43
Reduced fat	2.31	2.32	2.31	1.37

Source: *Euromonitor International from industry sources/national statistics*

Brazil: Retail sales of packaged foods for food intolerances by sector 2002-2004

Table: 4.176

% of total packaged food / as stated

	2002	2003	2004	% real change in value 2002-2004
Lactose-free	0.03	0.03	0.03	12.53

Source: *Euromonitor International from industry sources/national statistics*

Brazil: Retail sales of naturally healthy packaged foods by sector 2002-2004

Table: 4.177

% of total packaged food / as stated

	2002	2003	2004	% real change in value 2002-2004
High fibre	0.33	0.32	0.32	-0.74
Other naturally healthy food	0.70	0.67	0.67	-3.07
Soy-based dairy alternatives	0.18	0.19	0.20	13.11

Source: Euromonitor International from industry sources/national statistics

■ **Bulgaria**

Socio-economic Parameters

Bulgaria: Socio-economic parameters 1998-2004

Table: 4.178

As stated

	1998	1999	2000	2001	2002	2003	2004
Population: national estimates at January 1st ('000)	8,211.4	8,130.6	8,054.8	7,985.8	7,891.1	7,845.8	7,768.0
% aged 0-14 yrs	16.8	16.3	15.9	15.5	15.0	14.6	14.2
% aged 15-64 yrs	67.6	67.9	67.9	68.1	68.1	68.4	68.9
% aged 65+ yrs	15.6	15.9	16.2	16.3	16.9	17.0	16.9
% Male	48.9	48.9	48.8	48.8	48.7	48.6	48.6
% Female	51.1	51.1	51.2	51.2	51.3	51.4	51.4
% Urban	69.0	69.3	69.8	70.1	70.5	71.0	71.4
Occupants per household at January 1st (Number)	2.8	2.8	2.8	2.7	2.7	2.7	2.7
Households ('000)	2,934.9	2,930.4	2,924.8	2,921.9	2,918.4	2,915.1	2,912.0
Annual rates of inflation (% growth)	18.7	2.6	10.3	7.4	5.8	2.2	6.3
GDP (Lev million)	22,421.1	23,790.4	26,752.8	29,709.2	32,335.1	34,546.6	38,008.4
GDP (US$ million)	12,736.7	12,955.1	12,599.8	13,598.7	15,568.4	19,938.0	24,130.6
GDP (US$ per capita)	1,551.1	1,593.4	1,564.3	1,702.9	1,972.9	2,541.2	3,106.4

Source: Euromonitor International from International Monetary Fund (IMF), International Financial Statistics and World Economic Outlook/UN/national statistics

Life Expectancy

Bulgaria: Life expectancy 1998-2004

Table: 4.179

As stated

	1998	1999	2000	2001	2002	2003	2004	% change 1998-2004
Life expectancy at birth: total population (years)	71.6	71.6	71.6	71.5	71.9	72.2	72.3	1.07
Life expectancy at birth: total population: year on year growth	0.0	0.0	0.0	-0.1	0.6	0.3	0.3	
Healthy life expectancy at birth (years)	64.0			63.1	63.0			
Healthy life expectancy at birth: year on year growth					-0.2			

Source: Euromonitor International from World Bank

Sanitation

Bulgaria: Improved sanitary facilities and water source 2000

Table: 4.180

As stated

	2000
Population with access to improved sanitary facilities (% of population)	100.0
Population with access to improved water source (% of population)	100.0
Population with improved access to sanitation facilities, rural (% of rural population with access)	100.0
Population with improved access to sanitation facilities, urban (% of urban population with access)	100.0

Source: National statistics/World Bank

Health Expenditure

Bulgaria: Public health expenditure 1998-2004

Table: 4.181

As stated

	1998	1999	2000	2001	2002	2003	2004
Share of total health expenditure in GDP (% of total GDP)	3.9	5.0	4.8	4.8	4.7	4.8	4.7
Health expenditure (US$ per capita)	79.0	99.0	101.0	121.0	145.0	153.0	161.0

Source: Euromonitor International from OECD/national statistics

Bulgaria: Private health expenditure 1998-2004

Table: 4.182

As stated

	1998	1999	2000	2001	2002	2003	2004
Consumer expenditure on health goods and medical services (Lev million)	236.7	225.6	244.8	269.6	301.5	311.4	340.7
Consumer expenditure on health goods and medical services: real growth in national currency: 1990 = 100	117.9	109.6	107.8	110.6	116.9	118.1	121.6
Consumer expenditure on health goods and medical services as a percentage of total consumer expenditure	1.5	1.3	1.3	1.3	1.3	1.3	1.3

Source: National statistical offices/OECD/Eurostat/Euromonitor International

Bulgaria: Consumer expenditure on health goods and medical services by sector 1998-2004

Table: 4.183

% of total consumer expenditure on health goods and medical services

	1998	1999	2000	2001	2002	2003	2004
Pharmaceuticals, medical appliances/ equipment	26.0	17.2	16.5	16.5	15.9	16.2	16.1
Outpatient services	68.5	77.6	77.0	75.6	75.6	75.3	75.2
Hospital services	5.5	5.1	6.5	7.9	8.5	8.4	8.7
Total	100.0	100.0	100.0	100.0	100.0	100.0	100.0

Source: National statistical offices/OECD/Eurostat/Euromonitor International

Healthcare Infrastructure and Services

Bulgaria: Healthcare infrastructure and services by sector 1998-2004

Table: 4.184

As stated

	1998	1999	2000	2001	2002	2003	2004
Active pharmacists (number)	1,529	1,452	1,390	1,355	1,330	1,310	1,305
Dentists (number)	4,838	4,684	4,562	4,511	4,480	4,426	4,382
Doctors (number)	28,476	27,940	27,304	26,683	25,856	25,316	24,768
Hospital admissions (number)	1,331,831	1,298,709	1,261,151	1,212,167	1,294,645	1,289,482	1,298,391
Hospitals and clinics (number)	276	280	249	244	251	249	248
In-patient beds ('000)	81	73	67	63	56	45	44
Midwives (number)	5,826	5,459	5,292	5,165	5,057	4,992	4,942
Nurses (number)	47,343	44,114	43,435	42,707	41,829	41,325	40,950
Out-patient contacts (per capita)	6	5	5	5	5	5	5

Source: Euromonitor International from national statistics

Bulgaria: Healthcare infrastructure and services by sector: growth 1998-2004

Table: 4.185

Year on year growth: % change in stated unit

	1998	1999	2000	2001	2002	2003	2004
Active pharmacists (number)	-3.7	-5.0	-4.3	-2.5	-1.8	-1.5	-0.4
Dentists (number)	-7.7	-3.2	-2.6	-1.1	-0.7	-1.2	-1.0
Doctors (number)	-0.6	-1.9	-2.3	-2.3	-3.1	-2.1	-2.2
Hospital admissions (number)	2.5	-2.5	-2.9	-3.9	6.8	-0.4	0.7
Hospitals and clinics (number)	-4.2	1.4	-11.1	-2.0	2.9	-0.8	-0.4
In-patient beds (number)	-5.4	-9.3	-8.6	-6.6	-10.5	-19.6	-2.3
Midwives (number)	-1.6	-6.3	-3.1	-2.4	-2.1	-1.3	-1.0
Nurses (number)	-0.2	-6.8	-1.5	-1.7	-2.1	-1.2	-0.9
Out-patient contacts (per capita)	-3.5	-1.8	-3.2	-3.0	-7.3	2.1	-6.2

Source: Euromonitor International from national statistics

Immunisation

Bulgaria: Vaccination rates by disease type 1998-2004

Table: 4.186

%

	1998	1999	2000	2001	2002	2003	2004
Vaccination rate against DTP (diphtheria, tetanus, pertussis) 1 & 2 (%)			94.9	95.2	90.2	89.0	86.0
Vaccination rate against MMR (measles, mumps, rubella) (%)	95.5		88.6	90.0	92.1	94.0	95.0
Vaccination rate against polio (%)	97.0		98.3	94.3	93.6	92.0	90.0

Source: WHO

Infectious Diseases

Bulgaria: Incidence of disease by type 1998-2004

Table: 4.187

Number

	1998	1999	2000	2001	2002	2003	2004
Incidence of AIDS	3	11	16	14	13	5	6
Incidence of diphtheria	0	0	0	0	0		
Incidence of measles	80	24	46	8	0		
Incidence of polio	0	0	0	3	0		

Source: WHO

Bulgaria: Incidence of disease by type: growth 1998-2004

Table: 4.188

Year on year growth: %

	1998	1999	2000	2001	2002	2003	2004
Incidence of AIDS	-62.5	266.7	45.5	-12.5	-7.1	-61.5	20.0
Incidence of measles	247.8	-70.0	91.7	-82.6	-100.0		
Incidence of polio					-100.0		

Source: WHO

Causes of Death

Bulgaria: Deaths by disease 1998-2004

Table: 4.189

Number per 100,000 inhabitants

	1998	1999	2000	2001	2002	2003	2004
Deaths from heart disease	270.1	254.3	243.3	229.3	216.3	203.3	191.5
Deaths from lung cancer	35.8	37.3	35.6	35.8	35.3	34.6	34.3
Death by diseases of the digestive system	26.4	25.5	24.0	23.0	22.1	21.7	20.9
Deaths from chronic liver disease and cirrhosis	20.7	18.4	19.1	17.7	16.9	16.1	15.3
Deaths from ulcers of the stomach and duodenum	3.5	3.0	2.7	2.3	2.0	1.7	1.4

Source: WHO/Euromonitor International
Notes: Data is ranked in descending order by year 2004

Bulgaria: Deaths by disease: growth 1998-2004

Table: 4.190

% year on year growth

	1998	1999	2000	2001	2002	2003	2004
Deaths from lung cancer	-2.5	4.3	-4.6	0.5	-1.4	-2.0	-0.8
Death by diseases of the digestive system	-5.4	-3.4	-5.9	-4.2	-3.9	-1.8	-3.6
Deaths from chronic liver disease and cirrhosis	-0.7	-11.4	3.7	-7.1	-4.5	-4.7	-4.8
Deaths from heart disease	23.8	-5.9	-4.3	-5.8	-5.7	-6.0	-5.8
Deaths from ulcers of the stomach and duodenum	-23.4	-14.2	-8.6	-15.4	-13.0	-15.0	-15.0

Source: WHO/Euromonitor International
Notes: Data is ranked in descending order by year 2004

Smoking

Bulgaria: Smoking prevalence in population aged 15+ 1998-2004

Table: 4.191

% of population aged 15+

	1998	1999	2000	2001	2002	2003	2004
Smoking prevalence in population aged 15+ (% of population aged 15+)	36.5	37.1	37.4	37.5	38.2	38.5	38.9
Smoking prevalence in male population aged 15+ (% of male population)	49.9	50.4	50.5	51.4	51.7	52.5	52.9
Smoking prevalence in female population aged 15+ (% of female population)	23.9	24.6	25.2	24.6	25.7	25.4	25.9

Source: WHO/OECD/Euromonitor International

Nutrition and Obesity

Bulgaria: Nutrition and obesity 1998-2004

Table: 4.192

As stated

	1998	1999	2000	2001	2002	2003	2004
Availability of fruit and vegetables (kg/capita/year)	206.9	203.5	194.9	189.2	181.7	176.7	171.7
Average supply of calories per day (calories per capita)	2,787.4	2,823.3	2,802.7	2,751.0	2,847.9	2,852.6	2,875.6
Average supply of fat per day (grams per capita)	93.8	93.6	92.5	92.2	96.0	98.4	100.7
Average supply of protein per day (grams per capita)	88.4	89.0	85.9	84.3	88.4	89.6	90.1
Obese population (BMI 30kg/sq m or more) (% of population aged 15+)	13.3	13.6	13.9	13.9	14.1	14.1	14.1

Source: WHO/OECD/Euromonitor International

Bulgaria: Trends in OTC healthcare retail sales 1998-2004

Table: 4.193

As stated

	1998	1999	2000	2001	2002	2003	2004
OTC Healthcare (Lev million)	55.7	65.9	79.1	93.4	101.6	112.9	124.6
OTC Healthcare: real growth in national currency: 1998 = 100	100.0	115.2	125.5	138.0	141.8	154.3	160.1
OTC Healthcare: year on year (% real growth)	6.9	15.2	8.9	10.0	2.7	8.8	3.8
OTC Healthcare (Lev per capita)	6.8	8.1	9.8	11.7	12.9	14.4	16.0

Source: *Euromonitor International from industry sources/national statistics*

Bulgaria: OTC healthcare retail sales by sector 1998-2004

Table: 4.194

% of OTC retail value sales

	1998	1999	2000	2001	2002	2003	2004
Analgesics	36.5	34.7	34.1	33.2	32.1	31.8	31.6
Cough, cold and allergy (hay fever) remedies	18.3	19.9	20.3	20.7	21.4	21.8	22.3
Digestive remedies	4.9	5.2	5.9	6.1	6.2	6.3	6.2
Medicated skin care	7.4	8.0	8.5	8.6	8.3	8.1	8.0
Vitamins and dietary supplements	27.8	26.9	25.8	25.6	25.9	25.7	25.4

Source: *Euromonitor International from industry sources/national statistics*
Notes: *Only selected sectors are shown, so values are not expected to sum to 100*

■ Canada

Socio-economic Parameters

Canada: Socio-economic parameters 1998-2004

Table: 4.195

As stated

	1998	1999	2000	2001	2002	2003	2004
Population: national estimates at January 1st ('000)	30,157.1	30,403.9	30,689.0	31,021.3	31,361.6	31,629.7	31,931.7
% aged 0-14 yrs	19.8	19.5	19.2	18.9	18.6	18.3	18.0
% aged 15-64 yrs	67.9	68.1	68.3	68.5	68.7	68.9	69.2
% aged 65+ yrs	12.3	12.5	12.6	12.6	12.7	12.8	12.8
% Male	49.5	49.5	49.5	49.5	49.5	49.5	49.5
% Female	50.5	50.5	50.5	50.5	50.5	50.5	50.5
% Urban	76.9	77.0	77.1	77.2	77.3	77.5	77.6
Occupants per household at January 1st (Number)	2.7	2.7	2.7	2.7	2.7	2.7	2.7
Households ('000)	11,101.4	11,242.5	11,394.5	11,566.0	11,696.1	11,824.7	11,936.4
Annual rates of inflation (% growth)	1.0	1.7	2.7	2.5	2.2	2.8	1.8
GDP (C$ million)	914,973.0	982,441.0	1,075,570.0	1,108,200.0	1,157,968.0	1,218,772.0	1,293,289.0
GDP (US$ million)	616,783.1	661,251.4	724,235.9	715,540.2	737,878.8	869,899.0	994,057.7
GDP (US$ per capita)	20,452.3	21,748.9	23,599.2	23,066.1	23,528.1	27,502.6	31,130.8

Source: *Euromonitor International from International Monetary Fund (IMF), International Financial Statistics and World Economic Outlook/UN/national statistics*

Life Expectancy

Canada: Life expectancy 1998-2004

As stated

Table: 4.196

	1998	1999	2000	2001	2002	2003	2004	% change 1998-2004
Life expectancy at birth: total population (years)	79.0	79.1	79.1	79.3	79.8	80.0	80.3	1.61
Life expectancy at birth: total population: year on year growth	0.1	0.1	0.0	0.2	0.6	0.3	0.3	
Healthy life expectancy at birth (years)	72.0			69.7	69.9			
Healthy life expectancy at birth: year on year growth					0.2			

Source: Euromonitor International from World Bank

Sanitation

Canada: Improved sanitary facilities and water source 2000

As stated

Table: 4.197

	2000
Population with access to improved sanitary facilities (% of population)	100.0
Population with access to improved water source (% of population)	100.0
Population with improved access to sanitation facilities, rural (% of rural population with access)	99.0
Population with improved access to sanitation facilities, urban (% of urban population with access)	100.0

Source: National statistics/World Bank

Health Expenditure

Canada: Public health expenditure 1998-2004

As stated

Table: 4.198

	1998	1999	2000	2001	2002	2003	2004
Public expenditure on pharmaceuticals and other medical non-durables (C$ million)	4,026.0	4,578.0	5,335.0	6,116.0	6,822.0	7,551.0	8,573.9
Private insurance expenditure (% of total expenditure on health)	11.2	11.2	11.5	12.4	12.7	13.1	13.7
Share of total health expenditure in GDP (% of total GDP)	9.1	9.1	9.1	9.5	9.7	9.6	9.4
Health expenditure (US$ per capita)	1,842.0	1,916.0	2,064.0	2,124.0	2,222.0	2,324.0	2,411.0

Source: Euromonitor International from OECD/national statistics

Canada: Private health expenditure 1998-2004

As stated

Table: 4.199

	1998	1999	2000	2001	2002	2003	2004
Consumer expenditure on health goods and medical services (C$ million)	21,613.0	22,976.0	24,339.0	25,893.0	27,339.0	29,597.2	31,237.3
Consumer expenditure on health goods and medical services: real growth in national currency: 1990 = 100	142.3	148.7	153.3	159.1	164.3	173.1	179.4
Consumer expenditure on health goods and medical services as a percentage of total consumer expenditure	4.2	4.3	4.3	4.4	4.4	4.5	4.6

Source: National statistical offices/OECD/Eurostat/Euromonitor International

Canada: Consumer expenditure on health goods and medical services by sector 1998-2004

Table: 4.200

% of total consumer expenditure on health goods and medical services

	1998	1999	2000	2001	2002	2003	2004
Pharmaceuticals, medical appliances/ equipment	39.7	39.9	39.8	39.8	39.8	39.9	39.8
Outpatient services	54.7	54.6	54.8	54.8	54.8	54.9	55.0
Hospital services	5.6	5.5	5.5	5.4	5.4	5.2	5.2
Total	100.0	100.0	100.0	100.0	100.0	100.0	100.0

Source: National statistical offices/OECD/Eurostat/Euromonitor International

Healthcare Infrastructure and Services

Canada: Healthcare infrastructure and services by sector 1998-2004

Table: 4.201

As stated

	1998	1999	2000	2001	2002	2003	2004
Active pharmacists (number)	18,037	19,872	19,623	19,588	20,504	20,726	21,112
Consultations with GPs (general practitioners) (per capita)	6	6	6	6	6	6	6
Dentists (number)	16,490	16,908	17,314	17,691	17,961	18,326	18,676
Doctors (number)	62,937	63,651	64,454	65,226	66,289	67,193	68,132
Hospitals and clinics (number)	1,062	1,063	1,063	1,065	1,066	1,067	1,068
In-patient beds ('000)	105	98	98	98	98	98	98
Nurses (number)	307,087	306,967	310,887	310,234	292,212	287,593	284,307

Source: Euromonitor International from national statistics

Canada: Healthcare infrastructure and services by sector: growth 1998-2004

Table: 4.202

Year on year growth: % change in stated unit

	1998	1999	2000	2001	2002	2003	2004
Active pharmacists (number)	3.0	10.2	-1.3	-0.2	4.7	1.1	1.9
Consultations with GPs (general practitioners) (per capita)	0.0	0.0	0.0	-1.6	-1.6	-0.8	-1.1
Dentists (number)	1.6	2.5	2.4	2.2	1.5	2.0	1.9
Doctors (number)	1.6	1.1	1.3	1.2	1.6	1.4	1.4
Hospitals and clinics (number)	0.2	0.1	0.0	0.2	0.1	0.1	0.1
In-patient beds (number)	-3.0	-6.2	-0.3	-0.1	0.0	0.0	0.1
Nurses (number)	-1.3	0.0	1.3	-0.2	-5.8	-1.6	-1.1

Source: Euromonitor International from national statistics

Immunisation

Canada: Vaccination rates by disease type 1998-2004

Table: 4.203

%

	1998	1999	2000	2001	2002	2003	2004
Vaccination rate against MMR (measles, mumps, rubella) (%)	96.0						

Source: WHO

Infectious Diseases

Canada: Incidence of disease by type 1998-2004

Table: 4.204

Number

	1998	1999	2000	2001	2002	2003	2004
Incidence of AIDS	639	527	471	384	357	218	250
Incidence of diphtheria	0	1	0	1	2		
Incidence of measles	12	29	206	34	7		
Incidence of polio	0	0	0		0		

Source: WHO

Canada: Incidence of disease by type: growth 1998-2004

Table: 4.205

Year on year growth: %

	1998	1999	2000	2001	2002	2003	2004
Incidence of AIDS	-12.6	-17.5	-10.6	-18.5	-7.0	-38.9	14.7
Incidence of diphtheria	-100.0		-100.0		100.0		
Incidence of measles	-97.9	141.7	610.3	-83.5	-79.4		

Source: WHO

Causes of Death

Canada: Deaths by disease 1998-2004

Table: 4.206

Number per 100,000 inhabitants

	1998	1999	2000	2001	2002	2003	2004
Death by diseases of the circulatory system	216.0	211.0	208.0	206.0	198.0	190.0	184.5
Deaths from heart disease	142.2	139.2	136.2	133.3	130.3	127.5	123.5
Deaths from lung cancer	53.8	53.5	53.8	54.2	54.5	54.7	54.6
Death by diseases of the digestive system	21.2	20.7	20.3	19.8	19.4	19.1	18.8
Deaths from chronic liver disease and cirrhosis	7.2	7.0	7.1	7.1	7.1	7.1	7.1
Deaths from ulcers of the stomach and duodenum	1.6	1.5	1.5	1.5	1.4	1.4	1.4

Source: WHO/Euromonitor International
Notes: Data is ranked in descending order by year 2004

Canada: Deaths by disease: growth 1998-2004

Table: 4.207

% year on year growth

	1998	1999	2000	2001	2002	2003	2004
Deaths from chronic liver disease and cirrhosis	5.9	-2.2	1.4	0.0	0.0	0.0	0.5
Deaths from lung cancer	4.5	-0.5	0.6	0.7	0.6	0.4	-0.1
Deaths from ulcers of the stomach and duodenum	3.8	-3.9	0.0	0.0	-6.7	0.0	-1.4
Death by diseases of the digestive system	-2.3	-2.4	-1.9	-2.5	-2.0	-1.5	-1.6
Death by diseases of the circulatory system	-1.4	-2.3	-1.4	-1.0	-3.9	-4.0	-2.9
Deaths from heart disease	-1.9	-2.1	-2.2	-2.1	-2.3	-2.1	-3.2

Source: WHO/Euromonitor International
Notes: Data is ranked in descending order by year 2004

Canada: Other selected causes of death: 1998-2004

Table: 4.208

Number per 100,000 inhabitants

	1998	1999	2000	2001	2002	2003	2004
Death by motor traffic accidents	9.4						

Source: Euromonitor International from national statistics

Canada: Other selected causes of death: growth 1998-2004

Table: 4.209

% year on year growth

	1998	1999	2000	2001	2002	2003	2004
Death by motor traffic accidents	-4.1						

Source: Euromonitor International from national statistics

Smoking

Canada: Smoking prevalence in population aged 15+ 1998-2004

Table: 4.210

% of population aged 15+

	1998	1999	2000	2001	2002	2003	2004
Smoking prevalence in population aged 15+ (% of population aged 15+)	23.2	23.8	20.9	21.3	20.8	20.5	20.5
Smoking prevalence in male population aged 15+ (% of male population)	25.4	22.5	21.2	22.0	20.9	21.0	20.9
Smoking prevalence in female population aged 15+ (% of female population)	21.2	25.1	20.6	20.6	20.8	19.9	20.1

Source: WHO/OECD/Euromonitor International

Nutrition and Obesity

Canada: Nutrition and obesity 1998-2004

Table: 4.211

As stated

	1998	1999	2000	2001	2002	2003	2004
Average supply of calories per day (calories per capita)	3,454.4	3,513.0	3,546.9	3,545.2	3,589.3	3,625.2	3,656.6
Average supply of fat per day (grams per capita)	148.8	147.1	147.1	145.8	146.2	146.3	146.3
Average supply of protein per day (grams per capita)	102.8	106.2	107.0	106.3	105.0	104.1	103.2
Obese population (BMI 30kg/sq m or more) (% of population aged 15+)	14.6	14.6	14.8	14.9	15.2	15.7	16.0

Source: WHO/OECD/Euromonitor International

Over-the-Counter Healthcare

Canada: Trends in OTC healthcare retail sales 1998-2004

Table: 4.212

As stated

	1998	1999	2000	2001	2002	2003	2004
OTC Healthcare (C$ million)	2,269.0	2,398.9	2,529.5	2,635.8	2,766.0	2,836.2	2,903.3
OTC Healthcare: real growth in national currency: 1998 = 100	100.0	103.9	106.7	108.4	111.3	111.0	111.5
OTC Healthcare: year on year (% real growth)	5.1	3.9	2.6	1.6	2.6	-0.2	0.5
OTC Healthcare (C$ per capita)	75.2	78.9	82.4	85.0	88.2	89.7	90.9

Source: Euromonitor International from industry sources/national statistics

Canada: OTC healthcare retail sales by sector 1998-2004

Table: 4.213

% of OTC retail value sales

	1998	1999	2000	2001	2002	2003	2004
Analgesics	16.9	17.0	17.0	17.1	17.4	18.1	18.8
Cough, cold and allergy (hay fever) remedies	25.1	25.4	25.4	25.0	24.5	24.5	24.5
Digestive remedies	9.8	9.4	9.2	9.1	9.0	8.9	8.9
Medicated skin care	14.7	14.3	14.0	13.8	13.8	13.7	13.5
Vitamins and dietary supplements	27.7	27.4	27.0	26.5	25.7	25.5	25.2

Source: Euromonitor International from industry sources/national statistics
Notes: Only selected sectors are shown, so values are not expected to sum to 100

Health and Wellness

Canada: Retail sales of packaged foods by health and wellness category 2002-2004

Table: 4.214

C$ million

	2002	2003	2004
Packaged food: Total	33,851.8	35,167.7	36,517.5
Better for you	4,433.2	4,614.8	4,872.2
For food intolerance	281.4	297.0	305.1
Fortified/functional	297.2	314.8	353.3
Organic	464.8	527.6	582.6

Source: Euromonitor International from industry sources/national statistics

Canada: Per capita sales of packaged foods by health and wellness category 2002-2004

Table: 4.215

C$ per capita

	2002	2003	2004
Better for you	142.9	147.3	154.1
For food intolerance	9.1	9.5	9.7
Fortified/functional	9.6	10.1	11.2
Organic	15.0	16.8	18.4

Source: Euromonitor International from industry sources/national statistics

Canada: Retail sales of packaged food by health and wellness category: % share of total packaged food market 2002-2004

Table: 4.216

% value

	2002	2003	2004
Better for you	13.1	13.1	13.3
For food intolerance	0.8	0.8	0.8
Fortified/functional	0.9	0.9	1.0
Organic	1.4	1.5	1.6

Source: Euromonitor International from industry sources/national statistics

Canada: Retail sales of packaged food by health and wellness category: real growth index 2002-2004

Table: 4.217

2002 =100

	2002	2003	2004
Better for you	100.00	101.26	105.12
For food intolerance	100.00	102.65	103.71
Fortified/functional	100.00	103.04	113.70
Organic	100.00	110.41	119.90

Source: Euromonitor International from industry sources/national statistics

Canada: Retail sales of better-for-you packaged foods by sector 2002-2004

Table: 4.218

% of total packaged food / as stated

	2002	2003	2004	% real change in value 2002-2004
Combination	1.52	1.74	2.01	36.56
Reduced carb	0.03	0.04	0.10	207.23
Reduced fat	9.85	9.65	9.54	-0.07
Reduced salt	0.41	0.41	0.41	2.81

Source: *Euromonitor International from industry sources/national statistics*

Canada: Retail sales of packaged foods for food intolerances by sector 2002-2004

Table: 4.219

% of total packaged food / as stated

	2002	2003	2004	% real change in value 2002-2004
Diabetic	0.03	0.03	0.03	6.93
Gluten-free	0.00	0.00	0.00	2.44
Lactose-free	0.79	0.81	0.80	3.58

Source: *Euromonitor International from industry sources/national statistics*

Canada: Retail sales of naturally healthy packaged foods by sector 2002-2004

Table: 4.220

% of total packaged food / as stated

	2002	2003	2004	% real change in value 2002-2004
High fibre	0.55	0.55	0.56	5.32
Other naturally healthy food	0.61	0.61	0.61	3.46
Soy-based dairy alternatives	0.32	0.37	0.39	25.18

Source: *Euromonitor International from industry sources/national statistics*

■ Chile

Socio-economic Parameters

Chile: Socio-economic parameters 1998-2004

Table: 4.221

As stated

	1998	1999	2000	2001	2002	2003	2004
Population: national estimates at January 1st ('000)	14,821.7	15,017.8	15,211.3	15,402.0	15,589.1	15,773.5	15,955.6
% aged 0-14 yrs	28.8	28.6	28.5	28.1	27.7	27.3	27.0
% aged 15-64 yrs	64.2	64.3	64.4	64.6	64.9	65.2	65.4
% aged 65 + yrs	7.0	7.1	7.2	7.3	7.4	7.5	7.6
% Male	49.5	49.5	49.5	49.5	49.5	49.5	49.5
% Female	50.5	50.5	50.5	50.5	50.5	50.5	50.5
% Urban	85.2	85.4	84.6	85.0	85.3	85.1	85.3
Occupants per household at January 1st (Number)	3.9	3.9	3.9	3.8	3.8	3.7	3.7
Households ('000)	3,768.7	3,856.0	3,943.4	4,033.5	4,141.4	4,229.1	4,316.8
Annual rates of inflation (% growth)	5.1	3.3	3.8	3.6	2.5	2.8	1.1
GDP (CH$ million)	36,534,900.0	37,138,500.0	40,575,300.0	43,536,800.0	46,341,800.0	50,730,700.0	57,357,000.0
GDP (US$ million)	79,374.2	72,995.6	75,197.0	68,568.6	67,265.8	73,370.4	94,125.2
GDP (US$ per capita)	5,355.3	4,860.6	4,943.5	4,451.9	4,314.9	4,651.5	5,899.2

Source: *Euromonitor International from International Monetary Fund (IMF), International Financial Statistics and World Economic Outlook/UN/national statistics*

Life Expectancy

Chile: Life expectancy 1998-2004

Table: 4.222

As stated

	1998	1999	2000	2001	2002	2003	2004	% change 1998-2004
Life expectancy at birth: total population (years)	75.9	76.1	76.1	76.3	76.7	76.8	77.2	1.58
Life expectancy at birth: total population: year on year growth	0.2	0.2	0.0	0.3	0.5	0.2	0.4	
Healthy life expectancy at birth (years)	69.0			65.8	66.1			
Healthy life expectancy at birth: year on year growth					0.4			

Source: Euromonitor International from World Bank

Sanitation

Chile: Improved sanitary facilities and water source 2000

Table: 4.223

As stated

	2000
Population with access to improved sanitary facilities (% of population)	96.0
Population with access to improved water source (% of population)	93.0
Population with improved access to sanitation facilities, rural (% of rural population with access)	97.0
Population with improved access to sanitation facilities, urban (% of urban population with access)	96.0

Source: National statistics/World Bank

Health Expenditure

Chile: Public health expenditure 1998-2004

Table: 4.224

As stated

	1998	1999	2000	2001	2002	2003	2004
Share of total health expenditure in GDP (% of total GDP)	6.9	6.8	6.8	7.0	6.9	6.9	6.7
Health expenditure (US$ per capita)	325.0	293.0	281.0	253.0	246.0	236.0	225.0

Source: Euromonitor International from OECD/national statistics

Chile: Private health expenditure 1998-2004

Table: 4.225

As stated

	1998	1999	2000	2001	2002	2003	2004
Consumer expenditure on health goods and medical services (CH$ million)	2,002,128.1	2,161,535.2	2,490,313.2	2,792,918.3	3,122,772.8	3,248,550.5	3,407,647.6
Consumer expenditure on health goods and medical services: real growth in national currency: 1990 = 100	285.3	298.0	330.6	358.0	390.6	395.2	410.3
Consumer expenditure on health goods and medical services as a percentage of total consumer expenditure	9.1	9.8	10.4	11.1	11.8	11.8	11.9

Source: National statistical offices/OECD/Eurostat/Euromonitor International

Chile: Consumer expenditure on health goods and medical services by sector 1998-2004

Table: 4.226

% of total consumer expenditure on health goods and medical services

	1998	1999	2000	2001	2002	2003	2004
Pharmaceuticals, medical appliances/ equipment	59.3	59.0	58.7	58.6	58.2	58.2	58.3
Outpatient services	29.4	30.0	30.3	30.6	30.9	30.8	30.6
Hospital services	11.2	11.0	11.0	10.8	10.9	11.0	11.1
Total	100.0	100.0	100.0	100.0	100.0	100.0	100.0

Source: National statistical offices/OECD/Eurostat/Euromonitor International

Healthcare Infrastructure and Services

Chile: Healthcare infrastructure and services by sector 1998-2004

Table: 4.227

As stated

	1998	1999	2000	2001	2002	2003	2004
Active pharmacists (number)	323	321	320	322	324	326	328
Dentists (number)	1,078	1,355	1,367	1,372	1,386	1,396	1,403
Doctors (number)	8,308	10,552	11,707	12,356	12,835	12,982	13,049
Hospitals and clinics (number)	213	212	211	210	209	208	207
In-patient beds ('000)	42	42	41	40	40	40	40
Midwives (number)	2,133	2,171	2,213	2,254	2,291	2,331	2,372
Nurses (number)	3,479	3,677	3,841	4,001	4,117	4,214	4,283

Source: Euromonitor International from national statistics

Chile: Healthcare infrastructure and services by sector: growth 1998-2004

Table: 4.228

Year on year growth: % change in stated unit

	1998	1999	2000	2001	2002	2003	2004
Active pharmacists (number)	25.7	-0.6	-0.3	0.6	0.6	0.6	0.6
Dentists (number)	-90.3	25.7	0.9	0.4	1.0	0.7	0.5
Doctors (number)	5.3	27.0	10.9	5.5	3.9	1.1	0.5
Hospitals and clinics (number)	-0.5	-0.5	-0.5	-0.5	-0.5	-0.5	-0.5
In-patient beds (number)	35.2	1.3	-2.3	-2.5	-0.4	-0.2	-0.3
Midwives (number)	1.8	1.8	1.9	1.9	1.6	1.7	1.8
Nurses (number)	3.7	5.7	4.5	4.2	2.9	2.4	1.6

Source: Euromonitor International from national statistics

Immunisation

Chile: Vaccination rates by disease type 1998-2004

Table: 4.229

%

	1998	1999	2000	2001	2002	2003	2004
Vaccination rate against DTP (diphtheria, tetanus, pertussis) 1 & 2 (%)			97.9	99.0	99.0	99.0	99.0
Vaccination rate against MMR (measles, mumps, rubella) (%)	94.0	96.0	97.3	98.6	95.0	96.0	96.0
Vaccination rate against polio (%)	93.0	95.0	97.5	99.0	95.0	97.0	97.0

Source: WHO

Infectious Diseases

Chile: Incidence of disease by type 1998-2004

Table: 4.230

Number

	1998	1999	2000	2001	2002	2003	2004
Incidence of AIDS	492	553	553	654	536	204	250
Incidence of diphtheria	0	0	0	0			
Incidence of measles	6	31	0	0	0		
Incidence of polio	0	0	0	0			

Source: WHO

Chile: Incidence of disease by type: growth 1998-2004

Table: 4.231

Year on year growth: %

	1998	1999	2000	2001	2002	2003	2004
Incidence of AIDS	-10.7	12.4	0.0	18.3	-18.0	-61.9	22.5
Incidence of measles	-89.7	416.7	-100.0				

Source: WHO

Causes of Death

Chile: Deaths by disease 1998-2004

Table: 4.232

Number per 100,000 inhabitants

	1998	1999	2000	2001	2002	2003	2004
Deaths from heart disease	53.8	53.0	53.3	53.3	53.3	53.3	52.8
Death by diseases of the digestive system	24.0	24.4	24.6	25.5	25.4	25.5	25.6
Deaths from chronic liver disease and cirrhosis	22.7	20.5	19.3	17.8	16.4	15.0	13.7
Deaths from lung cancer	12.1	12.3	12.3	12.3	12.4	12.4	12.4
Deaths from ulcers of the stomach and duodenum	1.5	1.8	1.8	1.8	1.9	2.0	2.1

Source: WHO/Euromonitor International
Notes: Data is ranked in descending order by year 2004

Chile: Deaths by disease: growth 1998-2004

Table: 4.233

% year on year growth

	1998	1999	2000	2001	2002	2003	2004
Deaths from ulcers of the stomach and duodenum	-9.3	20.0	2.0	0.0	5.6	5.3	4.0
Death by diseases of the digestive system	1.3	1.7	0.8	3.7	-0.4	0.4	0.3
Deaths from lung cancer	-0.3	1.2	0.2	0.0	0.8	0.0	-0.2
Deaths from heart disease	1.8	-1.5	0.6	0.0	0.0	0.0	-0.9
Deaths from chronic liver disease and cirrhosis	-3.7	-9.6	-6.0	-7.8	-7.9	-8.5	-8.5

Source: WHO/Euromonitor International

Chile: Other selected causes of death: 1998-2004

Table: 4.234

Number per 100,000 inhabitants

	1998	1999	2000	2001	2002	2003	2004
Death by suicide and self-inflicted injury	6.2	6.4	6.6	6.7	6.7	6.8	6.8

Source: Euromonitor International from national statistics

Chile: Other selected causes of death: growth 1998-2004

Table: 4.235

% year on year growth

	1998	1999	2000	2001	2002	2003	2004
Death by suicide and self-inflicted injury	1.6	3.2	3.1	1.5	0.0	1.5	0.5

Source: *Euromonitor International from national statistics*
Notes: *Data is ranked in descending order by year 2004*

Smoking

Chile: Smoking prevalence in population aged 15+ 1998-2004

Table: 4.236

% of population aged 15+

	1998	1999	2000	2001	2002	2003	2004
Smoking prevalence in population aged 15+ (% of population aged 15+)	25.6	26.1	26.6	26.3	26.8	26.4	25.9
Smoking prevalence in male population aged 15+ (% of male population)	26.0	24.2	24.7	23.9	23.3	23.5	22.9
Smoking prevalence in female population aged 15+ (% of female population)	25.3	28.0	28.3	28.6	30.1	29.1	28.8

Source: *WHO/OECD/Euromonitor International*

Nutrition and Obesity

Chile: Nutrition and obesity 1998-2004

Table: 4.237

As stated

	1998	1999	2000	2001	2002	2003	2004
Average supply of calories per day (calories per capita)	2,796.5	2,800.1	2,824.8	2,847.5	2,863.2	2,880.4	2,898.6
Average supply of fat per day (grams per capita)	82.5	81.4	83.1	84.6	84.0	84.1	84.3
Average supply of protein per day (grams per capita)	76.5	75.9	77.4	78.1	78.4	78.9	79.4
Obese population (BMI 30kg/sq m or more) (% of population aged 15+)	16.1	17.8	18.1	18.4	18.9	19.1	19.5

Source: *WHO/OECD/Euromonitor International*

Over-the-Counter Healthcare

Chile: Trends in OTC healthcare retail sales 1998-2004

Table: 4.238

As stated

	1998	1999	2000	2001	2002	2003	2004
OTC Healthcare (CH$ million)	81,841.7	86,598.0	91,003.8	96,365.1	101,157.9	105,260.3	112,862.2
OTC Healthcare: real growth in national currency: 1998 = 100	100.0	102.4	103.6	105.9	108.5	109.8	116.5
OTC Healthcare: year on year (% real growth)	11.6	2.4	1.2	2.2	2.4	1.2	6.1
OTC Healthcare (CH$ per capita)	5,521.7	5,766.4	5,982.6	6,256.7	6,489.0	6,673.2	7,073.5

Source: *Euromonitor International from industry sources/national statistics*

Chile: OTC healthcare retail sales by sector 1998-2004

Table: 4.239

% of OTC retail value sales

	1998	1999	2000	2001	2002	2003	2004
Analgesics	25.9	26.0	26.0	26.4	27.3	26.6	26.3
Cough, cold and allergy (hay fever) remedies	19.8	20.4	19.9	21.4	20.5	20.6	23.3
Digestive remedies	12.6	12.5	12.8	12.1	13.0	12.8	11.5
Medicated skin care	16.3	16.2	16.4	16.0	16.1	16.3	15.8
Vitamins and dietary supplements	18.6	18.1	17.7	17.1	16.3	17.1	16.7

Source: *Euromonitor International from industry sources/national statistics*
Notes: *Only selected sectors are shown, so values are not expected to sum to 100*

■ **China**

Socio-economic Parameters

China: Socio-economic parameters 1998-2004

Table: 4.240

As stated

	1998	1999	2000	2001	2002	2003	2004
Population: national estimates at January 1st ('000)	1,248,099.8	1,258,540.0	1,268,239.6	1,276,290.9	1,285,535.9	1,295,229.4	1,304,129.8
% aged 0-14 yrs	24.3	23.9	23.5	22.6	21.3	20.5	19.5
% aged 15-64 yrs	68.3	68.4	69.1	69.7	70.6	71.4	72.4
% aged 65 + yrs	7.4	7.6	7.4	7.7	8.2	8.2	8.0
% Male	50.9	50.9	51.2	51.2	51.1	51.1	51.0
% Female	49.1	49.1	48.8	48.8	48.9	48.9	49.0
% Urban	31.1	31.6	32.1	32.5	33.0	34.1	34.8
Occupants per household at January 1st (Number)	3.6	3.7	3.6	3.6	3.5	3.5	3.4
Households ('000)	349,085.2	344,298.9	348,370.0	356,495.8	364,329.8	371,632.1	378,092.1
Annual rates of inflation (% growth)	-0.8	-1.4	0.3	0.5	-0.8	1.2	4.0
GDP (RMB million)	7,900,330.0	8,267,310.0	8,935,670.0	9,731,400.0	10,517,200.0	11,689,800.0	13,652,001.0
GDP (US$ million)	954,266.0	998,678.5	1,079,382.7	1,175,705.9	1,270,659.8	1,412,316.5	1,649,429.9
GDP (US$ per capita)	764.6	793.5	851.1	921.2	988.4	1,090.4	1,264.8

Source: *Euromonitor International from International Monetary Fund (IMF), International Financial Statistics and World Economic Outlook/UN/national statistics*

Life Expectancy

China: Life expectancy 1998-2004

Table: 4.241

As stated

	1998	1999	2000	2001	2002	2003	2004	% change 1998-2004
Life expectancy at birth: total population (years)	70.5	70.8	70.8	71.2	71.1	71.3	71.3	1.18
Life expectancy at birth: total population: year on year growth	0.4	0.4	0.0	0.6	-0.1	0.3	0.1	
Healthy life expectancy at birth (years)	62.0			62.8	63.2			
Healthy life expectancy at birth: year on year growth					0.6			

Source: *Euromonitor International from World Bank*

Sanitation

China: Improved sanitary facilities and water source 2000

Table: 4.242

As stated

	2000
Population with access to improved sanitary facilities (% of population)	40.0
Population with access to improved water source (% of population)	75.0
Population with improved access to sanitation facilities, rural (% of rural population with access)	27.0
Population with improved access to sanitation facilities, urban (% of urban population with access)	69.0

Source: National statistics/World Bank

Health Expenditure

China: Public health expenditure 1998-2004

Table: 4.243

As stated

	1998	1999	2000	2001	2002	2003	2004
Share of total health expenditure in GDP (% of total GDP)	4.8	5.1	5.3	5.5	5.5	5.7	5.9
Health expenditure (US$ per capita)	36.0	40.0	48.0	52.0	63.0	68.0	73.0

Source: Euromonitor International from OECD/national statistics

China: Private health expenditure 1998-2004

Table: 4.244

As stated

	1998	1999	2000	2001	2002	2003	2004
Consumer expenditure on health goods and medical services (RMB Million)	179,555.6	167,425.1	211,735.8	235,208.4	254,894.5	273,916.9	294,860.4
Consumer expenditure on health goods and medical services: real growth in national currency: 1990 = 100	662.0	626.1	789.8	873.3	953.7	1,013.1	1,048.6
Consumer expenditure on health goods and medical services as a percentage of total consumer expenditure	4.8	4.2	4.9	5.1	5.3	5.2	5.2

Source: National statistical offices/OECD/Eurostat/Euromonitor International

China: Consumer expenditure on health goods and medical services by sector 1998-2004

Table: 4.245

% of total consumer expenditure on health goods and medical services

	1998	1999	2000	2001	2002	2003	2004
Pharmaceuticals, medical appliances/ equipment	55.1	52.3	51.6	50.0	49.5	49.5	49.9
Outpatient services	21.9	24.6	25.0	26.5	28.1	28.3	28.0
Hospital services	23.0	23.1	23.3	23.5	22.4	22.3	22.1
Total	100.0	100.0	100.0	100.0	100.0	100.0	100.0

Source: National statistical offices/OECD/Eurostat/Euromonitor International

Healthcare Infrastructure and Services

China: Healthcare infrastructure and services by sector 1998-2004

Table: 4.246

As stated

	1998	1999	2000	2001	2002	2003	2004
Active pharmacists (number)	424,000	418,000	412,000	406,000	399,071	391,871	385,383
Doctors (number)	2,000,000	2,045,000	2,076,000	2,100,000	1,844,000	1,726,000	1,692,000
Hospitals and clinics (number)	67,081	66,935	66,509	65,424	64,548	63,319	62,290
In-patient beds ('000)	3,141	3,159	3,177	3,201	3,136	3,129	3,113
Midwives (number)	49,000	44,000	41,700	40,300	38,823	37,721	36,848
Nurses (number)	1,219,000	1,245,000	1,267,000	1,287,000	1,247,000	1,228,000	1,222,000

Source: Euromonitor International from national statistics

China: Healthcare infrastructure and services by sector: growth 1998-2004

Table: 4.247

Year on year growth: % change in stated unit

	1998	1999	2000	2001	2002	2003	2004
Active pharmacists (number)	-0.9	-1.4	-1.4	-1.5	-1.7	-1.8	-1.7
Doctors (number)	0.8	2.3	1.5	1.2	-12.2	-6.4	-2.0
Hospitals and clinics (number)	-1.2	-0.2	-0.6	-1.6	-1.3	-1.9	-1.6
In-patient beds (number)	0.2	0.6	0.6	0.8	-2.0	-0.2	-0.5
Midwives (number)	0.0	-10.2	-5.2	-3.4	-3.7	-2.8	-2.3
Nurses (number)	1.8	2.1	1.8	1.6	-3.1	-1.5	-0.5

Source: Euromonitor International from national statistics

Immunisation

China: Vaccination rates by disease type 1998-2004

Table: 4.248

%

	1998	1999	2000	2001	2002	2003	2004
Vaccination rate against DTP (diphtheria, tetanus, pertussis) 1 & 2 (%)				78.8	98.2	99.0	99.0
Vaccination rate against MMR (measles, mumps, rubella) (%)	97.0	85.0		78.7	97.9	99.0	99.0
Vaccination rate against polio (%)	98.0	85.0	90.0	79.1	98.4	95.0	98.0

Source: WHO

Infectious Diseases

China: Incidence of disease by type 1998-2004

Table: 4.249

Number

	1998	1999	2000	2001	2002	2003	2004
Incidence of AIDS	136	230	233	231	292	302	280
Incidence of diphtheria	40	16	19	12	11		
Incidence of measles	53,030	61,840	71,093	88,962	58,341		
Incidence of polio	0	1	0	0	0		

Source: WHO

China: Incidence of disease by type: growth 1998-2004

Table: 4.250

Year on year growth: %

	1998	1999	2000	2001	2002	2003	2004
Incidence of AIDS	7.9	69.1	1.3	-0.9	26.4	3.4	-7.3
Incidence of diphtheria	14.3	-60.0	18.8	-36.8	-8.3		
Incidence of measles	-33.4	16.6	15.0	25.1	-34.4		
Incidence of polio			-100.0				

Source: WHO

Causes of Death

China: Deaths by disease 1998-2004

Table: 4.251

Number per 100,000 inhabitants

	1998	1999	2000	2001	2002	2003	2004
Death by malignant neoplasms (cancers)	225.8	223.2	240.6	234.2	230.3	225.0	220.0
Death by diseases of the circulatory system	224.2	223.0	225.0	224.0	221.6	219.0	215.1
Death by diseases of the respiratory system	140.8	140.7	133.5	141.7	139.6	136.1	137.8
Deaths from heart disease	53.9	52.1	54.5	50.5	48.9	45.8	42.8
Deaths from lung cancer	45.1	43.1	40.7	40.8	41.5	41.6	42.3
Death by diseases of the digestive system	37.4	36.3	34.5	32.1	31.5	30.9	29.7
Deaths from ulcers of the stomach and duodenum	37.4	36.3	34.5	32.1	31.5	29.8	28.3
Deaths from chronic liver disease and cirrhosis	11.1	10.8	10.5	10.6	10.0	9.9	9.7

Source: WHO/Euromonitor International
Notes: Data is ranked in descending order by year 2004

China: Deaths by disease: growth 1998-2004

Table: 4.252

% year on year growth

	1998	1999	2000	2001	2002	2003	2004
Deaths from lung cancer	9.5	-4.4	-5.6	0.2	1.7	0.2	1.7
Death by diseases of the respiratory system	-0.1	-0.1	-5.1	6.1	-1.5	-2.5	1.2
Deaths from chronic liver disease and cirrhosis	-1.8	-2.7	-2.8	1.0	-5.7	-1.0	-1.7
Death by diseases of the circulatory system	-0.9	-0.5	0.9	-0.4	-1.1	-1.2	-1.8
Death by malignant neoplasms (cancers)	-0.6	-1.2	7.8	-2.7	-1.7	-2.3	-2.2
Death by diseases of the digestive system	-1.6	-2.9	-5.0	-7.0	-1.9	-1.9	-3.9
Deaths from ulcers of the stomach and duodenum	-1.6	-2.9	-5.0	-7.0	-1.9	-5.4	-5.1
Deaths from heart disease	0.6	-3.3	4.6	-7.3	-3.2	-6.3	-6.5

Source: WHO/Euromonitor International
Notes: Data is ranked in descending order by year 2004

China: Other selected causes of death: 1998-2004

Table: 4.253

Number per 100,000 inhabitants

	1998	1999	2000	2001	2002	2003	2004
Death by injury and poisoning	62.1	62.3	58.3	63.3	62.3	60.3	60.7
Death by suicide and self-inflicted injury	14.1	14.3	11.3	15.3	14.6	13.6	14.6
Death by motor traffic accidents	7.8	8.4	9.0	9.7	10.4	9.2	9.3

Source: Euromonitor International from national statistics
Notes: Data is ranked in descending order by year 2004

China: Other selected causes of death: growth 1998-2004

Table: 4.254

% year on year growth

	1998	1999	2000	2001	2002	2003	2004
Death by suicide and self-inflicted injury	-1.4	1.4	-21.0	35.4	-4.6	-6.8	7.1
Death by motor traffic accidents	5.4	7.7	7.1	7.8	7.2	-11.5	0.9
Death by injury and poisoning	0.5	0.3	-6.4	8.6	-1.6	-3.2	0.6

Source: Euromonitor International from national statistics
Notes: Data is ranked in descending order by year 2004

Smoking

China: Smoking prevalence in population aged 15+ 1998-2004

Table: 4.255

% of population aged 15+

	1998	1999	2000	2001	2002	2003	2004
Smoking prevalence in population aged 15+ (% of population aged 15+)	41.0	41.1	41.6	42.1	42.5	42.7	43.0
Smoking prevalence in male population aged 15+ (% of male population)	64.2	65.3	66.1	66.9	66.8	67.3	67.3
Smoking prevalence in female population aged 15+ (% of female population)	17.6	16.6	16.6	16.8	18.0	17.8	18.3

Source: WHO/OECD/Euromonitor International

Nutrition and Obesity

China: Nutrition and obesity 1998-2004

Table: 4.256

As stated

	1998	1999	2000	2001	2002	2003	2004
Average supply of calories per day (calories per capita)	2,977.4	2,960.9	2,969.1	2,953.3	2,951.0	2,947.6	2,941.5
Average supply of fat per day (grams per capita)	79.0	80.6	84.4	86.0	90.3	94.4	98.3
Average supply of protein per day (grams per capita)	81.0	80.9	82.7	82.3	81.5	81.2	80.8
Obese population (BMI 30kg/sq m or more) (% of population aged 15+)	4.0	4.0	4.1	4.2	4.3	4.4	4.5

Source: WHO/OECD/Euromonitor International

Over-the-Counter Healthcare

China: Trends in OTC healthcare retail sales 1998-2004

Table: 4.257

As stated

	1998	1999	2000	2001	2002	2003	2004
OTC Healthcare (RMB million)	44,120.1	36,637.3	30,657.6	27,772.3	29,167.2	33,326.3	38,429.7
OTC Healthcare: real growth in national currency: 1998 = 100	100.0	84.2	70.3	63.4	67.1	75.8	84.0
OTC Healthcare: year on year (% real growth)	-5.1	-15.8	-16.5	-9.8	5.8	13.0	10.9
OTC Healthcare (RMB per capita)	35.3	29.1	24.2	21.8	22.7	25.7	29.5

Source: Euromonitor International from industry sources/national statistics

China: OTC healthcare retail sales by sector 1998-2004

Table: 4.258

% of OTC retail value sales

	1998	1999	2000	2001	2002	2003	2004
Analgesics	1.2	1.7	2.4	3.1	3.3	3.2	3.1
Cough, cold and allergy (hay fever) remedies	5.5	7.7	10.6	13.4	14.7	14.6	14.2
Digestive remedies	1.3	1.7	2.3	2.9	3.2	3.1	3.0
Medicated skin care	1.4	2.0	2.8	3.6	3.9	3.7	3.6
Vitamins and dietary supplements	88.7	84.4	78.5	72.8	70.9	71.6	72.8

Source: Euromonitor International from industry sources/national statistics
Notes: Only selected sectors are shown, so values are not expected to sum to 100

Health and Wellness

China: Retail sales of packaged foods by health and wellness category 2002-2004

Table: 4.259

RMB million

	2002	2003	2004
Packaged food: Total	362,740.0	393,129.5	426,538.4
Better for you	1,215.3	1,394.8	1,586.9
For food intolerance	53.2	64.0	83.2
Fortified/functional	3,342.3	4,014.0	4,754.3
Organic	111.3	136.1	174.2

Source: Euromonitor International from industry sources/national statistics

China: Per capita sales of packaged foods by health and wellness category 2002-2004

Table: 4.260

RMB per capita

	2002	2003	2004
Better for you	0.9	1.1	1.2
For food intolerance	0.0	0.0	0.1
Fortified/functional	2.6	3.1	3.6
Organic	0.1	0.1	0.1

Source: Euromonitor International from industry sources/national statistics

China: Retail sales of packaged food by health and wellness category: % share of total packaged food market 2002-2004

Table: 4.261

% value

	2002	2003	2004
Better for you	0.3	0.4	0.4
For food intolerance	0.0	0.0	0.0
Fortified/functional	0.9	1.0	1.1
Organic	0.0	0.0	0.0

Source: Euromonitor International from industry sources/national statistics

China: Retail sales of packaged food by health and wellness category: real growth index 2002-2004

Table: 4.262

2002 =100

	2002	2003	2004
Better for you	100.00	113.85	127.63
For food intolerance	100.00	119.33	152.82
Fortified/functional	100.00	119.15	139.03
Organic	100.00	121.27	152.98

Source: Euromonitor International from industry sources/national statistics

China: Retail sales of better-for-you packaged foods by sector 2002-2004

Table: 4.263

% of total packaged food / as stated

	2002	2003	2004	% real change in value 2002-2004
Reduced fat	0.26	0.26	0.27	19.11
Reduced salt	0.00	0.00	0.00	5.04

Source: Euromonitor International from industry sources/national statistics

China: Retail sales of packaged foods for food intolerances by sector 2002-2004

Table: 4.264

% of total packaged food / as stated

	2002	2003	2004	% real change in value 2002-2004
Diabetic	0.01	0.02	0.02	52.85
Lactose-free	0.00	0.00	0.00	10.27

Source: Euromonitor International from industry sources/national statistics

China: Retail sales of naturally healthy packaged foods by sector 2002-2004

Table: 4.265

% of total packaged food / as stated

	2002	2003	2004	% real change in value 2002-2004
High fibre	0.03	0.04	0.04	47.47
Other naturally healthy food	1.07	1.06	1.04	12.19

Source: Euromonitor International from industry sources/national statistics

■ **Colombia**

Socio-economic Parameters

Colombia: Socio-economic parameters 1998-2004

Table: 4.266

As stated

	1998	1999	2000	2001	2002	2003	2004
Population: national estimates at January 1st ('000)	40,338.0	41,053.0	41,764.0	42,472.0	43,175.0	43,874.0	44,567.0
% aged 0-14 yrs	34.0	33.0	33.0	33.0	32.0	32.0	32.0
% aged 15-64 yrs	62.0	62.0	62.0	63.0	63.0	63.0	63.0
% aged 65 + yrs	5.0	5.0	5.0	5.0	5.0	5.0	5.0
% Male	49.0	49.0	49.0	49.0	49.0	49.0	49.0
% Female	51.0	51.0	51.0	51.0	51.0	51.0	51.0
% Urban	73.0	73.0	75.0	75.0	75.0	76.0	76.0
Occupants per household at January 1st (Number)	4.0	4.0	4.0	4.0	4.0	4.0	4.0
Households ('000)	9,003.0	9,421.0	9,854.0	10,297.0	10,761.0	11,194.0	11,604.0
Annual rates of inflation (% growth)	19.0	11.0	9.0	8.0	6.0	7.0	6.0
GDP (Col$ million)	140,483,000.0	151,565,000.0	174,896,000.0	188,559,000.0	204,530,000.0	230,091,000.0	255,984,000.0
GDP (US$ million)	98,513.0	86,301.0	83,766.0	81,995.0	81,673.0	79,958.0	97,384.0
GDP (US$ per capita)	2,442.0	2,102.0	2,006.0	1,931.0	1,892.0	1,822.0	2,185.0

Source: Euromonitor International from International Monetary Fund (IMF), International Financial Statistics and World Economic Outlook/UN/national statistics

Life Expectancy

Colombia: Life expectancy 1998-2004

Table: 4.267

As stated

	1998	1999	2000	2001	2002	2003	2004	% change 1998-2004
Life expectancy at birth: total population (years)	69.9	70.2	70.7	70.7	71.8	72.5	73.1	4.51
Life expectancy at birth: total population: year on year growth	0.5	0.4	0.7	0.0	1.6	0.9	0.9	
Healthy life expectancy at birth (years)	63.0			58.6	58.7			
Healthy life expectancy at birth: year on year growth					0.2			

Source: Euromonitor International from World Bank

Sanitation

Colombia: Improved sanitary facilities and water source 2000

Table: 4.268

As stated

	2000
Population with access to improved sanitary facilities (% of population)	86.0
Population with access to improved water source (% of population)	91.0
Population with improved access to sanitation facilities, rural (% of rural population with access)	56.0
Population with improved access to sanitation facilities, urban (% of urban population with access)	96.0

Source: National statistics/World Bank

Health Expenditure

Colombia: Public health expenditure 1998-2004

Table: 4.269

As stated

	1998	1999	2000	2001	2002	2003	2004
Share of total health expenditure in GDP (% of total GDP)	5.8	6.4	5.5	5.5	5.3	5.5	5.3
Health expenditure (US$ per capita)	240.0	203.0	158.0	159.0	151.0	142.0	139.0

Source: Euromonitor International from OECD/national statistics

Colombia: Private health expenditure 1998-2004

Table: 4.270

As stated

	1998	1999	2000	2001	2002	2003	2004
Consumer expenditure on health goods and medical services (Col$ million)	3,549,557.0	3,851,533.0	4,630,608.0	5,319,243.0	5,945,452.0	6,613,376.8	7,212,148.3
Consumer expenditure on health goods and medical services: real growth in national currency: 1990 = 100	112.8	110.4	121.5	129.3	135.9	141.1	145.3
Consumer expenditure on health goods and medical services as a percentage of total consumer expenditure	3.9	4.0	4.1	4.3	4.5	4.5	4.6

Source: National statistical offices/OECD/Eurostat/Euromonitor International

Colombia: Consumer expenditure on health goods and medical services by sector 1998-2004

Table: 4.271

% of total consumer expenditure on health goods and medical services

	1998	1999	2000	2001	2002	2003	2004
Pharmaceuticals, medical appliances/ equipment	75.5	72.1	74.4	73.5	72.8	72.0	71.4
Outpatient services	10.4	11.8	10.8	10.6	10.6	10.6	11.0
Hospital services	14.1	16.1	14.8	16.0	16.6	17.4	17.6
Total	100.0	100.0	100.0	100.0	100.0	100.0	100.0

Source: *National statistical offices/OECD/Eurostat/Euromonitor International*

Healthcare Infrastructure and Services

Colombia: Healthcare infrastructure and services by sector 1998-2004

Table: 4.272

As stated

	1998	1999	2000	2001	2002	2003	2004
Doctors (number)	40,551	40,632	40,618	40,605	40,486	40,334	40,240
In-patient beds ('000)	48	48	48	48	48	48	49

Source: *Euromonitor International from national statistics*

Colombia: Healthcare infrastructure and services by sector: growth 1998-2004

Table: 4.273

Year on year growth: % change in stated unit

	1998	1999	2000	2001	2002	2003	2004
Doctors (number)	0.5	0.2	0.0	0.0	-0.3	-0.4	-0.2
In-patient beds (number)	0.2	0.5	0.3	0.3	0.3	0.3	0.4

Source: *Euromonitor International from national statistics*

Immunisation

Colombia: Vaccination rates by disease type 1998-2004

Table: 4.274

%

	1998	1999	2000	2001	2002	2003	2004
Vaccination rate against DTP (diphtheria, tetanus, pertussis) 1 & 2 (%)			75.3	73.4	71.5	70.0	68.0
Vaccination rate against MMR (measles, mumps, rubella) (%)	73.0	75.0	75.4	90.2	93.1	96.0	99.0
Vaccination rate against polio (%)	72.0	75.0	78.4	83.1	82.8	87.0	90.0

Source: *WHO*

Infectious Diseases

Colombia: Incidence of disease by type 1998-2004

Table: 4.275

Number

	1998	1999	2000	2001	2002	2003	2004
Incidence of AIDS	1,125	906	867	1,157	1,602	1,406	1,503
Incidence of diphtheria	2	0	11	0	3		
Incidence of measles	61	44	1	3	139		
Incidence of polio	0	0	0	0	0		

Source: *WHO*

Colombia: Incidence of disease by type: growth 1998-2004

Table: 4.276

Year on year growth: %

	1998	1999	2000	2001	2002	2003	2004
Incidence of AIDS	-4.9	-19.5	-4.3	33.4	38.5	-12.2	6.9
Incidence of diphtheria	-33.3	-100.0		-100.0			
Incidence of measles	-9.0	-27.9	-97.7	200.0	4,533.3		

Source: WHO

Causes of Death

Colombia: Deaths by disease 1998-2004

Table: 4.277

Number per 100,000 inhabitants

	1998	1999	2000	2001	2002	2003	2004
Deaths from heart disease	53.7	54.0	53.1	52.3	51.3	50.0	49.2
Death by diseases of the digestive system	28.6	29.3	29.7	29.7	30.3	30.8	30.9
Deaths from lung cancer	7.4	7.1	6.5	6.3	6.1	5.9	5.7
Deaths from chronic liver disease and cirrhosis	4.3	4.3	4.3	4.2	4.1	4.1	4.1
Deaths from ulcers of the stomach and duodenum	2.5	2.5	2.7	2.8	2.8	2.9	3.0

Source: WHO/Euromonitor International
Notes: Data is ranked in descending order by year 2004

Colombia: Deaths by disease: growth 1998-2004

Table: 4.278

% year on year growth

	1998	1999	2000	2001	2002	2003	2004
Deaths from ulcers of the stomach and duodenum	14.7	1.0	8.0	3.7	0.0	3.6	1.9
Death by diseases of the digestive system	2.1	2.4	1.4	0.0	2.0	1.7	0.4
Deaths from chronic liver disease and cirrhosis	-0.3	0.9	0.0	-2.3	-2.4	0.0	-0.9
Deaths from heart disease	-1.2	0.5	-1.7	-1.5	-1.9	-2.5	-1.6
Deaths from lung cancer	2.5	-4.1	-8.5	-3.1	-3.2	-3.3	-2.7

Source: WHO/Euromonitor International
Notes: Data is ranked in descending order by year 2004

Smoking

Colombia: Smoking prevalence in population aged 15+ 1998-2004

Table: 4.279

% of population aged 15+

	1998	1999	2000	2001	2002	2003	2004
Smoking prevalence in population aged 15+ (% of population aged 15+)	22.3	22.8	23.2	23.2	23.2	22.8	23.3
Smoking prevalence in male population aged 15+ (% of male population)	24.1	24.5	25.2	25.6	26.3	26.8	27.4
Smoking prevalence in female population aged 15+ (% of female population)	20.6	21.2	21.3	20.9	20.3	19.1	19.4

Source: WHO/OECD/Euromonitor International

Nutrition and Obesity

Colombia: Nutrition and obesity 1998-2004

Table: 4.280

As stated

	1998	1999	2000	2001	2002	2003	2004
Average supply of calories per day (calories per capita)	2,533.9	2,556.8	2,574.8	2,576.6	2,584.6	2,593.7	2,600.6
Average supply of fat per day (grams per capita)	64.9	65.4	65.7	65.4	65.3	65.3	65.2
Average supply of protein per day (grams per capita)	60.2	59.9	60.2	60.7	60.6	60.7	60.9
Obese population (BMI 30kg/sq m or more) (% of population aged 15+)	19.7	21.0	21.0	21.0	21.0	21.3	21.4

Source: WHO/OECD/Euromonitor International

Over-the-Counter Healthcare

Colombia: Trends in OTC healthcare retail sales 1998-2004

Table: 4.281

As stated

	1998	1999	2000	2001	2002	2003	2004
OTC Healthcare (Col$ billion)	334.0	440.8	565.9	670.0	777.2	831.1	862.8
OTC Healthcare: real growth in national currency: 1998 = 100	100.0	119.0	139.9	153.5	167.4	167.1	163.6
OTC Healthcare: year on year (% real growth)	15.2	19.0	17.6	9.7	9.1	-0.2	-2.1
OTC Healthcare ('000 Col$ per capita)	8.3	10.7	13.6	15.8	18.0	18.9	19.4

Source: Euromonitor International from industry sources/national statistics

Colombia: OTC healthcare retail sales by sector 1998-2004

Table: 4.282

% of OTC retail value sales

	1998	1999	2000	2001	2002	2003	2004
Analgesics	27.0	28.2	29.4	29.5	29.7	28.6	28.3
Cough, cold and allergy (hay fever) remedies	28.0	26.4	25.2	24.2	23.7	22.9	22.9
Digestive remedies	16.2	15.8	15.1	14.6	14.5	15.8	15.8
Medicated skin care	11.8	11.2	10.6	10.1	9.7	9.4	9.3
Vitamins and dietary supplements	12.6	13.7	14.9	16.3	16.8	18.0	18.5

Source: Euromonitor International from industry sources/national statistics
Notes: Only selected sectors are shown, so values are not expected to sum to 100

■ Croatia

Socio-economic Parameters

Croatia: Socio-economic parameters 1998-2004

Table: 4.283

As stated

	1998	1999	2000	2001	2002	2003	2004
Population: national estimates at January 1st ('000)	4,501.2	4,553.8	4,473.8	4,437.5	4,439.2	4,440.9	4,442.1
% aged 0-14 yrs	19.9	19.8	17.1	17.0	16.9	16.8	16.7
% aged 15-64 yrs	67.8	67.9	67.0	66.9	66.7	66.6	66.5
% aged 65+ yrs	12.3	12.4	15.9	16.1	16.4	16.6	16.8
% Male	48.1	48.1	48.1	48.1	48.1	48.1	48.1
% Female	51.9	51.9	51.9	51.9	51.9	51.9	51.9
% Urban	56.9	57.3	57.5	57.9	58.3	58.8	59.3
Occupants per household at January 1st (Number)	3.0	3.1	3.0	3.0	3.0	3.0	3.0
Households ('000)	1,496.8	1,490.1	1,482.2	1,477.4	1,472.2	1,465.9	1,461.4
Annual rates of inflation (% growth)	6.4	3.5	5.3	4.8	1.7	0.1	3.7
GDP (HRK million)	137,604.0	141,579.0	152,519.0	165,639.0	179,390.0	193,067.0	206,923.0
GDP (US$ million)	21,628.1	19,905.8	18,427.8	19,860.8	22,798.1	28,800.8	34,282.4
GDP (US$ per capita)	4,805.0	4,371.3	4,119.1	4,475.7	5,135.6	6,485.3	7,717.5

Source: Euromonitor International from International Monetary Fund (IMF), International Financial Statistics and World Economic Outlook/UN/national statistics

Life Expectancy

Croatia: Life expectancy 1998-2004

Table: 4.284

As stated

	1998	1999	2000	2001	2002	2003	2004	% change 1998-2004
Life expectancy at birth: total population (years)	72.5	72.7	72.9	72.9	74.8	75.5	76.5	5.43
Life expectancy at birth: total population: year on year growth	0.3	0.2	0.2	0.1	2.6	0.9	1.3	
Healthy life expectancy at birth (years)	67.0			63.1	63.3			
Healthy life expectancy at birth: year on year growth					0.3			

Source: Euromonitor International from World Bank

Health Expenditure

Croatia: Public health expenditure 1998-2004

Table: 4.285

As stated

	1998	1999	2000	2001	2002	2003	2004
Share of total health expenditure in GDP (% of total GDP)	8.8	8.9	9.4	9.0	8.8	9.1	8.8
Health expenditure (US$ per capita)	387.0	387.0	374.0	366.0	369.0	363.0	359.0

Source: Euromonitor International from OECD/national statistics

Croatia: Private health expenditure 1998-2004

Table: 4.286

As stated

	1998	1999	2000	2001	2002	2003	2004
Consumer expenditure on health goods and medical services (HRK million)	1,378.7	1,555.5	1,711.1	1,786.6	1,945.0	2,122.6	2,282.7
Consumer expenditure on health goods and medical services: real growth in national currency: 1990 = 100	86.2	94.0	98.2	97.9	104.8	112.4	118.4
Consumer expenditure on health goods and medical services as a percentage of total consumer expenditure	1.7	1.9	1.9	1.9	2.0	2.0	2.0

Source: National statistical offices/OECD/Eurostat/Euromonitor International

Croatia: Consumer expenditure on health goods and medical services by sector 1998-2004

Table: 4.287

% of total consumer expenditure on health goods and medical services

	1998	1999	2000	2001	2002	2003	2004
Pharmaceuticals, medical appliances/ equipment	70.0	70.6	70.3	68.7	68.3	68.7	68.8
Outpatient services	24.0	23.9	24.6	26.4	26.9	26.7	26.6
Hospital services	6.0	5.5	5.0	4.9	4.8	4.6	4.5
Total	100.0	100.0	100.0	100.0	100.0	100.0	100.0

Source: National statistical offices/OECD/Eurostat/Euromonitor International

Healthcare Infrastructure and Services

Croatia: Healthcare infrastructure and services by sector 1998-2004

Table: 4.288

As stated

	1998	1999	2000	2001	2002	2003	2004
Active pharmacists (number)	1,550	1,502	1,493	1,575	1,620	1,662	1,703
Dentists (number)	1,121	769	664	615	548	523	499
Doctors (number)	8,600	8,046	7,751	7,779	7,790	7,808	7,824
Hospital admissions (number)	686,073	682,961	689,190	700,524	696,519	710,943	713,343
Hospitals and clinics (number)	78	78	77	78	79	79	80
In-patient beds ('000)	27	27	27	27	25	25	25
Nurses (number)	41,235	40,998	40,661	40,327	39,929	39,486	39,302
Out-patient contacts (per capita)	7	7	7	7	8	8	8

Source: Euromonitor International from national statistics

Croatia: Healthcare infrastructure and services by sector: growth 1998-2004

Table: 4.289

Year on year growth: % change in stated unit

	1998	1999	2000	2001	2002	2003	2004
Active pharmacists (number)	-3.8	-3.1	-0.6	5.5	2.9	2.6	2.5
Dentists (number)	-23.1	-31.4	-13.7	-7.4	-10.9	-4.6	-4.6
Doctors (number)	-7.7	-6.4	-3.7	0.4	0.1	0.2	0.2
Hospital admissions (number)	0.6	-0.5	0.9	1.6	-0.6	2.1	0.3
Hospitals and clinics (number)	0.0	0.0	-1.3	1.3	1.3	0.0	1.3
In-patient beds (number)	-0.7	-1.0	-0.2	-1.3	-5.4	-0.2	-0.5
Nurses (number)	-0.5	-0.6	-0.8	-0.8	-1.0	-1.1	-0.5
Out-patient contacts (per capita)	7.1	1.5	5.9	4.2	2.8	1.3	5.3

Source: Euromonitor International from national statistics

Immunisation

Croatia: Vaccination rates by disease type 1998-2004

Table: 4.290

%

	1998	1999	2000	2001	2002	2003	2004
Vaccination rate against DTP (diphtheria, tetanus, pertussis) 1 & 2 (%)				94.1	99.0	99.0	99.0
Vaccination rate against MMR (measles, mumps, rubella) (%)	93.0	92.0	93.2	94.4	94.7	95.0	96.0
Vaccination rate against polio (%)	93.0	93.0	93.5	94.1	94.7	95.0	96.0

Source: WHO

Infectious Diseases

Croatia: Incidence of disease by type 1998-2004

Table: 4.291

Number

	1998	1999	2000	2001	2002	2003	2004
Incidence of AIDS	12	16	19	7	20	1	5
Incidence of diphtheria	0	0	0	0	0		
Incidence of measles	648	31	9	8	6		
Incidence of polio	0	0	0	0	0		

Source: WHO

Croatia: Incidence of disease by type: growth 1998-2004

Table: 4.292

Year on year growth: %

	1998	1999	2000	2001	2002	2003	2004
Incidence of AIDS	-29.4	33.3	18.8	-63.2	185.7	-95.0	400.0
Incidence of measles	170.0	-95.2	-71.0	-11.1	-25.0		

Source: WHO

Causes of Death

Croatia: Deaths by disease 1998-2004

Table: 4.293

Number per 100,000 inhabitants

	1998	1999	2000	2001	2002	2003	2004
Deaths from heart disease	211.4	197.5	213.2	209.1	209.9	210.8	208.8
Deaths from lung cancer	57.1	54.8	56.5	55.6	55.4	55.1	54.7
Death by diseases of the digestive system	38.6	38.1	37.5	37.1	36.1	35.8	35.4
Deaths from chronic liver disease and cirrhosis	33.3	34.4	32.9	33.1	32.9	32.7	32.5
Deaths from ulcers of the stomach and duodenum	5.1	5.1	5.3	5.4	5.5	5.6	5.7
Death by malignant neoplasms (cancers)			267.7				
Death by diseases of the respiratory system			46.6				

Source: WHO/Euromonitor International
Notes: Data is ranked in descending order by year 2004

Croatia: Deaths by disease: growth 1998-2004

Table: 4.294

% year on year growth

	1998	1999	2000	2001	2002	2003	2004
Deaths from ulcers of the stomach and duodenum	-0.2	0.6	3.5	2.0	1.9	1.8	2.2
Deaths from chronic liver disease and cirrhosis	11.8	3.2	-4.4	0.7	-0.6	-0.6	-0.6
Deaths from lung cancer	6.5	-4.0	3.2	-1.7	-0.4	-0.5	-0.8
Deaths from heart disease	2.0	-6.6	7.9	-1.9	0.4	0.4	-1.0
Death by diseases of the digestive system	-1.5	-1.3	-1.6	-1.1	-2.7	-0.8	-1.0

Source: WHO/Euromonitor International
Notes: Data is ranked in descending order by year 2004

Croatia: Other selected causes of death: 1998-2004

Table: 4.295

Number per 100,000 inhabitants

	1998	1999	2000	2001	2002	2003	2004
Death by motor traffic accidents	14.9	15.0	16.4	17.9	18.7	18.9	20.0
Death by suicide and self-inflicted injury	22.9	21.7	21.1	20.7	20.6	19.7	19.4
Death by injury and poisoning			66.3				

Source: Euromonitor International from national statistics
Notes: Data is ranked in descending order by year 2004

Croatia: Other selected causes of death: growth 1998-2004

Table: 4.296

% year on year growth

	1998	1999	2000	2001	2002	2003	2004
Death by motor traffic accidents	0.7	9.3	9.1	4.5	1.1	5.7
Death by suicide and self-inflicted injury	-5.2	-2.8	-1.9	-0.5	-4.4	-1.8

Source: *Euromonitor International from national statistics*
Notes: *Data is ranked in descending order by year 2004*

Smoking

Croatia: Smoking prevalence in population aged 15+ 1998-2004

Table: 4.297

% of population aged 15+

	1998	1999	2000	2001	2002	2003	2004
Smoking prevalence in population aged 15+ (% of population aged 15+)	30.9	30.8	30.3	30.1	30.2	30.4	30.1
Smoking prevalence in male population aged 15+ (% of male population)	29.6	28.4	34.1	27.2	26.7	26.8	26.9
Smoking prevalence in female population aged 15+ (% of female population)	32.0	33.0	26.6	32.7	33.3	33.7	32.9

Source: *WHO/OECD/Euromonitor International*

Nutrition and Obesity

Croatia: Nutrition and obesity 1998-2004

Table: 4.298

As stated

	1998	1999	2000	2001	2002	2003	2004
Availability of fruit and vegetables (kg/capita/year)	186.4	199.4	187.5	186.9	188.0	186.6	184.4
Average supply of calories per day (calories per capita)	2,610.7	2,688.3	2,705.8	2,807.0	2,799.0	2,813.6	2,839.4
Average supply of fat per day (grams per capita)	70.1	89.6	92.0	92.7	81.3	83.3	84.6
Average supply of protein per day (grams per capita)	65.7	69.7	70.4	74.4	74.6	75.6	77.0
Microbiological food-borne diseases (per 100000 population)	44.0	39.0	77.0	92.0	83.0	89.0	93.0
Obese population (BMI 30kg/sq m or more) (% of population aged 15+)	7.8	8.0	8.3	9.0	9.2	9.6	10.0

Source: *WHO/OECD/Euromonitor International*

■ Czech Republic

Socio-economic Parameters

Czech Republic: Socio-economic parameters 1998-2004

Table: 4.299

As stated

	1998	1999	2000	2001	2002	2003	2004
Population: national estimates at January 1st ('000)	10,255.8	10,241.2	10,228.0	10,216.6	10,206.4	10,203.3	10,199.3
% aged 0-14 yrs	17.4	17.0	16.6	16.2	15.9	15.6	15.3
% aged 15-64 yrs	69.0	69.3	69.6	69.9	70.2	70.5	70.9
% aged 65+ yrs	13.6	13.7	13.8	13.9	13.9	13.9	13.8
% Male	48.7	48.7	48.7	48.7	48.7	48.7	48.7
% Female	51.3	51.3	51.3	51.3	51.3	51.3	51.3
% Urban	74.6	74.7	74.7	74.8	74.9	75.4	75.6
Occupants per household at January 1st (Number)	2.7	2.7	2.7	2.7	2.7	2.7	2.7
Households ('000)	3,870.0	3,851.1	3,836.5	3,827.7	3,817.1	3,804.3	3,791.6
Annual rates of inflation (% growth)	10.6	2.1	3.9	4.7	1.8	0.1	2.8
GDP (CK million)	1,962,480.0	2,041,350.0	2,150,060.0	2,315,250.0	2,414,670.0	2,550,750.0	2,751,070.0
GDP (US$ million)	60,793.3	59,051.1	55,703.3	60,871.1	73,756.3	90,423.3	107,046.8
GDP (US$ per capita)	5,927.7	5,766.0	5,446.2	5,958.1	7,226.4	8,862.2	10,495.5

Source: Euromonitor International from International Monetary Fund (IMF), International Financial Statistics and World Economic Outlook/UN/national statistics

Life Expectancy

Czech Republic: Life expectancy 1998-2004

Table: 4.300

As stated

	1998	1999	2000	2001	2002	2003	2004	% change 1998-2004
Life expectancy at birth: total population (years)	74.8	75.0	75.1	75.3	75.8	76.0	76.2	1.93
Life expectancy at birth: total population: year on year growth	0.3	0.3	0.2	0.3	0.6	0.2	0.3	
Healthy life expectancy at birth (years)	68.0				66.4	66.6		
Healthy life expectancy at birth: year on year growth					0.3			

Source: Euromonitor International from World Bank

Health Expenditure

Czech Republic: Public health expenditure 1998-2004

Table: 4.301

As stated

	1998	1999	2000	2001	2002	2003	2004
Public expenditure on pharmaceuticals and other medical non-durables (CK million)	27,200.0	24,211.0	24,314.0	26,719.0	29,445.0	31,954.0	35,820.0
Share of total health expenditure in GDP (% of total GDP)	7.1	7.1	7.1	7.4	7.4	7.5	7.4
Health expenditure (US$ per capita)	392.0	380.0	358.0	408.0	504.0	532.0	570.0

Source: Euromonitor International from OECD/national statistics

Czech Republic: Private health expenditure 1998-2004

Table: 4.302

As stated

	1998	1999	2000	2001	2002	2003	2004
Consumer expenditure on health goods and medical services (CK million)	10,413.0	11,289.0	13,810.0	16,912.0	18,020.0	20,006.8	20,940.5
Consumer expenditure on health goods and medical services: real growth in national currency: 1990 = 100	161.8	171.7	202.2	236.4	247.5	274.5	279.4
Consumer expenditure on health goods and medical services as a percentage of total consumer expenditure	1.1	1.1	1.3	1.5	1.5	1.7	1.7

Source: National statistical offices/OECD/Eurostat/Euromonitor International

Czech Republic: Consumer expenditure on health goods and medical services by sector 1998-2004

Table: 4.303

% of total consumer expenditure on health goods and medical services

	1998	1999	2000	2001	2002	2003	2004
Pharmaceuticals, medical appliances/equipment	73.4	73.3	76.3	78.3	78.5	78.7	78.9
Outpatient services	21.3	21.3	19.9	18.5	18.2	18.0	17.9
Hospital services	5.4	5.4	3.8	3.2	3.3	3.2	3.1
Total	100.0	100.0	100.0	100.0	100.0	100.0	100.0

Source: National statistical offices/OECD/Eurostat/Euromonitor International

Healthcare Infrastructure and Services

Czech Republic: Healthcare infrastructure and services by sector 1998-2004

Table: 4.304

As stated

	1998	1999	2000	2001	2002	2003	2004
Active pharmacists (number)	4,559	4,786	5,059	5,199	5,397	5,518	5,622
Consultations with GPs (general practitioners) (per capita)	12	12	13	13	13	13	13
Dentists (number)	6,386	6,426	6,658	6,698	6,697	6,791	6,836
Doctors (number)	31,192	31,653	34,604	35,222	35,750	36,752	37,182
Hospital admissions (number)	2,021,010	1,992,302	2,052,772	2,072,932	2,148,276	2,186,831	2,227,879
Hospitals and clinics (number)	207	203	211	202	201	200	198
In-patient beds ('000)	69	67	67	67	67	66	66
Nurses (number)	88,165	88,564	91,285	93,682	95,498	97,929	100,250
Out-patient contacts (per capita)	15	15	15	15	15	14	15

Source: Euromonitor International from national statistics

Czech Republic: Healthcare infrastructure and services by sector: growth 1998-2004

Table: 4.305

Year on year growth: % change in stated unit

	1998	1999	2000	2001	2002	2003	2004
Active pharmacists (number)	3.6	5.0	5.7	2.8	3.8	2.2	1.9
Consultations with GPs (general practitioners) (per capita)	-3.9	-0.8	2.4	0.8	1.6	1.6	1.5
Dentists (number)	-1.3	0.6	3.6	0.6	0.0	1.4	0.7
Doctors (number)	-2.7	1.5	9.3	1.8	1.5	2.8	1.2
Hospital admissions (number)	-3.0	-1.4	3.0	1.0	3.6	1.8	1.9
Hospitals and clinics (number)	1.0	-1.9	3.9	-4.3	-0.5	-0.5	-1.0
In-patient beds (number)	-1.4	-3.0	0.1	-0.9	-0.2	-0.3	-0.5
Nurses (number)	-0.1	0.5	3.1	2.6	1.9	2.5	2.4
Out-patient contacts (per capita)	-4.0	0.0	2.1	0.0	0.0	-2.7	3.5

Source: Euromonitor International from national statistics

Immunisation

Czech Republic: Vaccination rates by disease type 1998-2004

Table: 4.306

%

	1998	1999	2000	2001	2002	2003	2004
Vaccination rate against MMR (measles, mumps, rubella) (%)	95.0	97.0	99.0	99.0	99.0	99.0	99.0
Vaccination rate against polio (%)	97.0	98.0	97.4	97.2	97.1	97.0	96.0

Source: WHO

Infectious Diseases

Czech Republic: Incidence of disease by type 1998-2004

Table: 4.307

Number

	1998	1999	2000	2001	2002	2003	2004
Incidence of AIDS	8	16	13	3	8	4	6
Incidence of diphtheria	0	0	0	0	0		
Incidence of measles	19	2	9	6	4		
Incidence of polio	0	0	0	0	0		

Source: WHO

Czech Republic: Incidence of disease by type: growth 1998-2004

Table: 4.308

Year on year growth: %

	1998	1999	2000	2001	2002	2003	2004
Incidence of AIDS	-61.9	100.0	-18.8	-76.9	166.7	-50.0	50.0
Incidence of measles	35.7	-89.5	350.0	-33.3	-33.3		

Source: WHO

Causes of Death

Czech Republic: Deaths by disease 1998-2004

Table: 4.309

Number per 100,000 inhabitants

	1998	1999	2000	2001	2002	2003	2004
Death by diseases of the circulatory system	476.5	467.1	441.9	434.9	425.1	417.2	408.5
Death by malignant neoplasms (cancers)	225.0	223.5	224.2	224.0	223.2	223.8	224.8
Deaths from heart disease	233.5	238.5	227.6	227.3	224.4	221.5	218.0
Deaths from lung cancer	52.8	54.7	55.7	57.4	58.9	60.3	62.0
Death by diseases of the respiratory system	33.0	36.7	38.3	38.7	43.2	44.9	47.2
Death by diseases of the digestive system	33.2	33.3	33.0	29.6	28.4	30.7	29.9
Deaths from chronic liver disease and cirrhosis	18.5	18.1	18.0	17.7	17.5	17.2	16.8
Deaths from ulcers of the stomach and duodenum	5.0	5.1	5.9	6.3	6.7	7.2	7.7

Source: WHO/Euromonitor International
Notes: Data is ranked in descending order by year 2004

Czech Republic: Deaths by disease: growth 1998-2004

Table: 4.310

% year on year growth

	1998	1999	2000	2001	2002	2003	2004
Deaths from ulcers of the stomach and duodenum	-2.6	1.7	16.8	6.4	6.3	7.5	7.4
Death by diseases of the respiratory system	-5.4	11.2	4.4	1.0	11.6	3.9	5.1
Deaths from lung cancer	-2.2	3.6	1.9	3.0	2.6	2.4	2.9
Death by malignant neoplasms (cancers)	-1.2	-0.7	0.3	-0.1	-0.4	0.3	0.4
Deaths from heart disease	-7.9	2.1	-4.5	-0.2	-1.3	-1.3	-1.6
Deaths from chronic liver disease and cirrhosis	8.2	-2.5	-0.1	-1.9	-1.1	-1.7	-2.1
Death by diseases of the circulatory system	-5.6	-2.0	-5.4	-1.6	-2.3	-1.9	-2.1
Death by diseases of the digestive system	1.8	0.3	-0.9	-10.3	-4.1	8.1	-2.7

Source: WHO/Euromonitor International
Notes: Data is ranked in descending order by year 2004

Czech Republic: Other selected causes of death: 1998-2004

Table: 4.311

Number per 100,000 inhabitants

	1998	1999	2000	2001	2002	2003	2004
Death by injury and poisoning	59.5	58.6	59.2	59.0	58.7	58.5	58.9
Death by motor traffic accidents	8.1	14.1	14.1	15.1	20.2	20.6	23.2
Death by suicide and self-inflicted injury	13.7	13.6	13.8	13.8	13.7	13.8	13.8

Source: Euromonitor International from national statistics
Notes: Data is ranked in descending order by year 2004

Czech Republic: Other selected causes of death: growth 1998-2004

Table: 4.312

% year on year growth

	1998	1999	2000	2001	2002	2003	2004
Death by motor traffic accidents	-10.0	74.1	0.0	7.1	33.8	2.0	12.4
Death by injury and poisoning	-11.3	-1.5	1.0	-0.3	-0.5	-0.3	0.6
Death by suicide and self-inflicted injury	-3.5	-0.7	1.5	0.0	-0.7	0.7	0.1

Source: Euromonitor International from national statistics
Notes: Data is ranked in descending order by year 2004

Smoking

Czech Republic: Smoking prevalence in population aged 15+ 1998-2004

Table: 4.313

% of population aged 15+

	1998	1999	2000	2001	2002	2003	2004
Smoking prevalence in population aged 15+ (% of population aged 15+)	25.1	23.5	29.1	23.3	24.1	22.6	22.1
Smoking prevalence in male population aged 15+ (% of male population)	31.1	30.1	36.2	26.4	30.9	29.2	28.9
Smoking prevalence in female population aged 15+ (% of female population)	19.6	17.3	22.0	20.4	18.1	16.5	15.8

Source: WHO/OECD/Euromonitor International

Nutrition and Obesity

Czech Republic: Nutrition and obesity 1998-2004

Table: 4.314

As stated

	1998	1999	2000	2001	2002	2003	2004
Availability of fruit and vegetables (kg/capita/year)	151.6	154.6	145.4	142.0	138.6	136.2	131.8
Average supply of calories per day (calories per capita)	3,254.1	3,118.3	3,064.8	3,119.1	3,171.3	3,207.4	3,249.7
Average supply of fat per day (grams per capita)	115.8	112.9	111.1	115.0	118.0	120.4	123.3
Average supply of protein per day (grams per capita)	96.4	90.6	89.0	91.0	94.1	96.3	98.7
Microbiological food-borne diseases (per 100000 population)	207.0	183.0	187.0	139.0	162.0	157.0	142.0
Obese population (BMI 30kg/sq m or more) (% of population aged 15+)	13.3	14.2	14.4	14.6	14.8	15.0	15.2

Source: WHO/OECD/Euromonitor International

Over-the-Counter Healthcare

Czech Republic: Trends in OTC healthcare retail sales 1998-2004

Table: 4.315

As stated

	1998	1999	2000	2001	2002	2003	2004
OTC Healthcare (CK million)	4,390.4	4,855.6	5,217.5	5,623.4	5,865.1	6,098.8	6,328.4
OTC Healthcare: real growth in national currency: 1998 = 100	100.0	108.3	112.0	115.3	118.1	122.7	123.4
OTC Healthcare: year on year (% real growth)	-1.6	8.3	3.4	2.9	2.5	3.9	0.5
OTC Healthcare (CK per capita)	428.1	474.1	510.1	550.4	574.6	597.7	620.5

Source: Euromonitor International from industry sources/national statistics

Czech Republic: OTC healthcare retail sales by sector 1998-2004

Table: 4.316

% of OTC retail value sales

	1998	1999	2000	2001	2002	2003	2004
Analgesics	25.5	25.4	25.3	25.3	25.8	26.4	26.9
Cough, cold and allergy (hay fever) remedies	24.5	24.2	24.0	24.1	22.7	21.6	20.8
Digestive remedies	10.5	10.4	10.4	10.3	10.4	10.3	10.3
Medicated skin care	8.8	8.8	8.7	8.7	8.7	8.8	9.0
Vitamins and dietary supplements	23.6	23.9	24.3	24.7	25.3	25.8	26.0

Source: Euromonitor International from industry sources/national statistics
Notes: Only selected sectors are shown, so values are not expected to sum to 100

■ **Denmark**

Socio-economic Parameters

Denmark: Socio-economic parameters 1998-2004

Table: 4.317

As stated

	1998	1999	2000	2001	2002	2003	2004
Population: national estimates at January 1st ('000)	5,294.9	5,313.6	5,330.0	5,349.2	5,368.4	5,386.4	5,404.2
% aged 0-14 yrs	18.0	18.2	18.4	18.6	18.7	18.8	18.9
% aged 15-64 yrs	67.1	66.9	66.8	66.6	66.5	66.4	66.3
% aged 65 + yrs	14.9	14.9	14.8	14.8	14.8	14.8	14.8
% Male	49.4	49.4	49.4	49.4	49.4	49.5	49.5
% Female	50.6	50.6	50.6	50.6	50.6	50.5	50.5
% Urban	85.2	85.3	85.7	85.7	85.8	86.1	86.2
Occupants per household at January 1st (Number)	2.2	2.2	2.2	2.2	2.2	2.2	2.2
Households ('000)	2,407.0	2,423.2	2,434.1	2,444.7	2,456.1	2,466.7	2,473.00
Annual rates of inflation (% growth)	1.9	2.5	2.9	2.4	2.4	2.1	1.2
GDP (DKr million)	1,155,410.0	1,207,750.0	1,278,960.0	1,325,510.0	1,360,710.0	1,398,330.0	1,450,387.0
GDP (US$ million)	172,427.9	173,123.3	158,225.6	159,262.1	172,357.2	212,264.7	242,091.9
GDP (US$ per capita)	32,565.1	32,581.3	29,685.7	29,773.0	32,106.2	39,407.2	44,797.3

Source: *Euromonitor International from International Monetary Fund (IMF), International Financial Statistics and World Economic Outlook/UN/national statistics*

Life Expectancy

Denmark: Life expectancy 1998-2004

Table: 4.318

As stated

	1998	1999	2000	2001	2002	2003	2004	% change 1998-2004
Life expectancy at birth: total population (years)	76.7	76.9	76.9	77.2	77.2	77.3	77.3	0.69
Life expectancy at birth: total population: year on year growth	0.2	0.2	0.0	0.3	0.0	0.1	0.0	
Healthy life expectancy at birth (years)	69.0			69.8	70.1			
Healthy life expectancy at birth: year on year growth					0.3			

Source: *Euromonitor International from World Bank*

Sanitation

Denmark: Improved sanitary facilities and water source 2000

Table: 4.319

As stated

	2000
Population with access to improved water source (% of population)	100.0

Source: *National statistics/World Bank*

Health Expenditure

Denmark: Public health expenditure 1998-2004

Table: 4.320

As stated

	1998	1999	2000	2001	2002	2003	2004
Public expenditure on pharmaceuticals and other medical non-durables (DKr million)	4,255.0	4,415.0	4,584.0	5,110.0	5,835.0	6,536.0	7,415.0
Private insurance expenditure (% of total expenditure on health)	1.4	1.7	1.6	1.6	1.6	1.7	1.7
Share of total health expenditure in GDP (% of total GDP)	8.4	8.5	8.2	8.4	8.6	8.7	8.6
Health expenditure (US$ per capita)	2,725.0	2,767.0	2,476.0	2,568.0	2,831.0	2,866.0	2,931.0

Source: *Euromonitor International from OECD/national statistics*

Denmark: Private health expenditure 1998-2004

As stated

	1998	1999	2000	2001	2002	2003	2004
Consumer expenditure on health goods and medical services (DKr million)	14,283.0	14,820.0	15,373.0	16,414.0	17,249.0	18,220.0	19,339.8
Consumer expenditure on health goods and medical services: real growth in national currency: 1990 = 100	117.2	118.6	119.6	124.7	128.0	132.4	138.9
Consumer expenditure on health goods and medical services as a percentage of total consumer expenditure	2.5	2.5	2.6	2.7	2.7	2.8	2.9

Source: National statistical offices/OECD/Eurostat/Euromonitor International

Denmark: Consumer expenditure on health goods and medical services by sector 1998-2004

% of total consumer expenditure on health goods and medical services

	1998	1999	2000	2001	2002	2003	2004
Pharmaceuticals, medical appliances/ equipment	48.0	47.4	48.6	49.4	50.2	50.1	50.4
Outpatient services	40.7	41.2	39.7	39.1	38.7	38.8	39.0
Hospital services	11.3	11.4	11.7	11.5	11.1	11.1	10.7
Total	100.0	100.0	100.0	100.0	100.0	100.0	100.0

Source: National statistical offices/OECD/Eurostat/Euromonitor International

Healthcare Infrastructure and Services

Denmark: Healthcare infrastructure and services by sector 1998-2004

As stated

	1998	1999	2000	2001	2002	2003	2004
Active pharmacists (number)	2,404	2,643	2,666	2,685	2,638	2,695	2,705
Consultations with GPs (general practitioners) (per capita)	7	7	7	7	7	7	7
Dentists (number)	4,857	4,830	4,817	4,825	4,834	4,808	4,805
Doctors (number)	16,635	16,917	17,165	17,443	17,802	18,116	18,445
Hospital admissions (number)	966,354	989,442	1,004,516	1,015,059	1,028,623	1,040,390	1,054,240
Hospitals and clinics (number)	81	80	64	60	59	58	57
In-patient beds ('000)	18	18	21	21	21	21	21
In-patient surgical procedures (number)	408,057	406,654	406,421	404,717	403,590	403,428	399,644
Nurses (number)	49,474	50,178	50,905	51,529	51,990	52,597	53,173
Out-patient contacts (per capita)	6	6	6	6	6	6	6

Source: Euromonitor International from national statistics

Denmark: Healthcare infrastructure and services by sector: growth 1998-2004

Year on year growth: % change in stated unit

	1998	1999	2000	2001	2002	2003	2004
Active pharmacists (number)	-5.8	9.9	0.9	0.7	-1.8	2.2	0.4
Consultations with GPs (general practitioners) (per capita)	1.5	-2.9	4.5	1.4	1.4	2.8	2.2
Dentists (number)	-1.4	-0.6	-0.3	0.2	0.2	-0.5	-0.1
Doctors (number)	1.1	1.7	1.5	1.6	2.1	1.8	1.8
Hospital admissions (number)	0.7	2.4	1.5	1.0	1.3	1.1	1.3
Hospitals and clinics (number)	-1.2	-1.2	-20.0	-6.3	-1.7	-1.7	-1.7
In-patient beds (number)	-1.5	-1.7	17.0	-0.3	2.6	0.4	0.6
In-patient surgical procedures (number)	-0.3	-0.3	-0.1	-0.4	-0.3	0.0	-0.9
Nurses (number)	0.4	1.4	1.4	1.2	0.9	1.2	1.1
Out-patient contacts (per capita)	1.7	-3.3	5.2	1.6	0.0	-1.6	0.0

Source: Euromonitor International from national statistics

Immunisation

Denmark: Vaccination rates by disease type 1998-2004

Table: 4.325

%

	1998	1999	2000	2001	2002	2003	2004
Vaccination rate against DTP (diphtheria, tetanus, pertussis) 1 & 2 (%)				97.0	96.5	96.0	96.0
Vaccination rate against MMR (measles, mumps, rubella) (%)	91.0	92.0	93.0	94.0	99.0	99.0	99.0
Vaccination rate against polio (%)	99.0	99.0	95.9	97.0	98.1	99.0	99.0

Source: WHO

Infectious Diseases

Denmark: Incidence of disease by type 1998-2004

Table: 4.326

Number

	1998	1999	2000	2001	2002	2003	2004
Incidence of AIDS	71	73	60	19	43	34	25
Incidence of diphtheria			0	0	0		
Incidence of measles			14	11	32		
Incidence of polio	0	0	0	0	0		

Source: WHO

Denmark: Incidence of disease by type: growth 1998-2004

Table: 4.327

Year on year growth: %

	1998	1999	2000	2001	2002	2003	2004
Incidence of AIDS	-34.3	2.8	-17.8	-68.3	126.3	-20.9	-26.5
Incidence of measles				-21.4	190.9		

Source: WHO

Causes of Death

Denmark: Deaths by disease 1998-2004

Table: 4.328

Number per 100,000 inhabitants

	1998	1999	2000	2001	2002	2003	2004
Death by malignant neoplasms (cancers)	211.9	210.6	208.0	209.9	212.1	210.8	213.2
Death by diseases of the circulatory system	251.1	240.0	228.7	225.8	217.4	212.7	208.7
Deaths from heart disease	189.2	180.8	171.1	161.7	152.4	143.4	134.9
Death by diseases of the respiratory system	66.7	64.2	63.6	63.3	62.8	62.5	62.1
Deaths from lung cancer	61.6	60.8	59.2	57.6	55.9	54.1	52.6
Death by diseases of the digestive system	36.5	38.8	39.9	41.8	42.0	43.3	44.9
Deaths from chronic liver disease and cirrhosis	15.5	17.0	17.5	18.0	18.3	18.5	18.9
Deaths from ulcers of the stomach and duodenum	10.7	10.6	10.4	10.3	10.1	9.8	9.5

Source: WHO/Euromonitor International
Notes: Data is ranked in descending order by year 2004

Denmark: Deaths by disease: growth 1998-2004

Table: 4.329

% year on year growth

	1998	1999	2000	2001	2002	2003	2004
Death by diseases of the digestive system	-2.9	6.3	2.8	4.8	0.5	3.1	3.8
Deaths from chronic liver disease and cirrhosis	-9.4	9.4	2.9	2.9	1.7	1.1	2.4
Death by malignant neoplasms (cancers)	-1.6	-0.6	-1.2	0.9	1.0	-0.6	1.1
Death by diseases of the respiratory system	-1.9	-3.7	-0.9	-0.5	-0.8	-0.5	-0.7
Death by diseases of the circulatory system	-4.4	-4.4	-4.7	-1.3	-3.7	-2.2	-1.9
Deaths from ulcers of the stomach and duodenum	-2.2	-0.5	-1.9	-1.0	-1.9	-3.0	-2.7
Deaths from lung cancer	-5.0	-1.3	-2.6	-2.7	-3.0	-3.2	-2.8
Deaths from heart disease	-7.1	-4.4	-5.4	-5.5	-5.8	-5.9	-5.9

Source: WHO/Euromonitor International
Notes: Data is ranked in descending order by year 2004

Denmark: Other selected causes of death: 1998-2004

Table: 4.330

Number per 100,000 inhabitants

	1998	1999	2000	2001	2002	2003	2004
Death by injury and poisoning	48.2	47.9	46.2	46.6	50.2	51.7	53.4
Death by motor traffic accidents	9.4	8.9	8.9	9.1	9.2	9.4	9.7
Death by suicide and self-inflicted injury	12.1	11.9	10.9	10.1	9.9	9.6	9.1

Source: Euromonitor International from national statistics
Notes: Data is ranked in descending order by year 2004

Denmark: Other selected causes of death: growth 1998-2004

Table: 4.331

% year on year growth

	1998	1999	2000	2001	2002	2003	2004
Death by injury and poisoning	-4.7	-0.6	-3.5	0.9	7.7	3.0	3.2
Death by motor traffic accidents	3.3	-5.3	0.0	2.2	1.1	2.2	2.8
Death by suicide and self-inflicted injury	-8.3	-1.7	-8.4	-7.3	-2.0	-3.0	-4.7

Source: Euromonitor International from national statistics
Notes: Data is ranked in descending order by year 2004

Smoking

Denmark: Smoking prevalence in population aged 15+ 1998-2004

Table: 4.332

% of population aged 15+

	1998	1999	2000	2001	2002	2003	2004
Smoking prevalence in population aged 15+ (% of population aged 15+)	33.0	31.0	30.5	29.5	28.0	30.4	30.2
Smoking prevalence in male population aged 15+ (% of male population)	34.0	35.0	32.0	33.5	30.5	29.7	28.8
Smoking prevalence in female population aged 15+ (% of female population)	31.0	27.0	29.0	25.5	26.0	31.1	31.5

Source: WHO/OECD/Euromonitor International

Nutrition and Obesity

Denmark: Nutrition and obesity 1998-2004

Table: 4.333

As stated

	1998	1999	2000	2001	2002	2003	2004
Availability of fruit and vegetables (kg/capita/year)	168.5	195.3	203.0	195.4	212.7	219.7	231.0
Average supply of calories per day (calories per capita)	3,383.8	3,387.2	3,389.8	3,397.2	3,439.3	3,469.6	3,500.0
Average supply of fat per day (grams per capita)	133.6	136.6	138.8	140.4	139.5	139.5	139.6
Average supply of protein per day (grams per capita)	105.8	107.9	107.1	110.7	109.7	109.5	109.8
Microbiological food-borne diseases (per 100000 population)	77.0	57.0	32.0	37.0	36.0	39.0	41.0
Obese population (BMI 30kg/sq m or more) (% of population aged 15 +)	9.2	9.8	9.5	10.6	12.0	12.4	13.0

Source: WHO/OECD/Euromonitor International

Over-the-Counter Healthcare

Denmark: Trends in OTC healthcare retail sales 1998-2004

Table: 4.334

As stated

	1998	1999	2000	2001	2002	2003	2004
OTC Healthcare (DKr million)	1,933.2	1,997.3	2,082.9	2,156.7	2,211.0	2,265.3	2,298.9
OTC Healthcare: real growth in national currency: 1998 = 100	100.0	100.8	102.2	103.3	103.4	103.8	103.6
OTC Healthcare: year on year (% real growth)	2.2	0.8	1.3	1.2	0.1	0.4	-0.2
OTC Healthcare (DKr per capita)	365.1	375.9	390.8	403.2	411.9	420.6	425.4

Source: Euromonitor International from industry sources/national statistics

Denmark: OTC healthcare retail sales by sector 1998-2004

Table: 4.335

% of OTC retail value sales

	1998	1999	2000	2001	2002	2003	2004
Analgesics	22.0	21.4	20.7	20.3	19.7	19.1	18.9
Cough, cold and allergy (hay fever) remedies	15.5	15.5	15.5	15.3	14.9	14.6	14.4
Digestive remedies	8,342.6	7,967.4	7,496.4	7,166.3	6,917.6	6,708.6	6,499.4
Digestive remedies	12.2	11.9	11.4	11.1	11.0	10.8	10.7
Medicated skin care	8.7	8.8	8.9	8.9	9.1	9.3	9.4
Vitamins and dietary supplements	29.6	29.3	29.2	29.1	29.3	29.5	29.7

Source: Euromonitor International from industry sources/national statistics
Notes: Only selected sectors are shown, so values are not expected to sum to 100

Health and Wellness

Denmark: Retail sales of packaged foods by health and wellness category 2002-2004

Table: 4.336

DKr million

	2002	2003	2004
Packaged food: Total	59,200.2	60,455.6	61,164.7
Better for you	3,320.2	3,531.5	3,706.3
For food intolerance	49.4	57.4	63.9
Fortified/functional	561.3	590.6	616.9
Organic	1,445.1	1,660.4	1,859.2

Source: Euromonitor International from industry sources/national statistics

Denmark: Per capita sales of packaged foods by health and wellness category 2002-2004

Table: 4.337

DKr per capita

	2002	2003	2004
Better for you	618.4	655.5	685.7
For food intolerance	9.2	10.7	11.8
Fortified/functional	104.5	109.6	114.1
Organic	269.2	308.2	344.0

Source: *Euromonitor International from industry sources/national statistics*

Denmark: Retail sales of packaged food by health and wellness category: % share of total packaged food market 2002-2004

Table: 4.338

% value

	2002	2003	2004
Better for you	5.6	5.8	6.1
For food intolerance	0.1	0.1	0.1
Fortified/functional	0.9	1.0	1.0
Organic	2.4	2.7	3.0

Source: *Euromonitor International from industry sources/national statistics*

Denmark: Retail sales of packaged food by health and wellness category: real growth index 2002-2004

Table: 4.339

2002 =100

	2002	2003	2004
Better for you	100.00	103.77	106.77
For food intolerance	100.00	113.52	123.84
Fortified/functional	100.00	102.65	105.13
Organic	100.00	112.10	123.05

Source: *Euromonitor International from industry sources/national statistics*

Denmark: Retail sales of better-for-you packaged foods by sector 2002-2004

Table: 4.340

% of total packaged food / as stated

	2002	2003	2004	% real change in value 2002-2004
Combination	0.05	0.05	0.05	2.54
Reduced fat	4.65	4.89	5.09	8.22
Reduced salt	0.05	0.05	0.05	-3.25

Source: *Euromonitor International from industry sources/national statistics*

Denmark: Retail sales of packaged foods for food intolerances by sector 2002-2004

Table: 4.341

% of total packaged food / as stated

	2002	2003	2004	% real change in value 2002-2004
Gluten-free	0.08	0.10	0.10	23.84

Source: *Euromonitor International from industry sources/national statistics*

Denmark: Retail sales of naturally healthy packaged foods by sector 2002-2004

Table: 4.342

% of total packaged food / as stated

	2002	2003	2004	% real change in value 2002-2004
High fibre	4.45	4.52	4.76	5.59
Other naturally healthy food	1.39	1.38	1.37	-2.89
Soy-based dairy alternatives	0.08	0.09	0.09	11.44

Source: *Euromonitor International from industry sources/national statistics*

■ **Ecuador**

Socio-economic Parameters

Ecuador: Socio-economic parameters 1998-2004

Table: 4.343

As stated

	1998	1999	2000	2001	2002	2003	2004
Population: national estimates at January 1st ('000)	11,923.0	12,123.0	12,320.7	12,517.0	12,712.0	12,905.5	13,096.6
% aged 0-14 yrs	35.3	34.8	34.3	33.8	33.4	32.9	32.4
% aged 15-64 yrs	60.1	60.5	60.9	61.3	61.7	62.0	62.4
% aged 65 + yrs	4.6	4.7	4.8	4.9	5.0	5.1	5.2
% Male	50.2	50.2	50.2	50.2	50.2	50.2	50.2
% Female	49.8	49.8	49.8	49.8	49.8	49.8	49.8
% Urban	63.3	64.3	65.3	66.0	66.8	67.1	67.9
Occupants per household at January 1st (Number)	4.9	4.9	4.9	4.9	5.0	5.0	5.0
Households ('000)	2,434.3	2,476.3	2,509.1	2,538.0	2,566.0	2,594.2	2,618.9
Annual rates of inflation (% growth)	36.1	52.2	96.1	37.7	12.5	7.9	2.7
GDP (US$ million)	23,255.1	16,674.5	15,933.7	21,021.0	24,311.0	27,200.0	30,300.0
GDP (US$ per capita)	1,950.4	1,375.4	1,293.3	1,679.4	1,912.4	2,107.6	2,313.6

Source: *Euromonitor International from International Monetary Fund (IMF), International Financial Statistics and World Economic Outlook/UN/national statistics*

Life Expectancy

Ecuador: Life expectancy 1998-2004

Table: 4.344

As stated

	1998	1999	2000	2001	2002	2003	2004	% change 1998-2004
Life expectancy at birth: total population (years)	69.9	70.1	69.7	70.3	70.6	70.9	71.1	1.75
Life expectancy at birth: total population: year on year growth	0.3	0.3	-0.5	0.9	0.4	0.4	0.3	
Healthy life expectancy at birth (years)	61.0			56.4	56.7			
Healthy life expectancy at birth: year on year growth					0.4			

Source: *Euromonitor International from World Bank*

Sanitation

Ecuador: Improved sanitary facilities and water source 2000

Table: 4.345

As stated

	2000
Population with access to improved sanitary facilities (% of population)	86.0
Population with access to improved water source (% of population)	85.0
Population with improved access to sanitation facilities, rural (% of rural population with access)	74.0
Population with improved access to sanitation facilities, urban (% of urban population with access)	92.0

Source: *National statistics/World Bank*

Health Expenditure

Ecuador: Public health expenditure 1998-2004

Table: 4.346

As stated

	1998	1999	2000	2001	2002	2003	2004
Share of total health expenditure in GDP (% of total GDP)	4.4	3.7	4.1	4.5	4.5	4.3	4.1
Health expenditure (US$ per capita)	84.0	65.0	53.0	80.0	91.0	97.0	104.0

Source: Euromonitor International from OECD/national statistics

Ecuador: Private health expenditure 1998-2004

Table: 4.347

As stated

	1998	1999	2000	2001	2002	2003	2004
Consumer expenditure on health goods and medical services (US$ million)	374.7	246.9	239.7	320.9	356.3	373.8	386.4
Consumer expenditure on health goods and medical services as a percentage of total consumer expenditure	2.7	2.8	2.8	2.8	2.8	2.8	2.7

Source: National statistical offices/OECD/Eurostat/Euromonitor International

Ecuador: Consumer expenditure on health goods and medical services by sector 1998-2004

Table: 4.348

% of total consumer expenditure on health goods and medical services

	1998	1999	2000	2001	2002	2003	2004
Pharmaceuticals, medical appliances/ equipment	81.7	82.2	82.9	84.2	84.8	84.7	84.3
Outpatient services	14.6	14.3	13.7	12.7	12.1	12.2	12.4
Hospital services	3.7	3.5	3.4	3.1	3.0	3.2	3.3
Total	100.0	100.0	100.0	100.0	100.0	100.0	100.0

Source: National statistical offices/OECD/Eurostat/Euromonitor International

Healthcare Infrastructure and Services

Ecuador: Healthcare infrastructure and services by sector 1998-2004

Table: 4.349

As stated

	1998	1999	2000	2001	2002	2003	2004
Doctors (number)	16,588	17,075	18,335	19,376	20,109	20,360	20,597
Hospitals and clinics (number)	3,480	3,492	3,501	3,501	3,496	3,485	3,480
In-patient beds ('000)	18	18	18	20	20	20	21

Source: Euromonitor International from national statistics

Ecuador: Healthcare infrastructure and services by sector: growth 1998-2004

Table: 4.350

Year on year growth: % change in stated unit

	1998	1999	2000	2001	2002	2003	2004
Doctors (number)	4.6	2.9	7.4	5.7	3.8	1.2	1.2
Hospitals and clinics (number)	0.6	0.3	0.3	0.0	-0.1	-0.3	-0.1
In-patient beds (number)	-4.6	1.7	1.6	8.4	0.9	1.3	1.6

Source: Euromonitor International from national statistics

Immunisation

Ecuador: Vaccination rates by disease type 1998-2004

Table: 4.351

%

	1998	1999	2000	2001	2002	2003	2004
Vaccination rate against DTP (diphtheria, tetanus, pertussis) 1 & 2 (%)			99.0	99.0	99.0	99.0	99.0
Vaccination rate against MMR (measles, mumps, rubella) (%)	88.0	99.0	99.0	99.0	79.8	88.0	86.0
Vaccination rate against polio (%)	83.0	70.0	82.6	91.7	90.2	89.0	87.0

Source: WHO

Infectious Diseases

Ecuador: Incidence of disease by type 1998-2004

Table: 4.352

Number

	1998	1999	2000	2001	2002	2003	2004
Incidence of AIDS	186	325	313	299	325	326	282
Incidence of diphtheria	21	5	1	1	4		
Incidence of measles	0	0	0	2	0		
Incidence of polio	0	0	0	0	0		

Source: WHO

Ecuador: Incidence of disease by type: growth 1998-2004

Table: 4.353

Year on year growth: %

	1998	1999	2000	2001	2002	2003	2004
Incidence of AIDS	45.3	74.7	-3.7	-4.5	8.7	0.3	-13.5
Incidence of diphtheria	0.0	-76.2	-80.0	0.0	300.0		
Incidence of measles					-100.0		

Source: WHO

Causes of Death

Ecuador: Deaths by disease 1998-2004

Table: 4.354

Number per 100,000 inhabitants

	1998	1999	2000	2001	2002	2003	2004
Death by diseases of the digestive system	32.6	29.7	30.1	34.2	34.0	34.6	36.6
Deaths from heart disease	18.6	19.8	18.4	18.7	18.5	18.4	18.5
Deaths from chronic liver disease and cirrhosis	10.5	10.4	10.2	10.1	9.9	9.8	9.6
Deaths from lung cancer	3.7	3.5	3.6	3.4	3.3	3.2	3.1
Deaths from ulcers of the stomach and duodenum	2.5	2.1	2.1	1.8	1.6	1.4	1.2

Source: WHO/Euromonitor International
Notes: Data is ranked in descending order by year 2004

Ecuador: Deaths by disease: growth 1998-2004

Table: 4.355

% year on year growth

	1998	1999	2000	2001	2002	2003	2004
Death by diseases of the digestive system	2.8	-8.9	1.3	13.6	-0.6	1.8	5.8
Deaths from heart disease	14.4	6.5	-7.4	1.8	-1.1	-0.5	0.6
Deaths from chronic liver disease and cirrhosis	2.6	-1.2	-1.6	-1.2	-2.0	-1.0	-1.8
Deaths from lung cancer	2.1	-6.0	1.1	-4.5	-2.9	-3.0	-2.5
Deaths from ulcers of the stomach and duodenum	-13.0	-16.2	-0.7	-14.4	-11.1	-12.5	-13.1

Source: WHO/Euromonitor International
Notes: Data is ranked in descending order by year 2004

Smoking

Ecuador: Smoking prevalence in population aged 15+ 1998-2004

Table: 4.356

% of population aged 15+

	1998	1999	2000	2001	2002	2003	2004
Smoking prevalence in population aged 15+ (% of population aged 15+)	31.6	31.5	31.5	31.4	31.4	31.1	31.1
Smoking prevalence in male population aged 15+ (% of male population)	45.5	45.4	45.2	45.3	44.8	44.6	44.5
Smoking prevalence in female population aged 15+ (% of female population)	17.8	17.7	17.9	17.5	18.1	17.6	17.8

Source: WHO/OECD/Euromonitor International

Nutrition and Obesity

Ecuador: Nutrition and obesity 1998-2004

Table: 4.357

As stated

	1998	1999	2000	2001	2002	2003	2004
Average supply of calories per day (calories per capita)	2,687.1	2,704.4	2,702.1	2,755.2	2,754.0	2,762.9	2,777.0
Average supply of fat per day (grams per capita)	91.6	88.6	89.8	96.9	100.9	98.6	97.2
Average supply of protein per day (grams per capita)	56.4	55.9	55.8	56.4	57.9	58.0	58.2
Obese population (BMI 30kg/sq m or more) (% of population aged 15+)	13.2	13.6	13.6	13.8	14.0	14.2	14.4

Source: WHO/OECD/Euromonitor International

■ Egypt

Socio-economic Parameters

Egypt: Socio-economic parameters 1998-2004

Table: 4.358

As stated

	1998	1999	2000	2001	2002	2003	2004
Population: national estimates at January 1st ('000)	60,839.0	61,994.0	63,254.0	64,466.0	65,584.4	66,698.5	67,798.4
% aged 0-14 yrs	37.4	37.2	36.7	36.2	35.2	34.2	33.2
% aged 15-64 yrs	58.4	58.9	59.4	59.9	60.8	61.7	62.7
% aged 65+ yrs	4.2	3.9	3.8	3.9	4.0	4.1	4.1
% Male	50.8	51.2	51.2	51.2	51.1	51.1	51.1
% Female	49.2	48.8	48.8	48.8	48.9	48.9	48.9
% Urban	44.9	45.0	45.9	46.0	46.1	46.6	46.9
Occupants per household at January 1st (Number)	4.6	4.5	4.5	4.5	4.5	4.4	4.4
Households ('000)	13,328.1	13,653.1	13,995.7	14,356.2	14,730.8	15,127.0	15,535.5
Annual rates of inflation (% growth)	3.9	3.1	2.7	2.3	2.7	4.5	11.3
GDP (E£ million)	287,400.0	307,600.0	340,100.0	358,700.0	378,900.0	417,500.0	474,400.0
GDP (US$ million)	84,828.8	90,597.2	97,953.7	90,284.4	84,206.2	71,356.9	76,562.6
GDP (US$ per capita)	1,394.3	1,461.4	1,548.6	1,400.5	1,283.9	1,069.8	1,129.3

Source: Euromonitor International from International Monetary Fund (IMF), International Financial Statistics and World Economic Outlook/UN/national statistics

Life Expectancy

Egypt: Life expectancy 1998-2004

Table: 4.359

As stated

	1998	1999	2000	2001	2002	2003	2004	% change 1998-2004
Life expectancy at birth: total population (years)	65.5	65.9	66.3	66.5	67.1	67.5	68.0	3.94
Life expectancy at birth: total population: year on year growth	0.7	0.6	0.7	0.3	0.9	0.7	0.7	
Healthy life expectancy at birth (years)	58.0			59.0	59.5			
Healthy life expectancy at birth: year on year growth					0.8			

Source: Euromonitor International from World Bank

Sanitation

Egypt: Improved sanitary facilities and water source 2000

Table: 4.360

As stated

	2000
Population with access to improved sanitary facilities (% of population)	98.0
Population with access to improved water source (% of population)	97.0
Population with improved access to sanitation facilities, rural (% of rural population with access)	96.0
Population with improved access to sanitation facilities, urban (% of urban population with access)	100.0

Source: National statistics/World Bank

Health Expenditure

Egypt: Public health expenditure 1998-2004

Table: 4.361

As stated

	1998	1999	2000	2001	2002	2003	2004
Share of total health expenditure in GDP (% of total GDP)	3.9	3.9	3.8	3.9	4.0	4.1	4.3
Health expenditure (US$ per capita)	64.0	67.0	67.0	59.0	59.0	56.0	53.0

Source: Euromonitor International from OECD/national statistics

Egypt: Private health expenditure 1998-2004

Table: 4.362

As stated

	1998	1999	2000	2001	2002	2003	2004
Consumer expenditure on health goods and medical services (E£ million)	5,359.4	5,720.1	6,478.1	6,854.5	7,431.1	7,810.1	8,432.4
Consumer expenditure on health goods and medical services: real growth in national currency: 1990 = 100	135.4	140.2	154.7	160.0	168.8	169.8	164.8
Consumer expenditure on health goods and medical services as a percentage of total consumer expenditure	2.4	2.4	2.4	2.4	2.4	2.3	2.3

Source: *National statistical offices/OECD/Eurostat/Euromonitor International*

Egypt: Consumer expenditure on health goods and medical services by sector 1998-2004

Table: 4.363

% of total consumer expenditure on health goods and medical services

	1998	1999	2000	2001	2002	2003	2004
Pharmaceuticals, medical appliances/ equipment	27.2	27.1	25.9	24.6	24.1	24.7	25.1
Outpatient services	19.6	20.9	22.6	24.6	25.0	24.1	23.6
Hospital services	53.1	51.9	51.6	50.7	51.0	51.2	51.3
Total	100.0	100.0	100.0	100.0	100.0	100.0	100.0

Source: *National statistical offices/OECD/Eurostat/Euromonitor International*

Healthcare Infrastructure and Services

Egypt: Healthcare infrastructure and services by sector 1998-2004

Table: 4.364

As stated

	1998	1999	2000	2001	2002	2003	2004
Active pharmacists (number)	3,548	3,278	2,842	3,375	4,354	4,654	4,813
Dentists (number)	3,903	4,754	5,459	5,770	6,128	6,274	6,437
Doctors (number)	49,677	41,021	39,204	40,422	41,783	42,368	42,571
Hospitals and clinics (number)	331	321	333	327	326	324	322
In-patient beds ('000)	33	34	34	35	36	37	38
Nurses (number)	107,696	92,489	79,429	83,879	86,650	87,644	87,878

Source: *Euromonitor International from national statistics*

Egypt: Healthcare infrastructure and services by sector: growth 1998-2004

Table: 4.365

Year on year growth: % change in stated unit

	1998	1999	2000	2001	2002	2003	2004
Active pharmacists (number)	19.1	-7.6	-13.3	18.8	29.0	6.9	3.4
Dentists (number)	-3.2	21.8	14.8	5.7	6.2	2.4	2.6
Doctors (number)	-0.4	-17.4	-4.4	3.1	3.4	1.4	0.5
Hospitals and clinics (number)	-0.3	-3.0	3.7	-1.8	-0.3	-0.6	-0.6
In-patient beds (number)	1.7	1.0	2.7	2.3	2.0	2.3	2.2
Nurses (number)	8.7	-14.1	-14.1	5.6	3.3	1.1	0.3

Source: *Euromonitor International from national statistics*

Immunisation

Egypt: Vaccination rates by disease type 1998-2004

Table: 4.366

%

	1998	1999	2000	2001	2002	2003	2004
Vaccination rate against DTP (diphtheria, tetanus, pertussis) 1 & 2 (%)			98.2	97.7	97.9	98.0	98.0
Vaccination rate against MMR (measles, mumps, rubella) (%)	98.0	95.5	97.6	97.4	96.9	98.0	98.0
Vaccination rate against polio (%)	95.0	97.0	97.7	99.4	96.8	98.0	98.0

Source: WHO

Infectious Diseases

Egypt: Incidence of disease by type 1998-2004

Table: 4.367

Number

	1998	1999	2000	2001	2002	2003	2004
Incidence of AIDS	23	34	44	35	46	52	63
Incidence of diphtheria	3	2	0	0	0		
Incidence of measles	4,868	1,547	2,633	2,150	653		
Incidence of polio	35	9	4	5	7		

Source: WHO

Egypt: Incidence of disease by type: growth 1998-2004

Table: 4.368

Year on year growth: %

	1998	1999	2000	2001	2002	2003	2004
Incidence of AIDS	-8.0	47.8	29.4	-20.5	31.4	13.0	21.2
Incidence of diphtheria	200.0	-33.3	-100.0				
Incidence of measles	5.7	-68.2	70.2	-18.3	-69.6		
Incidence of polio	150.0	-74.3	-55.6	25.0	40.0		

Source: WHO

Smoking

Egypt: Smoking prevalence in population aged 15+ 1998-2004

Table: 4.369

% of population aged 15+

	1998	1999	2000	2001	2002	2003	2004
Smoking prevalence in population aged 15+ (% of population aged 15+)	36.5	36.6	37.0	37.2	37.2	37.6	37.7
Smoking prevalence in male population aged 15+ (% of male population)	56.5	56.9	56.9	56.4	56.8	56.5	56.6
Smoking prevalence in female population aged 15+ (% of female population)	16.1	15.7	16.3	17.3	16.8	17.8	17.7

Source: WHO/OECD/Euromonitor International

Nutrition and Obesity

Egypt: Nutrition and obesity 1998-2004

Table: 4.370

As stated

	1998	1999	2000	2001	2002	2003	2004
Average supply of calories per day (calories per capita)	3,336.0	3,348.6	3,336.0	3,349.0	3,338.0	3,331.9	3,328.8
Average supply of fat per day (grams per capita)	56.6	57.7	58.8	59.3	59.8	60.4	61.0
Average supply of protein per day (grams per capita)	93.5	94.1	94.7	94.9	95.4	95.9	96.3
Obese population (BMI 30kg/sq m or more) (% of population aged 15+)	5.6	5.6	5.6	5.7	5.7	5.8	5.9

Source: WHO/OECD/Euromonitor International

Over-the-Counter Healthcare

Egypt: Trends in OTC healthcare retail sales 1998-2004

Table: 4.371

As stated

	1998	1999	2000	2001	2002	2003	2004
OTC Healthcare (E£ million)	1,139.9	1,206.9	1,280.8	1,371.5	1,467.8	1,602.8	1,726.6
OTC Healthcare: real growth in national currency: 1998 = 100	100.0	102.7	106.2	111.2	115.8	121.3	124.2
OTC Healthcare: year on year (% real growth)	1.5	2.7	3.4	4.7	4.2	4.7	2.4
OTC Healthcare (E£ per capita)	18.7	19.5	20.2	21.3	22.4	24.0	25.5

Source: Euromonitor International from industry sources/national statistics

Egypt: OTC healthcare retail sales by sector 1998-2004

Table: 4.372

% of OTC retail value sales

	1998	1999	2000	2001	2002	2003	2004
Analgesics	17.1	17.5	18.0	18.3	18.7	19.2	19.3
Cough, cold and allergy (hay fever) remedies	20.5	20.5	20.6	20.8	21.3	22.4	23.2
Digestive remedies	17.8	18.3	18.6	18.3	18.1	17.4	17.4
Medicated skin care	13.1	12.9	12.8	12.6	12.4	12.0	11.7
Vitamins and dietary supplements	26.6	25.9	25.3	25.2	24.9	24.6	24.1

Source: Euromonitor International from industry sources/national statistics
Notes: Only selected sectors are shown, so values are not expected to sum to 100

■ Estonia

Socio-economic Parameters

Estonia: Socio-economic parameters 1998-2004

Table: 4.373

As stated

	1998	1999	2000	2001	2002	2003	2004
Population: national estimates at January 1st ('000)	1,393.1	1,379.2	1,372.1	1,367.0	1,361.2	1,356.0	1,350.6
% aged 0-14 yrs	19.6	18.9	18.3	17.7	17.2	16.6	16.0
% aged 15-64 yrs	65.9	66.3	66.8	67.0	67.3	67.5	67.9
% aged 65 + yrs	14.5	14.8	15.0	15.2	15.5	15.9	16.1
% Male	46.2	46.1	46.1	46.1	46.1	46.1	46.1
% Female	53.8	53.9	53.9	53.9	53.9	53.9	53.9
% Urban	69.1	68.9	68.6	68.6	68.7	69.5	69.8
Occupants per household at January 1st (Number)	2.5	2.4	2.4	2.4	2.4	2.4	2.3
Households ('000)	550.6	563.7	582.1	580.2	578.2	576.5	574.7
Annual rates of inflation (% growth)	8.2	3.3	4.0	5.7	3.6	1.3	3.0
GDP (Kroons million)	78,341.2	81,639.7	92,717.1	104,338.0	116,869.0	125,832.0	139,150.0
GDP (US$ million)	5,566.1	5,562.2	5,464.0	5,969.6	7,035.3	9,081.1	11,047.5
GDP (US$ per capita)	3,995.6	4,032.8	3,982.3	4,367.1	5,168.3	6,696.8	8,179.5

Source: Euromonitor International from International Monetary Fund (IMF), International Financial Statistics and World Economic Outlook/UN/national statistics

Life Expectancy

Estonia: Life expectancy 1998-2004

Table: 4.374

As stated

	1998	1999	2000	2001	2002	2003	2004	% change 1998-2004
Life expectancy at birth: total population (years)	70.5	70.7	71.0	71.2	71.1	71.3	71.3	1.16
Life expectancy at birth: total population: year on year growth	0.4	0.3	0.4	0.3	-0.1	0.2	0.1	
Healthy life expectancy at birth (years)	63.0			61.9	62.0			
Healthy life expectancy at birth: year on year growth					0.3			

Source: Euromonitor International from World Bank

Sanitation

Estonia: Improved sanitary facilities and water source 2000

Table: 4.375

As stated

	2000
Population with improved access to sanitation facilities, urban (% of urban population with access)	93.0

Source: National statistics/World Bank

Health Expenditure

Estonia: Public health expenditure 1998-2004

Table: 4.376

As stated

	1998	1999	2000	2001	2002	2003	2004
Share of total health expenditure in GDP (% of total GDP)	6.0	6.5	5.9	5.5	5.4	5.5	5.3
Health expenditure (US$ per capita)	223.0	244.0	221.0	224.0	263.0	269.0	280.0

Source: Euromonitor International from OECD/national statistics

Estonia: Private health expenditure 1998-2004

Table: 4.377

As stated

	1998	1999	2000	2001	2002	2003	2004
Consumer expenditure on health goods and medical services (Kroons million)	691.5	819.1	944.0	1,072.7	1,419.2	1,558.3	1,651.0
Consumer expenditure on health goods and medical services as a percentage of total consumer expenditure	1.4	1.7	1.7	1.8	2.1	2.2	2.1

Source: National statistical offices/OECD/Eurostat/Euromonitor International

Estonia: Consumer expenditure on health goods and medical services by sector 1998-2004

Table: 4.378

% of total consumer expenditure on health goods and medical services

	1998	1999	2000	2001	2002	2003	2004
Pharmaceuticals, medical appliances/ equipment	63.0	61.6	63.4	69.2	65.2	65.9	65.7
Outpatient services	36.2	36.4	33.0	27.4	32.7	32.0	32.2
Hospital services	0.8	2.0	3.6	3.4	2.1	2.1	2.2
Total	100.0	100.0	100.0	100.0	100.0	100.0	100.0

Source: National statistical offices/OECD/Eurostat/Euromonitor International

Healthcare Infrastructure and Services

Estonia: Healthcare infrastructure and services by sector 1998-2004

Table: 4.379

As stated

	1998	1999	2000	2001	2002	2003	2004
Active pharmacists (number)	1,315	1,367	1,400	1,440	1,484	1,525	1,569
Dentists (number)	985	1,012	1,015	1,095	1,135	1,170	1,201
Doctors (number)	4,311	4,426	4,414	4,293	4,208	4,138	4,050
Hospital admissions (number)	282,914	282,302	279,470	268,741	259,772	249,630	240,020
Hospitals and clinics (number)	78	78	68	68	51	50	49
In-patient beds ('000)	11	10	10	9	8	8	8
In-patient surgical procedures (number)	94,432	94,749	92,268	87,258	87,428	84,481	82,379
Midwives (number)	542	554	507	453	422	410	402
Nurses (number)	7,706	7,587	7,456	7,489	8,294	8,556	8,765
Out-patient contacts (per capita)	6	6	7	7	6	7	7

Source: Euromonitor International from national statistics

Estonia: Healthcare infrastructure and services by sector: growth 1998-2004

Table: 4.380

Year on year growth: % change in stated unit

	1998	1999	2000	2001	2002	2003	2004
Active pharmacists (number)	2.2	4.0	2.4	2.9	3.1	2.8	2.9
Dentists (number)	2.3	2.7	0.3	7.9	3.7	3.1	2.6
Doctors (number)	-1.1	2.7	-0.3	-2.7	-2.0	-1.7	-2.1
Hospital admissions (number)	5.8	-0.2	-1.0	-3.8	-3.3	-3.9	-3.8
Hospitals and clinics (number)	-1.3	0.0	-12.8	0.0	-25.0	-2.0	-2.0
In-patient beds (number)	-2.6	-1.4	-5.1	-5.2	-11.5	-3.0	0.0
In-patient surgical procedures (number)	8.8	0.3	-2.6	-5.4	0.2	-3.4	-2.5
Midwives (number)	-5.1	2.2	-8.5	-10.7	-6.8	-2.8	-2.0
Nurses (number)	-0.5	-1.5	-1.7	0.4	10.7	3.2	2.4
Out-patient contacts (per capita)	0.9	-1.6	6.3	-3.0	-0.9	2.5	3.0

Source: Euromonitor International from national statistics

Immunisation

Estonia: Vaccination rates by disease type 1998-2004

Table: 4.381

%

	1998	1999	2000	2001	2002	2003	2004
Vaccination rate against DTP (diphtheria, tetanus, pertussis) 1 & 2 (%)			0.0	89.0	90.0	90.0	91.0
Vaccination rate against MMR (measles, mumps, rubella) (%)	89.0	92.2	93.4	94.7	95.2	97.0	99.0
Vaccination rate against polio (%)	94.0	95.4	92.5	93.6	97.5	97.0	97.0

Source: WHO

Infectious Diseases

Estonia: Incidence of disease by type 1998-2004

Table: 4.382

Number

	1998	1999	2000	2001	2002	2003	2004
Incidence of AIDS	6	12	390	1,474	899	258	240
Incidence of diphtheria	0	0	2	2	0		
Incidence of measles	17	12	9	0	0		
Incidence of polio	0	0	0	0	0		

Source: WHO

Estonia: Incidence of disease by type: growth 1998-2004

Table: 4.383

Year on year growth: %

	1998	1999	2000	2001	2002	2003	2004
Incidence of AIDS	-33.3	100.0	3,150.0	277.9	-39.0	-71.3	-7.0
Incidence of diphtheria	-100.0			0.0	-100.0		
Incidence of measles	-5.6	-29.4	-25.0	-100.0			

Source: WHO

Causes of Death

Estonia: Deaths by disease 1998-2004

Table: 4.384

Number per 100,000 inhabitants

	1998	1999	2000	2001	2002	2003	2004
Death by diseases of the circulatory system	732.6	700.5	679.6	659.3	663.7	671.0	668.2
Deaths from heart disease	444.4	418.7	433.6	421.5	416.2	410.9	405.6
Death by malignant neoplasms (cancers)	235.0	224.8	216.1	207.7	207.9	208.3	204.3
Deaths from lung cancer	48.4	45.2	50.1	49.6	50.4	51.1	50.9
Death by diseases of the digestive system	31.5	29.8	33.5	32.7	33.6	32.4	32.2
Death by diseases of the respiratory system	41.6	35.9	34.1	33.5	32.7	29.2	27.9
Deaths from chronic liver disease and cirrhosis	18.9	16.2	19.9	19.2	19.6	20.1	20.3
Deaths from ulcers of the stomach and duodenum	6.3	4.9	6.0	5.4	5.2	5.0	4.7

Source: WHO/Euromonitor International
Notes: Data is ranked in descending order by year 2004

Estonia: Deaths by disease: growth 1998-2004

Table: 4.385

% year on year growth

	1998	1999	2000	2001	2002	2003	2004
Deaths from chronic liver disease and cirrhosis	25.2	-14.5	22.9	-3.3	2.1	2.6	1.1
Deaths from lung cancer	72.2	-6.6	10.9	-1.1	1.6	1.4	-0.4
Death by diseases of the circulatory system	6.1	-4.4	-3.0	-3.0	0.7	1.1	-0.4
Death by diseases of the digestive system	13.7	-5.4	12.4	-2.4	2.8	-3.6	-0.6
Deaths from heart disease	8.6	-5.8	3.6	-2.8	-1.3	-1.3	-1.3
Death by malignant neoplasms (cancers)	3.0	-4.3	-3.9	-3.9	0.1	0.2	-1.9
Death by diseases of the respiratory system	15.9	-13.7	-5.0	-1.8	-2.4	-10.7	-4.6
Deaths from ulcers of the stomach and duodenum	18.6	-23.5	23.3	-9.8	-3.7	-3.8	-5.6

Source: WHO/Euromonitor International
Notes: Data is ranked in descending order by year 2004

Estonia: Other selected causes of death: 1998-2004

Table: 4.386

Number per 100,000 inhabitants

	1998	1999	2000	2001	2002	2003	2004
Death by injury and poisoning	162.2	156.1	150.0	144.2	144.8	145.4	144.6

Source: Euromonitor International from national statistics

Estonia: Other selected causes of death: growth 1998-2004

Table: 4.387

% year on year growth

	1998	1999	2000	2001	2002	2003	2004
Death by injury and poisoning	2.3	-3.8	-3.9	-3.9	0.4	0.4	-0.5

Source: Euromonitor International from national statistics

Smoking

Estonia: Smoking prevalence in population aged 15+ 1998-2004

Table: 4.388

% of population aged 15+

	1998	1999	2000	2001	2002	2003	2004
Smoking prevalence in population aged 15+ (% of population aged 15+)	29.4	29.4	29.4	29.0	28.9	28.7	28.3
Smoking prevalence in male population aged 15+ (% of male population)	42.3	43.4	44.1	44.8	45.0	45.8	46.3
Smoking prevalence in female population aged 15+ (% of female population)	19.6	19.7	19.9	19.1	17.9	22.9	22.1

Source: WHO/OECD/Euromonitor International

Nutrition and Obesity

Estonia: Nutrition and obesity 1998-2004

Table: 4.389

As stated

	1998	1999	2000	2001	2002	2003	2004
Availability of fruit and vegetables (kg/capita/year)	133.5	139.2	147.5	154.1	161.0	168.8	178.1
Average supply of calories per day (calories per capita)	2,917.2	3,060.6	2,985.3	2,992.9	3,002.2	3,096.1	3,105.1
Average supply of fat per day (grams per capita)	100.6	103.3	88.6	90.9	91.0	93.5	95.7
Average supply of protein per day (grams per capita)	91.4	94.7	90.6	93.0	93.0	93.4	94.1
Microbiological food-borne diseases (per 100000 population)	1.0	1.0	9.0	4.0	5.0	5.0	6.0
Obese population (BMI 30kg/sq m or more) (% of population aged 15+)	15.0	15.5	15.9	16.3	16.8	17.2	17.6

Source: WHO/OECD/Euromonitor International

■ Finland

Socio-economic Parameters

Finland: Socio-economic parameters 1998-2004

Table: 4.390

As stated

	1998	1999	2000	2001	2002	2003	2004
Population: national estimates at January 1st ('000)	5,147.3	5,159.6	5,171.3	5,181.1	5,194.9	5,206.3	5,213.0
% aged 0-14 yrs	18.7	18.4	18.2	18.1	17.9	17.8	17.6
% aged 15-64 yrs	66.7	66.9	66.9	66.9	66.9	66.9	66.8
% aged 65+ yrs	14.6	14.7	14.8	15.0	15.2	15.3	15.5
% Male	48.7	48.8	48.8	48.8	48.8	48.9	48.9
% Female	51.3	51.2	51.2	51.2	51.2	51.1	51.1
% Urban	66.1	66.7	67.3	67.7	68.2	68.5	68.9
Occupants per household at January 1st (Number)	2.2	2.2	2.2	2.2	2.2	2.2	2.2
Households ('000)	2,355.0	2,365.0	2,382.0	2,382.0	2,396.2	2,404.1	2,413.5
Annual rates of inflation (% growth)	1.4	1.2	3.4	2.6	1.6	0.9	0.2
GDP (EUR million)	115,970.0	119,985.5	130,145.7	135,468.7	139,803.7	143,422.6	149,742.8
GDP (US$ million)	130,002.4	127,830.9	119,905.7	121,223.7	131,573.8	161,870.4	185,931.6
GDP (US$ per capita)	25,256.2	24,775.1	23,186.8	23,397.2	25,327.5	31,091.3	35,666.6

Source: Euromonitor International from International Monetary Fund (IMF), International Financial Statistics and World Economic Outlook/UN/national statistics

Life Expectancy

Finland: Life expectancy 1998-2004

Table: 4.391

As stated

	1998	1999	2000	2001	2002	2003	2004	% change 1998-2004
Life expectancy at birth: total population (years)	77.4	77.5	77.7	77.8	78.2	78.3	78.5	1.53
Life expectancy at birth: total population: year on year growth	0.3	0.2	0.2	0.2	0.4	0.3	0.3	
Healthy life expectancy at birth (years)	70.0			69.9	70.1			
Healthy life expectancy at birth: year on year growth					0.3			

Source: Euromonitor International from World Bank

Sanitation

Finland: Improved sanitary facilities and water source 2000

As stated

	2000
Population with access to improved sanitary facilities (% of population)	100.0
Population with access to improved water source (% of population)	100.0
Population with improved access to sanitation facilities, rural (% of rural population with access)	100.0
Population with improved access to sanitation facilities, urban (% of urban population with access)	100.0

Source: National statistics/World Bank

Health Expenditure

Finland: Public health expenditure 1998-2004

As stated

	1998	1999	2000	2001	2002	2003	2004
Public expenditure on pharmaceuticals and other medical non-durables (EUR million)	565.0	611.0	678.0	768.0	859.0	962.0	1,073.1
Private insurance expenditure (% of total expenditure on health)	2.6	2.7	2.6	2.5	2.4	2.4	2.4
Share of total health expenditure in GDP (% of total GDP)	6.9	6.9	6.6	7.0	7.3	7.0	7.0
Health expenditure (US$ per capita)	1,732.0	1,710.0	1,543.0	1,628.0	1,852.0	1,899.0	1,979.0

Source: Euromonitor International from OECD/national statistics

Finland: Private health expenditure 1998-2004

As stated

	1998	1999	2000	2001	2002	2003	2004
Consumer expenditure on health goods and medical services (EUR million)	1,997.0	2,106.0	2,355.0	2,541.0	2,697.0	2,756.0	2,783.9
Consumer expenditure on health goods and medical services: real growth in national currency: 1990 = 100	136.0	141.8	153.4	161.4	168.7	170.9	172.3
Consumer expenditure on health goods and medical services as a percentage of total consumer expenditure	3.6	3.6	3.8	3.9	3.9	3.9	4.0

Source: National statistical offices/OECD/Eurostat/Euromonitor International

Finland: Consumer expenditure on health goods and medical services by sector 1998-2004

% of total consumer expenditure on health goods and medical services

	1998	1999	2000	2001	2002	2003	2004
Pharmaceuticals, medical appliances/equipment	49.2	50.6	46.1	45.6	45.6	46.6	47.2
Outpatient services	33.6	32.0	37.0	38.5	38.5	37.9	37.7
Hospital services	17.2	17.4	16.9	15.9	15.9	15.5	15.1
Total	100.0	100.0	100.0	100.0	100.0	100.0	100.0

Source: National statistical offices/OECD/Eurostat/Euromonitor International

Healthcare Infrastructure and Services

Finland: Healthcare infrastructure and services by sector 1998-2004

Table: 4.396

As stated

	1998	1999	2000	2001	2002	2003	2004
Active pharmacists (number)	7,462	7,569	7,660	7,755	7,838	7,930	8,022
Consultations with GPs (general practitioners) (per capita)	4	4	4	4	4	4	4
Dentists (number)	4,833	4,826	4,794	4,731	4,636	4,574	4,503
Doctors (number)	15,436	15,794	15,905	16,110	16,272	16,435	16,616
Hospital admissions (number)	1,381,731	1,380,476	1,382,552	1,350,163	1,361,044	1,347,108	1,322,998
Hospitals and clinics (number)	343	363	389	390	391	394	398
In-patient beds ('000)	13,433	12,939	12,481	12,208	12,119	11,999	11,888
In-patient surgical procedures (number)	457,180	463,388	467,805	450,974	474,063	474,303	475,089
Midwives (number)	4,025	4,049	3,980	3,952	3,934	3,921	3,910
Nurses (number)	37,600	39,300	42,700	44,800	46,900	48,254	49,356
Out-patient contacts (per capita)	4	4	4	4	4	4	4

Source: Euromonitor International from national statistics

Finland: Healthcare infrastructure and services by sector: growth 1998-2004

Table: 4.397

Year on year growth: % change in stated unit

	1998	1999	2000	2001	2002	2003	2004
Active pharmacists (number)	1.3	1.4	1.2	1.2	1.1	1.2	1.2
Consultations with GPs (general practitioners) (per capita)	0.0	2.4	0.0	0.0	0.0	0.0	0.0
Dentists (number)	-0.1	-0.1	-0.7	-1.3	-2.0	-1.3	-1.6
Doctors (number)	1.6	2.3	0.7	1.3	1.0	1.0	1.1
Hospital admissions (number)	0.6	-0.1	0.2	-2.3	0.8	-1.0	-1.8
Hospitals and clinics (number)	-5.0	5.8	7.2	0.3	0.3	0.8	1.0
In-patient beds (number)	-5.2	-3.7	-3.5	-2.2	-0.7	-1.0	-0.9
In-patient surgical procedures (number)	6.3	1.4	1.0	-3.6	5.1	0.1	0.2
Midwives (number)	0.1	0.6	-1.7	-0.7	-0.5	-0.3	-0.3
Nurses (number)	0.8	4.5	8.7	4.9	4.7	2.9	2.3
Out-patient contacts (per capita)	0.0	2.4	0.0	0.0	-2.3	2.4	0.0

Source: Euromonitor International from national statistics

Immunisation

Finland: Vaccination rates by disease type 1998-2004

Table: 4.398

%

	1998	1999	2000	2001	2002	2003	2004
Vaccination rate against DTP (diphtheria, tetanus, pertussis) 1 & 2 (%)				98.8	98.8	99.0	99.0
Vaccination rate against MMR (measles, mumps, rubella) (%)				95.8	95.8	96.0	96.0
Vaccination rate against polio (%)				95.4	95.3	95.0	95.0

Source: WHO

Infectious Diseases

Finland: Incidence of disease by type 1998-2004

Table: 4.399

Number

	1998	1999	2000	2001	2002	2003	2004
Incidence of AIDS	20	10	16	10	21	12	15
Incidence of diphtheria	0			2	0		
Incidence of measles	1			1	0		
Incidence of polio	0	0	0	0	0		

Source: WHO

Finland: Incidence of disease by type: growth 1998-2004

Table: 4.400

Year on year growth: %

	1998	1999	2000	2001	2002	2003	2004
Incidence of AIDS	17.6	-50.0	60.0	-37.5	110.0	-42.9	25.0
Incidence of diphtheria					-100.0		
Incidence of measles					-100.0		

Source: WHO

Causes of Death

Finland: Deaths by disease 1998-2004

Table: 4.401

Number per 100,000 inhabitants

	1998	1999	2000	2001	2002	2003	2004
Death by diseases of the circulatory system	292.3	284.2	277.0	269.5	268.8	263.7	261.2
Deaths from heart disease	248.8	251.3	249.2	250.2	250.4	250.7	252.4
Death by malignant neoplasms (cancers)	150.5	147.4	145.3	143.0	142.6	140.9	138.5
Death by diseases of the respiratory system	54.0	53.9	54.1	54.1	54.0	54.0	54.5
Deaths from lung cancer	37.4	35.1	35.7	34.3	33.5	32.6	31.5
Death by diseases of the digestive system	27.9	27.0	27.9	26.7	26.9	26.2	25.9
Deaths from chronic liver disease and cirrhosis	12.7	12.1	13.0	13.0	13.2	13.4	13.4
Deaths from ulcers of the stomach and duodenum	4.5	5.0	5.2	5.6	5.9	6.2	6.6

Source: WHO/Euromonitor International
Notes: Data is ranked in descending order by year 2004

Finland: Deaths by disease: growth 1998-2004

Table: 4.402

% year on year growth

	1998	1999	2000	2001	2002	2003	2004
Deaths from ulcers of the stomach and duodenum	-14.6	10.0	4.5	7.8	5.4	5.1	6.7
Death by diseases of the respiratory system	0.2	-0.2	0.4	0.0	-0.2	0.0	0.9
Deaths from heart disease	1.4	1.0	-0.8	0.4	0.1	0.1	0.7
Deaths from chronic liver disease and cirrhosis	7.5	-4.5	8.0	-0.3	1.5	1.5	0.3
Death by diseases of the circulatory system	-2.4	-2.8	-2.5	-2.7	-0.3	-1.9	-0.9
Death by diseases of the digestive system	-2.8	-3.2	3.3	-4.3	0.7	-2.6	-1.2
Death by malignant neoplasms (cancers)	-1.1	-2.1	-1.4	-1.6	-0.3	-1.2	-1.7
Deaths from lung cancer	4.3	-6.2	1.7	-3.8	-2.3	-2.7	-3.4

Source: WHO/Euromonitor International
Notes: Data is ranked in descending order by year 2004

Finland: Other selected causes of death: 1998-2004

Table: 4.403

Number per 100,000 inhabitants

	1998	1999	2000	2001	2002	2003	2004
Death by injury and poisoning	68.6	67.0	65.4	63.9	63.7	62.7	62.4
Death by suicide and self-inflicted injury	21.5	21.2	20.4	19.3	19.5	18.8	18.4
Death by motor traffic accidents	8.6	8.5	7.5	7.3	7.2	7.1	7.0

Source: Euromonitor International from national statistics
Notes: Data is ranked in descending order by year 2004

Finland: Other selected causes of death: growth 1998-2004

Table: 4.404

% year on year growth

	1998	1999	2000	2001	2002	2003	2004
Death by injury and poisoning	-2.1	-2.3	-2.4	-2.3	-0.3	-1.6	-0.4
Death by motor traffic accidents	-3.4	-1.2	-11.8	-2.7	-1.4	-1.4	-0.8
Death by suicide and self-inflicted injury	-8.1	-1.4	-3.8	-5.4	1.0	-3.6	-1.9

Source: Euromonitor International from national statistics
Notes: Data is ranked in descending order by year 2004

Smoking

Finland: Smoking prevalence in population aged 15+ 1998-2004

Table: 4.405

% of population aged 15+

	1998	1999	2000	2001	2002	2003	2004
Smoking prevalence in population aged 15+ (% of population aged 15+)	25.0	23.0	23.0	24.0	23.4	23.4	23.6
Smoking prevalence in male population aged 15+ (% of male population)	30.0	27.0	27.0	29.0	27.5	26.5	26.2
Smoking prevalence in female population aged 15+ (% of female population)	20.0	20.0	20.0	20.0	19.9	20.6	21.2

Source: WHO/OECD/Euromonitor International

Nutrition and Obesity

Finland: Nutrition and obesity 1998-2004

Table: 4.406

As stated

	1998	1999	2000	2001	2002	2003	2004
Availability of fruit and vegetables (kg/capita/year)	136.5	158.3	155.6	163.8	165.9	167.8	169.7
Average supply of calories per day (calories per capita)	3,143.4	3,125.2	3,111.5	3,153.9	3,100.4	3,171.0	3,129.6
Average supply of fat per day (grams per capita)	130.3	125.3	119.6	123.5	123.0	122.3	122.5
Average supply of protein per day (grams per capita)	102.5	100.9	100.4	102.3	101.0	100.4	100.1
Microbiological food-borne diseases (per 100000 population)	95.0	89.0	76.0	58.0	38.0	40.0	42.0
Obese population (BMI 30kg/sq m or more) (% of population aged 15+)	9.5	10.1	11.2	11.4	12.8	13.5	13.9

Source: WHO/OECD/Euromonitor International

Over-the-Counter Healthcare

Finland: Trends in OTC healthcare retail sales 1998-2004

Table: 4.407

As stated

	1998	1999	2000	2001	2002	2003	2004
OTC Healthcare (EUR million)	285.9	297.4	305.8	318.9	326.6	336.9	351.1
OTC Healthcare: real growth in national currency: 1998 = 100	100.0	102.8	102.3	104.0	104.9	107.3	111.7
OTC Healthcare: year on year (% real growth)	-3.1	2.8	-0.5	1.7	0.8	2.3	4.1

Source: Euromonitor International from industry sources/national statistics

Finland: OTC healthcare retail sales by sector 1998-2004

Table: 4.408

% of OTC retail value sales

	1998	1999	2000	2001	2002	2003	2004
Analgesics	15.7	16.9	17.3	17.7	17.3	17.5	17.4
Cough, cold and allergy (hay fever) remedies	18.7	17.6	17.6	17.4	17.6	17.1	17.0
Digestive remedies	14.5	14.6	14.6	14.8	14.2	13.9	13.8
Medicated skin care	11.5	11.3	11.1	11.0	11.2	11.0	10.8
Vitamins and dietary supplements	29.8	29.1	28.4	27.8	27.6	27.4	27.0

Source: *Euromonitor International from industry sources/national statistics*
Notes: *Only selected sectors are shown, so values are not expected to sum to 100*

Health and Wellness

Finland: Retail sales of packaged foods by health and wellness category 2002-2004

Table: 4.409

EUR million

	2002	2003	2004
Packaged food: Total	6,232.5	6,405.5	6,576.3
Better for you	1,064.2	1,093.1	1,115.2
For food intolerance	39.6	51.2	56.3
Fortified/functional	151.1	168.1	183.0
Organic	39.0	43.0	47.3

Source: *Euromonitor International from industry sources/national statistics*

Finland: Per capita sales of packaged foods by health and wellness category 2002-2004

Table: 4.410

EUR per capita

	2002	2003	2004
Better for you	204.8	209.9	213.7
For food intolerance	7.6	9.8	10.8
Fortified/functional	29.1	32.3	35.1
Organic	7.5	8.3	9.1

Source: *Euromonitor International from industry sources/national statistics*

Finland: Retail sales of packaged food by health and wellness category: % share of total packaged food market 2002-2004

Table: 4.411

% value

	2002	2003	2004
Better for you	17.1	17.1	17.0
For food intolerance	0.6	0.8	0.9
Fortified/functional	2.4	2.6	2.8
Organic	0.6	0.7	0.7

Source: *Euromonitor International from industry sources/national statistics*

Finland: Retail sales of packaged food by health and wellness category: real growth index 2002-2004

Table: 4.412

2002 =100

	2002	2003	2004
Better for you	100.00	100.90	101.22
For food intolerance	100.00	127.21	137.29
Fortified/functional	100.00	109.30	117.02
Organic	100.00	108.35	117.15

Source: *Euromonitor International from industry sources/national statistics*

Finland: Retail sales of better-for-you packaged foods by sector 2002-2004

Table: 4.413

% of total packaged food / as stated

	2002	2003	2004	% real change in value 2002-2004
Combination	0.03	0.04	0.04	13.16
Reduced fat	14.50	14.51	14.42	1.40
Reduced salt	0.33	0.32	0.31	-4.01

Source: *Euromonitor International from industry sources/national statistics*

Finland: Retail sales of packaged foods for food intolerances by sector 2002-2004

Table: 4.414

% of total packaged food / as stated

	2002	2003	2004	% real change in value 2002-2004
Diabetic	0.14	0.16	0.17	23.53
Gluten-free	0.29	0.30	0.32	11.11
Lactose-free	0.20	0.34	0.37	84.34

Source: *Euromonitor International from industry sources/national statistics*

Finland: Retail sales of naturally healthy packaged foods by sector 2002-2004

Table: 4.415

% of total packaged food / as stated

	2002	2003	2004	% real change in value 2002-2004
High fibre	2.51	2.56	2.62	6.30
Other naturally healthy food	1.59	1.56	1.52	-2.47
Soy-based dairy alternatives	0.15	0.15	0.16	9.93

Source: *Euromonitor International from industry sources/national statistics*

■ **France**

Socio-economic Parameters

France: Socio-economic parameters 1998-2004

Table: 4.416

As stated

	1998	1999	2000	2001	2002	2003	2004
Population: national estimates at January 1st ('000)	58,299.0	58,496.6	58,748.7	59,038.5	59,344.0	59,663.3	59,978.8
% aged 0-14 yrs	19.0	18.9	18.9	18.8	18.7	18.7	18.7
% aged 15-64 yrs	65.2	65.2	65.1	65.1	65.0	65.1	65.2
% aged 65 + yrs	15.7	15.9	16.0	16.1	16.2	16.2	16.1
% Male	48.6	48.6	48.6	48.6	48.6	48.6	48.6
% Female	51.4	51.4	51.4	51.4	51.4	51.4	51.4
% Urban	75.2	75.4	75.6	75.8	76.0	76.2	76.5
Occupants per household at January 1st (Number)	2.5	2.5	2.4	2.4	2.4	2.4	2.4
Households ('000)	23,476.4	23,808.1	24,044.0	24,277.6	24,477.9	24,690.7	24,883.6
Annual rates of inflation (% growth)	0.7	0.5	1.7	1.7	1.9	2.1	2.1
GDP (EUR million)	1,306,294.6	1,354,294.5	1,421,693.4	1,475,761.0	1,528,222.0	1,558,702.0	1,623,159.0
GDP (US$ million)	1,464,356.2	1,442,846.3	1,309,833.6	1,320,579.7	1,438,258.9	1,759,189.8	2,015,432.8
GDP (US$ per capita)	25,118.0	24,665.5	22,295.5	22,368.1	24,236.0	29,485.3	33,602.4

Source: *Euromonitor International from International Monetary Fund (IMF), International Financial Statistics and World Economic Outlook/UN/national statistics*

Life Expectancy

France: Life expectancy 1998-2004

Table: 4.417

As stated

	1998	1999	2000	2001	2002	2003	2004	% change 1998-2004
Life expectancy at birth: total population (years)	78.8	78.9	79.1	79.3	79.7	80.2	80.4	2.08
Life expectancy at birth: total population: year on year growth	0.3	0.2	0.2	0.2	0.6	0.6	0.2	
Healthy life expectancy at birth (years)	73.0			71.1	71.3			
Healthy life expectancy at birth: year on year growth					0.2			

Source: Euromonitor International from World Bank

Health Expenditure

France: Public health expenditure 1998-2004

Table: 4.418

As stated

	1998	1999	2000	2001	2002	2003	2004
Public expenditure on pharmaceuticals and other medical non-durables (EUR million)	14,228.0	15,675.0	17,498.0	19,242.0	20,683.0	22,460.0	24,984.6
Private insurance expenditure (% of total expenditure on health)	12.6	12.6	12.6	12.9	13.2	13.2	13.3
Share of total health expenditure in GDP (% of total GDP)	9.3	9.3	9.4	9.6	9.9	10.1	10.5
Health expenditure (US$ per capita)	2,306.0	2,282.0	2,061.0	2,103.0	2,348.0	2,444.0	2,529.0

Source: Euromonitor International from OECD/national statistics

France: Private health expenditure 1998-2004

Table: 4.419

As stated

	1998	1999	2000	2001	2002	2003	2004
Consumer expenditure on health goods and medical services (EUR million)	25,623.0	26,578.0	27,645.0	28,770.0	30,505.0	31,993.0	33,949.6
Consumer expenditure on health goods and medical services: real growth in national currency: 1990 = 100	118.2	122.0	124.8	127.8	132.9	136.5	141.8
Consumer expenditure on health goods and medical services as a percentage of total consumer expenditure	3.6	3.6	3.5	3.5	3.6	3.7	3.8

Source: National statistical offices/OECD/Eurostat/Euromonitor International

France: Consumer expenditure on health goods and medical services by sector 1998-2004

Table: 4.420

% of total consumer expenditure on health goods and medical services

	1998	1999	2000	2001	2002	2003	2004
Pharmaceuticals, medical appliances/ equipment	39.9	40.6	42.0	43.0	43.0	43.0	42.8
Outpatient services	38.3	38.4	37.3	36.9	36.5	36.5	36.2
Hospital services	21.9	21.0	20.7	20.1	20.5	20.5	20.9
Total	100.0	100.0	100.0	100.0	100.0	100.0	100.0

Source: National statistical offices/OECD/Eurostat/Euromonitor International

Healthcare Infrastructure and Services

France: Healthcare infrastructure and services by sector 1998-2004

Table: 4.421

As stated

	1998	1999	2000	2001	2002	2003	2004
Active pharmacists (number)	61,712	63,038	64,338	65,526	67,937	69,655	71,525
Consultations with GPs (general practitioners) (per capita)	7	7	7	7	7	7	7
Dentists (number)	39,457	40,088	40,539	40,426	40,481	40,648	40,685
Doctors (number)	191,700	193,200	194,000	196,000	198,700	201,400	203,929
Hospital admissions (number)	13,497,976	13,509,484	13,541,664	13,568,676	13,595,688	13,568,209	13,758,910
Hospitals and clinics (number)	1,064	1,079	1,054	1,060	1,053	1,048	1,042
In-patient beds ('000)	410	402	392	393	395	396	397
Midwives (number)	10,165	13,921	14,353	14,725	15,153	15,520	15,796
Nurses (number)	373,938	381,047	397,279	412,231	425,981	439,115	454,019
Out-patient contacts (per capita)	7	7	7	7	7	7	7

Source: Euromonitor International from national statistics

France: Healthcare infrastructure and services by sector: growth 1998-2004

Table: 4.422

Year on year growth: % change in stated unit

	1998	1999	2000	2001	2002	2003	2004
Active pharmacists (number)	2.3	2.1	2.1	1.8	3.7	2.5	2.7
Consultations with GPs (general practitioners) (per capita)	3.1	0.0	4.5	0.0	0.0	0.0	0.0
Dentists (number)	0.0	1.6	1.1	-0.3	0.1	0.4	0.1
Doctors (number)	0.8	0.8	0.4	1.0	1.4	1.4	1.3
Hospital admissions (number)	0.3	0.1	0.2	0.2	0.2	-0.2	1.4
Hospitals and clinics (number)	1.8	1.4	-2.3	0.6	-0.7	-0.5	-0.6
In-patient beds (number)	-1.9	-1.8	-2.5	0.1	0.6	0.3	0.3
Midwives (number)	-2.4	37.0	3.1	2.6	2.9	2.4	1.8
Nurses (number)	3.6	1.9	4.3	3.8	3.3	3.1	3.4
Out-patient contacts (per capita)	1.4	1.3	1.3	1.3	0.7	-1.4	4.3

Source: Euromonitor International from national statistics

Immunisation

France: Vaccination rates by disease type 1998-2004

Table: 4.423

%

	1998	1999	2000	2001	2002	2003	2004
Vaccination rate against MMR (measles, mumps, rubella) (%)					85.0	88.0	88.0
Vaccination rate against polio (%)					98.0	98.0	98.0

Source: WHO

Infectious Diseases

France: Incidence of disease by type 1998-2004

Table: 4.424

Number

	1998	1999	2000	2001	2002	2003	2004
Incidence of AIDS	2,098	1,785	1,825	787	2,004	1,091	1,020
Incidence of diphtheria			0		1		
Incidence of measles			10,000		5,185		
Incidence of polio	0	0	0		0		

Source: WHO

France: Incidence of disease by type: growth 1998-2004

Table: 4.425

Year on year growth: %

	1998	1999	2000	2001	2002	2003	2004
Incidence of AIDS	-26.0	-14.9	2.2	-56.9	154.6	-45.6	-6.5

Source: WHO

Causes of Death

France: Deaths by disease 1998-2004

Table: 4.426

Number per 100,000 inhabitants

	1998	1999	2000	2001	2002	2003	2004
Death by malignant neoplasms (cancers)	179.9	178.2	179.1	178.4	176.5	175.8	173.0
Death by diseases of the circulatory system	168.4	163.6	162.3	160.9	159.3	158.6	156.0
Deaths from heart disease	78.0	76.9	76.8	76.5	76.2	75.9	75.4
Deaths from lung cancer	42.7	43.0	43.8	44.4	45.1	45.8	46.4
Death by diseases of the respiratory system	42.4	42.1	42.2	42.4	41.0	41.4	41.1
Death by diseases of the digestive system	30.5	29.3	28.4	27.6	27.2	27.0	26.4
Deaths from chronic liver disease and cirrhosis	16.3	15.8	15.6	15.3	15.0	14.7	14.5
Deaths from ulcers of the stomach and duodenum	2.6	2.5	2.5	2.5	2.5	2.5	2.5

Source: WHO/Euromonitor International
Notes: Data is ranked in descending order by year 2004

France: Deaths by disease: growth 1998-2004

Table: 4.427

% year on year growth

	1998	1999	2000	2001	2002	2003	2004
Deaths from lung cancer	2.5	0.7	1.9	1.4	1.6	1.6	1.3
Deaths from ulcers of the stomach and duodenum	3.4	-2.8	0.8	0.0	0.0	0.0	-0.2
Death by diseases of the respiratory system	4.2	-0.7	0.2	0.5	-3.3	1.0	-0.6
Deaths from heart disease	0.6	-1.4	-0.1	-0.4	-0.4	-0.4	-0.7
Deaths from chronic liver disease and cirrhosis	-0.3	-3.1	-1.2	-1.9	-2.0	-2.0	-1.3
Death by malignant neoplasms (cancers)	2.1	-0.9	0.5	-0.4	-1.1	-0.4	-1.6
Death by diseases of the circulatory system	1.6	-2.9	-0.8	-0.9	-1.0	-0.4	-1.7
Death by diseases of the digestive system	2.0	-3.9	-3.1	-2.8	-1.4	-0.7	-2.4

Source: WHO/Euromonitor International
Notes: Data is ranked in descending order by year 2004

France: Other selected causes of death: 1998-2004

Table: 4.428

Number per 100,000 inhabitants

	1998	1999	2000	2001	2002	2003	2004
Death by injury and poisoning	57.6	56.7	56.8	56.8	55.0	55.4	54.6
Death by suicide and self-inflicted injury	15.4	15.0	14.9	14.7	14.3	14.3	14.0
Death by motor traffic accidents	13.8	13.5	13.6	13.7	13.3	13.4	13.4

Source: Euromonitor International from national statistics
Notes: Data is ranked in descending order by year 2004

France: Other selected causes of death: growth 1998-2004

Table: 4.429

% year on year growth

	1998	1999	2000	2001	2002	2003	2004
Death by motor traffic accidents	7.8	-2.2	0.7	0.7	-2.9	0.8	-0.3
Death by injury and poisoning	1.9	-1.6	0.2	0.0	-3.2	0.7	-1.4
Death by suicide and self-inflicted injury	-4.9	-2.6	-0.7	-1.3	-2.7	0.0	-2.0

Source: Euromonitor International from national statistics
Notes: Data is ranked in descending order by year 2004

Smoking

France: Smoking prevalence in population aged 15+ 1998-2004

Table: 4.430

% of population aged 15+

	1998	1999	2000	2001	2002	2003	2004
Smoking prevalence in population aged 15+ (% of population aged 15+)	26.7	26.4	27.0	25.8	25.4	25.7	25.4
Smoking prevalence in male population aged 15+ (% of male population)	31.9	31.4	33.0	33.0	31.7	33.1	33.6
Smoking prevalence in female population aged 15+ (% of female population)	21.9	21.9	21.0	19.2	19.6	18.8	17.8

Source: WHO/OECD/Euromonitor International

Nutrition and Obesity

France: Nutrition and obesity 1998-2004

Table: 4.431

As stated

	1998	1999	2000	2001	2002	2003	2004
Availability of fruit and vegetables (kg/capita/year)	214.9	220.0	228.4	227.2	230.5	237.9	238.9
Average supply of calories per day (calories per capita)	3,591.3	3,588.8	3,600.9	3,646.4	3,653.9	3,669.0	3,689.4
Average supply of fat per day (grams per capita)	165.6	164.6	167.3	170.0	170.8	172.3	173.8
Average supply of protein per day (grams per capita)	117.2	116.8	117.5	118.9	119.2	119.8	120.5
Obese population (BMI 30kg/sq m or more) (% of population aged 15+)	8.6	9.0	9.0	10.0	12.6	14.5	15.2

Source: WHO/OECD/Euromonitor International

Over-the-Counter Healthcare

France: Trends in OTC healthcare retail sales 1998-2004

Table: 4.432

As stated

	1998	1999	2000	2001	2002	2003	2004
OTC Healthcare (EUR million)	2,272.4	2,324.1	2,390.4	2,443.1	2,458.9	2,517.2	2,561.3
OTC Healthcare: real growth in national currency: 1998 = 100	100.0	101.8	102.9	103.5	102.2	102.4	101.8
OTC Healthcare: year on year (% real growth)	1.1	1.8	1.1	0.5	-1.3	0.3	-0.6

Source: Euromonitor International from industry sources/national statistics

France: OTC healthcare retail sales by sector 1998-2004

Table: 4.433

% of OTC retail value sales

	1998	1999	2000	2001	2002	2003	2004
Analgesics	19.3	19.2	18.9	18.2	17.6	17.1	16.7
Cough, cold and allergy (hay fever) remedies	21.8	21.5	21.0	21.0	20.8	20.4	20.1
Digestive remedies	87,885.1	85,946.1	81,685.9	79,785.9	77,869.6	73,053.9	69,001.9
Digestive remedies	13.5	13.3	12.9	12.7	12.6	12.2	11.8
Medicated skin care	12.6	13.0	12.7	12.6	12.5	12.2	12.1
Vitamins and dietary supplements	20.9	20.9	20.9	20.9	21.5	21.8	22.2

Source: *Euromonitor International from industry sources/national statistics*
Notes: *Only selected sectors are shown, so values are not expected to sum to 100*

Health and Wellness

France: Retail sales of packaged foods by health and wellness category 2002-2004

Table: 4.434

EUR million

	2002	2003	2004
Packaged food: Total	53,654.3	55,348.7	56,568.3
Better for you	3,651.8	3,863.6	3,999.3
For food intolerance	99.5	111.8	125.2
Fortified/functional	673.2	774.0	855.4
Organic	399.5	438.2	480.2

Source: *Euromonitor International from industry sources/national statistics*

France: Per capita sales of packaged foods by health and wellness category 2002-2004

Table: 4.435

EUR per capita

	2002	2003	2004
Better for you	61.5	64.9	67.1
For food intolerance	1.7	1.9	2.1
Fortified/functional	11.3	13.0	14.3
Organic	6.7	7.4	8.1

Source: *Euromonitor International from industry sources/national statistics*

France: Retail sales of packaged food by health and wellness category: % share of total packaged food market 2002-2004

Table: 4.436

% value

	2002	2003	2004
Better for you	6.8	7.0	7.1
For food intolerance	0.2	0.2	0.2
Fortified/functional	1.3	1.4	1.5
Organic	0.7	0.8	0.8

Source: *Euromonitor International from industry sources/national statistics*

France: Retail sales of packaged food by health and wellness category: real growth index 2002-2004

Table: 4.437

2002 =100

	2002	2003	2004
Better for you	100.00	103.83	105.68
For food intolerance	100.00	110.21	121.42
Fortified/functional	100.00	112.83	122.61
Organic	100.00	107.63	115.97

Source: *Euromonitor International from industry sources/national statistics*

France: Retail sales of better-for-you packaged foods by sector 2002-2004

Table: 4.438

% of total packaged food / as stated

	2002	2003	2004	% real change in value 2002-2004
Combination	0.20	0.21	0.23	15.40
Reduced fat	5.91	6.02	6.03	3.79
Reduced salt	0.06	0.06	0.07	33.05

Source: Euromonitor International from industry sources/national statistics

France: Retail sales of packaged foods for food intolerances by sector 2002-2004

Table: 4.439

% of total packaged food / as stated

	2002	2003	2004	% real change in value 2002-2004
Diabetic	0.00	0.00	0.00	181.03
Gluten-free	0.17	0.18	0.20	17.75
Lactose-free	0.02	0.02	0.02	44.99

Source: Euromonitor International from industry sources/national statistics

France: Retail sales of naturally healthy packaged foods by sector 2002-2004

Table: 4.440

% of total packaged food / as stated

	2002	2003	2004	% real change in value 2002-2004
High fibre	0.10	0.11	0.12	13.13
Other naturally healthy food	0.99	0.98	0.98	-0.19
Soy-based dairy alternatives	0.26	0.27	0.29	13.14

Source: Euromonitor International from industry sources/national statistics

■ **Germany**

Socio-economic Parameters

Germany: Socio-economic parameters 1998-2004

Table: 4.441

As stated

	1998	1999	2000	2001	2002	2003	2004
Population: national estimates at January 1st ('000)	82,057.4	82,037.0	82,163.5	82,259.5	82,440.3	82,545.9	82,636.3
% aged 0-14 yrs	16.0	15.8	15.7	15.5	15.3	15.1	14.8
% aged 15-64 yrs	68.2	68.2	68.1	67.8	67.6	67.6	67.5
% aged 65 + yrs	15.8	15.9	16.2	16.6	17.1	17.3	17.7
% Male	48.7	48.8	48.8	48.8	48.9	48.9	48.9
% Female	51.3	51.2	51.2	51.2	51.1	51.1	51.1
% Urban	87.1	87.3	87.5	87.7	87.8	88.1	88.3
Occupants per household at January 1st (Number)	2.2	2.2	2.2	2.1	2.1	2.1	2.1
Households ('000)	37,532.0	37,795.0	38,124.0	38,456.0	38,720.0	38,930.9	39,166.1
Annual rates of inflation (% growth)	0.9	0.6	1.5	2.0	1.4	1.0	1.7
GDP (EUR million)	1,927,538.6	1,978,632.8	2,030,028.6	2,074,000.0	2,107,300.0	2,128,200.0	2,177,000.0
GDP (US$ million)	2,160,770.8	2,108,007.5	1,870,304.6	1,855,911.8	1,983,247.8	2,401,939.4	2,703,122.2
GDP (US$ per capita)	26,332.4	25,695.8	22,763.2	22,561.7	24,056.8	29,098.2	32,711.1

Source: Euromonitor International from International Monetary Fund (IMF), International Financial Statistics and World Economic Outlook/UN/national statistics

Life Expectancy

Germany: Life expectancy 1998-2004

Table: 4.442

As stated

	1998	1999	2000	2001	2002	2003	2004	% change 1998-2004
Life expectancy at birth: total population (years)	77.6	77.8	78.0	78.2	78.7	78.9	79.2	2.04
Life expectancy at birth: total population: year on year growth	0.3	0.2	0.2	0.3	0.6	0.3	0.4	
Healthy life expectancy at birth (years)	70.0			70.1	70.2			
Healthy life expectancy at birth: year on year growth					0.2			

Source: Euromonitor International from World Bank

Health Expenditure

Germany: Public health expenditure 1998-2004

Table: 4.443

As stated

	1998	1999	2000	2001	2002	2003	2004
Public expenditure on pharmaceuticals and other medical non-durables (EUR million)	18,722.0	20,301.0	21,257.0	23,528.0	24,910.0	26,525.0	28,877.6
Private insurance expenditure (% of total expenditure on health)	8.0	8.2	8.3	8.4	8.6	8.7	8.9
Share of total health expenditure in GDP (% of total GDP)	10.6	10.7	10.6	10.8	11.1	11.6	12.2
Health expenditure (US$ per capita)	2,772.0	2,727.0	2,398.0	2,418.0	2,631.0	2,748.0	2,864.0

Source: Euromonitor International from OECD/national statistics

Germany: Private health expenditure 1998-2004

Table: 4.444

As stated

	1998	1999	2000	2001	2002	2003	2004
Consumer expenditure on health goods and medical services (EUR million)	42,610.0	43,500.0	45,190.0	47,300.0	48,640.0	49,850.0	51,491.5
Consumer expenditure on health goods and medical services: real growth in national currency: 1990 = 100	151.3	153.6	157.2	161.4	163.7	166.0	168.7
Consumer expenditure on health goods and medical services as a percentage of total consumer expenditure	4.1	4.0	4.0	4.1	4.2	4.2	4.2

Source: National statistical offices/OECD/Eurostat/Euromonitor International

Germany: Consumer expenditure on health goods and medical services by sector 1998-2004

Table: 4.445

% of total consumer expenditure on health goods and medical services

	1998	1999	2000	2001	2002	2003	2004
Pharmaceuticals, medical appliances/equipment	35.0	35.4	34.3	34.5	34.5	34.3	35.2
Outpatient services	36.2	36.1	37.7	38.5	38.5	38.6	38.0
Hospital services	28.8	28.5	28.0	27.0	27.0	27.1	26.7
Total	100.0	100.0	100.0	100.0	100.0	100.0	100.0

Source: National statistical offices/OECD/Eurostat/Euromonitor International

Healthcare Infrastructure and Services

Germany: Healthcare infrastructure and services by sector 1998-2004

Table: 4.446

As stated

	1998	1999	2000	2001	2002	2003	2004
Active pharmacists (number)	45,465	46,064	46,078	45,869	46,513	46,742	46,981
Consultations with GPs (general practitioners) (per capita)	7	7	7	7	8	8	8
Dentists (number)	62,277	62,564	63,202	63,854	64,484	65,172	66,101
Doctors (number)	260,461	263,447	267,965	272,296	275,167	279,432	283,942
Hospital admissions (number)	18,604,298	18,994,362	19,317,636	19,418,936	19,668,219	19,800,984	20,233,442
Hospitals and clinics (number)	2,263	2,242	2,235	3,628	3,781	3,800	3,821
In-patient beds ('000)	534	529	523	516	511	506	502
In-patient surgical procedures (number)	5,904,209	6,368,877	6,711,483	7,074,601	7,411,953	7,769,795	8,192,310
Nurses (number)	769,715	779,005	790,899	801,237	815,639	830,947	846,904
Out-patient contacts (per capita)	7	7	7	8	8	8	8

Source: Euromonitor International from national statistics

Germany: Healthcare infrastructure and services by sector: growth 1998-2004

Table: 4.447

Year on year growth: % change in stated unit

	1998	1999	2000	2001	2002	2003	2004
Active pharmacists (number)	0.4	1.3	0.0	-0.5	1.4	0.5	0.5
Consultations with GPs (general practitioners) (per capita)	2.9	1.4	1.4	2.1	1.7	1.7	1.7
Dentists (number)	0.4	0.5	1.0	1.0	1.0	1.1	1.4
Doctors (number)	1.5	1.1	1.7	1.6	1.1	1.5	1.6
Hospital admissions (number)	3.3	2.1	1.7	0.5	1.3	0.7	2.2
Hospitals and clinics (number)	0.2	-0.9	-0.3	62.3	4.2	0.5	0.6
In-patient beds (number)	-1.3	-0.9	-1.1	-1.3	-1.0	-1.0	-0.9
In-patient surgical procedures (number)	4.6	7.9	5.4	5.4	4.8	4.8	5.4
Nurses (number)	1.5	1.2	1.5	1.3	1.8	1.9	1.9
Out-patient contacts (per capita)	3.1	3.0	2.9	2.8	4.1	3.8	2.4

Source: Euromonitor International from national statistics

Immunisation

Germany: Vaccination rates by disease type 1998-2004

Table: 4.448

%

	1998	1999	2000	2001	2002	2003	2004
Vaccination rate against MMR (measles, mumps, rubella) (%)			89.4	89.5	91.6	92.0	93.0
Vaccination rate against polio (%)			95.1	96.0	96.4	97.0	98.0

Source: WHO

Infectious Diseases

Germany: Incidence of disease by type 1998-2004

Table: 4.449

Number

	1998	1999	2000	2001	2002	2003	2004
Incidence of AIDS	943	578	1,474	484	1,008	837	752
Incidence of diphtheria	1	1	0	0	1		
Incidence of measles				6,024	4,657		
Incidence of polio	0	0	0	0	0		

Source: WHO

Germany: Incidence of disease by type: growth 1998-2004

Table: 4.450

Year on year growth: %

	1998	1999	2000	2001	2002	2003	2004
Incidence of AIDS	-33.4	-38.7	155.0	-67.2	108.3	-17.0	-10.2
Incidence of diphtheria	-66.7	0.0	-100.0				
Incidence of measles					-22.7		

Source: WHO

Causes of Death

Germany: Deaths by disease 1998-2004

Table: 4.451

Number per 100,000 inhabitants

	1998	1999	2000	2001	2002	2003	2004
Death by diseases of the circulatory system	301.3	291.9	290.6	286.0	279.0	270.0	265.6
Deaths from heart disease	217.9	213.3	211.9	209.7	207.5	205.3	204.0
Death by malignant neoplasms (cancers)	179.1	175.3	175.1	169.8	168.7	164.9	162.8
Deaths from lung cancer	46.3	45.9	46.3	46.5	46.7	46.9	46.9
Death by diseases of the respiratory system	37.0	38.2	39.6	37.5	38.2	37.1	36.2
Death by diseases of the digestive system	33.4	32.6	32.8	31.9	32.2	31.7	31.0
Deaths from chronic liver disease and cirrhosis	21.8	21.5	20.9	20.3	19.8	19.2	18.8
Deaths from ulcers of the stomach and duodenum	4.1	4.0	4.0	4.0	3.9	3.9	3.9

Source: WHO/Euromonitor International
Notes: Data is ranked in descending order by year 2004

Germany: Deaths by disease: growth 1998-2004

Table: 4.452

% year on year growth

	1998	1999	2000	2001	2002	2003	2004
Deaths from lung cancer	2.0	-0.9	1.0	0.4	0.4	0.4	0.0
Deaths from ulcers of the stomach and duodenum	0.5	-1.9	-0.3	0.0	-2.5	0.0	0.0
Deaths from heart disease	0.1	-2.1	-0.7	-1.0	-1.0	-1.1	-0.7
Death by malignant neoplasms (cancers)	-0.1	-2.1	-0.1	-3.0	-0.6	-2.3	-1.3
Death by diseases of the circulatory system	-2.2	-3.1	-0.4	-1.6	-2.4	-3.2	-1.6
Death by diseases of the digestive system	-2.3	-2.4	0.6	-2.7	0.9	-1.6	-2.1
Deaths from chronic liver disease and cirrhosis	-3.8	-1.4	-2.9	-2.9	-2.5	-3.0	-2.2
Death by diseases of the respiratory system	-3.9	3.2	3.7	-5.3	1.9	-2.9	-2.4

Source: WHO/Euromonitor International
Notes: Data is ranked in descending order by year 2004

Germany: Other selected causes of death: 1998-2004

Table: 4.453

Number per 100,000 inhabitants

	1998	1999	2000	2001	2002	2003	2004
Death by injury and poisoning	34.0	33.9	31.6	30.1	28.8	27.4	26.1
Death by motor traffic accidents	9.5	9.8	9.1	9.6	10.3	9.9	10.3
Death by suicide and self-inflicted injury	11.7	11.2	10.9	10.3	9.8	9.1	8.6

Source: Euromonitor International from national statistics
Notes: Data is ranked in descending order by year 2004

Germany: Other selected causes of death: growth 1998-2004

Table: 4.454

% year on year growth

	1998	1999	2000	2001	2002	2003	2004
Death by motor traffic accidents	-11.2	3.2	-7.1	5.5	7.3	-3.9	3.9
Death by injury and poisoning	-8.1	-0.3	-6.8	-4.7	-4.3	-4.9	-4.6
Death by suicide and self-inflicted injury	-4.9	-4.3	-2.7	-5.5	-4.9	-7.1	-5.0

Source: Euromonitor International from national statistics
Notes: Data is ranked in descending order by year 2004

Smoking

Germany: Smoking prevalence in population aged 15+ 1998-2004

Table: 4.455

% of population aged 15+

	1998	1999	2000	2001	2002	2003	2004
Smoking prevalence in population aged 15+ (% of population aged 15+)	31.4	23.5	34.5	32.4	34.6	34.8	32.5
Smoking prevalence in male population aged 15+ (% of male population)	38.6	30.9	28.2	27.6	27.9	27.6	27.5
Smoking prevalence in female population aged 15+ (% of female population)	22.1	16.5	19.5	18.0	16.8	17.2	16.6

Source: WHO/OECD/Euromonitor International

Nutrition and Obesity

Germany: Nutrition and obesity 1998-2004

Table: 4.456

As stated

	1998	1999	2000	2001	2002	2003	2004
Availability of fruit and vegetables (kg/capita/year)	204.7	207.5	223.1	212.3	221.1	225.6	228.7
Average supply of calories per day (calories per capita)	3,398.1	3,391.2	3,433.0	3,492.7	3,495.6	3,515.5	3,538.7
Average supply of fat per day (grams per capita)	147.1	144.0	145.5	141.8	146.4	149.1	151.2
Average supply of protein per day (grams per capita)	96.0	95.8	96.0	99.6	100.1	101.1	100.4
Obese population (BMI 30kg/sq m or more) (% of population aged 15+)	14.8	15.6	16.8	17.9	19.0	20.1	20.5

Source: WHO/OECD/Euromonitor International

Over-the-Counter Healthcare

Germany: Trends in OTC healthcare retail sales 1998-2004

Table: 4.457

As stated

	1998	1999	2000	2001	2002	2003	2004
OTC Healthcare (EUR million)	4,111.8	4,290.9	4,500.7	4,528.5	4,510.1	4,562.5	4,715.2
OTC Healthcare: real growth in national currency: 1998 = 100	100.0	103.8	107.3	105.8	104.0	104.1	105.7
OTC Healthcare: year on year (% real growth)	0.1	3.8	3.4	-1.3	-1.8	0.1	1.5

Source: Euromonitor International from industry sources/national statistics

Germany: OTC healthcare retail sales by sector 1998-2004

Table: 4.458

% of OTC retail value sales

	1998	1999	2000	2001	2002	2003	2004
Analgesics	16.9	16.9	16.9	17.0	16.9	16.6	16.1
Cough, cold and allergy (hay fever) remedies	23.3	23.4	23.3	23.1	22.6	23.0	22.8
Digestive remedies	11.2	11.2	11.3	11.3	11.2	11.0	10.7
Medicated skin care	15.9	15.9	16.1	16.1	16.6	16.6	16.9
Vitamins and dietary supplements	24.8	24.4	24.1	23.9	24.0	23.9	24.2

Source: *Euromonitor International from industry sources/national statistics*
Notes: *Only selected sectors are shown, so values are not expected to sum to 100*

Health and Wellness

Germany: Retail sales of packaged foods by health and wellness category 2002-2004

Table: 4.459

EUR million

	2002	2003	2004
Packaged food: Total	57,835.9	58,405.1	58,770.0
Better for you	4,906.1	5,089.2	5,183.8
For food intolerance	513.7	541.2	557.1
Fortified/functional	1,357.4	1,456.0	1,529.2
Organic	1,245.7	1,279.8	1,309.4

Source: *Euromonitor International from industry sources/national statistics*

Germany: Per capita sales of packaged foods by health and wellness category 2002-2004

Table: 4.460

EUR per capita

	2002	2003	2004
Better for you	59.9	62.2	63.3
For food intolerance	6.3	6.6	6.8
Fortified/functional	16.6	17.8	18.7
Organic	15.2	15.6	16.0

Source: *Euromonitor International from industry sources/national statistics*

Germany: Retail sales of packaged food by health and wellness category: % share of total packaged food market 2002-2004

Table: 4.461

% value

	2002	2003	2004
Better for you	8.5	8.7	8.8
For food intolerance	0.9	0.9	0.9
Fortified/functional	2.3	2.5	2.6
Organic	2.2	2.2	2.2

Source: *Euromonitor International from industry sources/national statistics*

Germany: Retail sales of packaged food by health and wellness category: real growth index 2002-2004

Table: 4.462

2002 =100

	2002	2003	2004
Better for you	100.00	102.70	103.99
For food intolerance	100.00	104.31	106.72
Fortified/functional	100.00	106.21	110.88
Organic	100.00	101.73	103.45

Source: *Euromonitor International from industry sources/national statistics*

Germany: Retail sales of better-for-you packaged foods by sector 2002-2004

Table: 4.463

% of total packaged food / as stated

	2002	2003	2004	% real change in value 2002-2004
Combination	0.01	0.01	0.01	49.11
Reduced carb	0.00	0.00	0.00	14.44
Reduced fat	7.35	7.57	7.66	4.15

Source: Euromonitor International from industry sources/national statistics

Germany: Retail sales of packaged foods for food intolerances by sector 2002-2004

Table: 4.464

% of total packaged food / as stated

	2002	2003	2004	% real change in value 2002-2004
Diabetic	0.11	0.10	0.11	-0.71
Gluten-free	0.04	0.04	0.04	9.23
Lactose-free	0.74	0.78	0.80	7.65

Source: Euromonitor International from industry sources/national statistics

Germany: Retail sales of naturally healthy packaged foods by sector 2002-2004

Table: 4.465

% of total packaged food / as stated

	2002	2003	2004	% real change in value 2002-2004
High fibre	5.29	5.22	5.20	-1.77
Other naturally healthy food	0.97	1.15	1.23	26.01
Soy-based dairy alternatives	0.19	0.23	0.29	53.73

Source: Euromonitor International from industry sources/national statistics

■ **Greece**

Socio-economic Parameters

Greece: Socio-economic parameters 1998-2004

Table: 4.466

As stated

	1998	1999	2000	2001	2002	2003	2004
Population: national estimates at January 1st ('000)	10,511.0	10,521.7	10,554.4	10,584.7	10,609.3	10,629.3	10,645.7
% aged 0-14 yrs	15.8	15.4	15.2	14.9	14.8	14.6	14.5
% aged 15-64 yrs	67.7	67.7	67.6	67.4	67.4	67.2	67.1
% aged 65 + yrs	16.5	16.9	17.3	17.6	17.9	18.1	18.4
% Male	49.3	49.3	49.3	49.3	49.3	49.3	49.3
% Female	50.7	50.7	50.7	50.7	50.7	50.7	50.7
% Urban	59.7	59.9	60.1	60.3	60.5	60.8	61.1
Occupants per household at January 1st (Number)	3.0	2.9	2.9	2.9	2.9	2.8	2.8
Households ('000)	3,540.6	3,579.2	3,627.6	3,664.4	3,706.5	3,746.4	3,786.0
Annual rates of inflation (% growth)	4.8	2.6	3.2	3.4	3.6	3.5	2.9
GDP (EUR million)	105,773.1	112,837.0	121,516.4	131,300.1	141,499.9	152,999.9	164,400.0
GDP (US$ million)	118,571.7	120,214.9	111,955.4	117,493.4	133,170.1	172,679.4	204,131.0
GDP (US$ per capita)	11,280.8	11,425.5	10,607.5	11,100.4	12,552.2	16,245.6	19,175.0

Source: Euromonitor International from International Monetary Fund (IMF), International Financial Statistics and World Economic Outlook/UN/national statistics

Life Expectancy

Greece: Life expectancy 1998-2004

Table: 4.467

As stated

	1998	1999	2000	2001	2002	2003	2004	% change 1998-2004
Life expectancy at birth: total population (years)	77.9	78.0	78.0	78.1	78.4	78.7	78.8	1.12
Life expectancy at birth: total population: year on year growth	0.1	0.1	0.0	0.1	0.4	0.3	0.1	
Healthy life expectancy at birth (years)	73.0			70.4	70.4			
Healthy life expectancy at birth: year on year growth					0.0			

Source: Euromonitor International from World Bank

Health Expenditure

Greece: Public health expenditure 1998-2004

Table: 4.468

As stated

	1998	1999	2000	2001	2002	2003	2004
Public expenditure on pharmaceuticals and other medical non-durables (EUR million)	961.0	1,098.0	1,278.0	1,362.0	1,474.0	1,611.0	1,806.0
Share of total health expenditure in GDP (% of total GDP)	9.4	9.6	9.4	9.4	9.1	9.5	9.5
Health expenditure (US$ per capita)	1,083.0	1,146.0	1,043.0	1,044.0	1,198.0	1,215.0	1,254.0

Source: Euromonitor International from OECD/national statistics

Greece: Private health expenditure 1998-2004

Table: 4.469

As stated

	1998	1999	2000	2001	2002	2003	2004
Consumer expenditure on health goods and medical services (EUR million)	4,421.0	4,643.0	4,516.0	4,897.0	5,319.0	5,635.0	6,082.7
Consumer expenditure on health goods and medical services: real growth in national currency: 1990 = 100	150.7	154.2	145.4	152.6	159.9	163.6	171.6
Consumer expenditure on health goods and medical services as a percentage of total consumer expenditure	5.5	5.5	5.0	5.1	5.2	5.2	5.3

Source: National statistical offices/OECD/Eurostat/Euromonitor International

Greece: Consumer expenditure on health goods and medical services by sector 1998-2004

Table: 4.470

% of total consumer expenditure on health goods and medical services

	1998	1999	2000	2001	2002	2003	2004
Pharmaceuticals, medical appliances/ equipment	10.8	10.3	10.8	10.3	10.2	10.2	10.2
Outpatient services	89.2	89.7	89.2	89.7	89.8	89.8	89.8
Total	100.0	100.0	100.0	100.0	100.0	100.0	100.0

Source: National statistical offices/OECD/Eurostat/Euromonitor International

Healthcare Infrastructure and Services

Greece: Healthcare infrastructure and services by sector 1998-2004

Table: 4.471

As stated

	1998	1999	2000	2001	2002	2003	2004
Active pharmacists (number)	8,767	8,928	8,977	9,057	9,181	9,297	9,424
Consultations with GPs (general practitioners) (per capita)	3	3	3	2	2	2	2
Dentists (number)	11,947	12,152	12,362	12,394	12,585	12,769	12,958
Doctors (number)	44,753	46,124	47,251	47,944	49,060	50,193	51,217
Hospital admissions (number)	1,620,768	1,688,596	1,756,424	1,824,252	1,892,080	1,946,189	2,015,570
Hospitals and clinics (number)	492	483	475	467	460	453	446
In-patient beds ('000)	42	42	42	42	42	43	43
Nurses (number)	40,932	41,151	42,129	42,919	43,663	44,666	45,595

Source: Euromonitor International from national statistics

Greece: Healthcare infrastructure and services by sector: growth 1998-2004

Table: 4.472

Year on year growth: % change in stated unit

	1998	1999	2000	2001	2002	2003	2004
Active pharmacists (number)	0.0	1.8	0.5	0.9	1.4	1.3	1.4
Consultations with GPs (general practitioners) (per capita)	-3.8	0.0	0.0	-4.0	0.0	-1.2	-1.3
Dentists (number)	2.7	1.7	1.7	0.3	1.5	1.5	1.5
Doctors (number)	4.0	3.1	2.4	1.5	2.3	2.3	2.0
Hospital admissions (number)	4.4	4.2	4.0	3.9	3.7	2.9	3.6
Hospitals and clinics (number)	-1.4	-1.8	-1.7	-1.7	-1.5	-1.5	-1.5
In-patient beds (number)	-0.3	-0.5	0.0	-0.1	0.8	1.2	0.7
Nurses (number)	1.8	0.5	2.4	1.9	1.7	2.3	2.1

Source: Euromonitor International from national statistics

Immunisation

Greece: Vaccination rates by disease type 1998-2004

Table: 4.473

%

	1998	1999	2000	2001	2002	2003	2004
Vaccination rate against MMR (measles, mumps, rubella) (%)		88.0					
Vaccination rate against polio (%)		87.0					

Source: WHO

Infectious Diseases

Greece: Incidence of disease by type 1998-2004

Table: 4.474

Number

	1998	1999	2000	2001	2002	2003	2004
Incidence of AIDS	146	137	143	44	91	35	29
Incidence of diphtheria	0	0	0	0	0		
Incidence of measles	66	69	56	12	5		
Incidence of polio	0	0	0	0	0		

Source: WHO

Greece: Incidence of disease by type: growth 1998-2004

Table: 4.475

Year on year growth: %

	1998	1999	2000	2001	2002	2003	2004
Incidence of AIDS	-38.9	-6.2	4.4	-69.2	106.8	-61.5	-17.1
Incidence of measles	-51.5	4.5	-18.8	-78.6	-58.3		

Source: WHO

Causes of Death

Greece: Deaths by disease 1998-2004

Table: 4.476

Number per 100,000 inhabitants

	1998	1999	2000	2001	2002	2003	2004
Death by diseases of the circulatory system	314.2	303.4	300.0	298.2	291.6	284.4	279.7
Death by malignant neoplasms (cancers)	150.4	154.0	151.8	153.4	154.0	152.5	153.0
Deaths from heart disease	116.7	120.9	117.0	115.2	113.4	111.6	109.1
Deaths from lung cancer	51.5	51.9	52.6	53.2	53.8	54.4	54.6
Death by diseases of the respiratory system	41.1	42.7	42.2	44.1	41.9	40.0	39.6
Death by diseases of the digestive system	15.1	15.3	15.1	14.9	14.5	15.0	14.9
Deaths from chronic liver disease and cirrhosis	5.7	6.1	6.3	6.5	6.7	6.9	7.1
Deaths from ulcers of the stomach and duodenum	2.7	2.6	2.8	2.9	3.0	3.1	3.2

Source: WHO/Euromonitor International
Notes: Data is ranked in descending order by year 2004

Greece: Deaths by disease: growth 1998-2004

Table: 4.477

% year on year growth

	1998	1999	2000	2001	2002	2003	2004
Deaths from ulcers of the stomach and duodenum	14.7	-4.7	8.1	3.6	3.4	3.3	3.9
Deaths from chronic liver disease and cirrhosis	0.8	6.7	2.8	3.2	3.1	3.0	2.6
Deaths from lung cancer	1.7	0.9	1.3	1.1	1.1	1.1	0.4
Death by malignant neoplasms (cancers)	-2.6	2.4	-1.4	1.1	0.4	-1.0	0.4
Death by diseases of the digestive system	-5.0	1.3	-1.3	-1.3	-2.7	3.4	-0.6
Death by diseases of the respiratory system	19.8	3.9	-1.2	4.5	-5.0	-4.5	-1.1
Death by diseases of the circulatory system	0.6	-3.4	-1.1	-0.6	-2.2	-2.5	-1.7
Deaths from heart disease	-6.4	3.6	-3.2	-1.5	-1.6	-1.6	-2.3

Source: WHO/Euromonitor International
Notes: Data is ranked in descending order by year 2004

Greece: Other selected causes of death: 1998-2004

Table: 4.478

Number per 100,000 inhabitants

	1998	1999	2000	2001	2002	2003	2004
Death by injury and poisoning	38.6	38.2	38.2	38.0	37.8	38.1	38.4
Death by motor traffic accidents	20.3	19.7	18.7	18.8	18.0	17.2	16.7
Death by suicide and self-inflicted injury	3.2	3.1	3.3	3.2	3.3	3.2	3.2

Source: Euromonitor International from national statistics
Notes: Data is ranked in descending order by year 2004

Greece: Other selected causes of death: growth 1998-2004

% year on year growth

	1998	1999	2000	2001	2002	2003	2004
Death by injury and poisoning	1.3	-1.0	0.0	-0.5	-0.5	0.8	0.7
Death by suicide and self-inflicted injury	3.2	-3.1	6.5	-3.0	3.1	-3.0	-1.2
Death by motor traffic accidents	-1.5	-3.0	-5.1	0.5	-4.3	-4.4	-3.1

Source: Euromonitor International from national statistics
Notes: Data is ranked in descending order by year 2004

Smoking

Greece: Smoking prevalence in population aged 15+ 1998-2004

Table: 4.480

% of population aged 15+

	1998	1999	2000	2001	2002	2003	2004
Smoking prevalence in population aged 15+ (% of population aged 15+)	38.2	37.9	37.6	37.4	37.1	36.8	36.6
Smoking prevalence in male population aged 15+ (% of male population)	47.9	47.5	46.8	45.5	45.0	44.7	44.7
Smoking prevalence in female population aged 15+ (% of female population)	27.6	28.4	29.0	29.0	28.5	28.3	28.1

Source: WHO/OECD/Euromonitor International

Nutrition and Obesity

Greece: Nutrition and obesity 1998-2004

Table: 4.481

As stated

	1998	1999	2000	2001	2002	2003	2004
Availability of fruit and vegetables (kg/capita/year)	402.5	452.5	454.3	417.3	442.8	449.2	453.3
Average supply of calories per day (calories per capita)	3,626.4	3,666.6	3,647.6	3,694.5	3,721.1	3,743.6	3,735.6
Average supply of fat per day (grams per capita)	151.5	151.3	147.0	148.5	152.7	155.1	157.7
Average supply of protein per day (grams per capita)	115.9	118.1	117.0	115.9	115.7	115.2	114.7
Microbiological food-borne diseases (per 100000 population)	1.0	3.0	3.0	4.0	5.0	5.0	6.0
Obese population (BMI 30kg/sq m or more) (% of population aged 15+)	8.0	8.5	9.2	10.1	10.3	11.0	11.4

Source: WHO/OECD/Euromonitor International

Over-the-Counter Healthcare

Greece: Trends in OTC healthcare retail sales 1998-2004

Table: 4.482

As stated

	1998	1999	2000	2001	2002	2003	2004
OTC Healthcare (EUR million)	110.3	116.0	123.1	131.7	142.9	152.6	159.7
OTC Healthcare: real growth in national currency: 1998 = 100	100.0	102.4	105.4	109.1	114.2	117.8	119.3
OTC Healthcare: year on year (% real growth)	-2.6	2.4	2.9	3.5	4.7	3.1	1.3

Source: Euromonitor International from industry sources/national statistics

Greece: OTC healthcare retail sales by sector 1998-2004

Table: 4.483

% of OTC retail value sales

	1998	1999	2000	2001	2002	2003	2004
Analgesics	13.5	13.1	12.8	13.3	14.2	14.6	15.4
Cough, cold and allergy (hay fever) remedies	24.9	24.9	24.4	23.6	23.2	23.3	23.2
Digestive remedies	7.0	7.0	7.0	6.9	6.7	6.5	6.3
Medicated skin care	19.7	19.4	19.4	19.2	18.6	18.6	18.5
Vitamins and dietary supplements	23.8	24.4	25.1	25.7	26.3	26.0	25.5

Source: *Euromonitor International from industry sources/national statistics*
Notes: *Only selected sectors are shown, so values are not expected to sum to 100*

Health and Wellness

Greece: Retail sales of packaged foods by health and wellness category 2002-2004

Table: 4.484

EUR million

	2002	2003	2004
Packaged food: Total	7,679.5	8,160.5	8,620.4
Better for you	420.2	477.9	533.1
For food intolerance	0.2	0.2	0.3
Fortified/functional	172.7	203.7	230.2
Organic	7.5	9.1	12.6

Source: *Euromonitor International from industry sources/national statistics*

Germany: Per capita sales of packaged foods by health and wellness category 2002-2004

Table: 4.485

EUR per capita

	2002	2003	2004
Better for you	59.9	62.2	63.3
For food intolerance	6.3	6.6	6.8
Fortified/functional	16.6	17.8	18.7
Organic	15.2	15.6	16.0

Source: *Euromonitor International from industry sources/national statistics*

Greece: Retail sales of packaged food by health and wellness category: % share of total packaged food market 2002-2004

Table: 4.486

% value

	2002	2003	2004
Better for you	5.5	5.9	6.2
For food intolerance	0.0	0.0	0.0
Fortified/functional	2.2	2.5	2.7
Organic	0.1	0.1	0.1

Source: *Euromonitor International from industry sources/national statistics*

Greece: Retail sales of packaged food by health and wellness category: real growth index 2002-2004

Table: 4.487

2002 =100

	2002	2003	2004
Better for you	100.00	109.55	118.64
For food intolerance	100.00	123.86	146.98
Fortified/functional	100.00	113.63	124.69
Organic	100.00	117.15	157.72

Source: *Euromonitor International from industry sources/national statistics*

Greece: Retail sales of better-for-you packaged foods by sector 2002-2004

Table: 4.488

% of total packaged food / as stated

	2002	2003	2004	% real change in value 2002-2004
Combination	0.07	0.09	0.15	144.50
Reduced fat	4.80	5.14	5.37	17.66

Source: *Euromonitor International from industry sources/national statistics*

Greece: Retail sales of packaged foods for food intolerances by sector 2002-2004

Table: 4.489

% of total packaged food / as stated

	2002	2003	2004	% real change in value 2002-2004
Diabetic	0.00	0.00	0.00	46.98

Source: *Euromonitor International from industry sources/national statistics*

Greece: Retail sales of naturally healthy packaged foods by sector 2002-2004

Table: 4.490

% of total packaged food / as stated

	2002	2003	2004	% real change in value 2002-2004
High fibre	1.02	1.08	1.12	15.28
Other naturally healthy food	1.91	2.04	2.16	18.85
Soy-based dairy alternatives	0.13	0.15	0.17	36.38

Source: *Euromonitor International from industry sources/national statistics*

■ **Hong Kong, China**

Socio-economic Parameters

Hong Kong, China: Socio-economic parameters 1998-2004

Table: 4.491

As stated

	1998	1999	2000	2001	2002	2003	2004
Population: national estimates at January 1st ('000)	6,543.7	6,606.5	6,665.0	6,724.9	6,787.0	6,878.3	6,957.9
% aged 0-14 yrs	17.7	17.5	16.9	16.4	16.1	15.8	15.5
% aged 15-64 yrs	71.7	71.8	72.1	72.4	72.4	72.6	72.8
% aged 65 + yrs	10.6	10.7	10.9	11.2	11.4	11.6	11.7
% Male	49.7	49.4	49.2	48.9	48.6	48.3	48.0
% Female	50.3	50.6	50.8	51.1	51.4	51.7	52.0
% Urban	100.0	100.0	100.0	100.0	100.0	100.0	100.0
Occupants per household at January 1st (Number)	3.4	3.4	3.3	3.3	3.3	3.2	3.2
Households ('000)	1,931.5	1,971.7	2,011.2	2,053.4	2,085.9	2,116.9	2,154.2
Annual rates of inflation (% growth)	2.9	-4.0	-3.7	-1.6	-3.0	-2.6	-0.4
GDP (HK$ million)	1,279,850.0	1,246,130.0	1,288,340.0	1,269,900.0	1,247,960.0	1,220,040.0	1,282,000.0
GDP (US$ million)	165,241.5	160,635.5	165,359.0	162,833.8	160,017.0	156,681.5	164,612.2
GDP (US$ per capita)	25,252.0	24,314.8	24,810.1	24,213.6	23,577.0	22,779.1	23,658.3

Source: *Euromonitor International from International Monetary Fund (IMF), International Financial Statistics and World Economic Outlook/UN/national statistics*

Life Expectancy

Hong Kong, China: Life expectancy 1998-2004

Table: 4.492

As stated

	1998	1999	2000	2001	2002	2003	2004	% change 1998-2004
Life expectancy at birth: total population (years)	79.4	79.5	79.6	79.8	80.0	80.1	80.3	1.14
Life expectancy at birth: total population: year on year growth	0.2	0.1	0.2	0.2	0.2	0.2	0.2	

Source: Euromonitor International from World Bank

Health Expenditure

Hong Kong, China: Public health expenditure 1998-2004

Table: 4.493

As stated

	1998	1999	2000	2001	2002	2003	2004
Share of total health expenditure in GDP (% of total GDP)	6.2	6.6	7.0	7.4	7.1	6.8	6.6
Health expenditure (US$ per capita)	1,577.6	1,726.0	1,874.4	2,022.8	2,173.0	2,327.0	2,480.0

Source: Euromonitor International from OECD/national statistics

Hong Kong, China: Private health expenditure 1998-2004

Table: 4.494

As stated

	1998	1999	2000	2001	2002	2003	2004
Consumer expenditure on health goods and medical services (HK$ million)	30,962.0	30,846.0	31,029.0	30,880.0	30,430.0	30,631.3	31,837.8
Consumer expenditure on health goods and medical services: real growth in national currency: 1990 = 100	128.4	133.2	139.3	140.9	143.2	147.9	154.4
Consumer expenditure on health goods and medical services as a percentage of total consumer expenditure	4.1	4.3	4.3	4.2	4.3	4.5	4.6

Source: National statistical offices/OECD/Eurostat/Euromonitor International

Hong Kong, China: Consumer expenditure on health goods and medical services by sector 1998-2004

Table: 4.495

% of total consumer expenditure on health goods and medical services

	1998	1999	2000	2001	2002	2003	2004
Pharmaceuticals, medical appliances/ equipment	17.7	17.7	17.9	18.1	18.3	18.3	18.6
Outpatient services	52.4	52.2	51.6	51.2	51.0	51.0	50.9
Hospital services	29.9	30.0	30.5	30.7	30.8	30.7	30.5
Total	100.0	100.0	100.0	100.0	100.0	100.0	100.0

Source: National statistical offices/OECD/Eurostat/Euromonitor International

Healthcare Infrastructure and Services

Hong Kong, China: Healthcare infrastructure and services by sector 1998-2004

Table: 4.496

As stated

	1998	1999	2000	2001	2002	2003	2004
Active pharmacists (number)	1,212	1,273	1,315	1,352	1,372	1,378	1,400
Dentists (number)	1,724	1,779	1,826	2,028	2,060	2,076	2,088
Doctors (number)	9,527	9,818	10,130	10,139	10,052	9,934	9,815
Hospitals and clinics (number)	102	105	102	104	107	110	113
In-patient beds ('000)	33	34	33	35	36	37	37
Midwives (number)	12,006	12,072	12,172	12,272	12,395	12,537	12,661
Nurses (number)	39,157	38,960	40,388	41,906	42,259	42,541	42,620

Source: Euromonitor International from national statistics

Hong Kong, China: Healthcare infrastructure and services by sector: growth 1998-2004

Table: 4.497

Year on year growth: % change in stated unit

	1998	1999	2000	2001	2002	2003	2004
Active pharmacists (number)	6.0	5.0	3.3	2.8	1.5	0.4	1.6
Dentists (number)	2.4	3.2	2.6	11.1	1.6	0.8	0.6
Doctors (number)	2.6	3.1	3.2	0.1	-0.9	-1.2	-1.2
Hospitals and clinics (number)	6.3	2.9	-2.9	2.0	2.9	2.8	2.7
In-patient beds (number)	6.6	4.4	-3.5	6.2	2.8	1.6	1.2
Midwives (number)	1.3	0.5	0.8	0.8	1.0	1.1	1.0
Nurses (number)	3.4	-0.5	3.7	3.8	0.8	0.7	0.2

Source: Euromonitor International from national statistics

Infectious Diseases

Hong Kong, China: Incidence of disease by type 1998-2004

Table: 4.498

Number

	1998	1999	2000	2001	2002	2003	2004
Incidence of AIDS	63	61	67	24	35	37	25

Source: WHO

Hong Kong, China: Incidence of disease by type: growth 1998-2004

Table: 4.499

Year on year growth: %

	1998	1999	2000	2001	2002	2003	2004
Incidence of AIDS	-1.6	-3.2	9.8	-64.2	45.8	5.7	-32.4

Source: WHO

Causes of Death

Hong Kong, China: Deaths by disease 1998-2004

Table: 4.500

Number per 100,000 inhabitants

	1998	1999	2000	2001	2002	2003	2004
Death by malignant neoplasms (cancers)	162.1	165.4	169.2	173.3	172.9	175.7	176.5
Death by diseases of the circulatory system	133.1	136.3	137.2	138.7	140.5	142.9	146.0
Death by diseases of the respiratory system	92.0	83.8	78.7	71.7	70.2	68.4	64.9
Deaths from heart disease	32.4	34.1	37.9	38.6	39.9	40.8	41.9
Deaths from lung cancer	22.9	22.1	20.7	21.8	21.6	22.3	22.9
Deaths from ulcers of the stomach and duodenum	20.3	19.1	20.6	21.1	20.9	21.1	21.5
Death by diseases of the digestive system	20.3	19.1	20.6	21.1	20.9	20.7	20.8
Deaths from chronic liver disease and cirrhosis	7.8	7.7	7.7	8.0	8.1	8.3	8.5

Source: WHO/Euromonitor International
Notes: Data is ranked in descending order by year 2004

Hong Kong, China: Deaths by disease: growth 1998-2004

Table: 4.501

% year on year growth

	1998	1999	2000	2001	2002	2003	2004
Deaths from lung cancer	-4.2	-3.5	-6.3	5.3	-0.9	3.2	2.8
Deaths from heart disease	-4.4	5.2	11.1	1.8	3.4	2.3	2.8
Deaths from chronic liver disease and cirrhosis	4.0	-1.3	0.0	3.9	1.2	2.5	2.3
Death by diseases of the circulatory system	6.1	2.4	0.7	1.1	1.3	1.7	2.2
Deaths from ulcers of the stomach and duodenum	-4.2	-5.9	7.9	2.4	-0.9	1.0	1.7
Death by diseases of the digestive system	-4.2	-5.9	7.9	2.4	-0.9	-1.0	0.5
Death by malignant neoplasms (cancers)	1.9	2.0	2.3	2.4	-0.2	1.6	0.5
Death by diseases of the respiratory system	-6.7	-8.9	-6.1	-8.9	-2.1	-2.6	-5.1

Source: WHO/Euromonitor International
Notes: Data is ranked in descending order by year 2004

Hong Kong, China: Other selected causes of death: 1998-2004

Table: 4.502

Number per 100,000 inhabitants

	1998	1999	2000	2001	2002	2003	2004
Death by motor traffic accidents	222.0	217.0	171.0	152.3	144.4	135.2	125.5
Death by injury and poisoning	28.7	30.5	30.4	31.3	31.3	31.5	31.9

Source: Euromonitor International from national statistics
Notes: Data is ranked in descending order by year 2004

Hong Kong, China: Other selected causes of death: growth 1998-2004

Table: 4.503

% year on year growth

	1998	1999	2000	2001	2002	2003	2004
Death by injury and poisoning	-1.4	6.3	-0.3	3.0	0.0	0.6	1.4
Death by motor traffic accidents		-2.3	-21.2	-10.9	-5.2	-6.4	-7.2

Source: Euromonitor International from national statistics
Notes: Data is ranked in descending order by year 2004

Smoking

Hong Kong, China: Smoking prevalence in population aged 15+ 1998-2004

Table: 4.504

% of population aged 15+

	1998	1999	2000	2001	2002	2003	2004
Smoking prevalence in population aged 15+ (% of population aged 15+)	19.1	18.6	17.9	18.1	17.6	17.8	18.2
Smoking prevalence in male population aged 15+ (% of male population)	27.1	26.6	25.6	25.9	25.4	25.4	25.4
Smoking prevalence in female population aged 15+ (% of female population)	11.4	10.9	10.7	10.7	10.5	10.9	11.7

Source: WHO/OECD/Euromonitor International

Nutrition and Obesity

Hong Kong, China: Nutrition and obesity 1998-2004

Table: 4.505

As stated

	1998	1999	2000	2001	2002	2003	2004
Average supply of calories per day (calories per capita)	3,331.6	3,367.8	3,388.3	3,441.1	3,476.3	3,511.9	3,551.6
Average supply of fat per day (grams per capita)	138.3	136.9	138.1	142.4	143.4	145.1	147.2
Average supply of protein per day (grams per capita)	105.7	108.2	112.1	110.7	114.1	116.8	119.0
Obese population (BMI 30kg/sq m or more) (% of population aged 15+)	5.2	5.2	5.2	5.2	5.2	5.2	5.2

Source: WHO/OECD/Euromonitor International

Over-the-Counter Healthcare

Hong Kong, China: Trends in OTC healthcare retail sales 1998-2004

Table: 4.506

As stated

	1998	1999	2000	2001	2002	2003	2004
OTC Healthcare (HK$ million)	1,675.8	1,725.7	1,807.2	1,853.0	1,903.1	1,977.4	2,007.1
OTC Healthcare: real growth in national currency: 1998 = 100	100.0	107.2	116.7	121.6	128.8	137.3	139.4
OTC Healthcare: year on year (% real growth)	-0.3	7.2	8.8	4.2	5.9	6.6	1.5
OTC Healthcare (HK$ per capita)	256.1	261.2	271.1	275.5	280.4	287.5	288.5

Source: Euromonitor International from industry sources/national statistics

Hong Kong, China: OTC healthcare retail sales by sector 1998-2004

Table: 4.507

% of OTC retail value sales

	1998	1999	2000	2001	2002	2003	2004
Analgesics	11.5	11.7	11.7	12.0	12.1	12.1	12.4
Cough, cold and allergy (hay fever) remedies	22.2	22.1	21.8	21.9	21.8	21.6	21.9
Digestive remedies	8.9	8.7	9.7	9.7	9.6	9.5	9.6
Medicated skin care	4.4	4.3	4.3	4.3	4.3	4.3	4.3
Vitamins and dietary supplements	50.0	50.1	49.5	49.2	49.1	49.5	48.7

Source: Euromonitor International from industry sources/national statistics
Notes: Only selected sectors are shown, so values are not expected to sum to 100

Health and Wellness

Hong Kong, China: Retail sales of packaged foods by health and wellness category 2002-2004

Table: 4.508

HK$ million

	2002	2003	2004
Packaged food: Total	18,230.9	18,748.5	19,303.0
Better for you	511.0	542.7	577.1
Fortified/functional	935.9	978.7	1,021.6
Organic	29.4	34.7	40.2

Source: Euromonitor International from industry sources/national statistics

Hong Kong, China: Per capita sales of packaged foods by health and wellness category 2002-2004

Table: 4.509

HK$ per capita

	2002	2003	2004
Better for you	70.8	73.2	75.8
Fortified/functional	129.7	131.9	134.1
Organic	4.1	4.7	5.3

Source: Euromonitor International from industry sources/national statistics

Hong Kong, China: Retail sales of packaged food by health and wellness category: % share of total packaged food market 2002-2004

Table: 4.510

% value

	2002	2003	2004
Better for you	2.8	2.9	3.0
Fortified/functional	5.1	5.2	5.3
Organic	0.2	0.2	0.2

Source: Euromonitor International from industry sources/national statistics

Hong Kong, China: Retail sales of packaged food by health and wellness category: real growth index 2002-2004

Table: 4.511

2002 = 100

	2002	2003	2004
Better for you	100.00	109.05	118.20
Fortified/functional	100.00	107.36	114.24
Organic	100.00	121.45	143.38

Source: Euromonitor International from industry sources/national statistics

Hong Kong, China: Retail sales of better-for-you packaged foods by sector 2002-2004

Table: 4.512

% of total packaged food / as stated

	2002	2003	2004	% real change in value 2002-2004
Reduced fat	1.55	1.61	1.66	18.48
Reduced salt	0.06	0.07	0.08	52.62

Source: Euromonitor International from industry sources/national statistics

Hong Kong, China: Retail sales of naturally healthy packaged foods by sector 2002-2004

Table: 4.513

% of total packaged food / as stated

	2002	2003	2004	% real change in value 2002-2004
High fibre	1.40	1.56	1.68	33.28
Other naturally healthy food	0.75	0.74	0.74	9.77
Soy-based dairy alternatives	2.08	2.13	2.17	15.61

Source: Euromonitor International from industry sources/national statistics

■ **Hungary**

Socio-economic Parameters

Hungary: Socio-economic parameters 1998-2004

Table: 4.514

As stated

	1998	1999	2000	2001	2002	2003	2004
Population: national estimates at January 1st ('000)	10,135.4	10,091.8	10,221.6	10,200.3	10,174.9	10,139.2	10,097.4
% aged 0-14 yrs	17.5	17.3	16.9	16.6	16.3	16.1	15.8
% aged 15-64 yrs	68.1	68.2	68.1	68.3	68.4	68.6	68.9
% aged 65+ yrs	14.4	14.5	15.0	15.1	15.3	15.3	15.3
% Male	47.8	47.7	47.6	47.6	47.5	47.5	47.5
% Female	52.2	52.3	52.4	52.4	52.5	52.5	52.5
% Urban	63.6	63.8	64.0	64.2	64.4	65.4	65.9
Occupants per household at January 1st (Number)	2.7	2.7	2.7	2.7	2.7	2.7	2.7
Households ('000)	3,735.2	3,729.0	3,783.3	3,720.7	3,714.4	3,711.0	3,697.2
Annual rates of inflation (% growth)	14.2	10.0	9.8	9.2	5.3	4.6	6.8
GDP (HuF million)	10,087,400.0	11,393,500.0	13,172,300.0	14,849,800.0	16,740,400.0	18,568,300.0	20,216,200.0
GDP (US$ million)	47,049.0	48,044.2	46,680.7	51,833.6	64,913.7	82,780.7	99,712.0
GDP (US$ per capita)	4,642.1	4,760.7	4,566.8	5,081.6	6,379.8	8,164.4	9,875.0

Source: Euromonitor International from International Monetary Fund (IMF), International Financial Statistics and World Economic Outlook/UN/national statistics

Life Expectancy

Hungary: Life expectancy 1998-2004

Table: 4.515

As stated

	1998	1999	2000	2001	2002	2003	2004	% change 1998-2004
Life expectancy at birth: total population (years)	71.0	71.3	71.5	71.7	72.6	73.0	73.6	3.63
Life expectancy at birth: total population: year on year growth	0.4	0.4	0.3	0.3	1.3	0.6	0.8	
Healthy life expectancy at birth (years)	64.0			61.6	61.8			
Healthy life expectancy at birth: year on year growth					0.2			

Source: Euromonitor International from World Bank

Sanitation

Hungary: Improved sanitary facilities and water source 2000

Table: 4.516

As stated

	2000
Population with access to improved sanitary facilities (% of population)	99.0
Population with access to improved water source (% of population)	99.0
Population with improved access to sanitation facilities, rural (% of rural population with access)	98.0
Population with improved access to sanitation facilities, urban (% of urban population with access)	100.0

Source: National statistics/World Bank

Health Expenditure

Hungary: Public health expenditure 1998-2004

Table: 4.517

As stated

	1998	1999	2000	2001	2002	2003	2004
Public expenditure on pharmaceuticals and other medical non-durables (HuF million)	145,474.0	150,561.0	165,253.0	191,015.0	224,505.0	260,320.0	322,872.2
Private insurance expenditure (% of total expenditure on health)		0.1	0.2	0.3	0.4	0.5	0.6
Share of total health expenditure in GDP (% of total GDP)	6.9	6.8	6.7	6.8	7.0	6.9	6.6
Health expenditure (US$ per capita)	335.0	345.0	326.0	375.0	496.0	521.0	554.0

Source: Euromonitor International from OECD/national statistics

Hungary: Private health expenditure 1998-2004

Table: 4.518

As stated

	1998	1999	2000	2001	2002	2003	2004
Consumer expenditure on health goods and medical services (HUF million)	164,550.0	208,256.0	246,790.0	302,877.0	342,613.0	388,004.3	428,385.8
Consumer expenditure on health goods and medical services: real growth in national currency: 1990 = 100	150.4	173.0	186.7	209.8	225.5	244.0	252.3
Consumer expenditure on health goods and medical services as a percentage of total consumer expenditure	3.0	3.3	3.4	3.6	3.8	4.0	4.0

Source: National statistical offices/OECD/Eurostat/Euromonitor International

Hungary: Consumer expenditure on health goods and medical services by sector 1998-2004

Table: 4.519

% of total consumer expenditure on health goods and medical services

	1998	1999	2000	2001	2002	2003	2004
Pharmaceuticals, medical appliances/ equipment	79.8	78.7	78.7	78.7	79.7	79.6	79.6
Outpatient services	15.1	16.7	17.3	17.2	16.3	16.3	16.2
Hospital services	5.1	4.6	4.0	4.0	3.9	4.1	4.3
Total	100.0	100.0	100.0	100.0	100.0	100.0	100.0

Source: National statistical offices/OECD/Eurostat/Euromonitor International

Healthcare Infrastructure and Services

Hungary: Healthcare infrastructure and services by sector 1998-2004

Table: 4.520

As stated

	1998	1999	2000	2001	2002	2003	2004
Active pharmacists (number)	4,789	4,762	4,905	5,024	5,070	5,123	5,141
Consultations with GPs (general practitioners) (per capita)	11	11	11	11	12	12	12
Dentists (number)	4,505	4,618	4,365	3,640	4,843	5,020	5,096
Doctors (number)	31,638	31,768	30,621	29,448	32,452	33,760	34,558
Hospital admissions (number)	2,344,708	2,357,854	2,405,460	2,429,504	2,498,987	2,520,410	2,592,696
Hospitals and clinics (number)	167	172	178	184	191	195	199
In-patient beds ('000)	66	65	64	61	60	60	59
In-patient surgical procedures (number)	1,310,949	1,264,598	1,271,293	1,238,119	1,245,486	1,237,176	1,229,312
Midwives (number)	2,277	2,279	2,113	2,059	2,020	1,997	1,975
Nurses (number)	82,843	50,415	81,210	84,947	86,853	88,519	90,189
Out-patient contacts (per capita)	11	11	11	11	12	12	12

Source: Euromonitor International from national statistics

Hungary: Healthcare infrastructure and services by sector: growth 1998-2004

Table: 4.521

Year on year growth: % change in stated unit

	1998	1999	2000	2001	2002	2003	2004
Active pharmacists (number)	0.5	-0.6	3.0	2.4	0.9	1.0	0.4
Consultations with GPs (general practitioners) (per capita)	-7.8	2.8	1.8	1.8	5.3	1.7	2.6
Dentists (number)	5.1	2.5	-5.5	-16.6	33.0	3.7	1.5
Doctors (number)	1.4	0.4	-3.6	-3.8	10.2	4.0	2.4
Hospital admissions (number)	1.7	0.6	2.0	1.0	2.9	0.9	2.9
Hospitals and clinics (number)	-0.6	3.0	3.5	3.5	3.7	2.1	2.1
In-patient beds (number)	0.5	-1.3	-0.8	-4.8	-1.2	-1.0	-1.2
In-patient surgical procedures (number)	-10.6	-3.5	0.5	-2.6	0.6	-0.7	-0.6
Midwives (number)	-6.9	0.1	-7.3	-2.6	-1.9	-1.1	-1.1
Nurses (number)	1.3	-39.1	61.1	4.6	2.2	1.9	1.9
Out-patient contacts (per capita)	-7.4	2.8	1.7	1.8	5.7	0.6	0.8

Source: Euromonitor International from national statistics

Immunisation

Hungary: Vaccination rates by disease type 1998-2004

Table: 4.522

%

	1998	1999	2000	2001	2002	2003	2004
Vaccination rate against DTP (diphtheria, tetanus, pertussis) 1 & 2 (%)			99.3	99.0	99.0	99.0	99.0
Vaccination rate against MMR (measles, mumps, rubella) (%)	99.0	99.0	99.0	99.0	99.0	99.0	99.0
Vaccination rate against polio (%)	99.0	99.0	99.0	99.0	99.0	99.0	99.0

Source: WHO

Infectious Diseases

Hungary: Incidence of disease by type 1998-2004

Table: 4.523

Number

	1998	1999	2000	2001	2002	2003	2004
Incidence of AIDS	36	37	27	12	26	13	18
Incidence of diphtheria	0	0	0	0	0		
Incidence of measles	23	1	1	20	0		
Incidence of polio	0	0	0	0			

Source: WHO

Hungary: Incidence of disease by type: growth 1998-2004

Table: 4.524

Year on year growth: %

	1998	1999	2000	2001	2002	2003	2004
Incidence of AIDS	16.1	2.8	-27.0	-55.6	116.7	-50.0	38.5
Incidence of measles	-4.2	-95.7	0.0	1,900.0	-100.0		

Source: WHO

Causes of Death

Hungary: Deaths by disease 1998-2004

Table: 4.525

Number per 100,000 inhabitants

	1998	1999	2000	2001	2002	2003	2004
Death by diseases of the circulatory system	556.5	470.7	412.9	477.7	472.0	476.0	503.6
Deaths from heart disease	310.9	312.8	297.2	293.4	286.6	279.9	274.1
Death by malignant neoplasms (cancers)	264.1	245.3	239.8	246.9	245.6	249.9	255.9
Deaths from lung cancer	78.1	78.3	78.0	78.1	77.9	77.7	76.8
Death by diseases of the digestive system	83.9	78.1	75.5	72.3	71.8	70.4	68.2
Deaths from chronic liver disease and cirrhosis	71.2	71.0	67.5	66.3	64.5	62.7	61.0
Death by diseases of the respiratory system	41.5	39.9	33.2	31.6	26.6	23.8	21.2
Deaths from ulcers of the stomach and duodenum	9.4	9.0	9.4	9.3	9.3	9.3	9.3

Source: WHO/Euromonitor International
Notes: Data is ranked in descending order by year 2004

Hungary: Deaths by disease: growth 1998-2004

Table: 4.526

% year on year growth

	1998	1999	2000	2001	2002	2003	2004
Death by diseases of the circulatory system	1.1	-15.4	-12.3	15.7	-1.2	0.8	5.8
Death by malignant neoplasms (cancers)	-0.1	-7.1	-2.2	3.0	-0.5	1.8	2.4
Deaths from ulcers of the stomach and duodenum	1.5	-4.0	4.3	-1.0	0.0	0.0	0.5
Deaths from lung cancer	2.2	0.3	-0.3	0.1	-0.3	-0.3	-1.1
Deaths from heart disease	2.2	0.6	-5.0	-1.3	-2.3	-2.3	-2.1
Deaths from chronic liver disease and cirrhosis	7.9	-0.2	-4.9	-1.8	-2.7	-2.8	-2.7
Death by diseases of the digestive system	5.5	-6.9	-3.3	-4.2	-0.7	-1.9	-3.2
Death by diseases of the respiratory system	-9.6	-3.9	-16.8	-4.8	-15.8	-10.5	-10.8

Source: WHO/Euromonitor International
Notes: Data is ranked in descending order by year 2004

Hungary: Other selected causes of death: 1998-2004

Table: 4.527

Number per 100,000 inhabitants

	1998	1999	2000	2001	2002	2003	2004
Death by injury and poisoning	86.3	77.5	70.4	74.9	71.7	73.6	75.1
Death by suicide and self-inflicted injury	27.3	27.7	26.5	24.3	23.8	22.8	21.8
Death by motor traffic accidents	15.4	14.1	13.3	13.6	13.2	13.2	13.1

Source: Euromonitor International from national statistics
Notes: Data is ranked in descending order by year 2004

Hungary: Other selected causes of death: growth 1998-2004

Table: 4.528

% year on year growth

	1998	1999	2000	2001	2002	2003	2004
Death by injury and poisoning	0.5	-10.2	-9.2	6.4	-4.3	2.6	2.0
Death by motor traffic accidents	0.7	-8.4	-5.7	2.3	-2.9	0.0	-0.8
Death by suicide and self-inflicted injury	1.1	1.5	-4.3	-8.3	-2.1	-4.2	-4.4

Source: Euromonitor International from national statistics
Notes: Data is ranked in descending order by year 2004

Smoking

Hungary: Smoking prevalence in population aged 15+ 1998-2004

Table: 4.529

% of population aged 15+

	1998	1999	2000	2001	2002	2003	2004
Smoking prevalence in population aged 15+ (% of population aged 15+)	32.5	32.5	30.6	32.1	32.6	32.6	32.3
Smoking prevalence in male population aged 15+ (% of male population)	40.2	44.0	38.2	38.3	37.3	37.7	36.8
Smoking prevalence in female population aged 15+ (% of female population)	25.7	21.0	21.0	23.0	28.4	28.0	28.3

Source: WHO/OECD/Euromonitor International

Nutrition and Obesity

Hungary: Nutrition and obesity 1998-2004

Table: 4.530

As stated

	1998	1999	2000	2001	2002	2003	2004
Availability of fruit and vegetables (kg/capita/year)	170.2	166.8	187.7	173.1	181.3	185.9	186.5
Average supply of calories per day (calories per capita)	3,348.5	3,344.8	3,487.2	3,441.6	3,483.2	3,528.2	3,557.2
Average supply of fat per day (grams per capita)	135.4	133.8	146.5	143.7	147.2	151.4	154.5
Average supply of protein per day (grams per capita)	86.0	88.2	94.0	94.8	96.8	99.4	101.7
Microbiological food-borne diseases (per 100000 population)	772.0	447.0	548.0	674.0	674.0	634.0	639.0
Obese population (BMI 30kg/sq m or more) (% of population aged 15+)	19.0	19.1	19.3	19.4	19.5	19.6	19.7

Source: WHO/OECD/Euromonitor International

Over-the-Counter Healthcare

Hungary: Trends in OTC healthcare retail sales 1998-2004

Table: 4.531

As stated

	1998	1999	2000	2001	2002	2003	2004
OTC Healthcare (HuF million)	25,942.9	30,471.2	34,501.3	38,581.6	41,477.4	44,033.7	47,044.2
OTC Healthcare: real growth in national currency: 1998 = 100	100.0	106.8	110.1	112.7	115.1	116.8	116.7
OTC Healthcare: year on year (% real growth)	9.7	6.8	3.1	2.4	2.1	1.5	-0.1
OTC Healthcare (HuF per capita)	2,559.6	3,019.4	3,375.3	3,782.4	4,076.5	4,342.9	4,659.1

Source: Euromonitor International from industry sources/national statistics

Hungary: OTC healthcare retail sales by sector 1998-2004

Table: 4.532

% of OTC retail value sales

	1998	1999	2000	2001	2002	2003	2004
Analgesics	23.1	23.8	23.7	23.4	23.3	23.0	22.6
Cough, cold and allergy (hay fever) remedies	25.8	25.2	24.9	25.0	24.9	24.9	24.7
Digestive remedies	14.2	14.0	14.0	14.0	14.0	14.1	13.9
Medicated skin care	9.9	9.8	9.7	9.7	9.6	9.6	9.4
Vitamins and dietary supplements	22.4	22.5	22.9	23.1	23.3	23.5	23.5

Source: Euromonitor International from industry sources/national statistics
Notes: Only selected sectors are shown, so values are not expected to sum to 100

Health and Wellness

Hungary: Retail sales of packaged foods by health and wellness category 2002-2004

Table: 4.533

HuF million

	2002	2003	2004
Packaged food: Total	1,099,916.8	1,188,830.5	1,273,766.7
Better for you	53,265.1	61,234.6	68,604.0
For food intolerance	5,049.7	5,975.6	6,534.8
Fortified/functional	7,389.3	8,988.3	10,432.4
Organic	5,593.5	6,893.7	8,612.0

Source: Euromonitor International from industry sources/national statistics

Hungary: Per capita sales of packaged foods by health and wellness category 2002-2004

Table: 4.534

HuF per capita

	2002	2003	2004
Better for you	5,307.2	6,112.6	6,861.2
For food intolerance	503.1	596.5	653.6
Fortified/functional	736.3	897.2	1,043.4
Organic	557.3	688.1	861.3

Source: Euromonitor International from industry sources/national statistics

Hungary: Retail sales of packaged food by health and wellness category: % share of total packaged food market 2002-2004

Table: 4.535

% value

	2002	2003	2004
Better for you	4.8	5.2	5.4
For food intolerance	0.5	0.5	0.5
Fortified/functional	0.7	0.8	0.8
Organic	0.5	0.6	0.7

Source: Euromonitor International from industry sources/national statistics

Hungary: Retail sales of packaged food by health and wellness category: real growth index 2002-2004

Table: 4.536

2002 = 100

	2002	2003	2004
Better for you	100.00	109.80	116.60
For food intolerance	100.00	113.02	117.16
Fortified/functional	100.00	116.18	127.82
Organic	100.00	117.71	139.39

Source: Euromonitor International from industry sources/national statistics

Hungary: Retail sales of better-for-you packaged foods by sector 2002-2004

Table: 4.537

% of total packaged food / as stated

	2002	2003	2004	% real change in value 2002-2004
Combination	0.02	0.03	0.05	132.28
Reduced carb	0.00	0.00	0.00	49.05
Reduced fat	3.81	4.09	4.27	17.65
Reduced salt	0.00	0.00	0.00	69.92

Source: Euromonitor International from industry sources/national statistics

Hungary: Retail sales of packaged foods for food intolerances by sector 2002-2004

Table: 4.538

% of total packaged food / as stated

	2002	2003	2004	% real change in value 2002-2004
Diabetic	0.25	0.26	0.26	9.49
Gluten-free	0.19	0.23	0.23	26.12
Lactose-free	0.02	0.02	0.02	29.60

Source: Euromonitor International from industry sources/national statistics

Hungary: Retail sales of naturally healthy packaged foods by sector 2002-2004

Table: 4.539

% of total packaged food / as stated

	2002	2003	2004	% real change in value 2002-2004
High fibre	1.22	1.24	1.27	9.39
Other naturally healthy food	0.85	0.87	0.89	10.09
Soy-based dairy alternatives	0.00	0.00	0.01	68.81

Source: Euromonitor International from industry sources/national statistics

■ India

Socio-economic Parameters

India: Socio-economic parameters 1998-2004

Table: 4.540

As stated

	1998	1999	2000	2001	2002	2003	2004
Population: national estimates at January 1st ('000)	974,492.9	991,634.5	1,008,548.8	1,025,165.8	1,041,471.3	1,057,505.0	1,073,344.7
% aged 0-14 yrs	35.0	34.7	34.3	33.9	33.5	33.1	32.6
% aged 15-64 yrs	60.2	60.5	60.8	61.1	61.5	61.8	62.2
% aged 65 + yrs	4.7	4.8	4.9	5.0	5.0	5.1	5.2
% Male	51.6	51.6	51.6	51.6	51.6	51.5	51.5
% Female	48.4	48.4	48.4	48.4	48.4	48.5	48.5
% Urban	27.8	28.1	28.4	28.7	29.1	29.6	30.0
Occupants per household at January 1st (Number)	5.4	5.4	5.4	5.3	5.3	5.3	5.3
Households ('000)	180,148.4	184,329.3	188,332.3	191,963.9	195,687.2	199,404.1	202,876.1
Annual rates of inflation (% growth)	13.2	4.7	4.0	3.7	4.4	3.8	3.8
GDP (Rs million)	17,409,900.0	19,368,300.0	20,895,000.0	22,821,400.0	24,695,600.0	27,721,900.0	29,946,072.0
GDP (US$ million)	421,962.0	449,846.0	464,936.7	483,643.6	508,032.2	595,103.8	660,820.5
GDP (US$ per capita)	433.0	453.6	461.0	471.8	487.8	562.7	615.7

Source: Euromonitor International from International Monetary Fund (IMF), International Financial Statistics and World Economic Outlook/UN/national statistics

Life Expectancy

India: Life expectancy 1998-2004

Table: 4.541

As stated

	1998	1999	2000	2001	2002	2003	2004	% change 1998-2004
Life expectancy at birth: total population (years)	59.8	60.2	60.6	60.8	61.0	61.3	61.5	2.95
Life expectancy at birth: total population: year on year growth	0.7	0.7	0.7	0.3	0.3	0.4	0.5	
Healthy life expectancy at birth (years)	53.0			51.2	51.4			
Healthy life expectancy at birth: year on year growth					0.4			

Source: Euromonitor International from World Bank

Sanitation

India: Improved sanitary facilities and water source 2000

Table: 4.542

As stated

	2000
Population with access to improved sanitary facilities (% of population)	28.0
Population with access to improved water source (% of population)	84.0
Population with improved access to sanitation facilities, rural (% of rural population with access)	15.0
Population with improved access to sanitation facilities, urban (% of urban population with access)	61.0

Source: National statistics/World Bank

Health Expenditure

India: Public health expenditure 1998-2004

Table: 4.543

As stated

	1998	1999	2000	2001	2002	2003	2004
Share of total health expenditure in GDP (% of total GDP)	5.0	5.2	5.1	5.1	4.9	5.0	5.1
Health expenditure (US$ per capita)	22.0	26.0	29.0	29.0	30.0	31.0	32.0

Source: Euromonitor International from OECD/national statistics

India: Private health expenditure 1998-2004

Table: 4.544

As stated

	1998	1999	2000	2001	2002	2003	2004
Consumer expenditure on health goods and medical services (Rs million)	441,616.9	628,286.8	835,170.0	981,680.0	1,158,123.0	1,257,536.1	1,368,092.4
Consumer expenditure on health goods and medical services: real growth in national currency: 1990 = 100	154.8	210.4	268.9	304.9	344.5	360.4	377.9
Consumer expenditure on health goods and medical services as a percentage of total consumer expenditure	3.9	5.0	6.5	6.9	7.6	7.7	7.8

Source: National statistical offices/OECD/Eurostat/Euromonitor International

India: Consumer expenditure on health goods and medical services by sector 1998-2004

Table: 4.545

% of total consumer expenditure on health goods and medical services

	1998	1999	2000	2001	2002	2003	2004
Pharmaceuticals, medical appliances/equipment	47.3	46.0	45.3	44.4	43.8	43.9	43.8
Outpatient services	37.2	38.3	39.0	39.7	39.5	39.3	39.3
Hospital services	15.5	15.7	15.7	15.9	16.6	16.8	16.8
Total	100.0	100.0	100.0	100.0	100.0	100.0	100.0

Source: National statistical offices/OECD/Eurostat/Euromonitor International

Healthcare Infrastructure and Services

India: Healthcare infrastructure and services by sector 1998-2004

Table: 4.546

As stated

	1998	1999	2000	2001	2002	2003	2004
Doctors (number)	503,947	493,582	483,117	472,719	462,294	451,879	441,922
Hospitals and clinics (number)	15,356	15,452	15,549	15,623	15,741	15,828	15,936
In-patient beds ('000)	922	933	948	969	978	997	1,009
Nurses (number)	583,531	592,352	595,326	597,663	598,325	605,872	609,438

Source: Euromonitor International from national statistics

India: Healthcare infrastructure and services by sector: growth 1998-2004

Table: 4.547

Year on year growth: % change in stated unit

	1998	1999	2000	2001	2002	2003	2004
Doctors (number)	-3.6	-2.1	-2.1	-2.2	-2.2	-2.3	-2.2
Hospitals and clinics (number)	0.6	0.6	0.6	0.5	0.8	0.6	0.7
In-patient beds (number)	2.2	1.2	1.6	2.2	0.9	1.9	1.2
Nurses (number)	1.6	1.5	0.5	0.4	0.1	1.3	0.6

Source: Euromonitor International from national statistics

Immunisation

India: Vaccination rates by disease type 1998-2004

Table: 4.548

%

	1998	1999	2000	2001	2002	2003	2004
Vaccination rate against DTP (diphtheria, tetanus, pertussis) 1 & 2 (%)				71.1	77.0	83.0	89.0
Vaccination rate against MMR (measles, mumps, rubella) (%)	84.3	87.0	88.5	55.6	67.0	57.0	50.0
Vaccination rate against polio (%)	90.4	93.4	95.1	70.4	70.0	75.0	76.0

Source: WHO

Infectious Diseases

India: Incidence of disease by type 1998-2004

Table: 4.549

Number

	1998	1999	2000	2001	2002	2003	2004
Incidence of AIDS	1,148	952	2,098	2,399	2,514	2,604	2,361
Incidence of diphtheria	1,378	1,786	3,094	5,101	5,472		
Incidence of measles	33,990	21,013	22,236	37,969	51,780		
Incidence of polio	4,322	2,817	265	268	1,600		

Source: WHO

India: Incidence of disease by type: growth 1998-2004

Table: 4.550

Year on year growth: %

	1998	1999	2000	2001	2002	2003	2004
Incidence of AIDS	-45.5	-17.1	120.4	14.3	4.8	3.6	-9.3
Incidence of diphtheria	3.9	29.6	73.2	64.9	7.3		
Incidence of measles	-44.3	-38.2	5.8	70.8	36.4		
Incidence of polio	90.0	-34.8	-90.6	1.1	497.0		

Source: WHO

Causes of Death

India: Deaths by disease 1998-2004

Table: 4.551

Number per 100,000 inhabitants

	1998	1999	2000	2001	2002	2003	2004
Deaths from heart disease	41.5	44.3	40.4	40.2	40.0	39.8	39.5
Deaths from lung cancer	35.7	36.1	36.9	35.8	37.2	36.9	37.3
Deaths from ulcers of the stomach and duodenum	27.6	25.9	27.7	25.8	25.8	24.6	23.6
Death by diseases of the digestive system	27.6	25.9	27.7	25.8	25.8	24.5	23.4
Deaths from chronic liver disease and cirrhosis	10.0	9.8	9.6	9.3	9.5	9.4	9.4

Source: WHO/Euromonitor International
Notes: Data is ranked in descending order by year 2004

India: Deaths by disease: growth 1998-2004

Table: 4.552

% year on year growth

	1998	1999	2000	2001	2002	2003	2004
Deaths from lung cancer	6.9	1.1	2.2	-3.0	3.9	-0.8	1.0
Deaths from chronic liver disease and cirrhosis	-1.0	-2.0	-2.0	-3.1	2.2	-1.1	-0.3
Deaths from heart disease	-5.7	6.7	-8.8	-0.5	-0.5	-0.5	-0.8
Deaths from ulcers of the stomach and duodenum	-1.1	-6.2	6.9	-6.9	0.0	-4.7	-4.0
Death by diseases of the digestive system	-1.1	-6.2	6.9	-6.9	0.0	-5.0	-4.6

Source: WHO/Euromonitor International
Notes: Data is ranked in descending order by year 2004

India: Other selected causes of death: 1998-2004

Table: 4.553

Number per 100,000 inhabitants

	1998	1999	2000	2001	2002	2003	2004
Death by suicide and self-inflicted injury	10.2	10.7	10.9	11.3	11.6	11.9	12.4

Source: Euromonitor International from national statistics

India: Other selected causes of death: growth 1998-2004

Table: 4.554

% year on year growth

	1998	1999	2000	2001	2002	2003	2004
Death by suicide and self-inflicted injury	1.0	4.9	1.9	3.7	2.7	2.6	3.8

Source: Euromonitor International from national statistics

Smoking

India: Smoking prevalence in population aged 15+ 1998-2004

Table: 4.555

% of population aged 15+

	1998	1999	2000	2001	2002	2003	2004
Smoking prevalence in population aged 15+ (% of population aged 15+)	35.9	36.0	36.2	36.1	37.2	37.3	38.0
Smoking prevalence in male population aged 15+ (% of male population)	57.2	57.0	56.3	57.7	57.4	58.1	58.8
Smoking prevalence in female population aged 15+ (% of female population)	13.2	13.8	14.9	13.3	15.8	15.3	15.9

Source: WHO/OECD/Euromonitor International

Nutrition and Obesity

India: Nutrition and obesity 1998-2004

Table: 4.556

As stated

	1998	1999	2000	2001	2002	2003	2004
Average supply of calories per day (calories per capita)	2,329.2	2,438.7	2,414.8	2,385.8	2,459.0	2,499.9	2,535.5
Average supply of fat per day (grams per capita)	44.6	51.2	52.1	50.0	49.6	49.2	48.6
Average supply of protein per day (grams per capita)	55.4	57.3	56.1	55.9	57.3	58.0	58.7
Obese population (BMI 30kg/sq m or more) (% of population aged 15+)	5.1	5.2	5.3	5.4	5.3	5.4	5.4

Source: WHO/OECD/Euromonitor International

Over-the-Counter Healthcare

India: Trends in OTC healthcare retail sales 1998-2004

Table: 4.557

As stated

	1998	1999	2000	2001	2002	2003	2004
OTC Healthcare (Rs million)	29,231.6	32,518.5	36,245.5	40,248.5	44,233.9	48,125.7	52,015.7
OTC Healthcare: real growth in national currency: 1998 = 100	100.0	106.3	113.9	122.0	128.4	134.6	138.9
OTC Healthcare: year on year (% real growth)	-1.6	6.3	7.2	7.1	5.3	4.8	3.2
OTC Healthcare (Rs per capita)	29.8	32.8	35.9	39.3	42.5	45.5	48.5

Source: Euromonitor International from industry sources/national statistics

India: OTC healthcare retail sales by sector 1998-2004

Table: 4.558

% of OTC retail value sales

	1998	1999	2000	2001	2002	2003	2004
Analgesics	21.3	21.6	21.7	21.9	22.1	22.3	22.4
Cough, cold and allergy (hay fever) remedies	19.3	19.8	20.4	21.1	21.6	22.0	22.3
Digestive remedies	11.7	11.6	11.5	11.3	11.2	11.0	10.7
Medicated skin care	10.3	9.9	9.6	9.3	9.0	8.9	8.7
Vitamins and dietary supplements	33.4	33.0	32.8	32.5	32.1	31.8	31.8

Source: Euromonitor International from industry sources/national statistics
Notes: Only selected sectors are shown, so values are not expected to sum to 100

■ **Indonesia**

Socio-economic Parameters

Indonesia: Socio-economic parameters 1998-2004

Table: 4.559

As stated

	1998	1999	2000	2001	2002	2003	2004
Population: national estimates at January 1st ('000)	204,468.7	207,320.4	210,149.2	212,956.7	215,742.9	218,506.5	221,246.5
% aged 0-14 yrs	32.1	31.6	31.1	30.6	30.2	29.7	29.3
% aged 15-64 yrs	63.4	63.7	64.1	64.5	64.8	65.1	65.4
% aged 65+ yrs	4.5	4.7	4.8	4.9	5.0	5.2	5.3
% Male	50.0	50.0	50.0	50.0	50.0	50.0	50.0
% Female	50.0	50.0	50.0	50.0	50.0	50.0	50.0
% Urban	38.8	39.8	40.2	41.1	42.2	43.1	44.2
Occupants per household at January 1st (Number)	4.1	4.1	4.0	4.0	3.9	3.9	3.9
Households ('000)	49,346.6	50,634.6	52,008.3	53,455.0	55,041.0	56,245.2	57,411.1
Annual rates of inflation (% growth)	58.4	20.5	3.7	11.5	11.9	6.6	6.2
GDP (Rp billion)	955,753.0	1,099,730.0	1,264,920.0	1,449,400.0	1,610,560.0	1,786,700.0	2,303,031.4
GDP (US$ million)	95,445.5	140,001.1	150,196.5	141,256.0	172,970.4	208,309.8	257,642.9
GDP (US$ per capita)	466.8	675.3	714.7	663.3	801.7	953.3	1,164.5

Source: Euromonitor International from International Monetary Fund (IMF), International Financial Statistics and World Economic Outlook/UN/national statistics

Life Expectancy

Indonesia: Life expectancy 1998-2004

Table: 4.560

As stated

	1998	1999	2000	2001	2002	2003	2004	% change 1998-2004
Life expectancy at birth: total population (years)	64.7	65.2	65.4	65.9	66.4	66.8	67.2	3.80
Life expectancy at birth: total population: year on year growth	0.7	0.7	0.4	0.8	0.8	0.6	0.6	
Healthy life expectancy at birth (years)	60.0			56.2	56.7			
Healthy life expectancy at birth: year on year growth					0.8			

Source: Euromonitor International from World Bank

Sanitation

Indonesia: Improved sanitary facilities and water source 2000

Table: 4.561

As stated

	2000
Population with access to improved sanitary facilities (% of population)	55.0
Population with access to improved water source (% of population)	78.0
Population with improved access to sanitation facilities, rural (% of rural population with access)	46.0
Population with improved access to sanitation facilities, urban (% of urban population with access)	69.0

Source: National statistics/World Bank

Health Expenditure

Indonesia: Public health expenditure 1998-2004

Table: 4.562

As stated

	1998	1999	2000	2001	2002	2003	2004
Share of total health expenditure in GDP (% of total GDP)	2.5	2.6	2.7	2.4	2.4	2.5	2.6
Health expenditure (US$ per capita)	12.0	18.0	20.0	21.0	26.0	27.0	29.0

Source: Euromonitor International from OECD/national statistics

Indonesia: Private health expenditure 1998-2004

Table: 4.563

As stated

	1998	1999	2000	2001	2002	2003	2004
Consumer expenditure on health goods and medical services (Rp million)	12,318,055.0	15,544,373.0	16,618,706.0	19,158,819.0	22,224,274.0	24,550,900.1	27,127,149.5
Consumer expenditure on health goods and medical services: real growth in national currency: 1990 = 100	231.0	241.9	249.4	257.8	267.3	277.1	288.2
Consumer expenditure on health goods and medical services as a percentage of total consumer expenditure	1.8	1.9	1.9	1.9	1.9	1.9	2.0

Source: National statistical offices/OECD/Eurostat/Euromonitor International

Indonesia: Consumer expenditure on health goods and medical services by sector 1998-2004

Table: 4.564

% of total consumer expenditure on health goods and medical services

	1998	1999	2000	2001	2002	2003	2004
Pharmaceuticals, medical appliances/ equipment	61.2	59.4	57.4	57.5	58.7	58.0	57.9
Outpatient services	29.1	30.2	31.7	31.4	30.2	30.8	31.0
Hospital services	9.8	10.4	10.9	11.1	11.1	11.2	11.1
Total	100.0	100.0	100.0	100.0	100.0	100.0	100.0

Source: National statistical offices/OECD/Eurostat/Euromonitor International

Healthcare Infrastructure and Services

Indonesia: Healthcare infrastructure and services by sector 1998-2004

Table: 4.565

As stated

	1998	1999	2000	2001	2002	2003	2004
Active pharmacists (number)				3,466	3,469	3,482	
Doctors (number)	19,291	25,535	21,467	20,912	20,738	20,632	20,486
Hospitals and clinics (number)	1,112	1,111	1,145	1,164	1,182	1,207	1,228
In-patient beds ('000)	123	123	126	127	128	130	131
Nurses (number)	162,060	162,014	163,412	164,241	165,772	166,242	166,641

Source: Euromonitor International from national statistics

Indonesia: Healthcare infrastructure and services by sector: growth 1998-2004

Table: 4.566

Year on year growth: % change in stated unit

	1998	1999	2000	2001	2002	2003	2004
Active pharmacists (number)					0.1	0.4	
Doctors (number)	1.4	32.4	-15.9	-2.6	-0.8	-0.5	-0.7
Hospitals and clinics (number)	2.0	-0.1	3.1	1.7	1.5	2.1	1.7
In-patient beds (number)	1.0	0.2	2.1	0.8	0.8	1.6	0.8
Nurses (number)	-1.6	0.0	0.9	0.5	0.9	0.3	0.2

Source: Euromonitor International from national statistics

Immunisation

Indonesia: Vaccination rates by disease type 1998-2004

Table: 4.567

%

	1998	1999	2000	2001	2002	2003	2004
Vaccination rate against DTP (diphtheria, tetanus, pertussis) 1 & 2 (%)			87.0	81.5	80.6	80.0	79.0
Vaccination rate against MMR (measles, mumps, rubella) (%)	90.9	88.3	73.0	75.7	43.7	42.0	32.0
Vaccination rate against polio (%)	92.6	90.3	74.0	76.7	74.5	76.0	76.0

Source: WHO

Infectious Diseases

Indonesia: Incidence of disease by type 1998-2004

Table: 4.568

Number

	1998	1999	2000	2001	2002	2003	2004
Incidence of AIDS	75	57	166	185	232	239	321
Incidence of diphtheria	14	114	23	34	51		
Incidence of measles	1,034	4,767	3,344	3,825	14,492		
Incidence of polio	49	39	35	0	0		

Source: WHO

Indonesia: Incidence of disease by type: growth 1998-2004

Table: 4.569

Year on year growth: %

	1998	1999	2000	2001	2002	2003	2004
Incidence of AIDS	120.6	-24.0	191.2	11.4	25.4	3.0	34.3
Incidence of diphtheria	-99.7	714.3	-79.8	47.8	50.0		
Incidence of measles	-93.2	361.0	-29.9	14.4	278.9		
Incidence of polio	-83.3	-20.4	-10.3	-100.0			

Source: WHO

Causes of Death

Indonesia: Deaths by disease 1998-2004

Table: 4.570

Number per 100,000 inhabitants

	1998	1999	2000	2001	2002	2003	2004
Deaths from heart disease	36.9	37.4	41.6	42.3	44.1	45.2	46.3
Deaths from ulcers of the stomach and duodenum	30.9	28.9	27.5	29.5	28.8	29.9	30.6
Death by diseases of the digestive system	30.9	28.9	27.5	29.5	28.8	29.8	30.4
Deaths from lung cancer	23.0	20.2	18.8	20.2	20.0	20.9	21.6
Deaths from chronic liver disease and cirrhosis	6.9	6.7	6.7	7.1	7.1	7.4	7.6

Source: WHO/Euromonitor International
Notes: Data is ranked in descending order by year 2004

Indonesia: Deaths by disease: growth 1998-2004

Table: 4.571

% year on year growth

	1998	1999	2000	2001	2002	2003	2004
Deaths from lung cancer	5.0	-12.2	-6.9	7.4	-1.0	4.5	3.3
Deaths from chronic liver disease and cirrhosis	4.5	-2.9	0.0	6.0	0.0	4.2	2.5
Deaths from heart disease	1.9	1.4	11.2	1.7	4.3	2.5	2.4
Deaths from ulcers of the stomach and duodenum	-1.6	-6.5	-4.8	7.3	-2.4	3.8	2.3
Death by diseases of the digestive system	-1.6	-6.5	-4.8	7.3	-2.4	3.5	1.9

Source: WHO/Euromonitor International
Notes: Data is ranked in descending order by year 2004

Smoking

Indonesia: Smoking prevalence in population aged 15+ 1998-2004

Table: 4.572

% of population aged 15+

	1998	1999	2000	2001	2002	2003	2004
Smoking prevalence in population aged 15+ (% of population aged 15+)	39.0	38.9	38.2	38.4	37.9	38.0	37.7
Smoking prevalence in male population aged 15+ (% of male population)	63.0	61.4	60.0	58.3	57.8	57.8	57.5
Smoking prevalence in female population aged 15+ (% of female population)	15.2	16.7	16.7	18.7	18.3	18.5	18.2

Source: WHO/OECD/Euromonitor International

Nutrition and Obesity

Indonesia: Nutrition and obesity 1998-2004

Table: 4.573

As stated

	1998	1999	2000	2001	2002	2003	2004
Average supply of calories per day (calories per capita)	2,864.1	2,895.7	2,919.7	2,911.4	2,903.9	2,902.9	2,898.5
Average supply of fat per day (grams per capita)	56.4	58.2	58.8	60.1	59.4	59.3	59.3
Average supply of protein per day (grams per capita)	62.0	66.2	65.9	64.2	64.2	63.9	63.4
Obese population (BMI 30kg/sq m or more) (% of population aged 15+)	5.7	5.8	5.8	5.8	5.7	5.7	5.7

Source: WHO/OECD/Euromonitor International

Over-the-Counter Healthcare

Indonesia: Trends in OTC healthcare retail sales 1998-2004

Table: 4.574

As stated

	1998	1999	2000	2001	2002	2003	2004
OTC Healthcare (Rp billion)	2,410.0	3,077.5	4,060.3	4,826.4	5,769.6	6,856.3	8,089.0
OTC Healthcare: real growth in national currency: 1998 = 100	100.0	106.1	128.1	135.2	146.9	166.2	184.1
OTC Healthcare: year on year (% real growth)	-24.2	6.1	20.7	5.6	8.6	13.1	10.8
OTC Healthcare ('000 Rp per capita)	11.8	14.8	19.3	22.7	26.7	31.4	36.6

Source: Euromonitor International from industry sources/national statistics

Indonesia: OTC healthcare retail sales by sector 1998-2004

Table: 4.575

% of OTC retail value sales

	1998	1999	2000	2001	2002	2003	2004
Analgesics	18.7	19.3	19.1	18.7	18.2	17.4	16.8
Cough, cold and allergy (hay fever) remedies	26.3	25.8	25.0	23.6	22.7	21.9	21.5
Digestive remedies	7.9	8.0	8.2	7.9	7.5	7.1	6.9
Medicated skin care	10.3	10.5	10.7	11.6	12.3	12.9	12.4
Vitamins and dietary supplements	27.8	27.6	28.4	30.2	31.7	33.5	35.4

Source: Euromonitor International from industry sources/national statistics
Notes: Only selected sectors are shown, so values are not expected to sum to 100

■ **Ireland**

Socio-economic Parameters

Ireland: Socio-economic parameters 1998-2004

Table: 4.576

As stated

	1998	1999	2000	2001	2002	2003	2004
Population: national estimates at January 1st ('000)	3,694.0	3,734.9	3,776.6	3,826.0	3,882.7	3,931.4	3,972.9
% aged 0-14 yrs	22.7	22.2	21.9	21.5	21.2	21.0	21.0
% aged 15-64 yrs	66.0	66.5	66.9	67.3	67.7	67.9	68.1
% aged 65+ yrs	11.4	11.3	11.2	11.2	11.2	11.1	11.0
% Male	49.6	49.6	49.7	49.7	49.7	49.7	49.7
% Female	50.4	50.4	50.3	50.3	50.3	50.3	50.3
% Urban	58.6	58.8	58.5	58.8	59.1	59.4	59.7
Occupants per household at January 1st (Number)	3.2	3.1	3.1	3.0	3.0	3.0	3.0
Households ('000)	1,172.2	1,198.8	1,225.5	1,255.8	1,288.0	1,316.7	1,343.1
Annual rates of inflation (% growth)	2.4	1.6	5.6	4.9	4.7	3.5	2.2
GDP (EUR million)	76,919.8	89,452.9	103,060.3	115,426.7	127,986.3	134,780.3	146,272.2
GDP (US$ million)	86,227.0	95,301.9	94,951.5	103,289.2	120,452.0	152,116.4	181,622.3
GDP (US$ per capita)	23,342.5	25,516.6	25,142.2	26,996.9	31,022.9	38,692.6	45,715.1

Source: Euromonitor International from International Monetary Fund (IMF), International Financial Statistics and World Economic Outlook/UN/national statistics

Life Expectancy

Ireland: Life expectancy 1998-2004

Table: 4.577

As stated

	1998	1999	2000	2001	2002	2003	2004	% change 1998-2004
Life expectancy at birth: total population (years)	76.0	76.2	76.3	76.5	77.1	77.4	77.8	2.24
Life expectancy at birth: total population: year on year growth	0.2	0.2	0.1	0.3	0.8	0.4	0.5	
Healthy life expectancy at birth (years)	70.0			68.9	69.0			
Healthy life expectancy at birth: year on year growth					0.1			

Source: Euromonitor International from World Bank

Health Expenditure

Ireland: Public health expenditure 1998-2004

Table: 4.578

As stated

	1998	1999	2000	2001	2002	2003	2004
Public expenditure on pharmaceuticals and other medical non-durables (EUR million)	419.0	484.0	557.0	714.0	867.0	1,053.0	1,326.8
Private insurance expenditure (% of total expenditure on health)	8.9	8.0	7.6	6.3	5.4	4.2	3.1
Share of total health expenditure in GDP (% of total GDP)	6.2	6.2	6.4	6.5	6.4	6.7	6.7
Health expenditure (US$ per capita)	1,454.0	1,589.0	1,579.0	1,839.0	2,255.0	2,477.0	2,677.0

Source: *Euromonitor International from OECD/national statistics*

Ireland: Private health expenditure 1998-2004

Table: 4.579

As stated

	1998	1999	2000	2001	2002	2003	2004
Consumer expenditure on health goods and medical services (EUR Million)	1,031.3	1,138.1	1,305.1	1,477.6	1,764.2	1,863.3	1,930.4
Consumer expenditure on health goods and medical services: real growth in national currency: 1990 = 100	145.9	158.4	172.1	185.7	211.9	216.3	219.2
Consumer expenditure on health goods and medical services as a percentage of total consumer expenditure	2.8	2.7	2.8	2.9	3.2	3.2	3.2

Source: *National statistical offices/OECD/Eurostat/Euromonitor International*

Ireland: Consumer expenditure on health goods and medical services by sector 1998-2004

Table: 4.580

% of total consumer expenditure on health goods and medical services

	1998	1999	2000	2001	2002	2003	2004
Pharmaceuticals, medical appliances/ equipment	18.4	20.7	19.8	22.9	24.4	24.4	24.2
Outpatient services	25.0	24.7	24.8	25.0	24.6	24.7	24.7
Hospital services	56.5	54.6	55.4	52.2	50.9	50.9	51.1
Total	100.0	100.0	100.0	100.0	100.0	100.0	100.0

Source: *National statistical offices/OECD/Eurostat/Euromonitor International*

Healthcare Infrastructure and Services

Ireland: Healthcare infrastructure and services by sector 1998-2004

Table: 4.581

As stated

	1998	1999	2000	2001	2002	2003	2004
Active pharmacists (number)	2,762	2,886	3,044	3,165	3,144	3,385	3,509
Dentists (number)	1,713	1,794	1,899	2,006	2,102	2,171	2,230
Doctors (number)	8,102	8,469	8,438	9,166	9,444	10,270	10,399
Hospital admissions (number)	547,389	541,484	561,529	570,653	566,829	582,037	584,796
In-patient beds ('000)	11	11	11	12	12	12	12
In-patient surgical procedures (number)	555,995	682,389	817,429	1,009,745	1,273,421	1,335,762	1,422,171
Nurses (number)	48,579	50,940	53,072	57,059	60,084	61,221	61,324

Source: *Euromonitor International from national statistics*

Ireland: Healthcare infrastructure and services by sector: growth 1998-2004

Table: 4.582

Year on year growth: % change in stated unit

	1998	1999	2000	2001	2002	2003	2004
Active pharmacists (number)	4.3	4.5	5.5	4.0	-0.7	7.7	3.7
Dentists (number)	2.5	4.7	5.9	5.6	4.8	3.3	2.7
Doctors (number)	3.9	4.5	-0.4	8.6	3.0	8.7	1.3
Hospital admissions (number)	0.3	-1.1	3.7	1.6	-0.7	2.7	0.5
In-patient beds (number)	-0.8	-0.6	1.1	1.1	2.1	2.5	0.8
In-patient surgical procedures (number)	14.3	22.7	19.8	23.5	26.1	4.9	6.5
Nurses (number)	3.0	4.9	4.2	7.5	5.3	1.9	0.2

Source: Euromonitor International from national statistics

Immunisation

Ireland: Vaccination rates by disease type 1998-2004

Table: 4.583

%

	1998	1999	2000	2001	2002	2003	2004
Vaccination rate against MMR (measles, mumps, rubella) (%)	77.0	77.0	77.0	73.0	72.5	71.0	70.0
Vaccination rate against polio (%)	85.0	86.0	85.0	84.0	82.5	82.0	80.0

Source: WHO

Infectious Diseases

Ireland: Incidence of disease by type 1998-2004

Table: 4.584

Number

	1998	1999	2000	2001	2002	2003	2004
Incidence of AIDS	41	41	21	4	13	5	6
Incidence of diphtheria	0	0		0	0		
Incidence of measles	204	147		241	243		
Incidence of polio	0	0	0	0	0		

Source: WHO

Ireland: Incidence of disease by type: growth 1998-2004

Table: 4.585

Year on year growth: %

	1998	1999	2000	2001	2002	2003	2004
Incidence of AIDS	36.7	0.0	-48.8	-81.0	225.0	-61.5	20.0
Incidence of measles	10.3	-27.9			0.8		

Source: WHO

Causes of Death

Ireland: Deaths by disease 1998-2004

Table: 4.586

Number per 100,000 inhabitants

	1998	1999	2000	2001	2002	2003	2004
Death by diseases of the circulatory system	324.6	322.9	309.0	298.0	282.0	275.0	262.7
Death by malignant neoplasms (cancers)	196.0	194.8	193.2	191.9	190.4	187.2	184.1
Deaths from heart disease	195.4	188.5	183.4	177.8	172.4	167.0	161.4
Death by diseases of the respiratory system	114.2	125.4	124.1	120.0	118.0	119.0	117.3
Deaths from lung cancer	41.1	38.7	39.9	40.1	40.3	40.4	40.9
Death by diseases of the digestive system	24.6	25.6	25.0	25.4	25.1	24.5	24.4
Deaths from chronic liver disease and cirrhosis	4.3	4.4	4.6	4.7	4.8	5.0	5.2
Deaths from ulcers of the stomach and duodenum	4.2	5.1	4.7	4.6	4.5	4.5	4.5

Source: WHO/Euromonitor International
Notes: Data is ranked in descending order by year 2004

Ireland: Deaths by disease: growth 1998-2004

Table: 4.587

% year on year growth

	1998	1999	2000	2001	2002	2003	2004
Deaths from chronic liver disease and cirrhosis	7.5	0.8	5.0	2.2	2.1	4.2	3.8
Deaths from lung cancer	8.3	-5.9	3.1	0.5	0.5	0.2	1.1
Death by diseases of the digestive system	-3.1	4.1	-2.3	1.6	-1.2	-2.4	-0.5
Deaths from ulcers of the stomach and duodenum	-20.2	21.1	-7.8	-2.1	-2.2	0.0	-0.7
Death by diseases of the respiratory system	-3.1	9.8	-1.0	-3.3	-1.7	0.8	-1.4
Death by malignant neoplasms (cancers)	-1.8	-0.6	-0.8	-0.7	-0.8	-1.7	-1.6
Deaths from heart disease	-2.2	-3.5	-2.7	-3.1	-3.0	-3.1	-3.4
Death by diseases of the circulatory system	-3.7	-0.5	-4.3	-3.6	-5.4	-2.5	-4.5

Source: WHO/Euromonitor International
Notes: Data is ranked in descending order by year 2004

Ireland: Other selected causes of death: 1998-2004

Table: 4.588

Number per 100,000 inhabitants

	1998	1999	2000	2001	2002	2003	2004
Death by injury and poisoning	41.3	40.1	41.3	40.9	40.9	39.6	39.2
Death by suicide and self-inflicted injury	13.2	11.1	12.1	11.0	10.5	11.2	11.0
Death by motor traffic accidents	11.5	10.4	10.2	9.4	8.8	9.7	9.5

Source: Euromonitor International from national statistics
Notes: Data is ranked in descending order by year 2004

Ireland: Other selected causes of death: growth 1998-2004

Table: 4.589

% year on year growth

	1998	1999	2000	2001	2002	2003	2004
Death by injury and poisoning	4.8	-2.9	3.0	-1.0	0.0	-3.2	-1.0
Death by suicide and self-inflicted injury	4.8	-15.9	9.0	-9.1	-4.5	6.7	-1.8
Death by motor traffic accidents	-2.5	-9.6	-1.9	-7.8	-6.4	10.2	-2.1

Source: Euromonitor International from national statistics
Notes: Data is ranked in descending order by year 2004

Ireland: Retail sales of packaged foods for food intolerances by sector 2002-2004

Table: 4.599

% of total packaged food / as stated

	2002	2003	2004	% real change in value 2002-2004
Diabetic	0.03	0.03	0.03	23.21
Gluten-free	0.11	0.11	0.11	10.37
Lactose-free	0.07	0.07	0.07	16.65

Source: Euromonitor International from industry sources/national statistics

Ireland: Retail sales of naturally healthy packaged foods by sector 2002-2004

Table: 4.600

% of total packaged food / as stated

	2002	2003	2004	% real change in value 2002-2004
High fibre	4.16	4.16	4.17	6.79
Other naturally healthy food	0.45	0.47	0.50	20.55
Soy-based dairy alternatives	0.05	0.05	0.06	30.70

Source: Euromonitor International from industry sources/national statistics

■ Israel

Socio-economic Parameters

Israel: Socio-economic parameters 1998-2004

Table: 4.601

As stated

	1998	1999	2000	2001	2002	2003	2004
Population: national estimates at January 1st ('000)	5,970.7	6,125.3	6,289.2	6,439.0	6,569.8	6,730.8	6,890.4
% aged 0-14 yrs	28.9	28.7	28.6	28.5	28.4	28.3	28.2
% aged 15-64 yrs	61.2	61.5	61.6	61.7	61.8	61.8	61.9
% aged 65+ yrs	9.9	9.8	9.8	9.8	9.9	9.9	9.9
% Male	49.3	49.3	49.3	49.3	49.3	49.3	49.3
% Female	50.7	50.7	50.7	50.7	50.7	50.7	50.7
% Urban	91.0	91.1	91.2	91.3	91.3	91.4	91.5
Occupants per household at January 1st (Number)	3.6	3.6	3.6	3.5	3.6	3.5	3.5
Households ('000)	1,650.6	1,699.5	1,752.3	1,815.3	1,849.8	1,902.7	1,956.6
Annual rates of inflation (% growth)	5.4	5.2	1.1	1.1	5.6	0.7	-0.4
GDP (NIS million)	394,136.0	429,918.0	470,733.0	477,797.0	493,707.0	501,984.0	526,852.0
GDP (US$ million)	103,718.1	103,852.0	115,451.3	113,608.4	104,205.5	110,226.1	117,548.9
GDP (US$ per capita)	17,371.2	16,954.7	18,357.1	17,643.7	15,861.3	16,376.3	17,059.7

Source: Euromonitor International from International Monetary Fund (IMF), International Financial Statistics and World Economic Outlook/UN/national statistics

Life Expectancy

Israel: Life expectancy 1998-2004

Table: 4.602

As stated

	1998	1999	2000	2001	2002	2003	2004	% change 1998-2004
Life expectancy at birth: total population (years)	78.1	78.2	78.5	78.5	79.3	79.8	80.2	2.73
Life expectancy at birth: total population: year on year growth	0.2	0.2	0.3	0.0	1.1	0.5	0.6	
Healthy life expectancy at birth (years)	70.0							

Source: Euromonitor International from World Bank

Health Expenditure

Israel: Public health expenditure 1998-2004

Table: 4.603

As stated

	1998	1999	2000	2001	2002	2003	2004
Share of total health expenditure in GDP (% of total GDP)	8.1	8.2	8.2	8.7	8.7	8.5	8.6
Health expenditure (US$ per capita)	1,511.0	1,498.0	1,617.0	1,754.0	1,496.0	1,436.0	1,375.0

Source: Euromonitor International from OECD/national statistics

Israel: Private health expenditure 1998-2004

Table: 4.604

As stated

	1998	1999	2000	2001	2002	2003	2004
Consumer expenditure on health goods and medical services (NIS million)	4,680.9	4,520.8	4,212.3	3,284.3	2,712.2	2,801.6	2,837.5
Consumer expenditure on health goods and medical services: real growth in national currency: 1990 = 100	196.4	180.3	166.1	128.1	100.1	102.7	104.5
Consumer expenditure on health goods and medical services as a percentage of total consumer expenditure	2.1	1.9	1.6	1.2	1.0	1.0	1.0

Source: National statistical offices/OECD/Eurostat/Euromonitor International

Israel: Consumer expenditure on health goods and medical services by sector 1998-2004

Table: 4.605

% of total consumer expenditure on health goods and medical services

	1998	1999	2000	2001	2002	2003	2004
Pharmaceuticals, medical appliances/ equipment	68.1	67.7	70.4	72.4	73.8	73.8	74.0
Outpatient services	25.4	25.5	23.5	21.8	20.7	20.8	20.7
Hospital services	6.5	6.8	6.2	5.7	5.5	5.4	5.3
Total	100.0	100.0	100.0	100.0	100.0	100.0	100.0

Source: National statistical offices/OECD/Eurostat/Euromonitor International

Healthcare Infrastructure and Services

Israel: Healthcare infrastructure and services by sector 1998-2004

Table: 4.606

As stated

	1998	1999	2000	2001	2002	2003	2004
Dentists (number)	6,834						
Doctors (number)	22,684						
Hospital admissions (number)	1,135,184	1,152,886	1,158,554	1,206,122	1,215,156	1,231,840	1,261,416
Hospitals and clinics (number)	317	327	343	354	363	372	377
In-patient beds ('000)	36	38	39	39	40	40	40
In-patient surgical procedures (number)	483,530	487,020	501,570	525,190	546,252	560,147	577,775
Nurses (number)	35,700						
Out-patient contacts (per capita)			7				

Source: Euromonitor International from national statistics

Israel: Healthcare infrastructure and services by sector: growth 1998-2004

Table: 4.607

Year on year growth: % change in stated unit

	1998	1999	2000	2001	2002	2003	2004
Hospital admissions (number)	3.1	1.6	0.5	4.1	0.7	1.4	2.4
Hospitals and clinics (number)	4.6	3.2	4.9	3.2	2.5	2.5	1.3
In-patient beds (number)	3.1	3.5	3.6	0.8	0.3	0.5	0.5
In-patient surgical procedures (number)	9.9	0.7	3.0	4.7	4.0	2.5	3.1

Source: Euromonitor International from national statistics

Immunisation

Israel: Vaccination rates by disease type 1998-2004

Table: 4.608

%

	1998	1999	2000	2001	2002	2003	2004
Vaccination rate against DTP (diphtheria, tetanus, pertussis) 1 & 2 (%)			97.0	97.0	97.0	99.0	99.0
Vaccination rate against MMR (measles, mumps, rubella) (%)	94.0	94.0	94.0	94.0	95.0	95.0	95.0
Vaccination rate against polio (%)	96.0		92.0	92.0	93.0	93.0	94.0

Source: WHO

Infectious Diseases

Israel: Incidence of disease by type 1998-2004

Table: 4.609

Number

	1998	1999	2000	2001	2002	2003	2004
Incidence of AIDS	36	137	50	39	78	22	32
Incidence of diphtheria	1	3	0	0	1		
Incidence of measles	8	14	36	19	2		
Incidence of polio	0	0	0	0	0		

Source: WHO

Israel: Incidence of disease by type: growth 1998-2004

Table: 4.610

Year on year growth: %

	1998	1999	2000	2001	2002	2003	2004
Incidence of AIDS	-20.0	280.6	-63.5	-22.0	100.0	-71.8	45.5
Incidence of diphtheria		200.0	-100.0				
Incidence of measles	-33.3	75.0	157.1	-47.2	-89.5		

Source: WHO

Causes of Death

Israel: Deaths by disease 1998-2004

Table: 4.611

Number per 100,000 inhabitants

	1998	1999	2000	2001	2002	2003	2004
Deaths from heart disease	113.0	116.7	121.2	125.8	130.5	135.3	140.2
Deaths from lung cancer	19.7	19.8	19.7	19.6	19.5	19.4	19.5
Death by diseases of the digestive system	17.4	17.9	16.4	15.2	14.0	14.1	13.5
Deaths from chronic liver disease and cirrhosis	4.9	4.3	4.1	3.7	3.4	3.1	2.8
Deaths from ulcers of the stomach and duodenum	1.6	1.6	1.5	1.4	1.5	1.3	1.2

Source: WHO/Euromonitor International
Notes: Data is ranked in descending order by year 2004

Israel: Deaths by disease: growth 1998-2004

Table: 4.612

% year on year growth

	1998	1999	2000	2001	2002	2003	2004
Deaths from heart disease	6.3	3.3	3.9	3.8	3.7	3.7	3.6
Deaths from lung cancer	-1.5	0.7	-0.5	-0.5	-0.5	-0.5	0.3
Death by diseases of the digestive system	3.6	2.9	-8.4	-7.3	-7.9	0.7	-4.4
Deaths from ulcers of the stomach and duodenum	-46.0	2.7	-6.3	-6.7	7.1	-13.3	-5.3
Deaths from chronic liver disease and cirrhosis	17.1	-13.0	-4.7	-9.8	-8.1	-8.8	-8.5

Source: WHO/Euromonitor International
Notes: Data is ranked in descending order by year 2004

Smoking

Israel: Smoking prevalence in population aged 15+ 1998-2004

Table: 4.613

% of population aged 15+

	1998	1999	2000	2001	2002	2003	2004
Smoking prevalence in population aged 15+ (% of population aged 15+)	28.0	27.6	27.0	36.3	36.4	36.9	37.2
Smoking prevalence in male population aged 15+ (% of male population)	33.0	31.0	30.0	40.5	40.6	40.6	40.5
Smoking prevalence in female population aged 15+ (% of female population)	25.0	24.4	24.0	32.3	32.3	33.5	34.1

Source: WHO/OECD/Euromonitor International

Nutrition and Obesity

Israel: Nutrition and obesity 1998-2004

Table: 4.614

As stated

	1998	1999	2000	2001	2002	2003	2004
Availability of fruit and vegetables (kg/capita/year)	369.2	374.9	370.6	360.2	363.4	355.6	352.9
Average supply of calories per day (calories per capita)	3,552.4	3,532.3	3,605.2	3,661.0	3,666.0	3,689.7	3,716.3
Average supply of fat per day (grams per capita)	126.0	123.6	135.0	141.4	139.0	140.6	142.4
Average supply of protein per day (grams per capita)	116.5	115.4	122.4	126.8	128.6	131.8	129.4
Microbiological food-borne diseases (per 100000 population)	35.0	51.0	38.0	54.0	65.0	67.0	72.0
Obese population (BMI 30kg/sq m or more) (% of population aged 15+)	17.8	17.9	17.8	17.8	17.8	18.0	18.1

Source: WHO/OECD/Euromonitor International

Over-the-Counter Healthcare

Israel: Trends in OTC healthcare retail sales 1998-2004

Table: 4.615

As stated

	1998	1999	2000	2001	2002	2003	2004
OTC Healthcare (NIS million)	506.7	536.3	559.7	599.4	729.8	802.4	859.6
OTC Healthcare: real growth in national currency: 1998 = 100	100.0	100.6	103.8	110.0	126.7	138.4	148.7
OTC Healthcare: year on year (% real growth)	4.2	0.6	3.2	5.9	15.3	9.2	7.4
OTC Healthcare (NIS per capita)	84.9	87.5	89.0	93.1	111.1	119.2	124.8

Source: Euromonitor International from industry sources/national statistics

Israel: OTC healthcare retail sales by sector 1998-2004

Table: 4.616

% of OTC retail value sales

	1998	1999	2000	2001	2002	2003	2004
Analgesics	17.9	17.3	16.9	16.7	16.3	15.9	16.0
Cough, cold and allergy (hay fever) remedies	15.5	15.2	15.1	14.1	13.1	12.6	12.4
Digestive remedies	10.4	10.2	10.2	10.1	11.0	10.8	10.7
Medicated skin care	12.8	12.2	12.0	12.1	13.1	12.9	13.1
Vitamins and dietary supplements	33.9	35.9	36.9	38.5	38.6	39.9	39.9

Source: Euromonitor International from industry sources/national statistics
Notes: Only selected sectors are shown, so values are not expected to sum to 100

■ Italy

Socio-economic Parameters

Italy: Socio-economic parameters 1998-2004

Table: 4.617

As stated

	1998	1999	2000	2001	2002	2003	2004
Population: national estimates at January 1st ('000)	57,563.4	57,612.6	57,679.9	57,844.0	58,008.7	58,143.4	58,250.5
% aged 0-14 yrs	14.6	14.5	14.4	14.4	14.4	14.4	14.3
% aged 15-64 yrs	68.0	67.8	67.6	67.4	67.3	67.2	67.1
% aged 65+ yrs	17.4	17.7	18.0	18.2	18.3	18.4	18.6
% Male	48.6	48.5	48.5	48.6	48.6	48.5	48.5
% Female	51.4	51.5	51.5	51.4	51.4	51.5	51.5
% Urban	66.8	66.9	67.0	67.1	67.3	67.5	67.6
Occupants per household at January 1st (Number)	2.7	2.6	2.6	2.6	2.6	2.5	2.5
Households ('000)	21,669.3	21,918.5	22,226.0	22,445.9	22,642.2	22,839.7	23,026.3
Annual rates of inflation (% growth)	2.0	1.7	2.5	2.8	2.5	2.7	2.2
GDP (EUR million)	1,072,872.1	1,107,996.3	1,166,547.0	1,218,535.0	1,260,428.0	1,300,926.0	1,351,794.0
GDP (US$ million)	1,202,689.6	1,180,443.7	1,074,762.3	1,090,401.9	1,186,229.4	1,468,257.4	1,678,486.2
GDP (US$ per capita)	20,893.3	20,489.3	18,633.2	18,850.7	20,449.2	25,252.3	28,814.9

Source: Euromonitor International from International Monetary Fund (IMF), International Financial Statistics and World Economic Outlook/UN/national statistics

Life Expectancy

Italy: Life expectancy 1998-2004

Table: 4.618

As stated

	1998	1999	2000	2001	2002	2003	2004	% change 1998-2004
Life expectancy at birth: total population (years)	78.9	79.0	79.1	79.3	79.7	79.9	80.1	1.48
Life expectancy at birth: total population: year on year growth	0.1	0.1	0.1	0.2	0.4	0.3	0.3	
Healthy life expectancy at birth (years)	73.0							

Source: Euromonitor International from World Bank

© Euromonitor International 2005

Health Expenditure

Italy: Public health expenditure 1998-2004

Table: 4.619

As stated

	1998	1999	2000	2001	2002	2003	2004
Public expenditure on pharmaceuticals and other medical non-durables (EUR million)	7,175.0	7,953.0	9,379.0	12,368.0	12,436.0	11,851.0	12,384.4
Private insurance expenditure (% of total expenditure on health)	0.9	0.9	0.9	0.9	0.9	0.9	0.9
Share of total health expenditure in GDP (% of total GDP)	7.7	7.8	8.2	8.4	8.0	8.4	8.8
Health expenditure (US$ per capita)	1,600.0	1,597.0	1,506.0	1,562.0	1,737.0	1,784.0	1,845.0

Source: Euromonitor International from OECD/national statistics

Italy: Private health expenditure 1998-2004

Table: 4.620

As stated

	1998	1999	2000	2001	2002	2003	2004
Consumer expenditure on health goods and medical services (EUR million)	21,055.4	21,624.1	22,363.6	21,677.8	23,079.9	23,680.0	24,506.7
Consumer expenditure on health goods and medical services: real growth in national currency: 1990 = 100	175.0	176.8	178.3	168.1	174.7	174.6	176.8
Consumer expenditure on health goods and medical services as a percentage of total consumer expenditure	3.3	3.2	3.1	2.9	3.0	3.0	3.0

Source: National statistical offices/OECD/Eurostat/Euromonitor International

Italy: Consumer expenditure on health goods and medical services by sector 1998-2004

Table: 4.621

% of total consumer expenditure on health goods and medical services

	1998	1999	2000	2001	2002	2003	2004
Pharmaceuticals, medical appliances/ equipment	51.8	52.6	52.5	48.2	50.5	51.0	50.5
Outpatient services	38.0	37.7	37.8	41.7	40.0	39.7	40.5
Hospital services	10.2	9.7	9.6	10.1	9.4	9.3	9.0
Total	100.0	100.0	100.0	100.0	100.0	100.0	100.0

Source: National statistical offices/OECD/Eurostat/Euromonitor International

Healthcare Infrastructure and Services

Italy: Healthcare infrastructure and services by sector 1998-2004

Table: 4.622

As stated

	1998	1999	2000	2001	2002	2003	2004
Active pharmacists (number)	60,974	61,326	62,862	63,008	64,130	64,576	64,860
Consultations with GPs (general practitioners) (per capita)	6	6	6	6	6	6	6
Dentists (number)	31,000	35,000	23,000	31,000	31,000	31,000	31,000
Doctors (number)	234,000	241,000	234,000	249,000	253,000	237,000	234,000
Hospital admissions (number)	10,182,892	9,672,963	9,279,501	9,255,297	8,803,602	8,435,061	8,111,174
Hospitals and clinics (number)	1,581	1,580	1,580	1,580	1,581	1,582	1,583
In-patient beds ('000)	285	261	251				
In-patient surgical procedures (number)	3,160,559	3,222,068	3,203,415	3,258,612	3,266,920	3,324,129	3,351,817
Nurses (number)	302,662	298,350	299,166	307,302	312,707	317,660	324,079
Out-patient contacts (per capita)		6					

Source: Euromonitor International from national statistics

Italy: Healthcare infrastructure and services by sector: growth 1998-2004

Table: 4.623

Year on year growth: % change in stated unit

	1998	1999	2000	2001	2002	2003	2004
Active pharmacists (number)	1.8	0.6	2.5	0.2	1.8	0.7	0.4
Consultations with GPs (general practitioners) (per capita)	-4.8	1.7	-2.5	-1.5	-1.5	-1.6	-1.6
Dentists (number)	10.7	12.9	-34.3	34.8	0.0	0.0	0.0
Doctors (number)	2.6	3.0	-2.9	6.4	1.6	-6.3	-1.3
Hospital admissions (number)	-0.6	-5.0	-4.1	-0.3	-4.9	-4.2	-3.8
Hospitals and clinics (number)	-0.5	-0.1	0.0	0.0	0.1	0.1	0.1
In-patient beds (number)	-4.8	-8.7	-3.9				
In-patient surgical procedures (number)		1.9	-0.6	1.7	0.3	1.8	0.8
Nurses (number)	1.0	-1.4	0.3	2.7	1.8	1.6	2.0

Source: Euromonitor International from national statistics

Immunisation

Italy: Vaccination rates by disease type 1998-2004

Table: 4.624

%

	1998	1999	2000	2001	2002	2003	2004
Vaccination rate against DTP (diphtheria, tetanus, pertussis) 1 & 2 (%)					98.0	98.0	98.0
Vaccination rate against MMR (measles, mumps, rubella) (%)	55.0	70.0	72.0	74.0	77.0	79.0	81.0
Vaccination rate against polio (%)	96.0	97.0	98.0	98.0	99.0	99.0	99.0

Source: WHO

Infectious Diseases

Italy: Incidence of disease by type 1998-2004

Table: 4.625

Number

	1998	1999	2000	2001	2002	2003	2004
Incidence of AIDS	2,483	2,201	1,903	989	1,753	894	762
Incidence of diphtheria	0	0	0		0		
Incidence of measles	4,072	2,908	1,457		9,385		
Incidence of polio	0	0	0	0	0		

Source: WHO

Italy: Incidence of disease by type: growth 1998-2004

Table: 4.626

Year on year growth: %

	1998	1999	2000	2001	2002	2003	2004
Incidence of AIDS	-34.3	-11.4	-13.5	-48.0	77.2	-49.0	-14.8
Incidence of measles	-90.1	-28.6	-49.9				

Source: WHO

Causes of Death

Italy: Deaths by disease 1998-2004

Table: 4.627

Number per 100,000 inhabitants

	1998	1999	2000	2001	2002	2003	2004
Death by diseases of the circulatory system	243.2	231.3	230.0	228.0	223.0	219.0	215.7
Death by malignant neoplasms (cancers)	174.6	170.6	169.1	167.8	165.4	162.1	159.5
Deaths from heart disease	136.1	131.7	133.3	133.3	133.4	133.4	133.8
Deaths from lung cancer	54.8	54.9	55.3	55.6	55.9	56.2	56.2
Death by diseases of the respiratory system	35.8	36.7	36.8	37.2	37.8	37.9	38.3
Death by diseases of the digestive system	28.7	27.2	25.8	25.0	23.1	22.9	22.0
Deaths from chronic liver disease and cirrhosis	20.8	19.9	19.1	18.3	17.4	16.6	16.0
Deaths from ulcers of the stomach and duodenum	3.5	3.3	3.3	3.2	3.2	3.1	3.1

Source: WHO/Euromonitor International
Notes: Data is ranked in descending order by year 2004

Italy: Deaths by disease: growth 1998-2004

Table: 4.628

% year on year growth

	1998	1999	2000	2001	2002	2003	2004
Death by diseases of the respiratory system	1.7	2.5	0.3	1.1	1.6	0.3	1.0
Deaths from heart disease	3.4	-3.2	1.2	0.0	0.1	0.0	0.3
Deaths from lung cancer	1.0	0.1	0.8	0.5	0.5	0.5	-0.1
Deaths from ulcers of the stomach and duodenum	1.3	-4.8	-0.5	-3.0	0.0	-3.1	-1.4
Death by diseases of the circulatory system	1.1	-4.9	-0.6	-0.9	-2.2	-1.8	-1.5
Death by malignant neoplasms (cancers)	-0.7	-2.3	-0.9	-0.8	-1.4	-2.0	-1.6
Deaths from chronic liver disease and cirrhosis	-3.8	-4.1	-4.2	-4.2	-4.9	-4.6	-3.8
Death by diseases of the digestive system	-0.7	-5.2	-5.1	-3.1	-7.6	-0.9	-4.1

Source: WHO/Euromonitor International
Notes: Data is ranked in descending order by year 2004

Italy: Other selected causes of death: 1998-2004

Table: 4.629

Number per 100,000 inhabitants

	1998	1999	2000	2001	2002	2003	2004
Death by injury and poisoning	35.6	34.3	34.0	32.9	32.0	33.6	33.5
Death by motor traffic accidents	13.0	12.6	13.0	12.9	12.8	12.4	12.1
Death by suicide and self-inflicted injury	6.3	5.7	5.5	5.4	5.0	4.6	4.3

Source: Euromonitor International from national statistics
Notes: Data is ranked in descending order by year 2004

Italy: Other selected causes of death: growth 1998-2004

Table: 4.630

% year on year growth

	1998	1999	2000	2001	2002	2003	2004
Death by injury and poisoning	-1.7	-3.7	-0.9	-3.2	-2.7	5.0	-0.4
Death by motor traffic accidents	4.8	-3.1	3.2	-0.8	-0.8	-3.1	-2.1
Death by suicide and self-inflicted injury	-4.5	-9.5	-3.5	-1.8	-7.4	-8.0	-6.3

Source: Euromonitor International from national statistics
Notes: Data is ranked in descending order by year 2004

Smoking

Italy: Smoking prevalence in population aged 15+ 1998-2004

Table: 4.631

% of population aged 15+

	1998	1999	2000	2001	2002	2003	2004
Smoking prevalence in population aged 15+ (% of population aged 15+)	24.7	24.7	24.4	24.1	23.5	22.4	22.6
Smoking prevalence in male population aged 15+ (% of male population)	32.6	32.8	31.9	31.6	29.8	29.4	29.5
Smoking prevalence in female population aged 15+ (% of female population)	17.5	17.3	17.4	17.1	17.6	16.0	16.2

Source: WHO/OECD/Euromonitor International

Nutrition and Obesity

Italy: Nutrition and obesity 1998-2004

Table: 4.632

As stated

	1998	1999	2000	2001	2002	2003	2004
Availability of fruit and vegetables (kg/capita/year)	294.5	320.1	329.4	317.8	334.6	342.5	348.6
Average supply of calories per day (calories per capita)	3,628.1	3,685.4	3,701.0	3,696.7	3,670.6	3,656.5	3,642.8
Average supply of fat per day (grams per capita)	154.8	157.6	157.2	157.7	158.1	158.3	158.6
Average supply of protein per day (grams per capita)	111.3	114.3	115.0	113.9	113.1	112.5	112.8
Obese population (BMI 30kg/sq m or more) (% of population aged 15+)	8.4	8.5	8.6	9.0	9.2	9.3	9.6

Source: WHO/OECD/Euromonitor International

Over-the-Counter Healthcare

Italy: Trends in OTC healthcare retail sales 1998-2004

Table: 4.633

As stated

	1998	1999	2000	2001	2002	2003	2004
OTC Healthcare (EUR million)	2,499.2	2,634.9	2,677.2	2,722.2	2,853.7	3,056.5	3,150.2
OTC Healthcare: real growth in national currency: 1998 = 100	100.0	103.7	102.8	101.7	104.0	108.5	109.5
OTC Healthcare: year on year (% real growth)	4.9	3.7	-0.9	-1.1	2.3	4.3	0.9

Source: Euromonitor International from industry sources/national statistics

Italy: OTC healthcare retail sales by sector 1998-2004

Table: 4.634

% of OTC retail value sales

	1998	1999	2000	2001	2002	2003	2004
Analgesics	16.0	15.8	16.0	16.0	15.8	15.1	14.7
Cough, cold and allergy (hay fever) remedies	21.7	21.0	20.1	18.7	18.7	18.3	17.4
Digestive remedies	14.4	13.8	13.6	13.5	13.3	12.7	11.9
Medicated skin care	12.0	12.5	12.4	12.5	12.1	11.9	11.7
Vitamins and dietary supplements	25.4	26.4	27.3	28.4	29.4	31.5	33.9

Source: Euromonitor International from industry sources/national statistics
Notes: Only selected sectors are shown, so values are not expected to sum to 100

Health and Wellness

Italy: Retail sales of packaged foods by health and wellness category 2002-2004

Table: 4.635

EUR million

	2002	2003	2004
Packaged food: Total	55,936.2	58,535.0	60,367.5
Better for you	2,788.2	2,906.8	3,003.3
For food intolerance	72.1	96.0	138.4
Fortified/functional	721.8	849.6	986.9
Organic	802.3	902.7	1,022.0

Source: Euromonitor International from industry sources/national statistics

Italy: Per capita sales of packaged foods by health and wellness category 2002-2004

Table: 4.636

EUR per capita

	2002	2003	2004
Better for you	48.2	50.1	51.7
For food intolerance	1.2	1.7	2.4
Fortified/functional	12.5	14.7	17.0
Organic	13.9	15.6	17.6

Source: Euromonitor International from industry sources/national statistics

Italy: Retail sales of packaged food by health and wellness category: % share of total packaged food market 2002-2004

Table: 4.637

% value

	2002	2003	2004
Better for you	5.0	5.0	5.0
For food intolerance	0.1	0.2	0.2
Fortified/functional	1.3	1.5	1.6
Organic	1.4	1.5	1.7

Source: Euromonitor International from industry sources/national statistics

Italy: Retail sales of packaged food by health and wellness category: real growth index 2002-2004

Table: 4.638

2002 =100

	2002	2003	2004
Better for you	100.00	101.51	102.73
For food intolerance	100.00	129.67	183.03
Fortified/functional	100.00	114.60	130.39
Organic	100.00	109.56	121.48

Source: Euromonitor International from industry sources/national statistics

Italy: Retail sales of better-for-you packaged foods by sector 2002-2004

Table: 4.639

% of total packaged food / as stated

	2002	2003	2004	% real change in value 2002-2004
Combination	0.00	0.00	0.01	23.71
Reduced fat	4.26	4.25	4.25	2.88
Reduced salt	0.11	0.11	0.11	-0.53

Source: Euromonitor International from industry sources/national statistics

Italy: Retail sales of packaged foods for food intolerances by sector 2002-2004

Table: 4.640

% of total packaged food / as stated

	2002	2003	2004	% real change in value 2002-2004
Diabetic	0.01	0.01	0.01	0.47
Gluten-free	0.07	0.08	0.10	34.86
Lactose-free	0.04	0.07	0.12	188.44

Source: *Euromonitor International from industry sources/national statistics*

Italy: Retail sales of naturally healthy packaged foods by sector 2002-2004

Table: 4.641

% of total packaged food / as stated

	2002	2003	2004	% real change in value 2002-2004
High fibre	0.27	0.27	0.27	0.60
Other naturally healthy food	2.05	2.11	2.15	7.68
Soy-based dairy alternatives	0.15	0.15	0.16	8.17

Source: *Euromonitor International from industry sources/national statistics*

■ Japan

Socio-economic Parameters

Japan: Socio-economic parameters 1998-2004

Table: 4.642

As stated

	1998	1999	2000	2001	2002	2003	2004
Population: national estimates at January 1st ('000)	126,479.0	126,686.0	126,929.0	127,291.0	127,435.0	127,593.9	127,738.1
% aged 0-14 yrs	15.1	14.8	14.6	14.4	14.2	14.1	14.0
% aged 15-64 yrs	68.7	68.5	68.1	67.7	67.3	67.1	66.9
% aged 65+ yrs	16.2	16.7	17.4	18.0	18.5	18.9	19.0
% Male	49.0	48.9	48.9	48.9	48.8	48.8	48.8
% Female	51.0	51.1	51.1	51.1	51.2	51.2	51.2
% Urban	78.5	78.7	78.9	79.0	79.2	79.4	79.6
Occupants per household at January 1st (Number)	2.8	2.7	2.7	2.7	2.7	2.7	2.6
Households ('000)	45,653.0	46,228.1	46,782.4	47,265.6	47,683.6	48,081.2	48,480.0
Annual rates of inflation (% growth)	0.7	-0.3	-0.7	-0.7	-0.9	-0.3	0.0
GDP (¥ million)	514,595,000.0	507,224,000.0	511,462,000.0	505,910,475.0	498,045,175.0	497,799,200.0	504,847,325.0
GDP (US$ million)	3,931,056.9	4,452,966.0	4,746,086.4	4,162,878.6	3,972,032.2	4,293,852.5	4,666,173.6
GDP (US$ per capita)	31,080.7	35,149.6	37,391.7	32,703.6	31,169.1	33,652.5	36,529.2

Source: *Euromonitor International from International Monetary Fund (IMF), International Financial Statistics and World Economic Outlook/UN/national statistics*

Life Expectancy

Japan: Life expectancy 1998-2004

Table: 4.643

As stated

	1998	1999	2000	2001	2002	2003	2004	% change 1998-2004
Life expectancy at birth: total population (years)	80.8	81.0	81.3	81.4	81.8	82.2	82.5	2.16
Life expectancy at birth: total population: year on year growth	0.3	0.3	0.4	0.1	0.6	0.4	0.4	
Healthy life expectancy at birth (years)	75.0							

Source: *Euromonitor International from World Bank*

Health Expenditure

Japan: Public health expenditure 1998-2004

Table: 4.644

As stated

	1998	1999	2000	2001	2002	2003	2004
Public expenditure on pharmaceuticals and other medical non-durables (¥ million)	4,452,831.0	4,481,475.0	4,760,467.0	5,087,824.0	5,327,662.0	5,611,430.0	5,907,246.8
Private insurance expenditure (% of total expenditure on health)	0.3	0.3	0.3	0.3	0.3	0.3	0.3
Share of total health expenditure in GDP (% of total GDP)	7.1	7.5	7.7	8.0	8.4	8.7	8.5
Health expenditure (US$ per capita)	2,222.0	2,601.0	2,827.0	2,558.0	2,476.0	2,434.0	2,369.0

Source: Euromonitor International from OECD/national statistics

Japan: Private health expenditure 1998-2004

Table: 4.645

As stated

	1998	1999	2000	2001	2002	2003	2004
Consumer expenditure on health goods and medical services (¥ million)	9,133,400.0	9,515,600.0	9,994,600.0	10,444,800.0	11,041,200.0	11,139,688.0	11,316,300.5
Consumer expenditure on health goods and medical services: real growth in national currency: 1990 = 100	114.4	119.6	126.5	133.2	142.1	143.7	146.0
Consumer expenditure on health goods and medical services as a percentage of total consumer expenditure	3.3	3.4	3.6	3.8	3.9	4.0	4.0

Source: National statistical offices/OECD/Eurostat/Euromonitor International

Japan: Consumer expenditure on health goods and medical services by sector 1998-2004

Table: 4.646

% of total consumer expenditure on health goods and medical services

	1998	1999	2000	2001	2002	2003	2004
Pharmaceuticals, medical appliances/ equipment	45.8	45.9	45.2	45.2	45.0	45.1	45.1
Outpatient services	34.5	34.4	34.5	34.3	34.3	34.2	34.0
Hospital services	19.7	19.7	20.3	20.5	20.7	20.8	20.9
Total	100.0	100.0	100.0	100.0	100.0	100.0	100.0

Source: National statistical offices/OECD/Eurostat/Euromonitor International

Healthcare Infrastructure and Services

Japan: Healthcare infrastructure and services by sector 1998-2004

Table: 4.647

As stated

	1998	1999	2000	2001	2002	2003	2004
Active pharmacists (number)	187,710	192,544	199,797	205,561	212,720	219,906	227,050
Consultations with GPs (general practitioners) (per capita)	15	15	14	15	14	14	14
Dentists (number)	86,847	87,786	89,668	90,583	91,783	93,156	94,349
Doctors (number)	246,548	249,852	253,469	259,342	260,500	264,157	267,826
Hospitals and clinics (number)	161,540	163,270	165,451	167,555	169,079	171,061	172,973
In-patient beds ('000)	1,892	1,873	1,864	1,856	1,839	1,828	1,816
Midwives (number)	24,202	24,457	24,694	24,972	25,252	25,544	25,734
Nurses (number)	985,821		1,042,468	1,071,438	1,096,967	1,107,428	1,130,002

Source: Euromonitor International from national statistics

Japan: Healthcare infrastructure and services by sector: growth 1998-2004

Table: 4.648

Year on year growth: % change in stated unit

	1998	1999	2000	2001	2002	2003	2004
Active pharmacists (number)	4.4	2.6	3.8	2.9	3.5	3.4	3.2
Consultations with GPs (general practitioners) (per capita)	1.4	0.0	-0.7	0.7	-0.2	0.0	0.0
Dentists (number)	0.9	1.1	2.1	1.0	1.3	1.5	1.3
Doctors (number)	1.6	1.3	1.4	2.3	0.4	1.4	1.4
Hospitals and clinics (number)	5.6	1.1	1.3	1.3	0.9	1.2	1.1
In-patient beds (number)	-8.3	-1.0	-0.4	-0.4	-0.9	-0.6	-0.7
Midwives (number)	1.2	1.1	1.0	1.1	1.1	1.2	0.7
Nurses (number)				2.8	2.4	1.0	2.0

Source: Euromonitor International from national statistics

Immunisation

Japan: Vaccination rates by disease type 1998-2004

Table: 4.649

%

	1998	1999	2000	2001	2002	2003	2004
Vaccination rate against DTP (diphtheria, tetanus, pertussis) 1 & 2 (%)			99.0	99.0	99.0	99.0	99.0
Vaccination rate against MMR (measles, mumps, rubella) (%)			96.4	97.6	99.0	99.0	99.0
Vaccination rate against polio (%)			98.5	81.1	99.0	99.0	99.0

Source: WHO

Infectious Diseases

Japan: Incidence of disease by type 1998-2004

Table: 4.650

Number

	1998	1999	2000	2001	2002	2003	2004
Incidence of AIDS	231	300	327	155	132	138	143
Incidence of diphtheria	1		1	1	0		
Incidence of measles	899		22,497	22,552	33,812		
Incidence of polio	0	0	0		0		

Source: WHO

Japan: Incidence of disease by type: growth 1998-2004

Table: 4.651

Year on year growth: %

	1998	1999	2000	2001	2002	2003	2004
Incidence of AIDS	-7.6	29.9	9.0	-52.6	-14.8	4.5	3.6
Incidence of diphtheria				0.0	-100.0		
Incidence of measles				0.2	49.9		

Source: WHO

Causes of Death

Japan: Deaths by disease 1998-2004

Table: 4.652

Number per 100,000 inhabitants

	1998	1999	2000	2001	2002	2003	2004
Death by malignant neoplasms (cancers)	155.7	154.6	153.4	154.4	153.4	153.1	154.5
Death by diseases of the circulatory system	151.3	150.6	145.8	145.0	142.8	139.8	137.6
Death by diseases of the respiratory system	61.1	67.8	67.7	72.2	75.6	68.9	68.8
Deaths from heart disease	57.2	58.9	59.4	60.1	60.9	61.6	62.7
Deaths from lung cancer	40.6	41.6	42.9	44.1	45.4	46.7	48.3
Death by diseases of the digestive system	19.7	20.0	18.4	17.9	16.9	15.6	14.6
Deaths from chronic liver disease and cirrhosis	11.2	11.4	11.2	11.1	11.0	10.9	10.7
Deaths from ulcers of the stomach and duodenum	3.1	3.2	3.3	3.3	3.4	3.5	3.5

Source: WHO/Euromonitor International
Notes: Data is ranked in descending order by year 2004

Japan: Deaths by disease: growth 1998-2004

Table: 4.653

% year on year growth

	1998	1999	2000	2001	2002	2003	2004
Deaths from lung cancer	3.6	2.4	3.1	2.8	2.9	2.9	3.4
Deaths from heart disease	-0.3	3.0	0.8	1.2	1.3	1.1	1.8
Deaths from ulcers of the stomach and duodenum	-0.4	4.6	2.1	0.0	3.0	2.9	1.3
Death by malignant neoplasms (cancers)	-0.1	-0.7	-0.8	0.7	-0.6	-0.2	0.9
Death by diseases of the respiratory system	-3.5	11.0	-0.1	6.6	4.7	-8.9	-0.2
Death by diseases of the circulatory system	-3.1	-0.5	-3.2	-0.5	-1.5	-2.1	-1.6
Deaths from chronic liver disease and cirrhosis	-3.3	2.1	-2.1	-0.9	-0.9	-0.9	-1.8
Death by diseases of the digestive system	-3.9	1.5	-8.0	-2.7	-5.6	-7.7	-6.1

Source: WHO/Euromonitor International
Notes: Data is ranked in descending order by year 2004

Japan: Other selected causes of death: 1998-2004

Table: 4.654

Number per 100,000 inhabitants

	1998	1999	2000	2001	2002	2003	2004
Death by injury and poisoning	46.6	46.2	48.6	49.2	50.2	48.1	47.5
Death by suicide and self-inflicted injury	20.4	20.0	22.9	23.6	24.9	22.4	22.1
Death by motor traffic accidents	9.2	8.8	8.4	8.0	7.6	8.4	8.4

Source: Euromonitor International from national statistics
Notes: Data is ranked in descending order by year 2004

Japan: Other selected causes of death: growth 1998-2004

Table: 4.655

% year on year growth

	1998	1999	2000	2001	2002	2003	2004
Death by motor traffic accidents	-4.2	-4.3	-4.5	-4.8	-5.0	10.5	-0.1
Death by suicide and self-inflicted injury	34.2	-2.0	14.5	3.1	5.5	-10.0	-1.1
Death by injury and poisoning	11.5	-0.9	5.2	1.2	2.0	-4.2	-1.3

Source: Euromonitor International from national statistics
Notes: Data is ranked in descending order by year 2004

Smoking

Japan: Smoking prevalence in population aged 15+ 1998-2004

Table: 4.656

% of population aged 15+

	1998	1999	2000	2001	2002	2003	2004
Smoking prevalence in population aged 15+ (% of population aged 15+)	35.3	34.3	34.3	33.6	33.4	33.0	32.7
Smoking prevalence in male population aged 15+ (% of male population)	55.2	54.0	53.5	52.0	52.0	51.0	50.4
Smoking prevalence in female population aged 15+ (% of female population)	16.5	15.7	16.2	16.3	15.8	16.1	16.1

Source: WHO/OECD/Euromonitor International

Nutrition and Obesity

Japan: Nutrition and obesity 1998-2004

Table: 4.657

As stated

	1998	1999	2000	2001	2002	2003	2004
Average supply of calories per day (calories per capita)	2,754.4	2,771.4	2,799.7	2,788.6	2,760.9	2,746.2	2,731.2
Average supply of fat per day (grams per capita)	80.7	81.9	86.6	86.8	84.6	84.0	83.3
Average supply of protein per day (grams per capita)	91.4	91.6	92.8	91.7	91.8	91.9	91.2
Obese population (BMI 30kg/sq m or more) (% of population aged 15+)	2.1	2.2	2.1	2.4	2.4	2.6	2.7

Source: WHO/OECD/Euromonitor International

Over-the-Counter Healthcare

Japan: Trends in OTC healthcare retail sales 1998-2004

Table: 4.658

As stated

	1998	1999	2000	2001	2002	2003	2004
OTC Healthcare (¥ billion)	2,030.2	2,118.8	2,144.6	2,178.2	2,195.9	2,239.8	2,254.3
OTC Healthcare: real growth in national currency: 1998 = 100	100.0	104.7	106.7	109.2	111.1	113.6	114.6
OTC Healthcare: year on year (% real growth)	-0.2	4.7	1.9	2.3	1.7	2.3	0.8
OTC Healthcare ('000 ¥ per capita)	16.1	16.7	16.9	17.1	17.2	17.6	17.6

Source: Euromonitor International from industry sources/national statistics

Japan: OTC healthcare retail sales by sector 1998-2004

Table: 4.659

% of OTC retail value sales

	1998	1999	2000	2001	2002	2003	2004
Analgesics	132,852.8	127,615.4	126,679.7	125,913.2	126,219.0	124,201.3	123,665.1
Analgesics	7.6	7.2	7.1	7.0	6.9	6.8	6.7
Cough, cold and allergy (hay fever) remedies	16.9	16.4	16.2	15.9	15.8	15.6	14.5
Digestive remedies	9.6	9.0	8.9	9.0	9.0	8.7	8.7
Medicated skin care	7.6	8.8	8.5	8.4	8.3	8.3	8.3
Vitamins and dietary supplements	52.2	52.8	53.6	53.9	54.0	54.6	55.6

Source: Euromonitor International from industry sources/national statistics
Notes: Only selected sectors are shown, so values are not expected to sum to 100

Health and Wellness

Japan: Retail sales of packaged foods by health and wellness category 2002-2004

YEN billion

	2002	2003	2004
Packaged food: Total	18,583.9	18,577.1	18,616.1
Better for you	429.5	449.8	465.1
For food intolerance	10.1	10.4	10.7
Fortified/functional	832.2	874.8	909.2
Organic	42.6	44.7	46.8

Source: Euromonitor International from industry sources/national statistics

Japan: Retail sales of packaged food by health and wellness category: % share of total packaged food market 2002-2004

% value

	2002	2003	2004
Better for you	2.3	2.4	2.5
For food intolerance	0.1	0.1	0.1
Fortified/functional	4.5	4.7	4.9
Organic	0.2	0.2	0.3

Source: Euromonitor International from industry sources/national statistics

Japan: Retail sales of packaged food by health and wellness category: real growth index 2002-2004

2002 =100

	2002	2003	2004
Better for you	100.00	105.03	109.28
For food intolerance	100.00	103.36	106.87
Fortified/functional	100.00	105.43	110.24
Organic	100.00	105.26	110.77

Source: Euromonitor International from industry sources/national statistics

Japan: Retail sales of better-for-you packaged foods by sector 2002-2004

% of total packaged food / as stated

	2002	2003	2004	% real change in value 2002-2004
Reduced fat	1.59	1.66	1.71	8.55
Reduced salt	0.11	0.11	0.12	11.69

Source: Euromonitor International from industry sources/national statistics

Japan: Retail sales of packaged foods for food intolerances by sector 2002-2004

% of total packaged food / as stated

	2002	2003	2004	% real change in value 2002-2004
Diabetic	0.03	0.03	0.03	8.10
Gluten-free	0.00	0.00	0.00	14.76
Lactose-free	0.02	0.02	0.02	3.66

Source: Euromonitor International from industry sources/national statistics

Japan: Retail sales of naturally healthy packaged foods by sector 2002-2004

Table: 4.665

% of total packaged food / as stated

	2002	2003	2004	% real change in value 2002-2004
High fibre	1.34	1.36	1.37	3.05
Other naturally healthy food	0.34	0.35	0.36	5.83
Soy-based dairy alternatives	0.14	0.17	0.21	52.53

Source: *Euromonitor International from industry sources/national statistics*

■ Jordan

Socio-economic Parameters

Jordan: Socio-economic parameters 1998-2004

Table: 4.666

As stated

	1998	1999	2000	2001	2002	2003	2004
Population: national estimates at January 1st ('000)	4,665.5	4,814.4	4,961.1	5,108.2	5,254.9	5,400.0	5,542.2
% aged 0-14 yrs	39.9	39.5	39.1	38.7	38.2	37.8	37.4
% aged 15-64 yrs	57.5	57.8	58.2	58.5	58.8	59.2	59.5
% aged 65+ yrs	2.6	2.7	2.8	2.9	2.9	3.0	3.1
% Male	52.2	52.2	52.1	52.1	52.1	52.1	52.0
% Female	47.8	47.8	47.9	47.9	47.9	47.9	48.0
% Urban	73.1	73.6	73.8	74.2	74.7	75.3	75.9
Occupants per household at January 1st (Number)	5.8	5.8	5.8	5.7	5.7	5.7	5.7
Households ('000)	804.3	833.5	862.5	891.1	920.2	948.7	976.7
Annual rates of inflation (% growth)	3.1	0.6	0.7	1.8	1.8	2.3	3.4
GDP (JOD million)	5,609.9	5,767.4	5,989.1	6,339.0	6,698.8	7,056.2	7,779.0
GDP (US$ million)	7,912.4	8,134.5	8,447.2	8,940.9	9,448.2	9,952.3	10,971.8
GDP (US$ per capita)	1,695.9	1,689.6	1,702.7	1,750.3	1,798.0	1,843.0	1,979.7

Source: *Euromonitor International from International Monetary Fund (IMF), International Financial Statistics and World Economic Outlook/UN/national statistics*

Life Expectancy

Jordan: Life expectancy 1998-2004

Table: 4.667

As stated

	1998	1999	2000	2001	2002	2003	2004	% change 1998-2004
Life expectancy at birth: total population (years)	70.3	70.6	70.7	70.8	70.8	71.0	71.1	1.11
Life expectancy at birth: total population: year on year growth	0.4	0.4	0.2	0.1	0.0	0.4	0.1	
Healthy life expectancy at birth (years)	60.0			73.5	73.6			
Healthy life expectancy at birth: year on year growth					0.1			

Source: *Euromonitor International from World Bank*

Sanitation

Jordan: Improved sanitary facilities and water source 2000

Table: 4.668

As stated

	2000
Population with access to improved sanitary facilities (% of population)	99.0
Population with access to improved water source (% of population)	96.0
Population with improved access to sanitation facilities, rural (% of rural population with access)	98.0
Population with improved access to sanitation facilities, urban (% of urban population with access)	100.0

Source: *National statistics/World Bank*

Health Expenditure

Jordan: Public health expenditure 1998-2004

Table: 4.669

As stated

	1998	1999	2000	2001	2002	2003	2004
Share of total health expenditure in GDP (% of total GDP)	8.1	8.6	9.2	9.5	9.9	9.5	9.8
Health expenditure (US$ per capita)	144.0	148.0	154.0	163.0	165.0	171.0	176.0

Source: Euromonitor International from OECD/national statistics

Jordan: Private health expenditure 1998-2004

Table: 4.670

As stated

	1998	1999	2000	2001	2002	2003	2004
Consumer expenditure on health goods and medical services (JOD million)	111.8	114.9	134.0	142.2	143.5	150.0	157.0
Consumer expenditure on health goods and medical services: real growth in national currency: 1990 = 100	214.9	219.6	254.5	265.3	262.9	268.5	271.9
Consumer expenditure on health goods and medical services as a percentage of total consumer expenditure	2.6	2.6	2.6	2.6	2.6	2.7	2.7

Source: National statistical offices/OECD/Eurostat/Euromonitor International

Jordan: Consumer expenditure on health goods and medical services by sector 1998-2004

Table: 4.671

% of total consumer expenditure on health goods and medical services

	1998	1999	2000	2001	2002	2003	2004
Pharmaceuticals, medical appliances/ equipment	28.2	28.9	30.4	30.9	31.1	30.9	31.0
Outpatient services	63.4	62.6	61.2	60.1	59.9	59.9	59.8
Hospital services	8.4	8.5	8.4	9.0	9.0	9.2	9.2
Total	100.0	100.0	100.0	100.0	100.0	100.0	100.0

Source: National statistical offices/OECD/Eurostat/Euromonitor International

Healthcare Infrastructure and Services

Jordan: Healthcare infrastructure and services by sector 1998-2004

Table: 4.672

As stated

	1998	1999	2000	2001	2002	2003	2004
Active pharmacists (number)	173	177	189	213	226	235	244
Dentists (number)	307	350	396	431	471	492	503
Doctors (number)	2,447	2,638	2,815	2,967	2,911	2,872	2,859
Hospitals and clinics (number)	83	84	86	91	95	97	99
In-patient beds ('000)	9	9	9	9	9	10	10
Midwives (number)	668	716	845	832	806	801	796
Nurses (number)	1,728	1,882	1,999	1,963	2,016	2,064	2,087

Source: Euromonitor International from national statistics

Jordan: Healthcare infrastructure and services by sector: growth 1998-2004

Table: 4.673

Year on year growth: % change in stated unit

	1998	1999	2000	2001	2002	2003	2004
Active pharmacists (number)	-5.5	2.3	6.8	12.7	6.1	4.0	3.8
Dentists (number)	-0.3	14.0	13.1	8.8	9.3	4.5	2.2
Doctors (number)	0.5	7.8	6.7	5.4	-1.9	-1.3	-0.5
Hospitals and clinics (number)	10.7	1.2	2.4	5.8	4.4	2.1	2.1
In-patient beds (number)	4.6	-4.1	-0.2	3.2	4.5	1.2	1.1
Midwives (number)	5.0	7.2	18.0	-1.5	-3.1	-0.6	-0.6
Nurses (number)	-3.8	8.9	6.2	-1.8	2.7	2.4	1.1

Source: Euromonitor International from national statistics

Immunisation

Jordan: Vaccination rates by disease type 1998-2004

Table: 4.674

%

	1998	1999	2000	2001	2002	2003	2004
Vaccination rate against DTP (diphtheria, tetanus, pertussis) 1 & 2 (%)			89.0	99.0	96.0	96.0	95.0
Vaccination rate against MMR (measles, mumps, rubella) (%)	86.0	83.0	94.0	99.0	95.0	97.0	98.0
Vaccination rate against polio (%)	91.0	85.0	94.0	97.0	95.0	96.0	97.0

Source: WHO

Infectious Diseases

Jordan: Incidence of disease by type 1998-2004

Table: 4.675

Number

	1998	1999	2000	2001	2002	2003	2004
Incidence of AIDS	11	3	14	7	8	8	9
Incidence of diphtheria	0	0	0	0	0		
Incidence of measles	428	115	32	61	19		
Incidence of polio	0	0	0	0	0		

Source: WHO

Jordan: Incidence of disease by type: growth 1998-2004

Table: 4.676

Year on year growth: %

	1998	1999	2000	2001	2002	2003	2004
Incidence of AIDS	-8.3	-72.7	366.7	-50.0	14.3	0.0	12.5
Incidence of measles	-93.9	-73.1	-72.2	90.6	-68.9		

Source: WHO

Causes of Death

Jordan: Other selected causes of death: 1998-2004

Table: 4.677

Number per 100,000 inhabitants

	1998	1999	2000	2001	2002	2003	2004
Death by suicide and self-inflicted injury	0.1	0.1	0.1	0.1	0.1	0.1	0.1

Source: Euromonitor International from national statistics

Jordan: Other selected causes of death: growth 1998-2004

Table: 4.678

% year on year growth

	1998	1999	2000	2001	2002	2003	2004
Death by suicide and self-inflicted injury	0.0	0.0	0.0	0.0	0.0	0.0	-0.7

Source: Euromonitor International from national statistics

Smoking

Jordan: Smoking prevalence in population aged 15+ 1998-2004

Table: 4.679

% of population aged 15+

	1998	1999	2000	2001	2002	2003	2004
Smoking prevalence in population aged 15+ (% of population aged 15+)	30.1	30.3	30.5	30.8	31.4	31.9	32.4
Smoking prevalence in male population aged 15+ (% of male population)	44.6	44.8	45.4	46.4	47.3	48.2	49.1
Smoking prevalence in female population aged 15+ (% of female population)	13.9	14.2	13.8	13.4	13.7	13.7	13.9

Source: WHO/OECD/Euromonitor International

Nutrition and Obesity

Jordan: Nutrition and obesity 1998-2004

Table: 4.680

As stated

	1998	1999	2000	2001	2002	2003	2004
Average supply of calories per day (calories per capita)	2,612.6	2,624.8	2,641.7	2,688.1	2,673.5	2,674.2	2,681.1
Average supply of fat per day (grams per capita)	80.1	75.6	77.6	84.2	81.5	81.3	81.9
Average supply of protein per day (grams per capita)	67.9	68.4	71.3	70.1	67.4	66.0	67.2
Obese population (BMI 30kg/sq m or more) (% of population aged 15+)	14.5	14.4	14.6	14.6	14.7	14.7	14.7

Source: WHO/OECD/Euromonitor International

Over-the-Counter Healthcare

Jordan: Trends in OTC healthcare retail sales 1998-2004

Table: 4.681

As stated

	1998	1999	2000	2001	2002	2003	2004
OTC Healthcare (US$ million)	2.8	3.3	3.2	3.3	3.0	3.2	3.5
OTC Healthcare (US$ per capita)	0.6	0.7	0.6	0.6	0.6	0.6	0.6

Source: Euromonitor International from industry sources/national statistics

Jordan: OTC healthcare retail sales by sector 1998-2004

Table: 4.682

% of OTC retail value sales

	1998	1999	2000	2001	2002	2003	2004
Analgesics	23.0	23.5	23.7	24.0	24.7	24.5	24.8
Cough, cold and allergy (hay fever) remedies	36.7	36.6	36.2	35.9	35.9	37.2	37.9
Digestive remedies	16.0	16.0	15.9	15.8	15.5	15.1	14.8
Medicated skin care	18.0	17.8	18.0	18.3	17.8	17.2	16.7
Vitamins and dietary supplements	4.3	4.2	4.2	4.1	4.1	4.0	3.9

Source: *Euromonitor International from industry sources/national statistics*
Notes: *Only selected sectors are shown, so values are not expected to sum to 100*

■ **Kazakhstan**

Socio-economic Parameters

Kazakhstan: Socio-economic parameters 1998-2004

Table: 4.683

As stated

	1998	1999	2000	2001	2002	2003	2004
Population: national estimates at January 1st ('000)	16,085.8	15,887.3	15,715.4	15,585.4	15,499.9	15,450.0	15,417.4
% aged 0-14 yrs	28.9	28.5	28.0	27.3	26.5	25.6	24.7
% aged 15-64 yrs	64.2	64.7	65.2	65.7	66.2	66.7	67.2
% aged 65+ yrs	6.9	6.8	6.8	7.0	7.3	7.7	8.1
% Male	48.4	48.3	48.2	48.1	48.1	48.0	48.0
% Female	51.6	51.7	51.8	51.9	51.9	52.0	52.0
% Urban	56.5	56.6	56.6	56.7	56.8	57.4	57.7
Occupants per household at January 1st (Number)	3.9	3.8	3.8	3.7	3.6	3.6	3.5
Households ('000)	4,103.9	4,152.7	4,161.5	4,235.0	4,299.8	4,335.7	4,358.7
Annual rates of inflation (% growth)	7.1	8.3	13.2	8.4	5.8	6.4	6.7
GDP (KZT million)	1,652,550.0	2,098,570.0	2,608,200.0	3,162,140.0	3,705,130.0	4,488,830.0	5,542,500.0
GDP (US$ million)	21,104.5	17,557.9	18,350.4	21,549.9	24,172.5	30,010.4	40,743.2
GDP (US$ per capita)	1,312.0	1,105.2	1,167.7	1,382.7	1,559.5	1,942.4	2,642.7

Source: *Euromonitor International from International Monetary Fund (IMF), International Financial Statistics and World Economic Outlook/UN/national statistics*

Life Expectancy

Kazakhstan: Life expectancy 1998-2004

Table: 4.684

As stated

	1998	1999	2000	2001	2002	2003	2004	% change 1998-2004
Life expectancy at birth: total population (years)	62.5	62.7	62.5	63.0	63.6	64.2	64.7	3.39
Life expectancy at birth: total population: year on year growth	0.3	0.3	-0.3	0.8	1.0	0.9	0.8	
Healthy life expectancy at birth (years)	56.0			58.5	58.5			
Healthy life expectancy at birth: year on year growth					0.1			

Source: *Euromonitor International from World Bank*

© **Euromonitor International 2005**

Sanitation

Kazakhstan: Improved sanitary facilities and water source 2000

As stated

	2000
Population with access to improved sanitary facilities (% of population)	99.0
Population with access to improved water source (% of population)	91.0
Population with improved access to sanitation facilities, rural (% of rural population with access)	98.0
Population with improved access to sanitation facilities, urban (% of urban population with access)	100.0

Source: National statistics/World Bank

Health Expenditure

Kazakhstan: Public health expenditure 1998-2004

As stated

	1998	1999	2000	2001	2002	2003	2004
Share of total health expenditure in GDP (% of total GDP)	3.5	3.5	3.3	3.1	3.0	2.9	2.8
Health expenditure (US$ per capita)	53.0	46.0	48.0	48.0	56.0	59.0	63.0

Source: Euromonitor International from OECD/national statistics

Kazakhstan: Private health expenditure 1998-2004

As stated

	1998	1999	2000	2001	2002	2003	2004
Consumer expenditure on health goods and medical services (KZT million)	52,534.2	58,871.1	65,904.5	78,381.3	89,608.3	92,882.3	102,580.4
Consumer expenditure on health goods and medical services as a percentage of total consumer expenditure	4.0	3.9	3.9	3.9	4.0	3.7	3.7

Source: National statistical offices/OECD/Eurostat/Euromonitor International

Kazakhstan: Consumer expenditure on health goods and medical services by sector 1998-2004

% of total consumer expenditure on health goods and medical services

	1998	1999	2000	2001	2002	2003	2004
Pharmaceuticals, medical appliances/ equipment	44.2	41.6	40.5	41.0	40.4	41.7	41.5
Outpatient services	50.5	53.8	55.4	54.9	55.1	54.0	54.1
Hospital services	5.3	4.6	4.1	4.1	4.5	4.4	4.4
Total	100.0	100.0	100.0	100.0	100.0	100.0	100.0

Source: National statistical offices/OECD/Eurostat/Euromonitor International

Healthcare Infrastructure and Services

Kazakhstan: Healthcare infrastructure and services by sector 1998-2004

Table: 4.689

As stated

	1998	1999	2000	2001	2002	2003	2004
Active pharmacists (number)	11,100	11,100	11,200	11,200	11,234	11,267	11,289
Dentists (number)	4,095						
Doctors (number)	53,200	50,600	49,000	51,300	53,700	54,600	54,900
Hospital admissions (number)	2,346,025	2,195,384	2,214,351	2,306,982	2,427,000	2,495,213	2,551,301
Hospitals and clinics (number)	991	917	938	981	1,005	1,029	1,051
In-patient beds ('000)	124	108	107	110	112	115	117
Nurses (number)	120,000	114,100	112,300	109,100	110,900	111,100	111,200
Out-patient contacts (per capita)	6	5	6	6	6	6	6

Source: Euromonitor International from national statistics

Kazakhstan: Healthcare infrastructure and services by sector: growth 1998-2004

Table: 4.690

Year on year growth: % change in stated unit

	1998	1999	2000	2001	2002	2003	2004
Active pharmacists (number)	1.8	0.0	0.9	0.0	0.3	0.3	0.2
Doctors (number)	-2.4	-4.9	-3.2	4.7	4.7	1.7	0.5
Hospital admissions (number)	-1.4	-6.4	0.9	4.2	5.2	2.8	2.2
Hospitals and clinics (number)	-1.5	-7.5	2.3	4.6	2.4	2.4	2.1
In-patient beds (number)	-9.5	-12.4	-1.2	3.1	1.5	2.6	2.1
Nurses (number)	-7.7	-4.9	-1.6	-2.8	1.6	0.2	0.1
Out-patient contacts (per capita)	3.6	-5.3	1.9	3.6	8.8	-1.6	1.6

Source: Euromonitor International from national statistics

Immunisation

Kazakhstan: Vaccination rates by disease type 1998-2004

Table: 4.691

%

	1998	1999	2000	2001	2002	2003	2004
Vaccination rate against DTP (diphtheria, tetanus, pertussis) 1 & 2 (%)			97.3	95.0	95.0	95.0	95.0
Vaccination rate against MMR (measles, mumps, rubella) (%)	99.0	99.0	99.0	95.0	95.0	94.0	93.0
Vaccination rate against polio (%)	99.0	99.0	97.2	95.0	95.0	93.0	92.0

Source: WHO

Infectious Diseases

Kazakhstan: Incidence of disease by type 1998-2004

Table: 4.692

Number

	1998	1999	2000	2001	2002	2003	2004
Incidence of AIDS	9	5	8	10	29	57	32
Incidence of diphtheria	75	17	13	14	14		
Incidence of measles	1,935	1,391	245	94	18		
Incidence of polio	0	0	0	0	0		

Source: WHO

Kazakhstan: Incidence of disease by type: growth 1998-2004

Table: 4.693

Year on year growth: %

	1998	1999	2000	2001	2002	2003	2004
Incidence of AIDS	12.5	-44.4	60.0	25.0	190.0	96.6	-43.9
Incidence of diphtheria	-53.7	-77.3	-23.5	7.7	0.0		
Incidence of measles	1,512.5	-28.1	-82.4	-61.6	-80.9		

Source: WHO

Causes of Death

Kazakhstan: Deaths by disease 1998-2004

Table: 4.694

Number per 100,000 inhabitants

	1998	1999	2000	2001	2002	2003	2004
Death by diseases of the circulatory system	498.6	489.4	500.5	499.0	498.0	498.0	492.7
Deaths from heart disease	250.1	244.1	243.0	240.6	238.2	235.7	233.8
Death by malignant neoplasms (cancers)	133.0	129.6	129.1	128.6	129.7	130.4	130.4
Death by diseases of the respiratory system	74.9	68.3	71.1	67.6	65.7	70.5	70.4
Death by diseases of the digestive system	40.4	38.0	41.4	37.3	36.5	35.3	33.8
Deaths from lung cancer	27.4	25.8	25.9	25.5	25.1	24.8	24.3
Deaths from chronic liver disease and cirrhosis	20.7	19.4	19.1	18.6	18.1	17.5	17.0
Deaths from ulcers of the stomach and duodenum	3.8	1.0	1.1	1.2	1.0	0.9	0.8

Source: WHO/Euromonitor International
Notes: Data is ranked in descending order by year 2004

Kazakhstan: Deaths by disease: growth 1998-2004

Table: 4.695

% year on year growth

	1998	1999	2000	2001	2002	2003	2004
Death by malignant neoplasms (cancers)	-0.9	-2.6	-0.4	-0.4	0.9	0.5	0.0
Death by diseases of the respiratory system	-9.9	-8.8	4.1	-4.9	-2.8	7.3	-0.1
Deaths from heart disease	0.6	-2.4	-0.4	-1.0	-1.0	-1.0	-0.8
Death by diseases of the circulatory system	0.2	-1.8	2.3	-0.3	-0.2	0.0	-1.1
Deaths from lung cancer	3.2	-5.7	0.3	-1.5	-1.6	-1.2	-1.9
Deaths from chronic liver disease and cirrhosis	0.6	-5.9	-1.7	-2.6	-2.7	-3.3	-2.6
Death by diseases of the digestive system	-6.7	-5.9	8.9	-9.9	-2.1	-3.3	-4.3
Deaths from ulcers of the stomach and duodenum	-1.9	-72.9	8.0	9.1	-16.7	-10.0	-7.1

Source: WHO/Euromonitor International
Notes: Data is ranked in descending order by year 2004

Kazakhstan: Other selected causes of death: 1998-2004

Table: 4.696

Number per 100,000 inhabitants

	1998	1999	2000	2001	2002	2003	2004
Death by injury and poisoning	138.7	126.0	140.7	137.1	138.1	138.0	138.3
Death by suicide and self-inflicted injury	28.7	26.8	29.9	29.7	30.3	29.5	29.6

Source: Euromonitor International from national statistics
Notes: Data is ranked in descending order by year 2004

Kazakhstan: Other selected causes of death: growth 1998-2004

Table: 4.697

% year on year growth

	1998	1999	2000	2001	2002	2003	2004
Death by suicide and self-inflicted injury	-5.6	-6.6	11.6	-0.7	2.0	-2.6	0.4
Death by injury and poisoning	-1.9	-9.2	11.7	-2.6	0.7	-0.1	0.3

Source: Euromonitor International from national statistics
Notes: Data is ranked in descending order by year 2004

Smoking

Kazakhstan: Smoking prevalence in population aged 15+ 1998-2004

Table: 4.698

% of population aged 15+

	1998	1999	2000	2001	2002	2003	2004
Smoking prevalence in population aged 15+ (% of population aged 15+)	31.1	31.7	28.0	23.9	21.7	20.6	20.4
Smoking prevalence in male population aged 15+ (% of male population)	56.8	57.9	58.9	46.5	44.3	42.7	41.2
Smoking prevalence in female population aged 15+ (% of female population)	8.0	8.3	8.6	7.6	6.8	6.4	5.7

Source: WHO/OECD/Euromonitor International

Nutrition and Obesity

Kazakhstan: Nutrition and obesity 1998-2004

Table: 4.699

As stated

	1998	1999	2000	2001	2002	2003	2004
Availability of fruit and vegetables (kg/capita/year)	77.2	84.6	102.5	116.2	119.2	128.5	135.2
Average supply of calories per day (calories per capita)	2,531.9	2,222.8	2,389.6	2,570.8	2,676.6	2,718.7	2,773.8
Average supply of fat per day (grams per capita)	62.3	63.6	71.6	74.1	76.0	79.3	80.4
Average supply of protein per day (grams per capita)	81.8	72.4	76.2	81.6	84.7	88.6	93.0
Microbiological food-borne diseases (per 100000 population)	1.0	2.0	7.0	6.0	6.0	6.0	6.0
Obese population (BMI 30kg/sq m or more) (% of population aged 15+)	5.6	5.8	5.3	5.4	5.5	5.6	5.7

Source: WHO/OECD/Euromonitor International

■ **Kuwait**

Socio-economic Parameters

Kuwait: Socio-economic parameters 1998-2004

Table: 4.700

As stated

	1998	1999	2000	2001	2002	2003	2004
Population: national estimates at January 1st ('000)	2,129.2	2,273.7	2,228.4	2,243.1	2,301.8	2,357.2	2,413.8
% aged 0-14 yrs	26.5	25.6	25.9	25.6	25.3	25.0	24.9
% aged 15-64 yrs	72.1	73.0	72.7	72.8	73.1	73.3	73.3
% aged 65+ yrs	1.4	1.4	1.5	1.6	1.6	1.7	1.8
% Male	60.6	61.1	60.8	60.4	60.3	60.2	60.1
% Female	39.4	38.9	39.2	39.6	39.7	39.8	39.9
% Urban	97.4	97.5	97.6	97.6	97.7	97.8	97.8
Occupants per household at January 1st (Number)	7.6	7.5	6.9	6.6	6.5	6.4	6.4
Households ('000)	280.5	302.6	322.3	339.0	353.4	365.8	377.7
Annual rates of inflation (% growth)	0.2	3.0	1.8	1.7	1.4	1.0	1.1
GDP (KWD million)	7,656.3	8,884.0	11,356.7	10,445.7	10,691.4	12,441.3	15,267.0
GDP (US$ million)	25,122.6	29,183.8	37,022.4	34,060.4	35,179.0	41,747.6	51,805.2
GDP (US$ per capita)	11,799.2	12,835.3	16,614.2	15,184.6	15,283.3	17,711.1	21,462.5

Source: Euromonitor International from International Monetary Fund (IMF), International Financial Statistics and World Economic Outlook/UN/national statistics

Life Expectancy

Kuwait: Life expectancy 1998-2004

Table: 4.701

As stated

	1998	1999	2000	2001	2002	2003	2004	% change 1998-2004
Life expectancy at birth: total population (years)	75.0	75.1	75.4	75.3	76.2	76.8	77.3	3.11
Life expectancy at birth: total population: year on year growth	0.2	0.2	0.4	-0.1	1.2	0.7	0.7	
Healthy life expectancy at birth (years)	63.0			52.1	52.4			
Healthy life expectancy at birth: year on year growth					0.7			

Source: Euromonitor International from World Bank

Health Expenditure

Kuwait: Public health expenditure 1998-2004

Table: 4.702

As stated

	1998	1999	2000	2001	2002	2003	2004
Share of total health expenditure in GDP (% of total GDP)	4.4	3.9	3.5	3.9	3.9	3.9	3.8
Health expenditure (US$ per capita)	557.0	531.0	516.0	539.0	547.0	552.0	564.0

Source: Euromonitor International from OECD/national statistics

Kuwait: Private health expenditure 1998-2004

Table: 4.703

As stated

	1998	1999	2000	2001	2002	2003	2004
Consumer expenditure on health goods and medical services (KWD million)	47.4	50.1	52.3	58.3	66.0	68.2	71.8
Consumer expenditure on health goods and medical services: real growth in national currency: 1990 = 100	120.7	123.8	126.9	139.4	155.6	159.1	165.6
Consumer expenditure on health goods and medical services as a percentage of total consumer expenditure	1.3	1.3	1.3	1.3	1.3	1.3	1.4

Source: National statistical offices/OECD/Eurostat/Euromonitor International

Kuwait: Consumer expenditure on health goods and medical services by sector 1998-2004

Table: 4.704

% of total consumer expenditure on health goods and medical services

	1998	1999	2000	2001	2002	2003	2004
Pharmaceuticals, medical appliances/ equipment	51.6	52.1	51.9	51.7	52.1	52.7	53.1
Outpatient services	42.7	42.1	41.8	41.5	40.9	40.8	40.4
Hospital services	5.8	5.8	6.3	6.8	7.1	6.5	6.5
Total	100.0	100.0	100.0	100.0	100.0	100.0	100.0

Source: *National statistical offices/OECD/Eurostat/Euromonitor International*

Healthcare Infrastructure and Services

Kuwait: Healthcare infrastructure and services by sector 1998-2004

Table: 4.705

As stated

	1998	1999	2000	2001	2002	2003	2004
Active pharmacists (number)	479	447	448	451	454	458	461
Dentists (number)	425	492	517	522	534	552	559
Doctors (number)	3,117	3,178	3,204	3,270	3,323	3,373	3,431
Hospitals and clinics (number)	85	86	90	91	92	94	95
In-patient beds ('000)	4	4	5	5	5	5	5
Nurses (number)	7,684	7,338	8,232	8,467	8,704	8,906	9,095

Source: *Euromonitor International from national statistics*

Kuwait: Healthcare infrastructure and services by sector: growth 1998-2004

Table: 4.706

Year on year growth: % change in stated unit

	1998	1999	2000	2001	2002	2003	2004
Active pharmacists (number)	-46.5	-6.7	0.2	0.7	0.7	0.9	0.7
Dentists (number)	4.4	15.8	5.1	1.0	2.3	3.4	1.3
Doctors (number)	3.4	2.0	0.8	2.1	1.6	1.5	1.7
Hospitals and clinics (number)	0.0	1.2	4.7	1.1	1.1	2.2	1.1
In-patient beds (number)	-1.3	1.0	3.2	4.9	2.1	2.0	2.0
Nurses (number)	0.9	-4.5	12.2	2.9	2.8	2.3	2.1

Source: *Euromonitor International from national statistics*

Immunisation

Kuwait: Vaccination rates by disease type 1998-2004

Table: 4.707

%

	1998	1999	2000	2001	2002	2003	2004
Vaccination rate against DTP (diphtheria, tetanus, pertussis) 1 & 2 (%)			97.0	97.0	97.0	97.0	97.0
Vaccination rate against MMR (measles, mumps, rubella) (%)	99.0	95.7	98.8	99.0	99.0	99.0	99.0
Vaccination rate against polio (%)	94.0	93.9	93.9	93.9	93.9	94.0	94.0

Source: *WHO*

Infectious Diseases

Kuwait: Incidence of disease by type 1998-2004

Table: 4.708

Number

	1998	1999	2000	2001	2002	2003	2004
Incidence of AIDS	19	4	12	5	9	10	7
Incidence of diphtheria	0	0	0				
Incidence of measles	90	13	6				
Incidence of polio	0	0	0	0			

Source: WHO

Kuwait: Incidence of disease by type: growth 1998-2004

Table: 4.709

Year on year growth: %

	1998	1999	2000	2001	2002	2003	2004
Incidence of AIDS	850.0	-78.9	200.0	-58.3	80.0	11.1	-30.0
Incidence of measles	246.2	-85.6	-53.8				

Source: WHO

Causes of Death

Kuwait: Deaths by disease 1998-2004

Table: 4.710

Number per 100,000 inhabitants

	1998	1999	2000	2001	2002	2003	2004
Deaths from heart disease	37.4	35.5	29.3	26.0	22.2	18.5	15.7
Deaths from lung cancer	3.3	2.6	3.3	3.1	2.9	2.7	2.5
Deaths from chronic liver disease and cirrhosis	1.8	1.5	1.6	1.4	1.2	1.0	0.9
Deaths from ulcers of the stomach and duodenum	0.2	0.2	0.3	0.3	0.4	0.4	0.4

Source: WHO/Euromonitor International
Notes: Data is ranked in descending order by year 2004

Kuwait: Deaths by disease: growth 1998-2004

Table: 4.711

% year on year growth

	1998	1999	2000	2001	2002	2003	2004
Deaths from ulcers of the stomach and duodenum	-28.6	20.3	34.7	-6.1	33.3	0.0	8.2
Deaths from lung cancer	-14.6	-21.0	27.7	-7.0	-6.5	-6.9	-6.6
Deaths from chronic liver disease and cirrhosis	22.3	-16.8	2.2	-9.8	-14.3	-16.7	-14.2
Deaths from heart disease	-9.0	-5.2	-17.4	-11.3	-14.6	-16.7	-14.9

Source: WHO/Euromonitor International
Notes: Data is ranked in descending order by year 2004

Smoking

Kuwait: Smoking prevalence in population aged 15+ 1998-2004

Table: 4.712

% of population aged 15+

	1998	1999	2000	2001	2002	2003	2004
Smoking prevalence in population aged 15+ (% of population aged 15+)	30.9	30.6	30.1	29.7	29.2	29.2	28.8
Smoking prevalence in male population aged 15+ (% of male population)	38.2	38.6	37.8	36.8	36.7	35.9	35.5
Smoking prevalence in female population aged 15+ (% of female population)	18.0	16.0	16.3	17.3	16.3	17.8	17.5

Source: WHO/OECD/Euromonitor International

Nutrition and Obesity

Kuwait: Nutrition and obesity 1998-2004

As stated

	1998	1999	2000	2001	2002	2003	2004
Average supply of calories per day (calories per capita)	3,102.2	3,054.3	3,084.0	3,062.9	3,010.0	2,978.0	2,945.0
Average supply of fat per day (grams per capita)	104.3	108.6	111.4	112.1	109.1	107.7	106.4
Average supply of protein per day (grams per capita)	92.9	88.9	86.6	84.0	79.8	76.4	73.2
Obese population (BMI 30kg/sq m or more) (% of population aged 15+)	33.8	35.3	35.5	36.2	36.5	37.1	37.6

Source: WHO/OECD/Euromonitor International

Over-the-Counter Healthcare

Kuwait: Trends in OTC healthcare retail sales 1998-2004

As stated

	1998	1999	2000	2001	2002	2003	2004
OTC Healthcare (US$ million)	8.1	8.1	8.8	9.5	10.4	11.8	12.5
OTC Healthcare (US$ per capita)	3.8	3.6	4.0	4.3	4.5	5.0	5.2

Source: Euromonitor International from industry sources/national statistics

Kuwait: OTC healthcare retail sales by sector 1998-2004

% of OTC retail value sales

	1998	1999	2000	2001	2002	2003	2004
Analgesics	6.0	5.6	5.3	5.0	5.0	4.8	5.1
Cough, cold and allergy (hay fever) remedies	7.4	6.9	6.7	6.2	5.8	5.5	5.5
Digestive remedies	3.7	3.5	3.4	3.3	3.6	3.6	3.6
Medicated skin care	5.0	4.6	4.4	4.3	4.7	4.7	4.8
Vitamins and dietary supplements	74.3	76.1	77.1	78.2	78.1	78.8	78.4

Source: Euromonitor International from industry sources/national statistics
Notes: Only selected sectors are shown, so values are not expected to sum to 100

■ **Latvia**

Socio-economic Parameters

Latvia: Socio-economic parameters 1998-2004

As stated

	1998	1999	2000	2001	2002	2003	2004
Population: national estimates at January 1st ('000)	2,420.8	2,399.2	2,381.7	2,364.3	2,345.8	2,331.5	2,318.9
% aged 0-14 yrs	19.4	18.7	18.0	17.3	16.6	16.0	15.4
% aged 15-64 yrs	66.2	66.7	67.2	67.4	67.8	68.2	68.5
% aged 65+ yrs	14.4	14.7	14.8	15.2	15.5	15.9	16.2
% Male	46.1	46.1	46.1	46.1	46.0	46.0	46.0
% Female	53.9	53.9	53.9	53.9	54.0	54.0	54.0
% Urban	69.1	69.0	69.0	69.0	69.1	70.0	70.3
Occupants per household at January 1st (Number)	3.0	3.0	3.0	3.0	3.0	2.9	2.9
Households ('000)	802.8	802.8	802.8	798.5	794.1	790.9	788.5
Annual rates of inflation (% growth)	4.7	2.4	2.7	2.5	1.9	2.9	6.2
GDP (Lats million)	3,902.9	4,224.2	4,685.7	5,168.3	5,691.1	6,322.5	7,238.0
GDP (US$ million)	6,617.0	7,218.8	7,725.8	8,230.8	9,206.0	11,063.4	13,397.9
GDP (US$ per capita)	2,733.4	3,008.8	3,243.8	3,481.4	3,924.5	4,745.2	5,777.7

Source: Euromonitor International from International Monetary Fund (IMF), International Financial Statistics and World Economic Outlook/UN/national statistics

Life Expectancy

Latvia: Life expectancy 1998-2004

Table: 4.717

As stated

	1998	1999	2000	2001	2002	2003	2004	% change 1998-2004
Life expectancy at birth: total population (years)	69.8	70.1	70.5	70.7	70.3	70.2	70.2	0.44
Life expectancy at birth: total population: year on year growth	0.4	0.4	0.5	0.3	-0.6	-0.1	-0.1	
Healthy life expectancy at birth (years)	62.0			59.9	60.0			
Healthy life expectancy at birth: year on year growth					0.2			

Source: Euromonitor International from World Bank

Health Expenditure

Latvia: Public health expenditure 1998-2004

Table: 4.718

As stated

	1998	1999	2000	2001	2002	2003	2004
Share of total health expenditure in GDP (% of total GDP)	6.8	6.9	6.3	6.4	6.5	6.5	6.2
Health expenditure (US$ per capita)	159.0	179.0	182.0	190.0	203.0	211.0	221.0

Source: Euromonitor International from OECD/national statistics

Latvia: Private health expenditure 1998-2004

Table: 4.719

As stated

	1998	1999	2000	2001	2002	2003	2004
Consumer expenditure on health goods and medical services (Lats million)	87.2	91.6	115.5	136.4	144.7	161.9	179.2
Consumer expenditure on health goods and medical services: real growth in national currency: 1990 = 100	194.6	199.6	245.3	282.7	294.3	320.0	333.2
Consumer expenditure on health goods and medical services as a percentage of total consumer expenditure	3.8	3.8	4.4	4.6	4.5	4.6	4.6

Source: National statistical offices/OECD/Eurostat/Euromonitor International

Latvia: Consumer expenditure on health goods and medical services by sector 1998-2004

Table: 4.720

% of total consumer expenditure on health goods and medical services

	1998	1999	2000	2001	2002	2003	2004
Pharmaceuticals, medical appliances/ equipment	60.6	63.3	63.2	62.3	62.1	62.2	62.3
Outpatient services	31.4	27.5	25.3	25.8	25.9	25.9	26.0
Hospital services	8.0	9.2	11.4	11.9	12.1	11.9	11.8
Total	100.0	100.0	100.0	100.0	100.0	100.0	100.0

Source: National statistical offices/OECD/Eurostat/Euromonitor International

Healthcare Infrastructure and Services

Latvia: Healthcare infrastructure and services by sector 1998-2004

Table: 4.721

As stated

	1998	1999	2000	2001	2002	2003	2004
Dentists (number)	1,064	1,026	1,278	1,350	1,392	1,416	1,435
Doctors (number)	7,964	8,041	8,134	7,744	7,921	7,883	7,824
Hospital admissions (number)	537,843	537,857	525,141	486,886	466,288	441,243	415,922
Hospitals and clinics (number)	150	151	142	140	129	131	132
In-patient beds ('000)	23	22	21	19	17	18	19
In-patient surgical procedures (number)	149,321	154,131	153,266	144,152	148,260	145,319	145,276
Nurses (number)	10,576	10,453	10,378	10,129	10,001	9,923	9,872
Out-patient contacts (per capita)	5	5	5	5	5	4	5

Source: Euromonitor International from national statistics

Latvia: Healthcare infrastructure and services by sector: growth 1998-2004

Table: 4.722

Year on year growth: % change in stated unit

	1998	1999	2000	2001	2002	2003	2004
Dentists (number)	-3.3	-3.6	24.6	5.6	3.1	1.7	1.3
Doctors (number)	-5.1	1.0	1.2	-4.8	2.3	-0.5	-0.7
Hospital admissions (number)	0.4	0.0	-2.4	-7.3	-4.2	-5.4	-5.7
Hospitals and clinics (number)	-3.8	0.7	-6.0	-1.4	-7.9	1.6	0.8
In-patient beds (number)	-2.8	-6.8	-4.3	-9.7	-7.9	6.9	0.9
In-patient surgical procedures (number)		3.2	-0.6	-5.9	2.8	-2.0	0.0
Nurses (number)	-2.1	-1.2	-0.7	-2.4	-1.3	-0.8	-0.5
Out-patient contacts (per capita)	2.2	6.5	-2.0	0.0	-4.2	-4.3	2.3

Source: Euromonitor International from national statistics

Immunisation

Latvia: Vaccination rates by disease type 1998-2004

Table: 4.723

%

	1998	1999	2000	2001	2002	2003	2004
Vaccination rate against DTP (diphtheria, tetanus, pertussis) 1 & 2 (%)			99.0	99.5	99.2	99.0	99.0
Vaccination rate against MMR (measles, mumps, rubella) (%)	97.0	97.0	97.4	97.9	98.3	99.0	99.0
Vaccination rate against polio (%)	94.0	99.0	96.3	97.3	97.5	98.0	99.0

Source: WHO

Infectious Diseases

Latvia: Incidence of disease by type 1998-2004

Table: 4.724

Number

	1998	1999	2000	2001	2002	2003	2004
Incidence of AIDS	11	17	24	42	55	58	50
Incidence of diphtheria	67	81	264	91	45		
Incidence of measles	3	0	0	1			
Incidence of polio	0	0	0	0	0		

Source: WHO

Latvia: Incidence of disease by type: growth 1998-2004

Table: 4.725

Year on year growth: %

	1998	1999	2000	2001	2002	2003	2004
Incidence of AIDS	266.7	54.5	41.2	75.0	31.0	5.5	-13.8
Incidence of diphtheria	59.5	20.9	225.9	-65.5	-50.5		
Incidence of measles	-25.0	-100.0					

Source: WHO

Causes of Death

Latvia: Deaths by disease 1998-2004

Table: 4.726

Number per 100,000 inhabitants

	1998	1999	2000	2001	2002	2003	2004
Death by diseases of the circulatory system	775.6	780.0	784.4	782.1	780.2	779.0	772.5
Deaths from heart disease	435.4	404.0	406.9	387.2	373.3	359.5	348.1
Death by malignant neoplasms (cancers)	231.8	235.0	238.2	241.4	244.7	244.4	245.8
Deaths from lung cancer	43.0	46.3	43.8	44.9	45.0	45.0	45.4
Death by diseases of the digestive system	29.7	31.1	31.8	28.5	29.2	30.8	30.3
Deaths from chronic liver disease and cirrhosis	15.4	13.9	14.5	13.8	13.3	12.9	12.3
Deaths from ulcers of the stomach and duodenum	6.0	5.1	6.6	6.4	6.6	6.8	6.9
Death by diseases of the respiratory system	34.6	33.8					

Source: WHO/Euromonitor International
Notes: Data is ranked in descending order by year 2004

Latvia: Deaths by disease: growth 1998-2004

Table: 4.727

% year on year growth

	1998	1999	2000	2001	2002	2003	2004
Deaths from ulcers of the stomach and duodenum	-9.0	-15.6	28.9	-2.6	3.1	3.0	1.0
Deaths from lung cancer	2.1	7.6	-5.4	2.5	0.2	0.0	0.8
Death by malignant neoplasms (cancers)		1.4	1.4	1.3	1.4	-0.1	0.6
Death by diseases of the circulatory system		0.6	0.6	-0.3	-0.2	-0.2	-0.8
Death by diseases of the digestive system	10.4	4.7	2.3	-10.4	2.5	5.5	-1.7
Deaths from heart disease	7.6	-7.2	0.7	-4.8	-3.6	-3.7	-3.2
Deaths from chronic liver disease and cirrhosis	19.5	-9.7	4.6	-5.1	-3.6	-3.0	-4.3
Death by diseases of the respiratory system		-2.3					

Source: WHO/Euromonitor International
Notes: Data is ranked in descending order by year 2004

Latvia: Other selected causes of death: 1998-2004

Table: 4.728

Number per 100,000 inhabitants

	1998	1999	2000	2001	2002	2003	2004
Death by suicide and self-inflicted injury	34.3	34.8	35.3	35.8	36.3	36.2	36.9
Death by motor traffic accidents	26.0	25.0	25.0	25.0	24.5	25.8	26.2
Death by injury and poisoning	73.9	71.0					

Source: Euromonitor International from national statistics
Notes: Data is ranked in descending order by year 2004

Latvia: Other selected causes of death: growth 1998-2004

Table: 4.729

% year on year growth

	1998	1999	2000	2001	2002	2003	2004
Death by suicide and self-inflicted injury		1.5	1.4	1.4	1.4	-0.3	1.9
Death by motor traffic accidents	18.2	-3.8	0.0	0.0	-2.0	5.3	1.7
Death by injury and poisoning		-3.9					

Source: Euromonitor International from national statistics
Notes: Data is ranked in descending order by year 2004

Smoking

Latvia: Smoking prevalence in population aged 15+ 1998-2004

Table: 4.730

% of population aged 15+

	1998	1999	2000	2001	2002	2003	2004
Smoking prevalence in population aged 15+ (% of population aged 15+)	37.3	29.2	36.9	36.2	35.4	34.7	33.9
Smoking prevalence in male population aged 15+ (% of male population)	58.0	49.1	57.5	56.8	56.1	56.4	55.7
Smoking prevalence in female population aged 15+ (% of female population)	20.4	13.0	20.0	19.3	18.4	16.9	16.0

Source: WHO/OECD/Euromonitor International

Nutrition and Obesity

Latvia: Nutrition and obesity 1998-2004

Table: 4.731

As stated

	1998	1999	2000	2001	2002	2003	2004
Availability of fruit and vegetables (kg/capita/year)	114.8	133.8	129.9	145.2	151.5	161.5	169.4
Average supply of calories per day (calories per capita)	2,872.2	2,882.7	2,920.1	3,016.8	2,938.0	2,909.4	2,893.3
Average supply of fat per day (grams per capita)	87.3	89.4	98.2	107.2	109.6	114.7	112.4
Average supply of protein per day (grams per capita)	79.2	79.3	79.4	79.9	80.2	80.5	80.8
Obese population (BMI 30kg/sq m or more) (% of population aged 15+)	9.0	9.3	10.0	11.5	13.0	13.5	13.8

Source: WHO/OECD/Euromonitor International

■ **Lithuania**

Socio-economic Parameters

Lithuania: Socio-economic parameters 1998-2004

Table: 4.732

As stated

	1998	1999	2000	2001	2002	2003	2004
Population: national estimates at January 1st ('000)	3,562.3	3,536.4	3,512.1	3,487.0	3,467.8	3,447.0	3,426.4
% aged 0-14 yrs	21.1	20.7	20.2	19.7	19.0	18.3	17.7
% aged 15-64 yrs	65.8	65.9	66.0	66.2	66.5	66.9	67.3
% aged 65 + yrs	13.2	13.5	13.7	14.1	14.4	14.7	15.0
% Male	46.9	46.9	46.8	46.8	46.7	46.7	46.7
% Female	53.1	53.1	53.2	53.2	53.3	53.3	53.3
% Urban	68.3	68.3	68.4	68.5	68.6	69.5	69.9
Occupants per household at January 1st (Number)	2.7	2.6	2.6	2.6	2.6	2.5	2.5
Households ('000)	1,335.8	1,342.0	1,349.0	1,356.8	1,357.0	1,361.7	1,363.9
Annual rates of inflation (% growth)	5.1	0.8	1.0	1.3	0.3	-1.2	1.2
GDP (Litai million)	44,377.4	43,359.4	45,525.9	48,378.7	51,642.9	56,179.1	61,897.7
GDP (US$ million)	11,094.4	10,839.9	11,381.5	12,094.7	14,045.0	18,354.0	22,260.6
GDP (US$ per capita)	3,114.4	3,065.2	3,240.7	3,468.5	4,050.1	5,324.6	6,496.7

Source: *Euromonitor International from International Monetary Fund (IMF), International Financial Statistics and World Economic Outlook/UN/national statistics*

Life Expectancy

Lithuania: Life expectancy 1998-2004

Table: 4.733

As stated

	1998	1999	2000	2001	2002	2003	2004	% change 1998-2004
Life expectancy at birth: total population (years)	72.1	72.4	72.6	72.9	71.9	71.8	71.3	-1.07
Life expectancy at birth: total population: year on year growth	0.4	0.3	0.3	0.4	-1.4	-0.2	-0.6	
Healthy life expectancy at birth (years)	64.0			60.8	61.1			
Healthy life expectancy at birth: year on year growth					0.5			

Source: *Euromonitor International from World Bank*

Health Expenditure

Lithuania: Public health expenditure 1998-2004

Table: 4.734

As stated

	1998	1999	2000	2001	2002	2003	2004
Share of total health expenditure in GDP (% of total GDP)	6.4	6.3	6.2	6.0	6.1	5.9	6.0
Health expenditure (US$ per capita)	194.0	194.0	212.0	220.0	241.0	257.0	272.0

Source: *Euromonitor International from OECD/national statistics*

Lithuania: Private health expenditure 1998-2004

Table: 4.735

As stated

	1998	1999	2000	2001	2002	2003	2004
Consumer expenditure on health goods and medical services (Litai million)	988.5	1,017.9	1,042.5	1,071.7	1,122.5	1,131.5	1,167.5
Consumer expenditure on health goods and medical services as a percentage of total consumer expenditure	3.7	3.6	3.6	3.4	3.5	3.5	3.4

Source: *National statistical offices/OECD/Eurostat/Euromonitor International*

Lithuania: Consumer expenditure on health goods and medical services by sector 1998-2004

Table: 4.736

% of total consumer expenditure on health goods and medical services

	1998	1999	2000	2001	2002	2003	2004
Pharmaceuticals, medical appliances/ equipment	68.4	71.8	73.4	80.6	83.4	84.0	84.0
Outpatient services	25.6	22.5	20.9	13.3	10.6	10.1	10.1
Hospital services	5.9	5.7	5.7	6.1	6.1	5.9	5.9
Total	100.0	100.0	100.0	100.0	100.0	100.0	100.0

Source: National statistical offices/OECD/Eurostat/Euromonitor International

Healthcare Infrastructure and Services

Lithuania: Healthcare infrastructure and services by sector 1998-2004

Table: 4.737

As stated

	1998	1999	2000	2001	2002	2003	2004
Active pharmacists (number)	2,895	2,970	2,995	3,020	3,056	3,098	3,131
Dentists (number)	2,259	2,306	2,446	2,490	2,309	2,372	2,421
Doctors (number)	14,622	14,578	14,034	14,031	13,856	13,682	13,567
Hospital admissions (number)	894,866	905,466	862,919	836,691	819,312	778,645	757,968
Hospitals and clinics (number)	187	186	187	189	188	191	192
In-patient beds ('000)	36	35	34	32	31	30	29
In-patient surgical procedures (number)	235,273	250,813	254,519	256,767	266,030	271,159	273,523
Midwives (number)	1,757	1,820	1,828	1,836	1,857	1,881	1,899
Nurses (number)	28,813	29,450	28,017	27,787	26,918	26,127	25,527
Out-patient contacts (per capita)	7	7	6	7	6	6	6

Source: Euromonitor International from national statistics

Lithuania: Healthcare infrastructure and services by sector: growth 1998-2004

Table: 4.738

Year on year growth: % change in stated unit

	1998	1999	2000	2001	2002	2003	2004
Active pharmacists (number)	-3.3	2.6	0.8	0.8	1.2	1.4	1.1
Dentists (number)	4.9	2.1	6.1	1.8	-7.3	2.7	2.1
Doctors (number)	-0.9	-0.3	-3.7	0.0	-1.2	-1.3	-0.8
Hospital admissions (number)	10.7	1.2	-4.7	-3.0	-2.1	-5.0	-2.7
Hospitals and clinics (number)	0.0	-0.5	0.5	1.1	-0.5	1.6	0.5
In-patient beds (number)	-2.3	-2.5	-1.6	-6.0	-3.3	-3.4	-3.3
In-patient surgical procedures (number)	9.8	6.6	1.5	0.9	3.6	1.9	0.9
Midwives (number)	-1.0	3.6	0.4	0.4	1.1	1.3	1.0
Nurses (number)	-0.6	2.2	-4.9	-0.8	-3.1	-2.9	-2.3
Out-patient contacts (per capita)	-8.0	0.0	-8.7	3.2	-1.5	0.0	-3.1

Source: Euromonitor International from national statistics

Immunisation

Lithuania: Vaccination rates by disease type 1998-2004

Table: 4.739

%

	1998	1999	2000	2001	2002	2003	2004
Vaccination rate against DTP (diphtheria, tetanus, pertussis) 1 & 2 (%)			98.6	98.5	98.1	98.0	98.0
Vaccination rate against MMR (measles, mumps, rubella) (%)	97.0	97.0	97.0	97.4	97.9	98.0	98.0
Vaccination rate against polio (%)	88.0	88.0	91.5	97.4	97.0	97.0	96.0

Source: WHO

Infectious Diseases

Lithuania: Incidence of disease by type 1998-2004

Table: 4.740

Number

	1998	1999	2000	2001	2002	2003	2004
Incidence of AIDS	8	7	8	7	9	6	7
Incidence of diphtheria	2	6	2	0	3		
Incidence of measles	18	23	19	7	103		
Incidence of polio	0	0	0	0	0		

Source: WHO

Lithuania: Incidence of disease by type: growth 1998-2004

Table: 4.741

Year on year growth: %

	1998	1999	2000	2001	2002	2003	2004
Incidence of AIDS	166.7	-12.5	14.3	-12.5	28.6	-33.3	16.7
Incidence of diphtheria	0.0	200.0	-66.7	-100.0			
Incidence of measles	-40.0	27.8	-17.4	-63.2	1,371.4		

Source: WHO

Causes of Death

Lithuania: Deaths by disease 1998-2004

Table: 4.742

Number per 100,000 inhabitants

	1998	1999	2000	2001	2002	2003	2004
Deaths from heart disease	379.0	360.1	341.3	322.6	304.0	285.6	267.8
Deaths from lung cancer	39.3	39.6	37.2	36.4	35.2	33.8	33.0
Death by diseases of the digestive system	23.9	24.9	25.7	23.8	23.7	24.1	23.7
Deaths from chronic liver disease and cirrhosis	16.5	14.6	15.1	14.1	13.4	12.7	12.0
Deaths from ulcers of the stomach and duodenum	4.3	4.3	4.5	4.6	4.6	4.6	4.6

Source: WHO/Euromonitor International
Notes: Data is ranked in descending order by year 2004

Lithuania: Deaths by disease: growth 1998-2004

Table: 4.743

% year on year growth

	1998	1999	2000	2001	2002	2003	2004
Deaths from ulcers of the stomach and duodenum	3.3	0.1	5.1	1.2	0.0	0.0	0.2
Death by diseases of the digestive system	-0.4	4.2	3.2	-7.4	-0.4	1.7	-1.6
Deaths from lung cancer	2.5	0.9	-6.1	-2.2	-3.3	-4.0	-2.3
Deaths from chronic liver disease and cirrhosis	29.9	-11.4	3.4	-6.8	-5.0	-5.2	-5.4
Deaths from heart disease	-8.0	-5.0	-5.2	-5.5	-5.8	-6.1	-6.2

Source: WHO/Euromonitor International
Notes: Data is ranked in descending order by year 2004

Smoking

Lithuania: Smoking prevalence in population aged 15+ 1998-2004

Table: 4.744

% of population aged 15+

	1998	1999	2000	2001	2002	2003	2004
Smoking prevalence in population aged 15+ (% of population aged 15+)	28.3	32.5	32.0	33.5	33.5	33.1	33.0
Smoking prevalence in male population aged 15+ (% of male population)	48.5	52.0	51.5	50.6	50.0	49.5	49.1
Smoking prevalence in female population aged 15+ (% of female population)	12.5	16.1	15.8	19.1	19.5	19.3	19.5

Source: WHO/OECD/Euromonitor International

Nutrition and Obesity

Lithuania: Nutrition and obesity 1998-2004

Table: 4.745

As stated

	1998	1999	2000	2001	2002	2003	2004
Availability of fruit and vegetables (kg/capita/year)	158.8	157.4	156.9	164.7	163.3	165.8	167.5
Average supply of calories per day (calories per capita)	3,260.8	3,192.0	3,353.6	3,400.3	3,324.5	3,310.7	3,397.2
Average supply of fat per day (grams per capita)	80.7	85.7	96.7	97.3	97.9	100.5	102.5
Average supply of protein per day (grams per capita)	98.5	99.5	104.7	107.7	111.0	109.3	106.4
Microbiological food-borne diseases (per 100000 population)	32.0						
Obese population (BMI 30kg/sq m or more) (% of population aged 15+)	8.8	9.6	10.8	12.9	14.0	14.5	14.9

Source: WHO/OECD/Euromonitor International

■ **Malaysia**

Socio-economic Parameters

Malaysia: Socio-economic parameters 1998-2004

Table: 4.746

As stated

	1998	1999	2000	2001	2002	2003	2004
Population: national estimates at January 1st ('000)	22,179.9	22,711.7	23,495.2	24,013.8	24,526.8	25,048.5	25,581.1
% aged 0-14 yrs	34.0	33.5	34.1	33.8	33.5	33.2	32.9
% aged 15-64 yrs	62.2	62.7	62.0	62.2	62.5	62.7	62.9
% aged 65 + yrs	3.7	3.8	4.0	4.0	4.1	4.1	4.2
% Male	51.2	51.2	50.9	50.9	50.9	50.9	50.9
% Female	48.8	48.8	49.1	49.1	49.1	49.1	49.1
% Urban	55.9	56.7	56.8	57.4	58.2	58.7	59.3
Occupants per household at January 1st (Number)	4.9	4.8	4.8	4.8	4.7	4.7	4.7
Households ('000)	4,563.5	4,725.8	4,910.9	5,054.6	5,195.7	5,329.1	5,456.0
Annual rates of inflation (% growth)	5.3	2.7	1.5	1.4	1.8	1.1	1.5
GDP (RM million)	283,243.0	300,764.0	343,215.0	334,404.0	361,624.0	394,200.0	447,547.0
GDP (US$ million)	72,175.4	79,148.4	90,319.7	88,001.1	95,164.2	103,736.8	117,775.5
GDP (US$ per capita)	3,254.1	3,484.9	3,844.2	3,664.6	3,880.0	4,141.4	4,604.0

Source: Euromonitor International from International Monetary Fund (IMF), International Financial Statistics and World Economic Outlook/UN/national statistics

Life Expectancy

Malaysia: Life expectancy 1998-2004

Table: 4.747

As stated

	1998	1999	2000	2001	2002	2003	2004	% change 1998-2004
Life expectancy at birth: total population (years)	71.3	71.5	71.7	71.7	72.0	72.3	72.6	1.88
Life expectancy at birth: total population: year on year growth	0.3	0.3	0.3	0.0	0.4	0.5	0.3	
Healthy life expectancy at birth (years)	61.0			63.8	63.8			
Healthy life expectancy at birth: year on year growth					-0.1			

Source: Euromonitor International from World Bank

Sanitation

Malaysia: Improved sanitary facilities and water source 2000

Table: 4.748

As stated

	2000
Population with improved access to sanitation facilities, rural (% of rural population with access)	98.0

Source: National statistics/World Bank

Health Expenditure

Malaysia: Public health expenditure 1998-2004

Table: 4.749

As stated

	1998	1999	2000	2001	2002	2003	2004
Share of total health expenditure in GDP (% of total GDP)	3.0	3.1	3.3	3.8	3.8	3.7	3.6
Health expenditure (US$ per capita)	99.0	109.0	129.0	143.0	149.0	158.0	164.0

Source: Euromonitor International from OECD/national statistics

Malaysia: Private health expenditure 1998-2004

As stated

	1998	1999	2000	2001	2002	2003	2004
Consumer expenditure on health goods and medical services (RM million)	2,584.0	2,816.0	3,306.0	3,442.8	3,620.6	3,861.2	4,065.0
Consumer expenditure on health goods and medical services: real growth in national currency: 1990 = 100	229.2	243.1	281.0	288.6	298.1	314.6	326.4
Consumer expenditure on health goods and medical services as a percentage of total consumer expenditure	2.2	2.2	2.2	2.3	2.3	2.3	2.4

Source: National statistical offices/OECD/Eurostat/Euromonitor International

Malaysia: Consumer expenditure on health goods and medical services by sector 1998-2004

% of total consumer expenditure on health goods and medical services

	1998	1999	2000	2001	2002	2003	2004
Pharmaceuticals, medical appliances/equipment	32.4	32.5	32.8	33.0	33.2	32.5	31.9
Outpatient services	42.0	41.7	41.3	40.8	40.5	40.9	41.2
Hospital services	25.7	25.8	26.0	26.2	26.3	26.6	26.9
Total	100.0	100.0	100.0	100.0	100.0	100.0	100.0

Source: National statistical offices/OECD/Eurostat/Euromonitor International

Healthcare Infrastructure and Services

Malaysia: Healthcare infrastructure and services by sector 1998-2004

As stated

	1998	1999	2000	2001	2002	2003	2004
Active pharmacists (number)	2,129						
Dentists (number)	2,058	1,909	2,144				
Doctors (number)	15,016	15,076	15,619				
Hospitals and clinics (number)	111	114	115				
In-patient beds ('000)	27	28	29				
Nurses (number)	18,134	20,914	23,255				

Source: Euromonitor International from national statistics

Malaysia: Healthcare infrastructure and services by sector: growth 1998-2004

Year on year growth: % change in stated unit

	1998	1999	2000	2001	2002	2003	2004
Active pharmacists (number)	21.9						
Dentists (number)	10.3	-7.2	12.3				
Doctors (number)	5.4	0.4	3.6				
Hospitals and clinics (number)	0.0	2.7	0.9				
In-patient beds (number)	-0.7	4.1	3.4				
Nurses (number)	12.9	15.3	11.2				

Source: Euromonitor International from national statistics

Immunisation

Malaysia: Vaccination rates by disease type 1998-2004

Table: 4.754

%

	1998	1999	2000	2001	2002	2003	2004
Vaccination rate against DTP (diphtheria, tetanus, pertussis) 1 & 2 (%)			94.5	94.5	95.3	96.0	96.0
Vaccination rate against MMR (measles, mumps, rubella) (%)	86.1	86.6	88.4	88.4	92.2	93.0	94.0
Vaccination rate against polio (%)	93.4	93.2	95.4	95.4	96.7	98.0	99.0

Source: WHO

Infectious Diseases

Malaysia: Incidence of disease by type 1998-2004

Table: 4.755

Number

	1998	1999	2000	2001	2002	2003	2004
Incidence of AIDS	875	1,200	1,168	1,302	1,193	1,076	1,082
Incidence of diphtheria	5	6	1	4	2		
Incidence of measles	483	2,576	6,187	2,198	408		
Incidence of polio	0	0	0	0	0		

Source: WHO

Malaysia: Incidence of disease by type: growth 1998-2004

Table: 4.756

Year on year growth: %

	1998	1999	2000	2001	2002	2003	2004
Incidence of AIDS	54.0	37.1	-2.7	11.5	-8.4	-9.8	0.6
Incidence of diphtheria	400.0	20.0	-83.3	300.0	-50.0		
Incidence of measles	-23.0	433.3	140.2	-64.5	-81.4		

Source: WHO

Causes of Death

Malaysia: Deaths by disease 1998-2004

Table: 4.757

Number per 100,000 inhabitants

	1998	1999	2000	2001	2002	2003	2004
Death by diseases of the circulatory system	60.9	62.6	63.6	64.2	64.7	61.3	60.9
Deaths from heart disease	32.7	33.4	33.9	34.4	35.5	36.2	37.2
Deaths from lung cancer	23.9	25.9	26.4	26.2	25.9	25.6	25.5
Death by malignant neoplasms (cancers)	19.8	21.3	21.2	20.9	20.8	20.0	19.4
Deaths from ulcers of the stomach and duodenum	18.9	19.2	18.4	18.8	18.6	18.8	19.1
Death by diseases of the digestive system	18.9	19.2	18.4	18.8	18.6	18.2	18.2
Deaths from chronic liver disease and cirrhosis	8.9	8.6	8.4	8.6	9.0	9.3	9.6

Source: WHO/Euromonitor International
Notes: Data is ranked in descending order by year 2004

Malaysia: Deaths by disease: growth 1998-2004

Table: 4.758

% year on year growth

	1998	1999	2000	2001	2002	2003	2004
Deaths from chronic liver disease and cirrhosis	1.1	-3.4	-2.3	2.4	4.7	3.3	3.8
Deaths from heart disease	9.0	2.1	1.5	1.5	3.2	2.0	2.7
Deaths from ulcers of the stomach and duodenum	-3.6	1.6	-4.2	2.2	-1.1	1.1	1.7
Deaths from lung cancer	-0.8	8.4	1.9	-0.8	-1.1	-1.2	-0.2
Death by diseases of the digestive system	-3.6	1.6	-4.2	2.2	-1.1	-2.2	-0.3
Death by diseases of the circulatory system	4.3	2.8	1.6	0.9	0.8	-5.3	-0.6
Death by malignant neoplasms (cancers)	-2.9	7.6	-0.5	-1.4	-0.5	-3.8	-2.9

Source: WHO/Euromonitor International
Notes: Data is ranked in descending order by year 2004

Malaysia: Other selected causes of death: 1998-2004

Table: 4.759

Number per 100,000 inhabitants

	1998	1999	2000	2001	2002	2003	2004
Death by motor traffic accidents	14.9	15.2	15.4	15.5	15.6	14.8	14.5
Death by suicide and self-inflicted injury	1.6	2.1	2.3	2.4	2.4	2.3	2.3

Source: Euromonitor International from national statistics
Notes: Data is ranked in descending order by year 2004

Malaysia: Other selected causes of death: growth 1998-2004

Table: 4.760

% year on year growth

	1998	1999	2000	2001	2002	2003	2004
Death by suicide and self-inflicted injury	100.0	31.3	9.5	4.3	0.0	-4.2	0.8
Death by motor traffic accidents	4.9	2.0	1.3	0.6	0.6	-5.1	-2.3

Source: Euromonitor International from national statistics
Notes: Data is ranked in descending order by year 2004

Smoking

Malaysia: Smoking prevalence in population aged 15+ 1998-2004

Table: 4.761

% of population aged 15+

	1998	1999	2000	2001	2002	2003	2004
Smoking prevalence in population aged 15+ (% of population aged 15+)	34.9	34.6	33.8	34.2	34.4	34.8	34.7
Smoking prevalence in male population aged 15+ (% of male population)	44.2	42.7	43.4	45.7	46.3	48.0	49.5
Smoking prevalence in female population aged 15+ (% of female population)	25.3	26.2	24.0	22.4	22.2	21.2	19.5

Source: WHO/OECD/Euromonitor International

Nutrition and Obesity

Malaysia: Nutrition and obesity 1998-2004

As stated

	1998	1999	2000	2001	2002	2003	2004
Average supply of calories per day (calories per capita)	2,846.1	2,856.8	2,899.9	2,892.1	2,881.1	2,880.9	2,877.0
Average supply of fat per day (grams per capita)	84.9	85.0	84.8	83.3	81.8	80.5	79.2
Average supply of protein per day (grams per capita)	74.6	76.2	76.6	75.7	76.3	76.6	76.7
Obese population (BMI 30kg/sq m or more) (% of population aged 15+)	6.2	6.5	6.5	6.5	6.5	6.7	6.7

Source: WHO/OECD/Euromonitor International

Over-the-Counter Healthcare

Malaysia: Trends in OTC healthcare retail sales 1998-2004

As stated

	1998	1999	2000	2001	2002	2003	2004
OTC Healthcare (RM million)	720.7	798.2	885.6	965.1	1,030.6	1,090.8	1,138.0
OTC Healthcare: real growth in national currency: 1998 = 100	100.0	107.8	117.8	126.6	132.7	139.0	141.9
OTC Healthcare: year on year (% real growth)	6.3	7.8	9.3	7.5	4.9	4.7	2.1
OTC Healthcare (RM per capita)	32.5	35.1	37.7	40.2	42.0	43.5	44.5

Source: Euromonitor International from industry sources/national statistics

Malaysia: OTC healthcare retail sales by sector 1998-2004

% of OTC retail value sales

	1998	1999	2000	2001	2002	2003	2004
Analgesics	13.9	13.5	13.1	13.0	12.8	12.6	12.5
Cough, cold and allergy (hay fever) remedies	21.2	20.4	20.2	19.3	18.9	18.5	18.4
Digestive remedies	4.9	5.0	4.8	4.8	4.7	4.7	4.7
Medicated skin care	8.1	8.1	8.0	7.9	7.8	7.8	7.7
Vitamins and dietary supplements	46.5	47.9	49.2	50.4	51.1	51.7	52.0

Source: Euromonitor International from industry sources/national statistics
Notes: Only selected sectors are shown, so values are not expected to sum to 100

Mexico: Healthcare infrastructure and services by sector: growth 1998-2004

Table: 4.772

Year on year growth: % change in stated unit

	1998	1999	2000	2001	2002	2003	2004
Consultations with GPs (general practitioners) (per capita)	0.0	9.0	-0.3	0.0	0.0	0.0	0.0
Dentists (number)	3.2	7.5	3.3	-1.1	2.3	2.3	2.1
Doctors (number)	1.7	10.2	4.7	7.6	3.4	2.9	2.2
Hospitals and clinics (number)	0.0	0.1	0.2	0.0	0.1	0.1	0.2
In-patient beds (number)	1.5	5.0	1.8	-0.5	1.5	1.1	1.0
Nurses (number)	4.0	5.2	-2.5	6.8	1.6	1.3	1.1

Source: Euromonitor International from national statistics

Immunisation

Mexico: Vaccination rates by disease type 1998-2004

Table: 4.773

%

	1998	1999	2000	2001	2002	2003	2004
Vaccination rate against DTP (diphtheria, tetanus, pertussis) 1 & 2 (%)			90.1	91.1	92.1	93.0	94.0
Vaccination rate against MMR (measles, mumps, rubella) (%)	96.0	95.0	95.9	95.2	95.7	97.0	98.0
Vaccination rate against polio (%)	96.0	96.0	89.3	89.3	91.5	92.0	93.0

Source: WHO

Infectious Diseases

Mexico: Incidence of disease by type 1998-2004

Table: 4.774

Number

	1998	1999	2000	2001	2002	2003	2004
Incidence of AIDS	4,758	4,372	4,855	4,297	4,854	4,922	3,828
Incidence of diphtheria	0	0	0	0			
Incidence of measles	0	0	30	3			
Incidence of polio	0	0	0	0			

Source: WHO

Mexico: Incidence of disease by type: growth 1998-2004

Table: 4.775

Year on year growth: %

	1998	1999	2000	2001	2002	2003	2004
Incidence of AIDS	29.6	-8.1	11.0	-11.5	13.0	1.4	-22.2
Incidence of measles				-90.0			

Source: WHO

Causes of Death

Mexico: Deaths by disease 1998-2004

Table: 4.776

Number per 100,000 inhabitants

	1998	1999	2000	2001	2002	2003	2004
Death by diseases of the digestive system	86.9	87.3	87.8	86.9	89.6	87.9	87.8
Deaths from heart disease	44.7	45.3	44.6	44.7	44.6	44.5	44.2
Deaths from chronic liver disease and cirrhosis	26.0	25.4	25.3	24.8	24.5	24.1	23.7
Deaths from lung cancer	6.5	6.6	6.3	6.3	6.2	6.2	6.2
Deaths from ulcers of the stomach and duodenum	3.1	3.0	2.8	2.7	2.5	2.3	2.2

Source: WHO/Euromonitor International
Notes: Data is ranked in descending order by year 2004

Mexico: Deaths by disease: growth 1998-2004

Table: 4.777

% year on year growth

	1998	1999	2000	2001	2002	2003	2004
Death by diseases of the digestive system	0.6	0.5	0.6	-1.0	3.1	-1.9	-0.1
Deaths from heart disease	-27.1	1.2	-1.5	0.3	-0.2	-0.2	-0.6
Deaths from lung cancer	-82.1	0.8	-3.1	-0.7	-1.6	0.0	-0.8
Deaths from chronic liver disease and cirrhosis		-2.4	-0.4	-1.9	-1.2	-1.6	-1.7
Deaths from ulcers of the stomach and duodenum		-3.5	-7.7	-3.6	-7.4	-8.0	-6.0

Source: WHO/Euromonitor International
Notes: Data is ranked in descending order by year 2004

Smoking

Mexico: Smoking prevalence in population aged 15+ 1998-2004

Table: 4.778

% of population aged 15+

	1998	1999	2000	2001	2002	2003	2004
Smoking prevalence in population aged 15+ (% of population aged 15+)	27.1	28.6	29.1	29.5	29.7	30.0	30.2
Smoking prevalence in male population aged 15+ (% of male population)	41.5	42.0	42.4	42.4	42.7	42.7	43.0
Smoking prevalence in female population aged 15+ (% of female population)	13.8	16.2	16.8	17.5	17.6	18.1	18.3

Source: WHO/OECD/Euromonitor International

Nutrition and Obesity

Mexico: Nutrition and obesity 1998-2004

Table: 4.779

As stated

	1998	1999	2000	2001	2002	2003	2004
Average supply of calories per day (calories per capita)	3,119.2	3,125.8	3,160.8	3,160.1	3,144.7	3,138.8	3,130.7
Average supply of fat per day (grams per capita)	87.1	86.9	86.8	86.0	87.5	88.3	88.9
Average supply of protein per day (grams per capita)	86.1	87.4	89.8	91.5	90.8	91.1	91.5
Obese population (BMI 30kg/sq m or more) (% of population aged 15+)	22.6	20.1	20.2	20.5	20.0	20.0	19.8

Source: WHO/OECD/Euromonitor International

Mexico: Trends in OTC healthcare retail sales 1998-2004

Table: 4.780

As stated

	1998	1999	2000	2001	2002	2003	2004
OTC Healthcare (MX$ million)	11,431.0	12,681.7	13,580.2	14,379.8	15,268.3	16,391.5	18,243.5
OTC Healthcare: real growth in national currency: 1998 = 100	100.0	95.2	93.1	92.6	93.7	96.2	102.5
OTC Healthcare: year on year (% real growth)	5.0	-4.8	-2.2	-0.4	1.1	2.7	6.6
OTC Healthcare (MX$ per capita)	120.2	131.3	138.3	144.2	150.9	159.6	175.1

Source: *Euromonitor International from industry sources/national statistics*

Mexico: OTC healthcare retail sales by sector 1998-2004

Table: 4.781

% of OTC retail value sales

	1998	1999	2000	2001	2002	2003	2004
Analgesics	18.3	18.3	18.1	17.5	17.0	16.4	16.0
Cough, cold and allergy (hay fever) remedies	31.9	31.1	30.7	30.7	30.4	30.3	33.3
Digestive remedies	17.4	16.3	15.5	15.1	14.6	14.5	13.1
Medicated skin care	12.0	12.9	13.4	13.3	13.0	13.2	12.9
Vitamins and dietary supplements	14.7	15.5	16.4	17.5	19.2	19.9	19.2

Source: *Euromonitor International from industry sources/national statistics*
Notes: *Only selected sectors are shown, so values are not expected to sum to 100*

Mexico: Retail sales of packaged foods by health and wellness category 2002-2004

Table: 4.782

MX$ million

	2002	2003	2004
Packaged food: Total	342,717.2	373,880.0	403,427.7
Better for you	12,037.3	13,201.0	15,451.0
For food intolerance	790.5	884.0	984.7
Fortified/functional	821.7	1,087.9	1,352.0
Organic	18.9	21.6	25.0

Source: *Euromonitor International from industry sources/national statistics*

Mexico: Per capita sales of packaged foods by health and wellness category 2002-2004

Table: 4.783

MX$ per capita

	2002	2003	2004
Better for you	118.2	127.8	147.5
For food intolerance	7.8	8.6	9.4
Fortified/functional	8.1	10.5	12.9
Organic	0.2	0.2	0.2

Source: *Euromonitor International from industry sources/national statistics*

Mexico: Retail sales of packaged food by health and wellness category: % share of total packaged food market 2002-2004

Table: 4.784

% value

	2002	2003	2004
Better for you	3.5	3.5	3.8
For food intolerance	0.2	0.2	0.2
Fortified/functional	0.2	0.3	0.3
Organic	0.0	0.0	0.0

Source: Euromonitor International from industry sources/national statistics

Mexico: Retail sales of packaged food by health and wellness category: real growth index 2002-2004

Table: 4.785

2002 =100

	2002	2003	2004
Better for you	100.00	104.84	118.68
For food intolerance	100.00	106.90	115.17
Fortified/functional	100.00	126.57	152.13
Organic	100.00	109.22	122.69

Source: Euromonitor International from industry sources/national statistics

Mexico: Retail sales of better-for-you packaged foods by sector 2002-2004

Table: 4.786

% of total packaged food / as stated

	2002	2003	2004	% real change in value 2002-2004
Combination	0.27	0.31	0.37	51.33
Reduced carb	0.00	0.00	0.00	33.81
Reduced fat	2.41	2.38	2.56	15.55
Reduced salt	0.00	0.00	0.00	80.24

Source: Euromonitor International from industry sources/national statistics

Mexico: Retail sales of packaged foods for food intolerances by sector 2002-2004

Table: 4.787

% of total packaged food / as stated

	2002	2003	2004	% real change in value 2002-2004
Diabetic	0.00	0.00	0.00	325.99
Lactose-free	0.23	0.24	0.24	14.40

Source: Euromonitor International from industry sources/national statistics

Mexico: Retail sales of naturally healthy packaged foods by sector 2002-2004

Table: 4.788

% of total packaged food / as stated

	2002	2003	2004	% real change in value 2002-2004
High fibre	0.96	1.07	1.15	30.46
Other naturally healthy food	0.20	0.19	0.19	4.21
Soy-based dairy alternatives	0.08	0.09	0.11	41.41

Source: Euromonitor International from industry sources/national statistics

■ **Morocco**

Socio-economic Parameters

Morocco: Socio-economic parameters 1998-2004

Table: 4.789

As stated

	1998	1999	2000	2001	2002	2003	2004
Population: national estimates at January 1st ('000)	27,956.8	28,411.3	28,873.7	29,345.6	29,827.5	30,317.9	30,814.3
% aged 0-14 yrs	34.6	33.9	33.3	32.6	32.1	31.5	31.0
% aged 15-64 yrs	61.3	61.9	62.5	63.1	63.6	64.1	64.5
% aged 65+ yrs	4.2	4.2	4.2	4.3	4.4	4.4	4.5
% Male	50.1	50.1	50.1	50.1	50.1	50.1	50.1
% Female	49.9	49.9	49.9	49.9	49.9	49.9	49.9
% Urban	54.5	55.3	55.1	55.8	56.7	57.1	57.8
Occupants per household at January 1st (Number)	5.7	5.5	5.4	5.3	5.3	5.2	5.2
Households ('000)	4,947.0	5,146.5	5,354.0	5,496.0	5,637.8	5,783.0	5,918.3
Annual rates of inflation (% growth)	2.8	0.7	1.9	0.6	2.8	1.2	2.0
GDP (Dh million)	344,010.0	345,590.0	354,210.0	383,180.0	397,780.0	418,660.0	441,773.0
GDP (US$ million)	35,817.9	35,248.4	33,335.5	33,900.7	36,094.2	43,727.1	49,816.4
GDP (US$ per capita)	1,281.2	1,240.6	1,154.5	1,155.2	1,210.1	1,442.3	1,616.7

Source: Euromonitor International from International Monetary Fund (IMF), International Financial Statistics and World Economic Outlook/UN/national statistics

Life Expectancy

Morocco: Life expectancy 1998-2004

Table: 4.790

As stated

	1998	1999	2000	2001	2002	2003	2004	% change 1998-2004
Life expectancy at birth: total population (years)	68.3	68.7	69.3	69.4	70.8	71.5	72.3	5.90
Life expectancy at birth: total population: year on year growth	0.6	0.6	0.8	0.1	2.0	0.9	1.3	
Healthy life expectancy at birth (years)	59.0			55.3	55.4			
Healthy life expectancy at birth: year on year growth					0.1			

Source: Euromonitor International from World Bank

Sanitation

Morocco: Improved sanitary facilities and water source 2000

Table: 4.791

As stated

	2000
Population with access to improved sanitary facilities (% of population)	68.0
Population with access to improved water source (% of population)	80.0
Population with improved access to sanitation facilities, rural (% of rural population with access)	44.0
Population with improved access to sanitation facilities, urban (% of urban population with access)	86.0

Source: National statistics/World Bank

Health Expenditure

Morocco: Public health expenditure 1998-2004

Table: 4.792

As stated

	1998	1999	2000	2001	2002	2003	2004
Share of total health expenditure in GDP (% of total GDP)	4.4	4.4	4.7	5.1	4.9	5.0	4.8
Health expenditure (US$ per capita)	56.0	54.0	54.0	53.0	55.0	55.0	56.0

Source: Euromonitor International from OECD/national statistics

Morocco: Private health expenditure 1998-2004

Table: 4.793

As stated

	1998	1999	2000	2001	2002	2003	2004
Consumer expenditure on health goods and medical services (Dh million)	14,124.0	13,914.0	14,688.0	15,877.0	16,548.0	17,067.4	18,215.5
Consumer expenditure on health goods and medical services: real growth in national currency: 1990 = 100	109.7	107.3	111.2	119.5	121.1	123.5	129.2
Consumer expenditure on health goods and medical services as a percentage of total consumer expenditure	5.7	5.8	5.8	5.8	5.8	5.6	5.9

Source: *National statistical offices/OECD/Eurostat/Euromonitor International*

Morocco: Consumer expenditure on health goods and medical services by sector 1998-2004

Table: 4.794

% of total consumer expenditure on health goods and medical services

	1998	1999	2000	2001	2002	2003	2004
Pharmaceuticals, medical appliances/ equipment	30.1	29.6	30.5	29.5	29.7	30.2	30.0
Outpatient services	51.5	50.8	50.3	50.8	50.5	49.7	49.7
Hospital services	18.5	19.7	19.2	19.7	19.8	20.1	20.4
Total	100.0	100.0	100.0	100.0	100.0	100.0	100.0

Source: *National statistical offices/OECD/Eurostat/Euromonitor International*

Healthcare Infrastructure and Services

Morocco: Healthcare infrastructure and services by sector 1998-2004

Table: 4.795

As stated

	1998	1999	2000	2001	2002	2003	2004
Active pharmacists (number)	5,026	4,298	5,197	6,375	8,640	9,037	9,258
Dentists (number)	1,964	2,111	2,299	2,453	2,578	2,665	2,750
Doctors (number)	10,771	11,907	12,439	12,955	13,955	14,437	14,657
Hospitals and clinics (number)	143	144	145	148	152	156	159
In-patient beds ('000)	26	25	26	26	28	29	30

Source: *Euromonitor International from national statistics*

Morocco: Healthcare infrastructure and services by sector: growth 1998-2004

Table: 4.796

Year on year growth: % change in stated unit

	1998	1999	2000	2001	2002	2003	2004
Active pharmacists (number)	60.5	-14.5	20.9	22.7	35.5	4.6	2.4
Dentists (number)	9.3	7.5	8.9	6.7	5.1	3.4	3.2
Doctors (number)	8.5	10.5	4.5	4.1	7.7	3.5	1.5
Hospitals and clinics (number)	0.0	0.7	0.7	2.1	2.7	2.6	1.9
In-patient beds (number)	-0.1	-1.1	0.8	3.2	6.0	3.6	3.4

Source: *Euromonitor International from national statistics*

Immunisation

Morocco: Vaccination rates by disease type 1998-2004

Table: 4.797

%

	1998	1999	2000	2001	2002	2003	2004
Vaccination rate against DTP (diphtheria, tetanus, pertussis) 1 & 2 (%)			97.0	98.0	94.5	94.0	93.0
Vaccination rate against MMR (measles, mumps, rubella) (%)	91.0	90.0	93.0	96.0	96.0	97.0	98.0
Vaccination rate against polio (%)	93.0	91.0	95.0	93.0	94.5	94.0	93.0

Source: WHO

Infectious Diseases

Morocco: Incidence of disease by type 1998-2004

Table: 4.798

Number

	1998	1999	2000	2001	2002	2003	2004
Incidence of AIDS	93	165	112	129	149	152	138
Incidence of diphtheria	0	0	0	0	0		
Incidence of measles	7,863	10,853	7,368	2,724	6,000		
Incidence of polio	0	0	0	0	0		

Source: WHO

Morocco: Incidence of disease by type: growth 1998-2004

Table: 4.799

Year on year growth: %

	1998	1999	2000	2001	2002	2003	2004
Incidence of AIDS	1.1	77.4	-32.1	15.2	15.5	2.0	-9.2
Incidence of measles	213.0	38.0	-32.1	-63.0	120.3		

Source: WHO

Causes of Death

Morocco: Deaths by disease 1998-2004

Table: 4.800

Number per 100,000 inhabitants

	1998	1999	2000	2001	2002	2003	2004
Death by diseases of the circulatory system	37.0	38.0	38.0	38.8	39.3	37.7	37.9
Death by malignant neoplasms (cancers)	10.5	10.0	10.0	9.9	9.9	9.7	9.7
Death by diseases of the respiratory system	7.0	7.0	7.0	7.0	7.1	6.8	6.7

Source: WHO/Euromonitor International
Notes: Data is ranked in descending order by year 2004

Morocco: Deaths by disease: growth 1998-2004

Table: 4.801

% year on year growth

	1998	1999	2000	2001	2002	2003	2004
Death by diseases of the circulatory system	2.8	2.7	0.0	2.1	1.3	-4.1	0.4
Death by malignant neoplasms (cancers)	0.0	-4.8	0.0	-1.0	0.0	-2.0	-0.4
Death by diseases of the respiratory system	0.0	0.0	0.0	0.0	1.4	-4.2	-1.3

Source: WHO/Euromonitor International
Notes: Data is ranked in descending order by year 2004

Morocco: Other selected causes of death: 1998-2004

Table: 4.802

Number per 100,000 inhabitants

	1998	1999	2000	2001	2002	2003	2004
Death by injury and poisoning	12.2	11.4	11.4	11.2	11.2	11.0	10.9

Source: Euromonitor International from national statistics

Morocco: Other selected causes of death: growth 1998-2004

Table: 4.803

% year on year growth

	1998	1999	2000	2001	2002	2003	2004
Death by injury and poisoning	0.0	-6.6	0.0	-1.8	0.0	-1.8	-0.9

Source: Euromonitor International from national statistics

Smoking

Morocco: Smoking prevalence in population aged 15+ 1998-2004

Table: 4.804

% of population aged 15+

	1998	1999	2000	2001	2002	2003	2004
Smoking prevalence in population aged 15+ (% of population aged 15+)	28.1	28.2	28.6	28.8	28.8	29.1	29.2
Smoking prevalence in male population aged 15+ (% of male population)	34.7	35.5	35.9	35.9	36.4	36.5	36.8
Smoking prevalence in female population aged 15+ (% of female population)	21.6	21.0	21.4	21.9	21.4	21.8	21.7

Source: WHO/OECD/Euromonitor International

Nutrition and Obesity

Morocco: Nutrition and obesity 1998-2004

Table: 4.805

As stated

	1998	1999	2000	2001	2002	2003	2004
Average supply of calories per day (calories per capita)	3,138.4	3,060.5	3,026.1	3,046.5	3,051.8	3,053.5	3,060.4
Average supply of fat per day (grams per capita)	61.6	61.5	60.0	59.7	58.2	56.9	55.8
Average supply of protein per day (grams per capita)	83.5	82.7	80.9	84.1	84.8	85.5	84.5
Obese population (BMI 30kg/sq m or more) (% of population aged 15+)	4.1	4.0	4.0	4.0	4.1	4.1	4.1

Source: WHO/OECD/Euromonitor International

Over-the-Counter Healthcare

Morocco: Trends in OTC healthcare retail sales 1998-2004

Table: 4.806

As stated

	1998	1999	2000	2001	2002	2003	2004
OTC Healthcare (Dh million)	1,583.2	1,711.8	1,858.4	2,021.3	2,195.1	2,325.6	2,471.7
OTC Healthcare: real growth in national currency: 1998 = 100	100.0	107.4	114.4	123.7	130.7	136.8	142.6
OTC Healthcare: year on year (% real growth)	5.0	7.4	6.5	8.1	5.6	4.7	4.2
OTC Healthcare (Dh per capita)	56.6	60.3	64.4	68.9	73.6	76.7	80.2

Source: Euromonitor International from industry sources/national statistics

Morocco: OTC healthcare retail sales by sector 1998-2004

Table: 4.807

% of OTC retail value sales

	1998	1999	2000	2001	2002	2003	2004
Analgesics	23.1	22.6	22.1	21.6	21.2	20.8	20.5
Cough, cold and allergy (hay fever) remedies	23.0	22.9	22.7	22.6	22.6	22.6	22.4
Digestive remedies	15.7	16.0	16.3	16.6	16.9	17.0	17.3
Medicated skin care	17.3	17.7	18.1	18.5	18.7	18.8	18.9
Vitamins and dietary supplements	12.4	12.5	12.5	12.6	12.7	12.8	12.8

Source: Euromonitor International from industry sources/national statistics
Notes: Only selected sectors are shown, so values are not expected to sum to 100

■ **Netherlands**

Socio-economic Parameters

Netherlands: Socio-economic parameters 1998-2004

Table: 4.808

As stated

	1998	1999	2000	2001	2002	2003	2004
Population: national estimates at January 1st ('000)	15,654.2	15,760.2	15,864.0	15,987.1	16,105.3	16,192.2	16,274.4
% aged 0-14 yrs	18.4	18.5	18.6	18.6	18.6	18.6	18.6
% aged 15-64 yrs	68.1	68.0	67.9	67.8	67.7	67.8	67.8
% aged 65+ yrs	13.5	13.5	13.6	13.6	13.7	13.6	13.7
% Male	49.4	49.4	49.5	49.5	49.5	49.5	49.5
% Female	50.6	50.6	50.5	50.5	50.5	50.5	50.5
% Urban	89.2	89.3	89.3	89.4	89.5	89.6	89.7
Occupants per household at January 1st (Number)	2.4	2.3	2.3	2.3	2.3	2.3	2.3
Households ('000)	6,655.9	6,745.4	6,801.0	6,867.0	6,934.3	7,002.0	7,058.0
Annual rates of inflation (% growth)	2.0	2.2	2.5	4.5	3.5	2.1	1.2
GDP (EUR million)	352,208.6	374,071.8	402,293.0	429,345.0	445,160.0	454,276.0	464,879.0
GDP (US$ million)	394,825.8	398,530.8	370,640.3	384,197.9	418,954.4	512,707.2	577,227.7
GDP (US$ per capita)	25,221.7	25,287.1	23,363.7	24,031.8	26,013.5	31,663.9	35,468.4

Source: Euromonitor International from International Monetary Fund (IMF), International Financial Statistics and World Economic Outlook/UN/national statistics

Life Expectancy

Netherlands: Life expectancy 1998-2004

Table: 4.809

As stated

	1998	1999	2000	2001	2002	2003	2004	% change 1998-2004
Life expectancy at birth: total population (years)	78.0	78.1	78.1	78.3	78.5	78.7	78.9	1.18
Life expectancy at birth: total population: year on year growth	0.1	0.1	0.0	0.2	0.4	0.2	0.3	
Healthy life expectancy at birth (years)	72.0			69.7	69.9			
Healthy life expectancy at birth: year on year growth					0.2			

Source: Euromonitor International from World Bank

Sanitation

Netherlands: Improved sanitary facilities and water source 2000

Table: 4.810

As stated

	2000
Population with access to improved sanitary facilities (% of population)	100.0
Population with access to improved water source (% of population)	100.0
Population with improved access to sanitation facilities, rural (% of rural population with access)	100.0
Population with improved access to sanitation facilities, urban (% of urban population with access)	100.0

Source: National statistics/World Bank

Health Expenditure

Netherlands: Public health expenditure 1998-2004

Table: 4.811

As stated

	1998	1999	2000	2001	2002	2003	2004
Public expenditure on pharmaceuticals and other medical non-durables (EUR million)	2,114.0	2,041.0	2,452.0	2,508.0	2,947.0	2,926.0	3,042.2
Private insurance expenditure (% of total expenditure on health)	16.6	16.9	16.1	16.5	17.1	17.6	18.1
Share of total health expenditure in GDP (% of total GDP)	8.6	8.7	8.6	8.9	8.8	8.5	8.3
Health expenditure (US$ per capita)	2,038.0	2,076.0	1,894.0	2,039.0	2,369.0	2,467.0	2,594.0

Source: Euromonitor International from OECD/national statistics

Netherlands: Private health expenditure 1998-2004

Table: 4.812

As stated

	1998	1999	2000	2001	2002	2003	2004
Consumer expenditure on health goods and medical services (EUR million)	6,477.0	7,250.0	7,539.0	8,114.0	8,465.0	9,541.3	9,734.6
Consumer expenditure on health goods and medical services: real growth in national currency: 1990 = 100	144.8	158.6	160.8	165.6	167.0	184.3	185.8
Consumer expenditure on health goods and medical services as a percentage of total consumer expenditure	3.7	3.9	3.8	3.9	3.9	4.2	4.2

Source: National statistical offices/OECD/Eurostat/Euromonitor International

Netherlands: Consumer expenditure on health goods and medical services by sector 1998-2004

Table: 4.813

% of total consumer expenditure on health goods and medical services

	1998	1999	2000	2001	2002	2003	2004
Pharmaceuticals, medical appliances/ equipment	33.2	33.1	33.5	33.5	33.6	35.8	35.8
Outpatient services	29.8	29.8	30.1	30.7	30.8	29.3	29.2
Hospital services	37.0	37.1	36.3	35.7	35.6	34.9	35.0
Total	100.0	100.0	100.0	100.0	100.0	100.0	100.0

Source: National statistical offices/OECD/Eurostat/Euromonitor International

Healthcare Infrastructure and Services

Netherlands: Healthcare infrastructure and services by sector 1998-2004

Table: 4.814

As stated

	1998	1999	2000	2001	2002	2003	2004
Active pharmacists (number)	2,922	2,965	3,069	3,148	3,224	3,298	3,372
Consultations with GPs (general practitioners) (per capita)	6	6	6	6	6	6	6
Dentists (number)	7,215	7,284	7,397	7,509	7,623	7,749	7,887
Doctors (number)	46,101	48,987	50,856	52,602	49,366	50,854	51,906
Hospital admissions (number)	1,556,788	1,526,068	1,488,812	1,487,033	1,453,045	1,421,251	1,412,163
Hospitals and clinics (number)	698	693	685	690	690	690	689	688
In-patient beds ('000)	58	57	55	53	52	51	50
Midwives (number)	1,422	1,507	1,576	1,627	1,725	1,825	1,883
Nurses (number)	197,000	200,500	213,100	205,800	198,274	194,754	192,924
Out-patient contacts (per capita)	6	6	6	6	6	6	6

Source: Euromonitor International from national statistics

Netherlands: Healthcare infrastructure and services by sector: growth 1998-2004

Table: 4.815

Year on year growth: % change in stated unit

	1998	1999	2000	2001	2002	2003	2004
Active pharmacists (number)	7.5	1.5	3.5	2.6	2.4	2.3	2.2
Consultations with GPs (general practitioners) (per capita)	-5.1	3.6	2.3	-2.3	-3.4	0.0	-1.3
Dentists (number)	1.7	1.0	1.6	1.5	1.5	1.7	1.8
Doctors (number)		6.3	3.8	3.4	-6.2	3.0	2.1
Hospital admissions (number)	1.4	-2.0	-2.4	-0.1	-2.3	-2.2	-0.6
Hospitals and clinics (number)	1.0	-0.7	-1.2	0.7	0.0	-0.1	-0.1
In-patient beds (number)	-0.6	-1.0	-3.1	-4.0	-2.3	-1.9	-2.0
Midwives (number)	4.8	6.0	4.6	3.2	6.0	5.8	3.2
Nurses (number)	9.4	1.8	6.3	-3.4	-3.7	-1.8	-0.9
Out-patient contacts (per capita)	-3.4	1.8	1.7	-1.7	-3.4	3.6	-5.2

Source: Euromonitor International from national statistics

Immunisation

Netherlands: Vaccination rates by disease type 1998-2004

Table: 4.816

%

	1998	1999	2000	2001	2002	2003	2004
Vaccination rate against MMR (measles, mumps, rubella) (%)	96.1	96.0	96.0	96.0	96.0	96.0	96.0
Vaccination rate against polio (%)	97.3				97.5	98.0	98.0

Source: WHO

Infectious Diseases

Netherlands: Incidence of disease by type 1998-2004

Table: 4.817

Number

	1998	1999	2000	2001	2002	2003	2004
Incidence of AIDS	291	234	192	76	234	61	75
Incidence of diphtheria	0	1	0		0		
Incidence of measles	9	2,368	1,019		3		
Incidence of polio	0	0	0	0	0		

Source: WHO

Netherlands: Incidence of disease by type: growth 1998-2004

Table: 4.818

Year on year growth: %

	1998	1999	2000	2001	2002	2003	2004
Incidence of AIDS	-14.9	-19.6	-17.9	-60.4	207.9	-73.9	23.0
Incidence of diphtheria	-100.0		-100.0				
Incidence of measles	-57.1	26,211.1	-57.0				

Source: WHO

Causes of Death

Netherlands: Deaths by disease 1998-2004

Table: 4.819

Number per 100,000 inhabitants

	1998	1999	2000	2001	2002	2003	2004
Death by diseases of the circulatory system	235.2	229.7	221.9	215.7	218.1	209.3	207.3
Death by malignant neoplasms (cancers)	192.4	194.2	191.1	191.3	190.6	188.3	188.7
Deaths from heart disease	121.7	115.8	112.3	108.4	104.5	100.6	96.3
Death by diseases of the respiratory system	63.9	64.1	63.9	65.2	65.7	66.4	67.4
Deaths from lung cancer	55.0	55.2	55.0	54.9	54.7	54.4	54.5
Death by diseases of the digestive system	23.6	23.3	22.6	22.2	21.8	22.3	22.2
Deaths from chronic liver disease and cirrhosis	5.3	5.3	5.3	5.2	5.2	5.1	5.0
Deaths from ulcers of the stomach and duodenum	2.3	2.3	2.3	2.2	2.1	2.1	2.0

Source: WHO/Euromonitor International
Notes: Data is ranked in descending order by year 2004

Netherlands: Deaths by disease: growth 1998-2004

Table: 4.820

% year on year growth

	1998	1999	2000	2001	2002	2003	2004
Death by diseases of the respiratory system	4.8	0.3	-0.3	2.0	0.8	1.1	1.5
Deaths from lung cancer	-0.3	0.2	-0.3	-0.2	-0.4	-0.5	0.2
Death by malignant neoplasms (cancers)	-1.2	0.9	-1.6	0.1	-0.4	-1.2	0.2
Death by diseases of the digestive system	-1.3	-1.3	-3.0	-1.8	-1.8	2.3	-0.2
Death by diseases of the circulatory system	-1.5	-2.3	-3.4	-2.8	1.1	-4.0	-0.9
Deaths from chronic liver disease and cirrhosis	-1.5	0.4	-0.2	-1.9	0.0	-1.9	-1.8
Deaths from ulcers of the stomach and duodenum	-5.8	0.7	-2.0	-4.3	-4.5	0.0	-2.4
Deaths from heart disease	-1.9	-4.9	-3.0	-3.5	-3.6	-3.7	-4.3

Source: WHO/Euromonitor International
Notes: Data is ranked in descending order by year 2004

Netherlands: Other selected causes of death: 1998-2004

Table: 4.821

Number per 100,000 inhabitants

	1998	1999	2000	2001	2002	2003	2004
Death by injury and poisoning	26.5	27.6	26.2	26.5	26.3	26.1	26.1
Death by suicide and self-inflicted injury	8.5	8.5	8.2	8.2	8.0	8.1	8.1
Death by motor traffic accidents	6.8	7.2	6.7	6.7	6.7	6.7	6.8

Source: Euromonitor International from national statistics
Notes: Data is ranked in descending order by year 2004

Netherlands: Other selected causes of death: growth 1998-2004

Table: 4.822

% year on year growth

	1998	1999	2000	2001	2002	2003	2004
Death by motor traffic accidents	-8.1	5.9	-6.9	0.0	0.0	0.0	0.9
Death by suicide and self-inflicted injury	-5.6	0.0	-3.5	0.0	-2.4	1.2	0.5
Death by injury and poisoning	-6.0	4.2	-5.1	1.1	-0.8	-0.8	0.2

Source: Euromonitor International from national statistics
Notes: Data is ranked in descending order by year 2004

Smoking

Netherlands: Smoking prevalence in population aged 15+ 1998-2004

Table: 4.823

% of population aged 15+

	1998	1999	2000	2001	2002	2003	2004
Smoking prevalence in population aged 15+ (% of population aged 15+)	34.6	33.8	32.4	34.5	33.5	32.9	32.8
Smoking prevalence in male population aged 15+ (% of male population)	38.5	36.0	35.9	38.9	37.9	34.9	34.0
Smoking prevalence in female population aged 15+ (% of female population)	30.7	31.7	29.2	30.2	29.2	31.0	31.6

Source: WHO/OECD/Euromonitor International

Nutrition and Obesity

Netherlands: Nutrition and obesity 1998-2004

Table: 4.824

As stated

	1998	1999	2000	2001	2002	2003	2004
Availability of fruit and vegetables (kg/capita/year)	192.0	226.2	212.4	219.0	213.1	209.0	203.4
Average supply of calories per day (calories per capita)	3,207.1	3,252.9	3,374.1	3,326.1	3,362.3	3,400.0	3,424.6
Average supply of fat per day (grams per capita)	141.7	141.5	145.7	145.1	144.3	144.3	144.1
Average supply of protein per day (grams per capita)	104.8	103.4	109.3	110.7	107.5	109.8	113.0
Obese population (BMI 30kg/sq m or more) (% of population aged 15+)	8.4	9.0	9.1	10.8	11.0	11.3	12.5

Source: WHO/OECD/Euromonitor International

Over-the-Counter Healthcare

Netherlands: Trends in OTC healthcare retail sales 1998-2004

Table: 4.825

As stated

	1998	1999	2000	2001	2002	2003	2004
OTC Healthcare (EUR million)	384.7	409.2	438.0	469.3	506.5	538.4	561.2
OTC Healthcare: real growth in national currency: 1998 = 100	100.0	104.1	108.6	111.3	116.2	120.9	124.3
OTC Healthcare: year on year (% real growth)	3.4	4.1	4.4	2.5	4.3	4.1	2.8

Source: Euromonitor International from industry sources/national statistics

Netherlands: OTC healthcare retail sales by sector 1998-2004

Table: 4.826

% of OTC retail value sales

	1998	1999	2000	2001	2002	2003	2004
Analgesics	15.5	15.2	15.0	14.7	14.4	14.6	14.1
Cough, cold and allergy (hay fever) remedies	32.5	31.3	30.6	30.0	29.3	28.4	27.9
Digestive remedies	7.6	7.4	7.2	7.2	7.1	7.2	7.1
Medicated skin care	7.1	7.1	7.0	6.9	6.9	6.8	6.7
Vitamins and dietary supplements	25.5	27.6	29.2	30.6	32.0	33.0	34.4

Source: *Euromonitor International from industry sources/national statistics*
Notes: *Only selected sectors are shown, so values are not expected to sum to 100*

Health and Wellness

Netherlands: Retail sales of packaged foods by health and wellness category 2002-2004

Table: 4.827

EUR million

	2002	2003	2004
Packaged food: Total	13,746.8	14,298.1	14,822.6
Better for you	1,196.2	1,273.1	1,344.8
For food intolerance	53.0	54.8	56.4
Fortified/functional	233.0	266.7	311.1
Organic	242.5	266.4	295.0

Source: *Euromonitor International from industry sources/national statistics*

Netherlands: Per capita sales of packaged foods by health and wellness category 2002-2004

Table: 4.828

EUR per capita

	2002	2003	2004
Better for you	74.4	78.6	82.5
For food intolerance	3.3	3.4	3.5
Fortified/functional	14.5	16.5	19.1
Organic	15.1	16.4	18.1

Source: *Euromonitor International from industry sources/national statistics*

Netherlands: Retail sales of packaged food by health and wellness category: % share of total packaged food market 2002-2004

Table: 4.829

% value

	2002	2003	2004
Better for you	8.7	8.9	9.1
For food intolerance	0.4	0.4	0.4
Fortified/functional	1.7	1.9	2.1
Organic	1.8	1.9	2.0

Source: *Euromonitor International from industry sources/national statistics*

Netherlands: Retail sales of packaged food by health and wellness category: real growth index 2002-2004

Table: 4.830

2002 =100

	2002	2003	2004
Better for you	100.00	103.73	107.43
For food intolerance	100.00	100.69	101.71
Fortified/functional	100.00	111.58	127.60
Organic	100.00	107.05	116.21

Source: *Euromonitor International from industry sources/national statistics*

Netherlands: Retail sales of better-for-you packaged foods by sector 2002-2004

Table: 4.831

% of total packaged food / as stated

	2002	2003	2004	% real change in value 2002-2004
Combination	0.17	0.18	0.18	6.69
Reduced carb	0.02	0.02	0.02	-0.78
Reduced fat	6.71	6.90	7.06	8.38
Reduced salt	0.43	0.43	0.40	-4.28

Source: Euromonitor International from industry sources/national statistics

Netherlands: Retail sales of packaged foods for food intolerances by sector 2002-2004

Table: 4.832

% of total packaged food / as stated

	2002	2003	2004	% real change in value 2002-2004
Diabetic	0.25	0.26	0.26	5.67
Gluten-free	0.04	0.04	0.04	7.33
Lactose-free	0.10	0.09	0.08	-10.94

Source: Euromonitor International from industry sources/national statistics

Netherlands: Retail sales of naturally healthy packaged foods by sector 2002-2004

Table: 4.833

% of total packaged food / as stated

	2002	2003	2004	% real change in value 2002-2004
High fibre	5.88	5.80	5.80	1.59
Other naturally healthy food	0.42	0.43	0.45	11.79
Soy-based dairy alternatives	0.11	0.12	0.13	20.95

Source: Euromonitor International from industry sources/national statistics

■ **New Zealand**

Socio-economic Parameters

New Zealand: Socio-economic parameters 1998-2004

Table: 4.834

As stated

	1998	1999	2000	2001	2002	2003	2004
Population: national estimates at January 1st ('000)	3,816.0	3,836.0	3,858.7	3,880.5	3,939.1	3,975.9	4,011.8
% aged 0-14 yrs	23.0	22.9	22.8	22.6	22.3	22.1	21.8
% aged 15-64 yrs	65.4	65.4	65.5	65.5	65.8	66.1	66.4
% aged 65+ yrs	11.6	11.7	11.8	11.9	11.9	11.8	11.8
% Male	49.2	49.1	49.1	49.0	49.1	49.1	49.1
% Female	50.8	50.9	50.9	51.0	50.9	50.9	50.9
% Urban	85.6	85.7	86.9	86.8	86.7	87.3	87.5
Occupants per household at January 1st (Number)	2.8	2.7	2.7	2.7	2.7	2.7	2.7
Households ('000)	1,381.4	1,400.4	1,422.4	1,440.5	1,458.4	1,481.5	1,502.2
Annual rates of inflation (% growth)	1.3	-0.1	2.6	2.6	2.7	1.8	2.3
GDP (NZ$ million)	102,465.0	108,570.0	114,842.0	121,825.0	127,831.0	134,814.0	146,037.0
GDP (US$ million)	54,845.4	57,456.3	52,173.6	51,213.9	59,121.1	78,284.7	96,797.9
GDP (US$ per capita)	14,372.7	14,978.2	13,521.1	13,197.9	15,008.7	19,690.0	24,128.1

Source: Euromonitor International from International Monetary Fund (IMF), International Financial Statistics and World Economic Outlook/UN/national statistics

Life Expectancy

New Zealand: Life expectancy 1998-2004

Table: 4.835

As stated

	1998	1999	2000	2001	2002	2003	2004	% change 1998-2004
Life expectancy at birth: total population (years)	78.1	78.2	78.3	78.5	78.9	79.2	79.4	1.71
Life expectancy at birth: total population: year on year growth	0.2	0.2	0.1	0.3	0.5	0.3	0.3	
Healthy life expectancy at birth (years)	69.0			70.1	70.3			
Healthy life expectancy at birth: year on year growth					0.3			

Source: Euromonitor International from World Bank

Sanitation

New Zealand: Improved sanitary facilities and water source 2000

Table: 4.836

As stated

	2000
Population with improved access to sanitation facilities, rural (% of rural population with access)	100.0

Source: National statistics/World Bank

Health Expenditure

New Zealand: Public health expenditure 1998-2004

Table: 4.837

As stated

	1998	1999	2000	2001	2002	2003	2004
Public expenditure on pharmaceuticals and other medical non-durables (NZ$ million)	813.0	903.0	925.0	996.0	1,054.0	1,102.0	1,175.6
Private insurance expenditure (% of total expenditure on health)	6.4	6.2	6.3	6.3	5.7	5.5	5.2
Share of total health expenditure in GDP (% of total GDP)	7.9	8.0	8.0	8.3	8.2	8.4	8.8
Health expenditure (US$ per capita)	1,125.0	1,155.0	1,055.0	1,056.0	1,255.0	1,288.0	1,351.0

Source: Euromonitor International from OECD/national statistics

New Zealand: Private health expenditure 1998-2004

Table: 4.838

As stated

	1998	1999	2000	2001	2002	2003	2004
Consumer expenditure on health goods and medical services (NZ$ million)	1,717.0	1,830.0	1,939.0	2,119.0	2,359.0	2,438.0	2,562.9
Consumer expenditure on health goods and medical services: real growth in national currency: 1990 = 100	116.7	124.6	128.6	136.9	148.5	150.8	155.0
Consumer expenditure on health goods and medical services as a percentage of total consumer expenditure	2.9	2.9	3.0	3.1	3.3	3.3	3.4

Source: National statistical offices/OECD/Eurostat/Euromonitor International

New Zealand: Consumer expenditure on health goods and medical services by sector 1998-2004

Table: 4.839

% of total consumer expenditure on health goods and medical services

	1998	1999	2000	2001	2002	2003	2004
Pharmaceuticals, medical appliances/ equipment	24.7	24.6	24.7	24.5	27.0	27.1	27.1
Outpatient services	47.6	47.1	46.9	46.5	44.6	44.4	44.3
Hospital services	27.7	28.3	28.5	29.0	28.4	28.5	28.6
Total	100.0	100.0	100.0	100.0	100.0	100.0	100.0

Source: National statistical offices/OECD/Eurostat/Euromonitor International

Healthcare Infrastructure and Services

New Zealand: Healthcare infrastructure and services by sector 1998-2004

Table: 4.840

As stated

	1998	1999	2000	2001	2002	2003	2004
Active pharmacists (number)	2,944	3,405	3,733	3,843	3,927	3,999	4,026
Consultations with GPs (general practitioners) (per capita)				4			
Dentists (number)	1,496	1,558	1,591	1,601	1,645	1,685	1,710
Doctors (number)	8,491	8,616	8,615	8,491	8,403	8,395	8,383
Hospitals and clinics (number)	387	412	433	444	453	462	470
In-patient beds ('000)	24	24	24	24	24	24	24
Nurses (number)	36,736	36,770	36,976	37,303	37,097	36,514	36,504

Source: Euromonitor International from national statistics

New Zealand: Healthcare infrastructure and services by sector: growth 1998-2004

Table: 4.841

Year on year growth: % change in stated unit

	1998	1999	2000	2001	2002	2003	2004
Active pharmacists (number)	13.4	15.7	9.6	2.9	2.2	1.8	0.7
Dentists (number)	1.6	4.1	2.1	0.6	2.7	2.4	1.5
Doctors (number)	3.2	1.5	0.0	-1.4	-1.0	-0.1	-0.1
Hospitals and clinics (number)	2.1	6.5	5.1	2.5	2.0	2.0	1.7
In-patient beds (number)	3.3	0.7	0.3	-0.7	0.7	1.3	0.8
Nurses (number)	8.0	0.1	0.6	0.9	-0.6	-1.6	0.0

Source: Euromonitor International from national statistics

Immunisation

New Zealand: Vaccination rates by disease type 1998-2004

Table: 4.842

%

	1998	1999	2000	2001	2002	2003	2004
Vaccination rate against DTP (diphtheria, tetanus, pertussis) 1 & 2 (%)			89.1	89.1	89.1	89.0	89.0
Vaccination rate against MMR (measles, mumps, rubella) (%)	81.0	83.0	85.2	85.2	87.3	89.0	90.0
Vaccination rate against polio (%)	82.0	85.0	82.4	82.4	82.0	82.0	82.0

Source: WHO

Infectious Diseases

New Zealand: Incidence of disease by type 1998-2004

Table: 4.843

Number

	1998	1999	2000	2001	2002	2003	2004
Incidence of AIDS	29	33	27	26	22	20	25
Incidence of diphtheria	1	0	0	0	1		
Incidence of measles	164	106	65	65	21		
Incidence of polio	0	0	0	0	0		

Source: WHO

New Zealand: Incidence of disease by type: growth 1998-2004

Table: 4.844

Year on year growth: %

	1998	1999	2000	2001	2002	2003	2004
Incidence of AIDS	-32.6	13.8	-18.2	-3.7	-15.4	-9.1	25.0
Incidence of diphtheria		-100.0					
Incidence of measles	-92.0	-35.4	-38.7	0.0	-67.7		

Source: WHO

Causes of Death

New Zealand: Deaths by disease 1998-2004

Table: 4.845

Number per 100,000 inhabitants

	1998	1999	2000	2001	2002	2003	2004
Deaths from heart disease	163.6	175.3	175.4	178.4	181.4	184.4	186.4
Death by diseases of the circulatory system	247.4	240.0	237.0	215.0	200.0	185.0	172.0
Death by malignant neoplasms (cancers)	189.1	184.0	182.0	178.0	174.0	172.0	168.3
Deaths from lung cancer	36.4	38.5	38.9	39.8	40.7	41.5	42.4
Death by diseases of the respiratory system	49.2	45.0	38.0	33.0	29.0	25.0	21.6
Death by diseases of the digestive system	14.3	13.5	12.0	11.0	9.0	7.5	6.4
Deaths from chronic liver disease and cirrhosis	2.9	3.8	3.8	4.1	4.3	4.6	4.9
Deaths from ulcers of the stomach and duodenum	2.9	2.6	2.1	2.3	2.1	1.9	1.8

Source: WHO/Euromonitor International
Notes: Data is ranked in descending order by year 2004

New Zealand: Deaths by disease: growth 1998-2004

Table: 4.846

% year on year growth

	1998	1999	2000	2001	2002	2003	2004
Deaths from chronic liver disease and cirrhosis	-12.6	30.4	-0.4	7.9	4.9	7.0	5.9
Deaths from lung cancer	-1.1	5.7	1.0	2.3	2.3	2.0	2.1
Deaths from heart disease	-3.4	7.2	0.0	1.7	1.7	1.7	1.1
Death by malignant neoplasms (cancers)	1.6	-2.7	-1.1	-2.2	-2.2	-1.1	-2.2
Deaths from ulcers of the stomach and duodenum	-14.2	-10.9	-18.0	9.5	-8.7	-9.5	-3.7
Death by diseases of the circulatory system	-7.7	-3.0	-1.3	-9.3	-7.0	-7.5	-7.0
Death by diseases of the respiratory system	-27.0	-8.5	-15.6	-13.2	-12.1	-13.8	-13.5
Death by diseases of the digestive system	-17.3	-5.6	-11.1	-8.3	-18.2	-16.7	-14.8

Source: WHO/Euromonitor International
Notes: Data is ranked in descending order by year 2004

New Zealand: Other selected causes of death: 1998-2004

Table: 4.847

Number per 100,000 inhabitants

	1998	1999	2000	2001	2002	2003	2004
Death by injury and poisoning	43.5	42.3	41.9	40.5	39.2	38.6	37.9
Death by suicide and self-inflicted injury	15.2	15.5	15.8	16.1	16.5	17.0	17.5
Death by motor traffic accidents	14.5	14.4	14.3	14.1	14.0	13.8	13.6

Source: Euromonitor International from national statistics
Notes: Data is ranked in descending order by year 2004

New Zealand: Other selected causes of death: growth 1998-2004

Table: 4.848

% year on year growth

	1998	1999	2000	2001	2002	2003	2004
Death by suicide and self-inflicted injury	1.3	2.0	1.9	1.9	2.5	3.0	3.2
Death by motor traffic accidents	-2.0	-0.7	-0.7	-1.4	-0.7	-1.4	-1.2
Death by injury and poisoning	-6.5	-2.8	-0.9	-3.3	-3.2	-1.5	-1.9

Source: Euromonitor International from national statistics
Notes: Data is ranked in descending order by year 2004

Smoking

New Zealand: Smoking prevalence in population aged 15+ 1998-2004

Table: 4.849

% of population aged 15+

	1998	1999	2000	2001	2002	2003	2004
Smoking prevalence in population aged 15+ (% of population aged 15+)	26.0	25.0	26.0	25.0	23.9	23.7	22.9
Smoking prevalence in male population aged 15+ (% of male population)	26.0	26.0	25.0	25.1	24.8	24.8	24.7
Smoking prevalence in female population aged 15+ (% of female population)	26.0	24.1	26.9	24.9	23.2	22.6	21.2

Source: WHO/OECD/Euromonitor International

Nutrition and Obesity

New Zealand: Nutrition and obesity 1998-2004

Table: 4.850

As stated

	1998	1999	2000	2001	2002	2003	2004
Average supply of calories per day (calories per capita)	3,172.2	3,197.3	3,228.1	3,213.8	3,219.2	3,226.0	3,229.9
Average supply of fat per day (grams per capita)	113.3	114.9	112.6	112.4	115.3	116.9	118.4
Average supply of protein per day (grams per capita)	95.0	98.1	95.0	97.7	99.9	101.3	103.2
Obese population (BMI 30kg/sq m or more) (% of population aged 15+)	16.1	16.3	16.3	16.4	16.5	16.6	16.7

Source: WHO/OECD/Euromonitor International

Over-the-Counter Healthcare

New Zealand: Trends in OTC healthcare retail sales 1998-2004

Table: 4.851

As stated

	1998	1999	2000	2001	2002	2003	2004
OTC Healthcare (NZ$ million)	164.3	176.6	189.8	197.6	205.0	211.8	218.6
OTC Healthcare: real growth in national currency: 1998 = 100	100.0	107.6	112.7	114.4	115.5	117.3	118.2
OTC Healthcare: year on year (% real growth)	4.6	7.6	4.8	1.4	1.0	1.6	0.8
OTC Healthcare (NZ$ per capita)	43.1	46.0	49.2	50.9	52.0	53.3	54.5

Source: *Euromonitor International from industry sources/national statistics*

New Zealand: OTC healthcare retail sales by sector 1998-2004

Table: 4.852

% of OTC retail value sales

	1998	1999	2000	2001	2002	2003	2004
Analgesics	11.1	10.9	10.7	10.7	10.7	10.8	10.8
Cough, cold and allergy (hay fever) remedies	25.0	24.6	24.2	24.0	24.1	24.2	24.3
Digestive remedies	2.8	2.7	2.7	2.6	2.6	2.6	2.6
Medicated skin care	13.2	12.7	12.3	12.4	12.4	12.4	12.6
Vitamins and dietary supplements	33.0	34.4	35.4	35.2	35.1	34.5	34.0

Source: *Euromonitor International from industry sources/national statistics*
Notes: *Only selected sectors are shown, so values are not expected to sum to 100*

■ Nigeria

Socio-economic Parameters

Nigeria: Socio-economic parameters 1998-2004

Table: 4.853

As stated

	1998	1999	2000	2001	2002	2003	2004
Population: national estimates at January 1st ('000)	107,124.7	110,157.0	113,212.7	116,283.6	119,366.2	122,459.2	125,562.4
% aged 0-14 yrs	45.5	45.3	45.1	44.9	44.7	44.5	44.3
% aged 15-64 yrs	51.5	51.7	51.8	52.0	52.2	52.4	52.6
% aged 65 + yrs	3.0	3.0	3.0	3.1	3.1	3.1	3.1
% Male	50.3	50.3	50.3	50.3	50.3	50.4	50.4
% Female	49.7	49.7	49.7	49.7	49.7	49.6	49.6
% Urban	42.2	43.1	43.4	44.2	45.0	45.8	46.7
Occupants per household at January 1st (Number)	4.8	4.8	4.8	4.8	4.8	4.8	4.8
Households ('000)	22,149.5	22,794.7	23,447.2	24,120.7	24,766.6	25,448.2	26,100.5
Annual rates of inflation (% growth)	10.3	4.8	14.5	13.0	12.9	14.0	15.0
GDP (NGN million)	2,881,310.0	3,320,640.0	4,980,960.0	4,864,450.0	5,602,570.0	7,191,050.0	8,553,280.0
GDP (US$ million)	33,503.9	35,961.8	48,978.4	43,732.9	46,464.3	55,648.8	64,364.6
GDP (US$ per capita)	312.8	326.5	432.6	376.1	389.3	454.4	512.6

Source: *Euromonitor International from International Monetary Fund (IMF), International Financial Statistics and World Economic Outlook/UN/national statistics*

Life Expectancy

Nigeria: Life expectancy 1998-2004

Table: 4.854

As stated

	1998	1999	2000	2001	2002	2003	2004	% change 1998-2004
Life expectancy at birth: total population (years)	51.1	51.3	51.6	51.6	48.8	48.0	46.6	-8.88
Life expectancy at birth: total population: year on year growth	0.4	0.3	0.6	0.0	-5.4	-1.7	-2.8	
Healthy life expectancy at birth (years)	38.0			41.9	41.9			
Healthy life expectancy at birth: year on year growth					-0.1			

Source: Euromonitor International from World Bank

Sanitation

Nigeria: Improved sanitary facilities and water source 2000

Table: 4.855

As stated

	2000
Population with access to improved sanitary facilities (% of population)	54.0
Population with access to improved water source (% of population)	62.0
Population with improved access to sanitation facilities, rural (% of rural population with access)	45.0
Population with improved access to sanitation facilities, urban (% of urban population with access)	66.0

Source: National statistics/World Bank

Health Expenditure

Nigeria: Public health expenditure 1998-2004

Table: 4.856

As stated

	1998	1999	2000	2001	2002	2003	2004
Share of total health expenditure in GDP (% of total GDP)	3.1	3.0	3.0	3.4	3.4	3.5	3.4
Health expenditure (US$ per capita)	17.0	17.0	18.0	20.0	19.0	20.0	20.0

Source: Euromonitor International from OECD/national statistics

Nigeria: Private health expenditure 1998-2004

Table: 4.857

As stated

	1998	1999	2000	2001	2002	2003	2004
Consumer expenditure on health goods and medical services (NGN million)	90,702.2	60,817.9	81,455.5	128,209.9	168,509.6	229,631.2	270,562.8
Consumer expenditure on health goods and medical services: real growth in national currency: 1990 = 100	223.4	143.0	167.2	233.0	269.4	322.0	329.9
Consumer expenditure on health goods and medical services as a percentage of total consumer expenditure	3.2	2.9	3.2	3.6	3.5	3.7	3.6

Source: National statistical offices/OECD/Eurostat/Euromonitor International

Nigeria: Consumer expenditure on health goods and medical services by sector 1998-2004

Table: 4.858

% of total consumer expenditure on health goods and medical services

	1998	1999	2000	2001	2002	2003	2004
Pharmaceuticals, medical appliances/ equipment	40.5	37.5	34.2	29.8	31.0	31.1	31.5
Outpatient services	52.4	55.0	57.2	60.4	59.4	59.4	58.9
Hospital services	7.1	7.5	8.6	9.8	9.7	9.6	9.7
Total	100.0	100.0	100.0	100.0	100.0	100.0	100.0

Source: National statistical offices/OECD/Eurostat/Euromonitor International

Healthcare Infrastructure and Services

Nigeria: Healthcare infrastructure and services by sector 1998-2004

Table: 4.859

As stated

	1998	1999	2000	2001	2002	2003	2004
Active pharmacists (number)	7,230	7,316	7,330	7,381	7,396	7,405	7,438
Dentists (number)	1,596	1,635	1,696	1,750	1,778	1,802	1,829
Doctors (number)	22,481	22,495	22,504	22,534	22,568	22,609	22,653
Midwives (number)	71,681	73,240	74,699	76,401	78,122	79,521	80,946
Nurses (number)	99,716	103,322	106,828	110,833	114,342	117,912	120,898

Source: Euromonitor International from national statistics

Nigeria: Healthcare infrastructure and services by sector: growth 1998-2004

Table: 4.860

Year on year growth: % change in stated unit

	1998	1999	2000	2001	2002	2003	2004
Active pharmacists (number)	0.2	1.2	0.2	0.7	0.2	0.1	0.4
Dentists (number)	4.0	2.4	3.7	3.2	1.6	1.3	1.5
Doctors (number)	0.4	0.1	0.0	0.1	0.2	0.2	0.2
Midwives (number)	2.4	2.2	2.0	2.3	2.3	1.8	1.8
Nurses (number)	3.9	3.6	3.4	3.7	3.2	3.1	2.5

Source: Euromonitor International from national statistics

Immunisation

Nigeria: Vaccination rates by disease type 1998-2004

Table: 4.861

%

	1998	1999	2000	2001	2002	2003	2004
Vaccination rate against DTP (diphtheria, tetanus, pertussis) 1 & 2 (%)			48.0	52.0	56.0	60.0	64.0
Vaccination rate against MMR (measles, mumps, rubella) (%)	26.0		30.0				
Vaccination rate against polio (%)	22.0		38.0	40.0	45.0	42.0	38.0

Source: WHO

Infectious Diseases

Nigeria: Incidence of disease by type 1998-2004

Table: 4.862

Number

	1998	1999	2000	2001	2002	2003	2004
Incidence of AIDS	18,490	16,188	9,715	3,661	3,989	2,026	1,756
Incidence of diphtheria	708		3,995	2,468	790		
Incidence of measles	143,098		212,183	168,107	42,007		
Incidence of polio	312	981	638	56	202		

Source: WHO

Nigeria: Incidence of disease by type: growth 1998-2004

Table: 4.863

Year on year growth: %

	1998	1999	2000	2001	2002	2003	2004
Incidence of AIDS	384.7	-12.4	-40.0	-62.3	9.0	-49.2	-13.3
Incidence of diphtheria				-38.2	-68.0		
Incidence of measles	569.2			-20.8	-75.0		
Incidence of polio	-18.5	214.4	-35.0	-91.2	260.7		

Source: WHO

Smoking

Nigeria: Smoking prevalence in population aged 15+ 1998-2004

Table: 4.864

% of population aged 15+

	1998	1999	2000	2001	2002	2003	2004
Smoking prevalence in population aged 15+ (% of population aged 15+)	15.2	15.5	14.8	14.9	14.6	14.9	14.4
Smoking prevalence in male population aged 15+ (% of male population)	15.4	15.5	15.2	15.4	16.0	17.0	16.9
Smoking prevalence in female population aged 15+ (% of female population)	15.0	15.5	14.4	14.4	13.2	12.8	11.9

Source: WHO/OECD/Euromonitor International

Nutrition and Obesity

Nigeria: Nutrition and obesity 1998-2004

Table: 4.865

As stated

	1998	1999	2000	2001	2002	2003	2004
Average supply of calories per day (calories per capita)	2,773.5	2,765.3	2,704.0	2,684.4	2,725.5	2,739.0	2,751.1
Average supply of fat per day (grams per capita)	64.8	64.8	62.6	61.7	62.0	61.7	61.4
Average supply of protein per day (grams per capita)	62.9	62.6	62.1	60.3	61.1	61.2	61.1
Obese population (BMI 30kg/sq m or more) (% of population aged 15+)	18.7	18.5	18.8	19.7	19.9	20.6	21.1

Source: WHO/OECD/Euromonitor International

■ **Norway**

Socio-economic Parameters

Norway: Socio-economic parameters 1998-2004

Table: 4.866

As stated

	1998	1999	2000	2001	2002	2003	2004
Population: national estimates at January 1st ('000)	4,417.6	4,445.3	4,478.5	4,503.4	4,524.1	4,555.5	4,581.7
% aged 0-14 yrs	19.8	19.9	20.0	20.0	20.0	20.0	19.8
% aged 15-64 yrs	64.6	64.7	64.8	64.9	65.0	65.2	65.4
% aged 65+ yrs	15.7	15.5	15.3	15.1	14.9	14.8	14.7
% Male	49.5	49.5	49.5	49.5	49.6	49.6	49.6
% Female	50.5	50.5	50.5	50.5	50.4	50.4	50.4
% Urban	74.8	75.1	74.2	74.7	75.2	75.0	75.2
Occupants per household at January 1st (Number)	2.3	2.3	2.3	2.3	2.3	2.3	2.3
Households ('000)	1,901.3	1,922.6	1,946.4	1,961.5	1,978.7	1,998.0	2,015.9
Annual rates of inflation (% growth)	2.3	2.3	3.1	3.0	1.3	2.5	0.5
GDP (NKr million)	1,132,130.0	1,233,040.0	1,469,070.0	1,526,230.0	1,519,130.0	1,561,910.0	1,685,550.0
GDP (US$ million)	150,048.4	158,098.9	166,904.9	169,738.6	190,277.0	220,601.9	250,050.8
GDP (US$ per capita)	33,966.0	35,565.2	37,268.1	37,690.9	42,058.9	48,425.0	54,576.6

Source: *Euromonitor International from International Monetary Fund (IMF), International Financial Statistics and World Economic Outlook/UN/national statistics*

Life Expectancy

Norway: Life expectancy 1998-2004

Table: 4.867

As stated

	1998	1999	2000	2001	2002	2003	2004	% change 1998-2004
Life expectancy at birth: total population (years)	78.3	78.5	78.7	78.8	79.0	79.3	79.5	1.45
Life expectancy at birth: total population: year on year growth	0.2	0.2	0.3	0.1	0.4	0.3	0.3	
Healthy life expectancy at birth (years)	72.0			70.7	70.8			
Healthy life expectancy at birth: year on year growth					0.1			

Source: *Euromonitor International from World Bank*

Sanitation

Norway: Improved sanitary facilities and water source 2000

Table: 4.868

As stated

	2000
Population with access to improved water source (% of population)	100.0
Population with improved access to sanitation facilities, rural (% of rural population with access)	100.0
Population with improved access to sanitation facilities, urban (% of urban population with access)	100.0

Source: *National statistics/World Bank*

Health Expenditure

Norway: Public health expenditure 1998-2004

Table: 4.869

As stated

	1998	1999	2000	2001	2002	2003	2004
Public expenditure on pharmaceuticals and other medical non-durables (NKr million)							
Share of total health expenditure in GDP (% of total GDP)	8.5	8.5	7.6	8.0	8.1	7.9	7.9
Health expenditure (US$ per capita)	2,865.0	3,024.0	2,850.0	3,031.0	3,647.0	3,855.0	4,078.0

Source: *Euromonitor International from OECD/national statistics*

Norway: Private health expenditure 1998-2004

Table: 4.870

As stated

	1998	1999	2000	2001	2002	2003	2004
Consumer expenditure on health goods and medical services (NKr million)	14,165.0	15,067.0	16,441.0	17,650.0	18,806.0	19,337.8	19,499.0
Consumer expenditure on health goods and medical services: real growth in national currency: 1990 = 100	144.8	150.5	159.3	166.0	174.7	175.3	175.9
Consumer expenditure on health goods and medical services as a percentage of total consumer expenditure	2.7	2.7	2.8	2.9	2.9	2.9	2.8

Source: *National statistical offices/OECD/Eurostat/Euromonitor International*

Norway: Consumer expenditure on health goods and medical services by sector 1998-2004

Table: 4.871

% of total consumer expenditure on health goods and medical services

	1998	1999	2000	2001	2002	2003	2004
Pharmaceuticals, medical appliances/equipment	41.4	42.3	43.7	43.6	43.1	46.0	46.0
Outpatient services	57.1	56.2	54.8	54.7	55.3	52.4	52.4
Hospital services	1.5	1.5	1.5	1.7	1.6	1.6	1.6
Total	100.0	100.0	100.0	100.0	100.0	100.0	100.0

Source: *National statistical offices/OECD/Eurostat/Euromonitor International*

Healthcare Infrastructure and Services

Norway: Healthcare infrastructure and services by sector 1998-2004

Table: 4.872

As stated

	1998	1999	2000	2001	2002	2003	2004
Active pharmacists (number)					1,595	1,610	1,622
Consultations with GPs (general practitioners) (per capita)	5	5	5	5	5	6	6
Dentists (number)	3,642	3,635	3,608	3,628	3,853	3,984	4,111
Doctors (number)	12,110	12,473	12,813	13,388	15,586	16,279	16,882
Hospital admissions (number)	712,883	730,568	749,394	787,584	805,840	830,963	851,008
In-patient beds ('000)	14	14	14	14	14	14	14
Nurses (number)	43,638	45,133	46,128	46,877	47,991	49,120	50,191

Source: *Euromonitor International from national statistics*

Norway: Healthcare infrastructure and services by sector: growth 1998-2004

Table: 4.873

Year on year growth: % change in stated unit

	1998	1999	2000	2001	2002	2003	2004
Active pharmacists (number)						0.9	0.7
Consultations with GPs (general practitioners) (per capita)	3.7	3.1	6.7	-1.1	3.8	2.5	1.3
Dentists (number)	-1.4	-0.2	-0.7	0.6	6.2	3.4	3.2
Doctors (number)	9.0	3.0	2.7	4.5	16.4	4.4	3.7
Hospital admissions (number)	2.9	2.5	2.6	5.1	2.3	3.1	2.4
In-patient beds (number)	-0.2	-1.3	-1.6	0.0	0.4	0.6	0.3
Nurses (number)	3.6	3.4	2.2	1.6	2.4	2.4	2.2

Source: *Euromonitor International from national statistics*

Immunisation

Norway: Vaccination rates by disease type 1998-2004

%

	1998	1999	2000	2001	2002	2003	2004
Vaccination rate against DTP (diphtheria, tetanus, pertussis) 1 & 2 (%)					92.0	92.0	92.0
Vaccination rate against MMR (measles, mumps, rubella) (%)	93.0	93.0	93.0	93.0	88.0	90.0	89.0
Vaccination rate against polio (%)				95.0	91.0	90.0	90.0

Source: WHO

Infectious Diseases

Norway: Incidence of disease by type 1998-2004

Number

	1998	1999	2000	2001	2002	2003	2004
Incidence of AIDS	36	23	38	6	33	3	8
Incidence of diphtheria			0	0	0		
Incidence of measles			0	4	5		
Incidence of polio	0	0	0	0	0		

Source: WHO

Norway: Incidence of disease by type: growth 1998-2004

Year on year growth: %

	1998	1999	2000	2001	2002	2003	2004
Incidence of AIDS	5.9	-36.1	65.2	-84.2	450.0	-90.9	166.7
Incidence of measles					25.0		

Source: WHO

Causes of Death

Norway: Deaths by disease 1998-2004

Number per 100,000 inhabitants

	1998	1999	2000	2001	2002	2003	2004
Death by diseases of the circulatory system	258.3	252.1	246.6	240.8	235.2	242.5	239.2
Deaths from heart disease	199.1	196.0	189.9	184.7	179.5	174.3	167.7
Death by malignant neoplasms (cancers)	168.0	168.3	164.2	163.1	161.2	162.2	163.2
Death by diseases of the respiratory system	50.4	55.3	54.5	57.4	59.4	54.5	54.7
Deaths from lung cancer	38.0	38.3	37.4	36.8	36.2	35.6	35.3
Death by diseases of the digestive system	19.5	19.4	18.9	18.9	18.8	18.8	18.8
Deaths from ulcers of the stomach and duodenum	5.2	6.4	6.8	7.3	7.8	8.3	8.9
Deaths from chronic liver disease and cirrhosis	5.9	5.2	5.2	5.0	4.8	4.7	4.6

Source: WHO/Euromonitor International
Notes: Data is ranked in descending order by year 2004

Norway: Deaths by disease: growth 1998-2004

Table: 4.878

% year on year growth

	1998	1999	2000	2001	2002	2003	2004
Deaths from ulcers of the stomach and duodenum	-0.1	23.9	5.7	7.4	6.8	6.4	6.7
Death by malignant neoplasms (cancers)	-4.2	0.2	-2.4	-0.7	-1.2	0.6	0.6
Death by diseases of the respiratory system	-3.1	9.7	-1.4	5.3	3.5	-8.2	0.4
Death by diseases of the digestive system	-1.5	-0.5	-2.6	0.0	-0.5	0.0	0.0
Deaths from lung cancer	-3.5	0.6	-2.2	-1.6	-1.6	-1.7	-0.8
Death by diseases of the circulatory system	-2.0	-2.4	-2.2	-2.4	-2.3	3.1	-1.4
Deaths from chronic liver disease and cirrhosis	5.5	-11.3	-0.4	-3.8	-4.0	-2.1	-2.6
Deaths from heart disease	-3.7	-1.6	-3.1	-2.7	-2.8	-2.9	-3.8

Source: WHO/Euromonitor International
Notes: Data is ranked in descending order by year 2004

Norway: Other selected causes of death: 1998-2004

Table: 4.879

Number per 100,000 inhabitants

	1998	1999	2000	2001	2002	2003	2004
Death by injury and poisoning	40.8	42.4	43.1	44.3	45.4	42.5	42.0
Death by suicide and self-inflicted injury	11.8	12.7	13.0	13.7	14.3	12.9	12.8
Death by motor traffic accidents	8.7	7.8	8.8	8.5	8.5	8.3	8.2

Source: Euromonitor International from national statistics
Notes: Data is ranked in descending order by year 2004

Norway: Other selected causes of death: growth 1998-2004

Table: 4.880

% year on year growth

	1998	1999	2000	2001	2002	2003	2004
Death by suicide and self-inflicted injury	5.4	7.6	2.4	5.4	4.4	-9.8	-1.1
Death by motor traffic accidents	17.6	-10.3	12.8	-3.4	0.0	-2.4	-1.1
Death by injury and poisoning	0.5	3.9	1.7	2.8	2.5	-6.4	-1.3

Source: Euromonitor International from national statistics
Notes: Data is ranked in descending order by year 2004

Smoking

Norway: Smoking prevalence in population aged 15+ 1998-2004

Table: 4.881

% of population aged 15+

	1998	1999	2000	2001	2002	2003	2004
Smoking prevalence in population aged 15+ (% of population aged 15+)	32.9	32.3	31.2	29.6	29.6	31.9	31.9
Smoking prevalence in male population aged 15+ (% of male population)	33.5	32.4	31.3	29.5	29.5	30.9	30.6
Smoking prevalence in female population aged 15+ (% of female population)	32.3	32.2	31.1	29.7	29.7	32.8	33.2

Source: WHO/OECD/Euromonitor International

Nutrition and Obesity

Norway: Nutrition and obesity 1998-2004

Table: 4.882

As stated

	1998	1999	2000	2001	2002	2003	2004
Availability of fruit and vegetables (kg/capita/year)	163.1	171.2	166.9	173.0	171.1	173.8	172.6
Average supply of calories per day (calories per capita)	3,352.4	3,393.5	3,363.6	3,425.5	3,484.2	3,528.0	3,579.3
Average supply of fat per day (grams per capita)	137.1	137.9	137.2	141.2	145.4	148.8	145.6
Average supply of protein per day (grams per capita)	104.2	104.8	104.3	106.6	107.6	108.6	109.8
Obese population (BMI 30kg/sq m or more) (% of population aged 15 +)	8.0	8.7	9.2	10.3	11.5	11.9	12.2

Source: WHO/OECD/Euromonitor International

Over-the-Counter Healthcare

Norway: Trends in OTC healthcare retail sales 1998-2004

Table: 4.883

As stated

	1998	1999	2000	2001	2002	2003	2004
OTC Healthcare (NKr million)	2,471.9	2,597.7	2,752.8	2,887.7	3,029.7	3,191.2	3,362.9
OTC Healthcare: real growth in national currency: 1998 = 100	100.0	102.7	105.6	107.5	111.3	114.4	120.0
OTC Healthcare: year on year (% real growth)	2.9	2.7	2.8	1.8	3.6	2.8	4.9
OTC Healthcare (NKr per capita)	559.6	584.4	614.7	641.2	669.7	700.5	734.0

Source: Euromonitor International from industry sources/national statistics

Norway: OTC healthcare retail sales by sector 1998-2004

Table: 4.884

% of OTC retail value sales

	1998	1999	2000	2001	2002	2003	2004
Analgesics	14.6	14.5	14.3	14.1	14.1	14.3	14.7
Cough, cold and allergy (hay fever) remedies	19.3	19.0	18.4	17.2	16.5	15.6	15.2
Digestive remedies	7.8	7.5	7.2	7.1	6.9	6.8	6.8
Medicated skin care	8.0	7.9	7.7	7.5	7.4	7.1	7.0
Vitamins and dietary supplements	41.5	42.4	43.8	45.3	46.2	46.5	46.6

Source: Euromonitor International from industry sources/national statistics
Notes: Only selected sectors are shown, so values are not expected to sum to 100

Health and Wellness

Norway: Retail sales of packaged foods by health and wellness category 2002-2004

Table: 4.885

NKr million

	2002	2003	2004
Packaged food: Total	53,682.6	56,138.3	58,816.9
Better for you	6,657.3	6,885.8	7,177.0
For food intolerance	145.2	175.5	198.8
Fortified/functional	857.8	922.5	967.2
Organic	283.3	319.8	358.3

Source: Euromonitor International from industry sources/national statistics

Norway: Per capita sales of packaged foods by health and wellness category 2002-2004

Table: 4.886

NKr per capita

	2002	2003	2004
Better for you	1,470.3	1,511.7	1,566.3
For food intolerance	32.1	38.5	43.4
Fortified/functional	189.5	202.5	211.1
Organic	62.6	70.2	78.2

Source: *Euromonitor International from industry sources/national statistics*

Norway: Retail sales of packaged food by health and wellness category: % share of total packaged food market 2002-2004

Table: 4.887

% value

	2002	2003	2004
Better for you	12.4	12.3	12.2
For food intolerance	0.3	0.3	0.3
Fortified/functional	1.6	1.6	1.6
Organic	0.5	0.6	0.6

Source: *Euromonitor International from industry sources/national statistics*

Norway: Retail sales of packaged food by health and wellness category: real growth index 2002-2004

Table: 4.888

2002 = 100

	2002	2003	2004
Better for you	100.00	100.71	103.93
For food intolerance	100.00	117.67	131.99
Fortified/functional	100.00	104.72	108.70
Organic	100.00	109.93	121.95

Source: *Euromonitor International from industry sources/national statistics*

Norway: Retail sales of better-for-you packaged foods by sector 2002-2004

Table: 4.889

% of total packaged food / as stated

	2002	2003	2004	% real change in value 2002-2004
Reduced carb	0.05	0.15	0.30	502.94
Reduced fat	10.10	9.81	9.56	-0.03
Reduced salt	0.05	0.05	0.05	10.85

Source: *Euromonitor International from industry sources/national statistics*

Norway: Retail sales of packaged foods for food intolerances by sector 2002-2004

Table: 4.890

% of total packaged food / as stated

	2002	2003	2004	% real change in value 2002-2004
Gluten-free	0.16	0.18	0.19	25.91
Lactose-free	0.11	0.13	0.15	41.05

Source: *Euromonitor International from industry sources/national statistics*

Norway: Retail sales of naturally healthy packaged foods by sector 2002-2004

Table: 4.891

% of total packaged food / as stated

	2002	2003	2004	% real change in value 2002-2004
High fibre	4.82	4.76	4.88	6.98
Other naturally healthy food	0.46	0.47	0.46	3.86
Soy-based dairy alternatives	0.03	0.03	0.03	-2.82

Source: Euromonitor International from industry sources/national statistics

■ **Pakistan**

Socio-economic Parameters

Pakistan: Socio-economic parameters 1998-2004

Table: 4.892

As stated

	1998	1999	2000	2001	2002	2003	2004
Population: national estimates at January 1st ('000)	133,591.4	137,198.5	140,835.2	144,465.0	148,093.2	151,743.5	155,445.8
% aged 0-14 yrs	42.7	42.4	42.2	41.9	41.6	41.4	41.1
% aged 15-64 yrs	53.7	54.0	54.2	54.4	54.7	54.9	55.1
% aged 65 + yrs	3.6	3.6	3.6	3.6	3.7	3.7	3.7
% Male	51.2	51.2	51.2	51.2	51.2	51.2	51.2
% Female	48.8	48.8	48.8	48.8	48.8	48.8	48.8
% Urban	35.9	36.5	37.0	37.5	38.1	38.7	39.4
Occupants per household at January 1st (Number)	7.2	7.2	7.2	7.3	7.2	7.2	7.2
Households ('000)	18,673.6	19,136.3	19,492.2	19,755.0	20,430.5	21,069.2	21,532.9
Annual rates of inflation (% growth)	6.2	4.1	4.4	3.1	3.3	2.9	7.4
GDP (PKR million)	2,677,700.0	2,938,400.0	3,793,440.0	4,162,650.0	4,401,700.0	4,821,300.0	5,458,060.0
GDP (US$ million)	59,442.8	59,360.8	70,709.5	67,218.4	73,700.9	83,482.8	93,687.9
GDP (US$ per capita)	445.0	432.7	502.1	465.3	497.7	550.2	602.7

Source: Euromonitor International from International Monetary Fund (IMF), International Financial Statistics and World Economic Outlook/UN/national statistics

Life Expectancy

Pakistan: Life expectancy 1998-2004

Table: 4.893

As stated

	1998	1999	2000	2001	2002	2003	2004	% change 1998-2004
Life expectancy at birth: total population (years)	60.2	60.6	61.2	61.3	61.4	61.5	61.9	2.79
Life expectancy at birth: total population: year on year growth	0.7	0.7	1.0	0.1	0.2	0.3	0.5	
Healthy life expectancy at birth (years)	56.0			50.9	50.9			
Healthy life expectancy at birth: year on year growth					0.1			

Source: Euromonitor International from World Bank

Sanitation

Pakistan: Improved sanitary facilities and water source 2000

Table: 4.894

As stated

	2000
Population with access to improved sanitary facilities (% of population)	62.0
Population with access to improved water source (% of population)	90.0
Population with improved access to sanitation facilities, rural (% of rural population with access)	43.0
Population with improved access to sanitation facilities, urban (% of urban population with access)	95.0

Source: National statistics/World Bank

Health Expenditure

Pakistan: Public health expenditure 1998-2004

Table: 4.895

As stated

	1998	1999	2000	2001	2002	2003	2004
Share of total health expenditure in GDP (% of total GDP)	3.9	4.0	4.1	3.9	4.0	3.9	3.9
Health expenditure (US$ per capita)	16.0	15.0	14.0	12.0	13.0	12.0	12.0

Source: *Euromonitor International from OECD/national statistics*

Pakistan: Private health expenditure 1998-2004

Table: 4.896

As stated

	1998	1999	2000	2001	2002	2003	2004
Consumer expenditure on health goods and medical services (PKR million)	106,081.3	121,151.4	125,368.4	134,644.1	142,226.5	151,324.8	166,074.4
Consumer expenditure on health goods and medical services: real growth in national currency: 1990 = 100	256.2	280.9	278.5	290.0	296.8	306.9	313.6
Consumer expenditure on health goods and medical services as a percentage of total consumer expenditure	5.2	5.2	5.1	5.0	4.9	4.7	4.7

Source: *National statistical offices/OECD/Eurostat/Euromonitor International*

Pakistan: Consumer expenditure on health goods and medical services by sector 1998-2004

Table: 4.897

% of total consumer expenditure on health goods and medical services

	1998	1999	2000	2001	2002	2003	2004
Pharmaceuticals, medical appliances/equipment	38.6	38.2	39.0	40.7	41.4	40.7	40.1
Outpatient services	1.2	1.1	1.2	1.1	1.0	1.1	1.1
Hospital services	60.2	60.7	59.8	58.2	57.5	58.2	58.7
Total	100.0	100.0	100.0	100.0	100.0	100.0	100.0

Source: *National statistical offices/OECD/Eurostat/Euromonitor International*

Healthcare Infrastructure and Services

Pakistan: Healthcare infrastructure and services by sector 1998-2004

Table: 4.898

As stated

	1998	1999	2000	2001	2002	2003	2004
Dentists (number)	3,444	3,867	4,175	4,622	4,821	4,999	5,108
Doctors (number)	82,682	87,105	91,823	96,248	99,378	102,003	104,723
Hospitals and clinics (number)	872	879	876	907	920	933	947
In-patient beds ('000)	91	92	94	98	99	99	100
Midwives (number)	22,103	22,401	22,525	22,711	22,985	23,231	23,523
Nurses (number)	32,938	35,979	37,528	40,019	41,599	42,277	43,040

Source: *Euromonitor International from national statistics*

Pakistan: Healthcare infrastructure and services by sector: growth 1998-2004

Table: 4.899

Year on year growth: % change in stated unit

	1998	1999	2000	2001	2002	2003	2004
Dentists (number)	9.0	12.3	8.0	10.7	4.3	3.7	2.2
Doctors (number)	5.4	5.3	5.4	4.8	3.3	2.6	2.7
Hospitals and clinics (number)	0.8	0.8	-0.3	3.5	1.4	1.4	1.5
In-patient beds (number)	0.8	1.7	1.9	4.3	0.7	0.7	0.3
Midwives (number)	1.2	1.3	0.6	0.8	1.2	1.1	1.3
Nurses (number)	14.9	9.2	4.3	6.6	3.9	1.6	1.8

Source: Euromonitor International from national statistics

Immunisation

Pakistan: Vaccination rates by disease type 1998-2004

Table: 4.900

%

	1998	1999	2000	2001	2002	2003	2004
Vaccination rate against DTP (diphtheria, tetanus, pertussis) 1 & 2 (%)			88.0	86.0	76.9	73.0	67.0
Vaccination rate against MMR (measles, mumps, rubella) (%)	76.0	81.0	75.0	75.0	63.0	68.0	66.0
Vaccination rate against polio (%)	79.0	80.0	74.0	74.0	70.7	72.0	70.0

Source: WHO

Infectious Diseases

Pakistan: Incidence of disease by type 1998-2004

Table: 4.901

Number

	1998	1999	2000	2001	2002	2003	2004
Incidence of AIDS	23	17	15	8	10	10	9
Incidence of diphtheria	20	12	13	19	22		
Incidence of measles	2,333	2,940	2,064	3,849	3,903		
Incidence of polio	341	558	199	116	90		

Source: WHO

Pakistan: Incidence of disease by type: growth 1998-2004

Table: 4.902

Year on year growth: %

	1998	1999	2000	2001	2002	2003	2004
Incidence of AIDS	21.1	-26.1	-11.8	-46.7	25.0	0.0	-10.0
Incidence of diphtheria	-23.1	-40.0	8.3	46.2	15.8		
Incidence of measles	26.2	26.0	-29.8	86.5	1.4		
Incidence of polio	-70.3	63.6	-64.3	-41.7	-22.4		

Source: WHO

Causes of Death

Pakistan: Deaths by disease 1998-2004

Table: 4.903

Number per 100,000 inhabitants

	1998	1999	2000	2001	2002	2003	2004
Deaths from heart disease	32.4	33.3	31.5	31.4	30.5	30.1	29.9
Death by diseases of the digestive system	26.4	28.9	29.2	28.0	27.5	26.9	26.3
Deaths from ulcers of the stomach and duodenum	26.4	28.9	29.2	28.0	27.5	26.6	25.7
Deaths from lung cancer	28.9	24.8	26.6	25.7	25.7	25.1	24.4
Deaths from chronic liver disease and cirrhosis	8.3	8.1	7.9	7.6	7.7	7.5	7.4

Source: WHO/Euromonitor International
Notes: Data is ranked in descending order by year 2004

Pakistan: Deaths by disease: growth 1998-2004

Table: 4.904

% year on year growth

	1998	1999	2000	2001	2002	2003	2004
Deaths from heart disease	0.6	2.8	-5.4	-0.3	-2.9	-1.3	-0.6
Deaths from chronic liver disease and cirrhosis	-2.4	-2.4	-2.5	-3.8	1.3	-2.6	-1.9
Death by diseases of the digestive system	-4.3	9.5	1.0	-4.1	-1.8	-2.2	-2.3
Deaths from lung cancer	11.2	-14.2	7.3	-3.4	0.0	-2.3	-2.8
Deaths from ulcers of the stomach and duodenum	-4.3	9.5	1.0	-4.1	-1.8	-3.3	-3.3

Source: WHO/Euromonitor International
Notes: Data is ranked in descending order by year 2004

Smoking

Pakistan: Smoking prevalence in population aged 15+ 1998-2004

Table: 4.905

% of population aged 15+

	1998	1999	2000	2001	2002	2003	2004
Smoking prevalence in population aged 15+ (% of population aged 15+)	24.4	24.8	25.0	25.7	26.2	27.0	27.6
Smoking prevalence in male population aged 15+ (% of male population)	34.6	34.7	36.0	36.6	38.0	38.8	39.0
Smoking prevalence in female population aged 15+ (% of female population)	13.7	14.5	13.5	14.4	13.9	14.7	15.8

Source: WHO/OECD/Euromonitor International

Nutrition and Obesity

Pakistan: Nutrition and obesity 1998-2004

Table: 4.906

As stated

	1998	1999	2000	2001	2002	2003	2004
Average supply of calories per day (calories per capita)	2,445.8	2,455.5	2,447.1	2,425.7	2,418.8	2,410.1	2,399.9
Average supply of fat per day (grams per capita)	65.2	67.8	65.0	65.4	65.1	64.5	64.1
Average supply of protein per day (grams per capita)	63.2	62.6	62.4	61.8	61.9	61.8	61.7
Obese population (BMI 30kg/sq m or more) (% of population aged 15+)	5.6	5.6	5.7	5.8	5.7	5.8	5.8

Source: WHO/OECD/Euromonitor International

■ **Peru**

Socio-economic Parameters

Peru: Socio-economic parameters 1998-2004

As stated

	1998	1999	2000	2001	2002	2003	2004
Population: national estimates at January 1st ('000)	24,896.7	25,322.0	25,742.6	26,156.4	26,563.7	26,966.1	27,366.3
% aged 0-14 yrs	35.5	35.1	34.7	34.3	33.9	33.4	32.9
% aged 15-64 yrs	60.0	60.3	60.6	60.9	61.2	61.6	61.9
% aged 65 + yrs	4.5	4.6	4.7	4.8	4.9	5.0	5.1
% Male	50.3	50.3	50.3	50.3	50.3	50.3	50.3
% Female	49.7	49.7	49.7	49.7	49.7	49.7	49.7
% Urban	72.0	72.4	72.6	72.9	73.3	73.6	74.0
Occupants per household at January 1st (Number)	4.8	4.7	4.7	4.7	4.7	4.8	4.8
Households ('000)	5,232.9	5,335.4	5,436.0	5,516.1	5,596.0	5,665.9	5,737.3
Annual rates of inflation (% growth)	7.2	3.5	3.8	2.0	0.2	2.3	3.7
GDP (n/s million)	165,893.0	173,881.0	185,426.0	188,313.0	198,657.0	210,747.0	233,432.0
GDP (US$ million)	56,618.8	51,393.4	53,130.7	53,698.9	56,492.8	60,586.1	68,391.6
GDP (US$ per capita)	2,274.1	2,029.6	2,063.9	2,053.0	2,126.7	2,246.8	2,499.1

Source: Euromonitor International from International Monetary Fund (IMF), International Financial Statistics and World Economic Outlook/UN/national statistics

Life Expectancy

Peru: Life expectancy 1998-2004

As stated

	1998	1999	2000	2001	2002	2003	2004	% change 1998-2004
Life expectancy at birth: total population (years)	67.8	68.1	68.1	68.5	69.7	70.3	71.0	4.74
Life expectancy at birth: total population: year on year growth	0.5	0.4	0.0	0.6	1.8	0.9	1.0	
Healthy life expectancy at birth (years)	59.0			57.1	57.4			
Healthy life expectancy at birth: year on year growth					0.6			

Source: Euromonitor International from World Bank

Sanitation

Peru: Improved sanitary facilities and water source 2000

As stated

	2000
Population with access to improved sanitary facilities (% of population)	71.0
Population with access to improved water source (% of population)	80.0
Population with improved access to sanitation facilities, rural (% of rural population with access)	49.0
Population with improved access to sanitation facilities, urban (% of urban population with access)	79.0

Source: National statistics/World Bank

Health Expenditure

Peru: Public health expenditure 1998-2004

As stated

	1998	1999	2000	2001	2002	2003	2004
Share of total health expenditure in GDP (% of total GDP)	4.6	4.9	4.7	4.7	4.7	4.7	4.7
Health expenditure (US$ per capita)	102.0	98.0	96.0	94.0	93.0	91.0	90.0

Source: Euromonitor International from OECD/national statistics

Peru: Private health expenditure 1998-2004

Table: 4.911

As stated

	1998	1999	2000	2001	2002	2003	2004
Consumer expenditure on health goods and medical services (n/s million)	6,336.7	6,476.1	6,991.7	7,280.6	7,575.6	7,870.3	8,321.2
Consumer expenditure on health goods and medical services: real growth in national currency: 1990 = 100	125.0	123.5	128.5	131.2	136.2	138.4	141.1
Consumer expenditure on health goods and medical services as a percentage of total consumer expenditure	5.3	5.3	5.3	5.3	5.3	5.1	5.0

Source: National statistical offices/OECD/Eurostat/Euromonitor International

Peru: Consumer expenditure on health goods and medical services by sector 1998-2004

Table: 4.912

% of total consumer expenditure on health goods and medical services

	1998	1999	2000	2001	2002	2003	2004
Pharmaceuticals, medical appliances/ equipment	37.0	37.8	37.8	38.0	38.3	38.2	38.1
Outpatient services	50.3	49.8	50.0	49.9	49.6	49.6	49.5
Hospital services	12.7	12.3	12.3	12.1	12.1	12.3	12.3
Total	100.0	100.0	100.0	100.0	100.0	100.0	100.0

Source: National statistical offices/OECD/Eurostat/Euromonitor International

Healthcare Infrastructure and Services

Peru: Healthcare infrastructure and services by sector 1998-2004

Table: 4.913

As stated

	1998	1999	2000	2001	2002	2003	2004
Doctors (number)	27,880	28,775	30,108	31,743	32,395	33,156	33,731
Hospitals and clinics (number)	472	475	503	483	478	477	476
In-patient beds ('000)	42	46	44	42	43	43	43
Nurses (number)			20,587				

Source: Euromonitor International from national statistics

Peru: Healthcare infrastructure and services by sector: growth 1998-2004

Table: 4.914

Year on year growth: % change in stated unit

	1998	1999	2000	2001	2002	2003	2004
Doctors (number)	6.7	3.2	4.6	5.4	2.1	2.3	1.7
Hospitals and clinics (number)	-0.4	0.6	5.9	-4.0	-1.0	-0.2	-0.2
In-patient beds (number)	-1.3	7.7	-4.1	-4.3	1.6	0.3	0.0

Source: Euromonitor International from national statistics

Immunisation

Peru: Vaccination rates by disease type 1998-2004

Table: 4.915

%

	1998	1999	2000	2001	2002	2003	2004
Vaccination rate against DTP (diphtheria, tetanus, pertussis) 1 & 2 (%)			91.3	91.0	90.9	91.0	90.0
Vaccination rate against MMR (measles, mumps, rubella) (%)	93.0	92.0	93.0	97.3	95.2	97.0	98.0
Vaccination rate against polio (%)	96.0	96.0	95.0	91.8	94.5	92.0	92.0

Source: WHO

Infectious Diseases

Peru: Incidence of disease by type 1998-2004

Table: 4.916

Number

	1998	1999	2000	2001	2002	2003	2004
Incidence of AIDS	1,031	1,009	615	775	893	902	802
Incidence of diphtheria	2	8	0	0	0		
Incidence of measles	10	12	1	0	0		
Incidence of polio	0	0	0	0	0		

Source: WHO

Peru: Incidence of disease by type: growth 1998-2004

Table: 4.917

Year on year growth: %

	1998	1999	2000	2001	2002	2003	2004
Incidence of AIDS	-4.4	-2.1	-39.0	26.0	15.2	1.0	-11.1
Incidence of diphtheria	0.0	300.0	-100.0				
Incidence of measles	-89.5	20.0	-91.7	-100.0			

Source: WHO

Causes of Death

Peru: Deaths by disease 1998-2004

Table: 4.918

Number per 100,000 inhabitants

	1998	1999	2000	2001	2002	2003	2004
Deaths from heart disease		7.1	13.4	15.1	21.4	27.4	34.7
Death by diseases of the digestive system	28.1	30.4	31.8	31.4	31.8	31.7	32.0
Deaths from lung cancer		2.0	4.3	4.2	6.2	7.8	9.5
Deaths from chronic liver disease and cirrhosis	12.9	10.3	10.4	10.4	8.8	8.7	8.3
Deaths from ulcers of the stomach and duodenum		1.5	1.4	1.3	1.3	1.2	1.1

Source: WHO/Euromonitor International
Notes: Data is ranked in descending order by year 2004

Peru: Deaths by disease: growth 1998-2004

Table: 4.919

% year on year growth

	1998	1999	2000	2001	2002	2003	2004
Deaths from heart disease			89.2	12.3	41.7	28.0	26.5
Deaths from lung cancer			116.4	-3.4	47.6	25.8	21.6
Death by diseases of the digestive system	-5.4	8.2	4.6	-1.3	1.3	-0.3	0.9
Deaths from chronic liver disease and cirrhosis	2.4	-20.1	0.7	0.2	-15.4	-1.1	-4.8
Deaths from ulcers of the stomach and duodenum			-4.2	-10.1	0.0	-7.7	-5.4

Source: WHO/Euromonitor International
Notes: Data is ranked in descending order by year 2004

Smoking

Peru: Smoking prevalence in population aged 15+ 1998-2004

Table: 4.920

% of population aged 15+

	1998	1999	2000	2001	2002	2003	2004
Smoking prevalence in population aged 15+ (% of population aged 15+)	33.7	31.5	31.7	32.2	33.1	33.3	33.3
Smoking prevalence in male population aged 15+ (% of male population)	47.3	48.9	48.3	50.6	50.0	49.9	49.8
Smoking prevalence in female population aged 15+ (% of female population)	20.2	14.1	15.1	13.8	16.2	16.8	16.8

Source: WHO/OECD/Euromonitor International

Nutrition and Obesity

Peru: Nutrition and obesity 1998-2004

Table: 4.921

As stated

	1998	1999	2000	2001	2002	2003	2004
Average supply of calories per day (calories per capita)	2,512.7	2,510.1	2,529.1	2,550.2	2,570.9	2,591.5	2,612.6
Average supply of fat per day (grams per capita)	44.2	45.4	47.7	47.3	48.0	48.8	49.4
Average supply of protein per day (grams per capita)	63.4	63.6	65.6	66.6	67.1	68.0	68.9
Obese population (BMI 30kg/sq m or more) (% of population aged 15+)	10.1	8.1	8.1	8.2	9.3	9.7	10.2

Source: WHO/OECD/Euromonitor International

■ Philippines

Socio-economic Parameters

Philippines: Socio-economic parameters 1998-2004

Table: 4.922

As stated

	1998	1999	2000	2001	2002	2003	2004
Population: national estimates at January 1st ('000)	73,147.8	74,745.8	76,504.1	78,055.5	79,612.2	81,168.2	82,715.7
% aged 0-14 yrs	37.4	37.1	36.8	36.5	36.2	35.9	35.5
% aged 15-64 yrs	58.9	59.1	59.3	59.5	59.8	60.0	60.3
% aged 65 + yrs	3.8	3.8	3.9	4.0	4.0	4.1	4.2
% Male	50.4	50.4	50.4	50.3	50.3	50.3	50.3
% Female	49.6	49.6	49.6	49.7	49.7	49.7	49.7
% Urban	56.8	57.7	58.2	58.9	59.6	60.4	61.1
Occupants per household at January 1st (Number)	5.0	5.0	5.0	5.0	5.0	5.0	4.9
Households ('000)	14,519.3	14,901.3	15,271.5	15,645.0	16,009.8	16,391.5	16,758.8
Annual rates of inflation (% growth)	9.7	6.7	4.4	6.1	3.0	3.0	5.9
GDP (Ps million)	2,665,060.0	2,976,900.0	3,354,730.0	3,631,470.0	3,959,650.0	4,299,930.0	4,843,450.0
GDP (US$ million)	65,171.5	76,157.0	75,912.3	71,215.6	76,732.0	79,329.7	86,428.6
GDP (US$ per capita)	891.0	1,018.9	992.3	912.4	963.8	977.3	1,044.9

Source: *Euromonitor International from International Monetary Fund (IMF), International Financial Statistics and World Economic Outlook/UN/national statistics*

Life Expectancy

Philippines: Life expectancy 1998-2004

Table: 4.923

As stated

	1998	1999	2000	2001	2002	2003	2004	% change 1998-2004
Life expectancy at birth: total population (years)	67.1	67.4	67.4	67.7	68.3	68.8	69.1	2.99
Life expectancy at birth: total population: year on year growth	0.5	0.4	0.0	0.4	0.9	0.7	0.5	
Healthy life expectancy at birth (years)	59.0			55.2	55.5			
Healthy life expectancy at birth: year on year growth					0.5			

Source: *Euromonitor International from World Bank*

Sanitation

Philippines: Improved sanitary facilities and water source 2000

Table: 4.924

As stated

	2000
Population with access to improved sanitary facilities (% of population)	83.0
Population with access to improved water source (% of population)	86.0
Population with improved access to sanitation facilities, rural (% of rural population with access)	69.0
Population with improved access to sanitation facilities, urban (% of urban population with access)	93.0

Source: *National statistics/World Bank*

Health Expenditure

Philippines: Public health expenditure 1998-2004

Table: 4.925

As stated

	1998	1999	2000	2001	2002	2003	2004
Share of total health expenditure in GDP (% of total GDP)	3.5	3.5	3.4	3.3	3.1	3.2	3.1
Health expenditure (US$ per capita)	32.0	36.0	34.0	29.0	28.0	27.0	25.0

Source: *Euromonitor International from OECD/national statistics*

Philippines: Private health expenditure 1998-2004

Table: 4.926

As stated

	1998	1999	2000	2001	2002	2003	2004
Consumer expenditure on health goods and medical services (Ps million)	37,333.6	40,723.0	43,997.7	45,188.4	46,301.0	48,227.5	52,108.6
Consumer expenditure on health goods and medical services: real growth in national currency: 1990 = 100	127.1	129.9	134.5	130.2	129.5	131.0	133.6
Consumer expenditure on health goods and medical services as a percentage of total consumer expenditure	1.9	1.9	1.9	1.8	1.6	1.6	1.6

Source: National statistical offices/OECD/Eurostat/Euromonitor International

Philippines: Consumer expenditure on health goods and medical services by sector 1998-2004

Table: 4.927

% of total consumer expenditure on health goods and medical services

	1998	1999	2000	2001	2002	2003	2004
Pharmaceuticals, medical appliances/ equipment	27.1	27.2	27.3	27.2	27.2	27.2	27.2
Outpatient services	54.6	54.1	54.1	53.8	53.6	53.6	53.6
Hospital services	18.4	18.7	18.6	19.0	19.2	19.1	19.2
Total	100.0	100.0	100.0	100.0	100.0	100.0	100.0

Source: National statistical offices/OECD/Eurostat/Euromonitor International

Healthcare Infrastructure and Services

Philippines: Healthcare infrastructure and services by sector 1998-2004

Table: 4.928

As stated

	1998	1999	2000	2001	2002	2003	2004
Dentists (number)	1,713	2,027	2,280	2,465	2,533	2,574	2,598
Doctors (number)	2,848	2,948	2,985	2,999	2,960	2,877	2,826
Hospitals and clinics (number)	1,713	1,794	1,712	1,740	1,741	1,745	1,752
In-patient beds ('000)	82	84	81				
Midwives (number)	14,962	16,173	17,176	17,522	17,409	16,768	16,698
Nurses (number)	4,389	4,945	5,303	5,580	5,643	5,704	5,745

Source: Euromonitor International from national statistics

Philippines: Healthcare infrastructure and services by sector: growth 1998-2004

Table: 4.929

Year on year growth: % change in stated unit

	1998	1999	2000	2001	2002	2003	2004
Dentists (number)	25.0	18.3	12.5	8.1	2.8	1.6	0.9
Doctors (number)	10.3	3.5	1.3	0.5	-1.3	-2.8	-1.8
Hospitals and clinics (number)	-5.7	4.7	-4.6	1.6	0.1	0.2	0.4
In-patient beds (number)	0.1	1.9	-3.0				
Midwives (number)	12.7	8.1	6.2	2.0	-0.6	-3.7	-0.4
Nurses (number)	7.2	12.7	7.2	5.2	1.1	1.1	0.7

Source: Euromonitor International from national statistics

Immunisation

Philippines: Vaccination rates by disease type 1998-2004

Table: 4.930

%

	1998	1999	2000	2001	2002	2003	2004
Vaccination rate against DTP (diphtheria, tetanus, pertussis) 1 & 2 (%)			81.0	58.0	75.0	65.0	62.0
Vaccination rate against MMR (measles, mumps, rubella) (%)	87.0		80.0	75.0	73.0	69.0	66.0
Vaccination rate against polio (%)	87.0		75.0	90.0	70.0	73.0	71.0

Source: WHO

Infectious Diseases

Philippines: Incidence of disease by type 1998-2004

Table: 4.931

Number

	1998	1999	2000	2001	2002	2003	2004
Incidence of AIDS	45	78	40	56	44	47	45
Incidence of diphtheria	83	64	88	73	62		
Incidence of measles	1,984	2,981	7,120	7,360	7,003		
Incidence of polio	0	0	0	3	0		

Source: WHO

Philippines: Incidence of disease by type: growth 1998-2004

Table: 4.932

Year on year growth: %

	1998	1999	2000	2001	2002	2003	2004
Incidence of AIDS	95.7	73.3	-48.7	40.0	-21.4	6.8	-4.3
Incidence of diphtheria	-39.9	-22.9	37.5	-17.0	-15.1		
Incidence of measles	-78.5	50.3	138.8	3.4	-4.9		
Incidence of polio					-100.0		

Source: WHO

Causes of Death

Philippines: Deaths by disease 1998-2004

Table: 4.933

Number per 100,000 inhabitants

	1998	1999	2000	2001	2002	2003	2004
Deaths from heart disease	61.5	59.0	64.9	67.2	67.3	68.8	70.9
Deaths from ulcers of the stomach and duodenum	31.9	30.9	29.9	32.4	32.0	33.6	34.9
Death by diseases of the digestive system	31.9	30.9	29.9	32.4	32.0	31.1	31.8
Deaths from lung cancer	29.9	28.8	26.9	28.3	27.5	28.1	28.7
Deaths from chronic liver disease and cirrhosis	12.4	12.3	12.2	12.7	13.2	13.7	14.4
Death by malignant neoplasms (cancers)	43.2						

Source: WHO/Euromonitor International
Notes: Data is ranked in descending order by year 2004

Philippines: Deaths by disease: growth 1998-2004

Table: 4.934

% year on year growth

	1998	1999	2000	2001	2002	2003	2004
Deaths from chronic liver disease and cirrhosis	3.3	-0.8	-0.8	4.1	3.9	3.8	5.0
Deaths from ulcers of the stomach and duodenum	-4.5	-3.1	-3.2	8.4	-1.2	5.0	3.9
Deaths from heart disease	2.2	-4.1	10.0	3.5	0.1	2.2	3.0
Death by diseases of the digestive system	-4.5	-3.1	-3.2	8.4	-1.2	-2.8	2.3
Deaths from lung cancer	-4.2	-3.7	-6.6	5.2	-2.8	2.2	2.2
Death by malignant neoplasms (cancers)	18.0						

Source: *WHO/Euromonitor International*
Notes: *Data is ranked in descending order by year 2004*

Smoking

Philippines: Smoking prevalence in population aged 15+ 1998-2004

Table: 4.935

% of population aged 15+

	1998	1999	2000	2001	2002	2003	2004
Smoking prevalence in population aged 15+ (% of population aged 15+)	35.2	35.2	35.7	35.4	35.7	35.8	35.9
Smoking prevalence in male population aged 15+ (% of male population)	57.6	58.3	57.2	57.4	57.3	57.3	57.4
Smoking prevalence in female population aged 15+ (% of female population)	12.9	12.2	14.3	13.5	14.1	14.2	14.4

Source: *WHO/OECD/Euromonitor International*

Nutrition and Obesity

Philippines: Nutrition and obesity 1998-2004

Table: 4.936

As stated

	1998	1999	2000	2001	2002	2003	2004
Average supply of calories per day (calories per capita)	2,330.8	2,374.4	2,375.5	2,371.3	2,379.3	2,383.4	2,387.1
Average supply of fat per day (grams per capita)	43.6	49.4	48.9	46.1	48.4	49.5	50.2
Average supply of protein per day (grams per capita)	54.8	54.7	55.2	56.2	56.1	56.3	56.6
Obese population (BMI 30kg/sq m or more) (% of population aged 15+)	5.1	4.0	3.9	4.3	5.5	5.7	5.8

Source: *WHO/OECD/Euromonitor International*

Over-the-Counter Healthcare

Philippines: Trends in OTC healthcare retail sales 1998-2004

Table: 4.937

As stated

	1998	1999	2000	2001	2002	2003	2004
OTC Healthcare (Ps million)	11,769.0	14,350.0	17,991.5	21,096.0	23,840.6	27,655.3	31,324.7
OTC Healthcare: real growth in national currency: 1998 = 100	100.0	114.3	137.3	151.7	166.5	187.5	201.5
OTC Healthcare: year on year (% real growth)	3.1	14.3	20.1	10.5	9.8	12.6	7.5
OTC Healthcare (Ps per capita)	160.9	192.0	235.2	270.3	299.5	340.7	378.7

Source: *Euromonitor International from industry sources/national statistics*

Philippines: OTC healthcare retail sales by sector 1998-2004

% of OTC retail value sales

	1998	1999	2000	2001	2002	2003	2004
Analgesics	20.6	20.9	20.8	22.5	24.6	25.3	26.7
Cough, cold and allergy (hay fever) remedies	32.7	31.7	30.6	26.0	24.5	24.7	24.5
Digestive remedies	9.4	8.5	7.8	7.7	7.8	6.8	6.3
Medicated skin care	10.3	10.6	10.4	10.6	10.2	9.2	8.5
Vitamins and dietary supplements	24.2	25.6	27.6	30.9	30.6	31.9	32.2

Source: Euromonitor International from industry sources/national statistics
Notes: Only selected sectors are shown, so values are not expected to sum to 100

▪ Poland

Socio-economic Parameters

Poland: Socio-economic parameters 1998-2004

As stated

	1998	1999	2000	2001	2002	2003	2004
Population: national estimates at January 1st ('000)	38,660.0	38,667.0	38,653.6	38,644.2	38,632.5	38,621.7	38,588.9
% aged 0-14 yrs	21.1	20.3	19.6	18.8	18.2	17.6	17.0
% aged 15-64 yrs	67.2	67.8	68.4	68.9	69.3	69.7	70.2
% aged 65 + yrs	11.7	11.9	12.1	12.3	12.5	12.7	12.8
% Male	48.6	48.6	48.6	48.6	48.6	48.6	48.6
% Female	51.4	51.4	51.4	51.4	51.4	51.4	51.4
% Urban	64.8	65.2	65.4	65.7	66.1	66.5	67.0
Occupants per household at January 1st (Number)	3.0	3.0	2.9	2.9	2.9	2.9	2.9
Households ('000)	12,885.9	13,006.8	13,123.1	13,239.3	13,337.0	13,425.9	13,511.2
Annual rates of inflation (% growth)	11.7	7.3	10.1	5.5	1.9	0.7	3.5
GDP (PLN million)	553,560.0	640,378.0	723,886.0	760,595.0	781,112.0	814,698.0	883,656.0
GDP (US$ million)	159,279.5	161,421.8	166,561.1	185,787.4	191,447.6	209,484.0	241,591.8
GDP (US$ per capita)	4,120.0	4,174.7	4,309.1	4,807.6	4,955.6	5,424.0	6,260.7

Source: Euromonitor International from International Monetary Fund (IMF), International Financial Statistics and World Economic Outlook/UN/national statistics

Life Expectancy

Poland: Life expectancy 1998-2004

As stated

	1998	1999	2000	2001	2002	2003	2004	% change 1998-2004
Life expectancy at birth: total population (years)	73.4	73.6	73.9	74.0	74.7	75.0	75.4	2.72
Life expectancy at birth: total population: year on year growth	0.3	0.3	0.4	0.1	0.9	0.5	0.5	
Healthy life expectancy at birth (years)	66.0			64.3	64.3			
Healthy life expectancy at birth: year on year growth					0.1			

Source: Euromonitor International from World Bank

Health Expenditure

Poland: Public health expenditure 1998-2004

Table: 4.941

As stated

	1998	1999	2000	2001	2002	2003	2004
Public expenditure on pharmaceuticals and other medical non-durables (PLN million)	2,910.0	3,531.0	4,510.0	5,186.0	5,466.0	6,052.0	6,937.5
Share of total health expenditure in GDP (% of total GDP)	6.4	6.2	5.8	6.1	6.2	6.2	5.9
Health expenditure (US$ per capita)	264.0	249.0	244.0	289.0	301.0	318.0	338.0

Source: Euromonitor International from OECD/national statistics

Poland: Private health expenditure 1998-2004

Table: 4.942

As stated

	1998	1999	2000	2001	2002	2003	2004
Consumer expenditure on health goods and medical services (PLN million)	14,004.0	16,420.0	19,113.0	21,331.0	22,769.0	23,152.9	24,725.7
Consumer expenditure on health goods and medical services: real growth in national currency: 1990 = 100	168.8	184.4	194.9	206.2	216.0	218.1	225.0
Consumer expenditure on health goods and medical services as a percentage of total consumer expenditure	4.0	4.2	4.3	4.5	4.6	4.6	4.6

Source: National statistical offices/OECD/Eurostat/Euromonitor International

Poland: Consumer expenditure on health goods and medical services by sector 1998-2004

Table: 4.943

% of total consumer expenditure on health goods and medical services

	1998	1999	2000	2001	2002	2003	2004
Pharmaceuticals, medical appliances/equipment	65.9	66.8	66.4	70.1	70.7	69.7	69.6
Outpatient services	32.4	31.0	31.5	27.8	26.8	28.1	28.1
Hospital services	1.7	2.1	2.0	2.1	2.4	2.2	2.2
Total	100.0	100.0	100.0	100.0	100.0	100.0	100.0

Source: National statistical offices/OECD/Eurostat/Euromonitor International

Healthcare Infrastructure and Services

Poland: Healthcare infrastructure and services by sector 1998-2004

Table: 4.944

As stated

	1998	1999	2000	2001	2002	2003	2004
Active pharmacists (number)	20,572	21,857	22,161	23,774	24,421	24,653	24,855
Consultations with GPs (general practitioners) (per capita)	5	5	5	6	6	6	6
Dentists (number)	17,323	13,260	11,758	10,124	10,775	10,924	11,084
Doctors (number)	90,086	87,524	85,031	86,706	88,070	90,512	92,979
Hospital admissions (number)	5,339,126	5,685,288	6,007,091	6,336,215	6,670,198	6,994,503	7,296,147
Hospitals and clinics (number)	715	698	716	736	739	747	758
In-patient beds ('000)	213	205	191	188	188	187	185
Midwives (number)	24,434	24,221	21,997	21,843	21,743	21,538	21,406
Nurses (number)	213,127	197,153	189,632	186,491	185,892	183,990	182,103
Out-patient contacts (per capita)	5	5	5	6	5	6	6

Source: Euromonitor International from national statistics

Poland: Healthcare infrastructure and services by sector: growth 1998-2004

Table: 4.945

Year on year growth: % change in stated unit

	1998	1999	2000	2001	2002	2003	2004
Active pharmacists (number)	-0.4	6.2	1.4	7.3	2.7	1.0	0.8
Consultations with GPs (general practitioners) (per capita)	1.9	-1.4	0.7	2.6	1.8	2.3	2.1
Dentists (number)	-1.7	-23.5	-11.3	-13.9	6.4	1.4	1.5
Doctors (number)	-1.1	-2.8	-2.8	2.0	1.6	2.8	2.7
Hospital admissions (number)	2.5	6.5	5.7	5.5	5.3	4.9	4.3
Hospitals and clinics (number)	-0.3	-2.4	2.6	2.8	0.4	1.1	1.5
In-patient beds (number)	1.6	-3.9	-6.8	-1.4	-0.1	-0.7	-0.8
Midwives (number)	-1.6	-0.9	-9.2	-0.7	-0.5	-0.9	-0.6
Nurses (number)	-1.9	-7.5	-3.8	-1.7	-0.3	-1.0	-1.0
Out-patient contacts (per capita)	1.9	-1.9	1.9	1.9	-3.6	5.7	3.6

Source: Euromonitor International from national statistics

Immunisation

Poland: Vaccination rates by disease type 1998-2004

Table: 4.946

%

	1998	1999	2000	2001	2002	2003	2004
Vaccination rate against MMR (measles, mumps, rubella) (%)		97.0	97.4	97.2	97.6	98.0	98.0
Vaccination rate against polio (%)		98.0	98.2	97.7	97.9	98.0	98.0

Source: WHO

Infectious Diseases

Poland: Incidence of disease by type 1998-2004

Table: 4.947

Number

	1998	1999	2000	2001	2002	2003	2004
Incidence of AIDS	132	113	109	56	130	62	75
Incidence of diphtheria	0	0	1	0	0		
Incidence of measles	2,255	99	77	133	33		
Incidence of polio	0	0	0	0	0		

Source: WHO

Poland: Incidence of disease by type: growth 1998-2004

Table: 4.948

Year on year growth: %

	1998	1999	2000	2001	2002	2003	2004
Incidence of AIDS	12.8	-14.4	-3.5	-48.6	132.1	-52.3	21.0
Incidence of diphtheria				-100.0			
Incidence of measles	567.2	-95.6	-22.2	72.7	-75.2		

Source: WHO

Causes of Death

Poland: Deaths by disease 1998-2004

Table: 4.949

Number per 100,000 inhabitants

	1998	1999	2000	2001	2002	2003	2004
Death by diseases of the circulatory system	379.8	446.2	421.9	427.9	428.8	417.1	412.2
Death by malignant neoplasms (cancers)	170.1	198.7	202.5	212.8	208.9	206.7	209.8
Deaths from heart disease	137.8	147.6	143.8	142.9	140.1	137.7	136.8
Deaths from lung cancer	48.6	49.8	51.8	52.3	53.8	55.0	56.6
Death by diseases of the respiratory system	29.6	44.4	44.3	44.1	41.4	40.8	39.9
Death by diseases of the digestive system	31.8	34.9	34.6	38.0	36.6	35.2	35.1
Deaths from chronic liver disease and cirrhosis	13.6	15.1	14.3	14.6	14.2	14.0	14.0
Deaths from ulcers of the stomach and duodenum	3.8	3.8	3.9	4.1	4.2	4.4	4.6

Source: WHO/Euromonitor International
Notes: Data is ranked in descending order by year 2004

Poland: Deaths by disease: growth 1998-2004

Table: 4.950

% year on year growth

	1998	1999	2000	2001	2002	2003	2004
Deaths from ulcers of the stomach and duodenum	2.7	0.9	2.9	4.0	2.4	4.8	4.7
Deaths from lung cancer	0.4	2.4	4.0	1.1	2.9	2.2	3.0
Death by malignant neoplasms (cancers)	5.1	16.8	1.9	5.1	-1.8	-1.1	1.5
Deaths from chronic liver disease and cirrhosis	7.1	10.7	-4.7	1.8	-2.7	-1.4	-0.1
Death by diseases of the digestive system	-0.6	9.7	-0.9	9.8	-3.7	-3.8	-0.2
Deaths from heart disease	13.0	7.1	-2.6	-0.6	-2.0	-1.7	-0.6
Death by diseases of the circulatory system	1.1	17.5	-5.4	1.4	0.2	-2.7	-1.2
Death by diseases of the respiratory system	-15.7	50.0	-0.2	-0.5	-6.1	-1.4	-2.2

Source: WHO/Euromonitor International
Notes: Data is ranked in descending order by year 2004

Poland: Other selected causes of death: 1998-2004

Table: 4.951

Number per 100,000 inhabitants

	1998	1999	2000	2001	2002	2003	2004
Death by injury and poisoning	68.0	65.8	61.3	61.7	58.3	55.0	52.5
Death by motor traffic accidents	16.9	17.5	16.5	16.6	16.4	16.8	16.8
Death by suicide and self-inflicted injury	13.1	13.7	13.8	14.6	14.2	13.6	13.6

Source: Euromonitor International from national statistics
Notes: Data is ranked in descending order by year 2004

Poland: Other selected causes of death: growth 1998-2004

Table: 4.952

% year on year growth

	1998	1999	2000	2001	2002	2003	2004
Death by suicide and self-inflicted injury	0.8	4.6	0.7	5.8	-2.7	-4.2	0.0
Death by motor traffic accidents	-0.6	3.6	-5.7	0.6	-1.2	2.4	-0.2
Death by injury and poisoning	-4.1	-3.2	-6.8	0.7	-5.5	-5.7	-4.5

Source: Euromonitor International from national statistics
Notes: Data is ranked in descending order by year 2004

Smoking

Poland: Smoking prevalence in population aged 15+ 1998-2004

Table: 4.953

% of population aged 15+

	1998	1999	2000	2001	2002	2003	2004
Smoking prevalence in population aged 15+ (% of population aged 15+)	29.8	29.5	32.0	32.0	32.0	28.7	28.4
Smoking prevalence in male population aged 15+ (% of male population)	39.0	39.5	40.0	40.0	40.0	36.9	36.8
Smoking prevalence in female population aged 15+ (% of female population)	21.3	20.3	25.0	25.0	25.0	21.1	20.7

Source: WHO/OECD/Euromonitor International

Nutrition and Obesity

Poland: Nutrition and obesity 1998-2004

Table: 4.954

As stated

	1998	1999	2000	2001	2002	2003	2004
Availability of fruit and vegetables (kg/capita/year)	188.1	173.4	175.7	174.1	174.9	176.5	177.0
Average supply of calories per day (calories per capita)	3,355.9	3,353.7	3,382.4	3,369.8	3,374.5	3,380.2	3,383.6
Average supply of fat per day (grams per capita)	112.0	112.6	111.7	111.4	112.8	113.5	114.1
Average supply of protein per day (grams per capita)	99.7	99.5	99.5	98.7	99.4	99.7	99.8
Obese population (BMI 30kg/sq m or more) (% of population aged 15+)	11.5	12.0	12.2	12.5	12.7	13.0	13.3

Source: WHO/OECD/Euromonitor International

Over-the-Counter Healthcare

Poland: Trends in OTC healthcare retail sales 1998-2004

Table: 4.955

As stated

	1998	1999	2000	2001	2002	2003	2004
OTC Healthcare (PLN million)	1,510.3	1,804.5	2,195.1	2,520.1	2,775.0	3,027.5	3,276.2
OTC Healthcare: real growth in national currency: 1998 = 100	100.0	111.3	123.0	133.8	144.6	156.7	163.5
OTC Healthcare: year on year (% real growth)	22.8	11.3	10.5	8.8	8.1	8.3	4.4
OTC Healthcare (PLN per capita)	39.1	46.7	56.8	65.2	71.8	78.4	84.9

Source: Euromonitor International from industry sources/national statistics

Poland: OTC healthcare retail sales by sector 1998-2004

Table: 4.956

% of OTC retail value sales

	1998	1999	2000	2001	2002	2003	2004
Analgesics	22.0	22.2	23.5	23.3	23.2	23.3	24.2
Cough, cold and allergy (hay fever) remedies	22.2	22.1	21.7	21.4	21.4	21.3	21.3
Digestive remedies	9.7	10.3	10.5	10.9	11.2	11.2	11.4
Medicated skin care	7.4	7.6	7.7	7.9	7.9	7.8	7.7
Vitamins and dietary supplements	26.5	25.5	24.6	24.5	24.3	24.4	23.4

Source: Euromonitor International from industry sources/national statistics
Notes: Only selected sectors are shown, so values are not expected to sum to 100

Health and Wellness

Poland: Retail sales of packaged foods by health and wellness category 2002-2004

Table: 4.957

PLN million

	2002	2003	2004
Packaged food: Total	36,513.1	37,959.1	39,358.0
Better for you	1,196.3	1,248.2	1,304.3
For food intolerance	14.8	17.2	19.7
Fortified/functional	234.3	278.1	320.1
Organic	33.3	43.1	50.8

Source: *Euromonitor International from industry sources/national statistics*

Poland: Per capita sales of packaged foods by health and wellness category 2002-2004

Table: 4.958

PLN per capita

	2002	2003	2004
Better for you	30.9	32.2	33.7
For food intolerance	0.4	0.4	0.5
Fortified/functional	6.1	7.2	8.3
Organic	0.9	1.1	1.3

Source: *Euromonitor International from industry sources/national statistics*

Poland: Retail sales of packaged food by health and wellness category: % share of total packaged food market 2002-2004

Table: 4.959

% value

	2002	2003	2004
Better for you	3.3	3.3	3.3
For food intolerance	0.0	0.0	0.0
Fortified/functional	0.6	0.7	0.8
Organic	0.1	0.1	0.1

Source: *Euromonitor International from industry sources/national statistics*

Poland: Retail sales of packaged food by health and wellness category: real growth index 2002-2004

Table: 4.960

2002 = 100

	2002	2003	2004
Better for you	100.00	103.51	105.84
For food intolerance	100.00	115.56	129.13
Fortified/functional	100.00	117.74	132.62
Organic	100.00	128.36	148.12

Source: *Euromonitor International from industry sources/national statistics*

Poland: Retail sales of better-for-you packaged foods by sector 2002-2004

Table: 4.961

% of total packaged food / as stated

	2002	2003	2004	% real change in value 2002-2004
Combination	0.00	0.00	0.00	104.16
Reduced carb	0.04	0.04	0.05	51.06
Reduced fat	2.04	2.01	2.01	3.06
Reduced salt	0.00	0.00	0.00	50.56

Source: *Euromonitor International from industry sources/national statistics*

Poland: Retail sales of packaged foods for food intolerances by sector 2002-2004

Table: 4.962

% of total packaged food / as stated

	2002	2003	2004	% real change in value 2002-2004
Diabetic	0.01	0.01	0.01	30.65
Gluten-free	0.03	0.03	0.04	28.58

Source: *Euromonitor International from industry sources/national statistics*

Poland: Retail sales of naturally healthy packaged foods by sector 2002-2004

Table: 4.963

% of total packaged food / as stated

	2002	2003	2004	% real change in value 2002-2004
High fibre	0.31	0.33	0.35	21.08
Other naturally healthy food	1.88	1.90	1.89	5.25
Soy-based dairy alternatives	0.01	0.01	0.01	9.09

Source: *Euromonitor International from industry sources/national statistics*

■ **Portugal**

Socio-economic Parameters

Portugal: Socio-economic parameters 1998-2004

Table: 4.964

As stated

	1998	1999	2000	2001	2002	2003	2004
Population: national estimates at January 1st ('000)	10,107.9	10,150.1	10,198.2	10,262.9	10,335.6	10,393.8	10,445.3
% aged 0-14 yrs	16.7	16.4	16.1	16.0	16.0	16.0	16.0
% aged 15-64 yrs	67.8	67.8	67.8	67.6	67.5	67.4	67.3
% aged 65 + yrs	15.5	15.8	16.1	16.4	16.5	16.6	16.7
% Male	48.2	48.2	48.2	48.3	48.3	48.3	48.3
% Female	51.8	51.8	51.8	51.7	51.7	51.7	51.7
% Urban	60.7	62.5	64.4	65.4	66.5	67.0	67.5
Occupants per household at January 1st (Number)	2.9	2.9	2.8	2.8	2.8	2.8	2.7
Households ('000)	3,480.6	3,534.5	3,592.4	3,650.8	3,707.8	3,757.9	3,808.8
Annual rates of inflation (% growth)	2.7	2.3	2.8	4.4	3.5	3.3	2.4
GDP (EUR million)	95,997.1	108,029.6	115,546.0	123,053.9	129,279.9	130,448.6	135,035.1
GDP (US$ million)	107,612.8	115,093.3	106,454.8	110,114.4	121,669.5	147,227.6	167,669.4
GDP (US$ per capita)	10,646.4	11,339.1	10,438.6	10,729.4	11,771.9	14,164.9	16,052.1

Source: *Euromonitor International from International Monetary Fund (IMF), International Financial Statistics and World Economic Outlook/UN/national statistics*

Life Expectancy

Portugal: Life expectancy 1998-2004

Table: 4.965

As stated

	1998	1999	2000	2001	2002	2003	2004	% change 1998-2004
Life expectancy at birth: total population (years)	75.9	76.1	76.4	76.5	77.0	77.3	77.8	2.42
Life expectancy at birth: total population: year on year growth	0.3	0.2	0.4	0.1	0.7	0.4	0.5	
Healthy life expectancy at birth (years)	69.0			66.8	66.8			
Healthy life expectancy at birth: year on year growth					0.0			

Source: *Euromonitor International from World Bank*

Health Expenditure

Portugal: Public health expenditure 1998-2004

Table: 4.966

As stated

	1998	1999	2000	2001	2002	2003	2004
Public expenditure on pharmaceuticals and other medical non-durables (EUR million)							
Private insurance expenditure (% of total expenditure on health)	1.5	1.5	1.6	1.6	1.7	1.7	1.7
Share of total health expenditure in GDP (% of total GDP)	8.6	8.7	9.1	9.2	8.7	8.5	8.1
Health expenditure (US$ per capita)	932.0	985.0	951.0	994.0	1,092.0	1,128.0	1,175.0

Source: Euromonitor International from OECD/national statistics

Portugal: Private health expenditure 1998-2004

Table: 4.967

As stated

	1998	1999	2000	2001	2002	2003	2004
Consumer expenditure on health goods and medical services (EUR million)	2,782.0	3,043.0	3,272.0	3,492.0	3,620.0	3,714.0	3,860.7
Consumer expenditure on health goods and medical services: real growth in national currency: 1990 = 100	86.1	92.0	96.2	98.4	98.5	97.8	99.4
Consumer expenditure on health goods and medical services as a percentage of total consumer expenditure	4.3	4.4	4.5	4.5	4.6	4.6	4.6

Source: National statistical offices/OECD/Eurostat/Euromonitor International

Portugal: Consumer expenditure on health goods and medical services by sector 1998-2004

Table: 4.968

% of total consumer expenditure on health goods and medical services

	1998	1999	2000	2001	2002	2003	2004
Pharmaceuticals, medical appliances/ equipment	29.2	30.7	30.7	30.2	30.1	29.6	29.5
Outpatient services	70.8	69.3	69.3	69.8	69.9	70.4	70.5
Total	100.0	100.0	100.0	100.0	100.0	100.0	100.0

Source: National statistical offices/OECD/Eurostat/Euromonitor International

Healthcare Infrastructure and Services

Portugal: Healthcare infrastructure and services by sector 1998-2004

Table: 4.969

As stated

	1998	1999	2000	2001	2002	2003	2004
Active pharmacists (number)	7,505	7,797	8,056	8,322	8,565	8,789	9,018
Consultations with GPs (general practitioners) (per capita)	3	4	4	4	4	4	4
Dentists (number)	3,322	3,769	4,370	4,799	4,841	4,922	5,024
Doctors (number)	31,087	31,758	32,498	33,233	34,015	34,833	35,454
Hospital admissions (number)	1,196,282	1,221,699	1,144,549	1,169,020	1,143,154	1,126,133	1,110,255
Hospitals and clinics (number)	1,115	1,123	1,116	1,122	1,146	1,154	1,166
In-patient beds ('000)	33	34	35	36	36	37	38
In-patient surgical procedures (number)	596,441	597,606	580,680	607,184	609,582	616,230	627,241
Nurses (number)	37,747	37,487	37,477	39,529	40,210	40,892	41,421
Out-patient contacts (per capita)	3	3	4	4	4	4	4

Source: Euromonitor International from national statistics

Portugal: Healthcare infrastructure and services by sector: growth 1998-2004

Table: 4.970

Year on year growth: % change in stated unit

	1998	1999	2000	2001	2002	2003	2004
Active pharmacists (number)	2.3	3.9	3.3	3.3	2.9	2.6	2.6
Consultations with GPs (general practitioners) (per capita)	0.0	2.9	0.0	2.9	0.9	1.4	1.4
Dentists (number)	9.8	13.5	15.9	9.8	0.9	1.7	2.1
Doctors (number)	2.2	2.2	2.3	2.3	2.4	2.4	1.8
Hospital admissions (number)	2.2	2.1	-6.3	2.1	-2.2	-1.5	-1.4
Hospitals and clinics (number)	6.6	0.7	-0.6	0.5	2.1	0.7	1.0
In-patient beds (number)	4.0	3.5	3.0	1.0	1.4	2.8	2.7
In-patient surgical procedures (number)	6.0	0.2	-2.8	4.6	0.4	1.1	1.8
Nurses (number)	3.2	-0.7	0.0	5.5	1.7	1.7	1.3
Out-patient contacts (per capita)	0.0	0.0	2.9	2.9	0.0	5.6	-2.6

Source: Euromonitor International from national statistics

Immunisation

Portugal: Vaccination rates by disease type 1998-2004

Table: 4.971

%

	1998	1999	2000	2001	2002	2003	2004
Vaccination rate against MMR (measles, mumps, rubella) (%)	96.0	96.0	96.0	96.0	91.9	93.0	92.0
Vaccination rate against polio (%)	96.0				93.8	94.0	94.0

Source: WHO

Infectious Diseases

Portugal: Incidence of disease by type 1998-2004

Table: 4.972

Number

	1998	1999	2000	2001	2002	2003	2004
Incidence of AIDS	874	1,010	1,123	931	822	289	245
Incidence of diphtheria	0	0	0		0		
Incidence of measles	96	50	45		8		
Incidence of polio	0	0	0	0	0		

Source: WHO

Portugal: Incidence of disease by type: growth 1998-2004

Table: 4.973

Year on year growth: %

	1998	1999	2000	2001	2002	2003	2004
Incidence of AIDS	-2.1	15.6	11.2	-17.1	-11.7	-64.8	-15.2
Incidence of measles	-25.6	-47.9	-10.0				

Source: WHO

Causes of Death

Portugal: Deaths by disease 1998-2004

Table: 4.974

Number per 100,000 inhabitants

	1998	1999	2000	2001	2002	2003	2004
Death by diseases of the circulatory system	316.6	309.3	289.4	290.0	278.0	264.5	256.2
Death by malignant neoplasms (cancers)	162.8	161.3	159.9	159.1	158.4	157.0	157.6
Death by diseases of the respiratory system	70.8	83.2	72.6	77.3	78.2	76.0	76.7
Deaths from heart disease	94.2	92.1	88.3	85.6	82.6	79.6	76.6
Death by diseases of the digestive system	35.4	33.4	31.2	31.8	31.6	30.8	30.5
Deaths from lung cancer	28.5	27.3	28.1	27.5	27.2	26.8	26.5
Deaths from chronic liver disease and cirrhosis	20.8	19.3	17.8	16.4	15.1	13.8	12.7
Deaths from ulcers of the stomach and duodenum	3.9	4.1	3.4	3.3	3.0	2.8	2.6

Source: WHO/Euromonitor International
Notes: Data is ranked in descending order by year 2004

Portugal: Deaths by disease: growth 1998-2004

Table: 4.975

% year on year growth

	1998	1999	2000	2001	2002	2003	2004
Death by diseases of the respiratory system	2.6	17.5	-12.7	6.5	1.2	-2.8	0.9
Death by malignant neoplasms (cancers)	0.7	-0.9	-0.9	-0.5	-0.4	-0.9	0.4
Death by diseases of the digestive system	-1.4	-5.6	-6.6	1.9	-0.6	-2.5	-0.9
Deaths from lung cancer	7.1	-4.3	3.0	-2.2	-1.1	-1.5	-1.1
Death by diseases of the circulatory system	-0.1	-2.3	-6.4	0.2	-4.1	-4.9	-3.1
Deaths from heart disease	2.1	-2.3	-4.1	-3.1	-3.5	-3.6	-3.8
Deaths from ulcers of the stomach and duodenum	0.5	4.9	-17.9	-2.0	-9.1	-6.7	-5.5
Deaths from chronic liver disease and cirrhosis	-4.6	-7.5	-7.3	-8.1	-7.9	-8.6	-8.1

Source: WHO/Euromonitor International
Notes: Data is ranked in descending order by year 2004

Portugal: Other selected causes of death: 1998-2004

Table: 4.976

Number per 100,000 inhabitants

	1998	1999	2000	2001	2002	2003	2004
Death by injury and poisoning	47.0	44.3	40.7	40.6	37.7	34.6	32.5
Death by motor traffic accidents	18.7	15.6	13.0	12.8	10.1	7.3	6.1
Death by suicide and self-inflicted injury	4.7	4.5	4.2	4.2	4.0	3.9	3.8

Source: Euromonitor International from national statistics
Notes: Data is ranked in descending order by year 2004

Portugal: Other selected causes of death: growth 1998-2004

Table: 4.977

% year on year growth

	1998	1999	2000	2001	2002	2003	2004
Death by suicide and self-inflicted injury	-11.3	-4.3	-6.7	0.0	-4.8	-2.5	-2.7
Death by injury and poisoning	-5.6	-5.7	-8.1	-0.2	-7.1	-8.2	-5.9
Death by motor traffic accidents	-5.6	-16.6	-16.7	-1.5	-21.1	-27.7	-16.8

Source: Euromonitor International from national statistics
Notes: Data is ranked in descending order by year 2004

Smoking

Portugal: Smoking prevalence in population aged 15+ 1998-2004

Table: 4.978

% of population aged 15+

	1998	1999	2000	2001	2002	2003	2004
Smoking prevalence in population aged 15+ (% of population aged 15+)	20.7	20.5	21.1	20.9	21.1	22.2	22.7
Smoking prevalence in male population aged 15+ (% of male population)	32.9	32.8	32.5	32.5	32.2	31.8	31.6
Smoking prevalence in female population aged 15+ (% of female population)	9.6	9.5	10.8	10.4	11.1	13.5	14.5

Source: WHO/OECD/Euromonitor International

Nutrition and Obesity

Portugal: Nutrition and obesity 1998-2004

Table: 4.979

As stated

	1998	1999	2000	2001	2002	2003	2004
Availability of fruit and vegetables (kg/capita/year)	313.6	326.9	311.9	319.5	310.5	308.6	304.9
Average supply of calories per day (calories per capita)	3,604.9	3,735.7	3,750.9	3,754.7	3,740.9	3,733.5	3,727.4
Average supply of fat per day (grams per capita)	130.8	138.3	139.6	139.2	139.8	140.4	140.9
Average supply of protein per day (grams per capita)	115.2	118.9	118.4	120.2	118.4	117.4	116.7
Obese population (BMI 30kg/sq m or more) (% of population aged 15+)	14.0	14.2	14.4	14.8	15.4	15.9	16.2

Source: WHO/OECD/Euromonitor International

Over-the-Counter Healthcare

Portugal: Trends in OTC healthcare retail sales 1998-2004

Table: 4.980

As stated

	1998	1999	2000	2001	2002	2003	2004
OTC Healthcare (EUR million)	175.0	181.4	185.7	196.4	214.0	228.4	236.9
OTC Healthcare: real growth in national currency: 1998 = 100	100.0	101.3	100.8	102.1	107.5	111.1	112.4
OTC Healthcare: year on year (% real growth)	-0.9	1.3	-0.5	1.3	5.2	3.4	1.2

Source: Euromonitor International from industry sources/national statistics

Portugal: OTC healthcare retail sales by sector 1998-2004

Table: 4.981

% of OTC retail value sales

	1998	1999	2000	2001	2002	2003	2004
Analgesics	23.2	23.4	22.9	23.6	24.8	25.6	26.3
Cough, cold and allergy (hay fever) remedies	19.1	18.6	18.5	17.9	17.7	17.6	17.7
Digestive remedies	20.5	20.7	20.7	20.2	18.9	18.1	17.7
Medicated skin care	15.1	15.0	15.1	14.8	14.9	14.9	15.2
Vitamins and dietary supplements	11.0	11.4	11.9	11.9	12.0	12.3	11.7

Source: Euromonitor International from industry sources/national statistics
Notes: Only selected sectors are shown, so values are not expected to sum to 100

■ Romania

Socio-economic Parameters

Romania: Socio-economic parameters 1998-2004

Table: 4.982

As stated

	1998	1999	2000	2001	2002	2003	2004
Population: national estimates at January 1st ('000)	22,526.1	22,488.6	22,455.5	22,430.5	22,375.2	22,315.9	22,254.6
% aged 0-14 yrs	19.2	19.0	18.5	18.0	17.5	16.9	16.4
% aged 15-64 yrs	68.0	68.1	68.3	68.5	68.8	69.2	69.5
% aged 65+ yrs	12.7	13.0	13.2	13.5	13.7	13.9	14.1
% Male	49.0	48.9	48.9	48.9	48.9	48.8	48.8
% Female	51.0	51.1	51.1	51.1	51.1	51.2	51.2
% Urban	55.7	55.9	56.2	56.5	56.7	57.6	58.1
Occupants per household at January 1st (Number)	3.2	3.2	3.1	3.1	3.1	3.0	2.9
Households ('000)	6,950.5	7,036.1	7,131.1	7,222.9	7,320.2	7,458.9	7,553.8
Annual rates of inflation (% growth)	59.1	45.8	45.7	34.5	22.5	15.3	11.9
GDP (Leu billion)	373,798.0	545,730.0	803,773.0	1,167,690.0	1,514,750.0	1,903,350.0	2,387,910.0
GDP (US$ million)	42,115.3	35,592.3	37,025.4	40,180.9	45,824.6	57,329.6	73,166.6
GDP (US$ per capita)	1,869.6	1,582.7	1,648.8	1,791.4	2,048.0	2,569.0	3,287.7

Source: Euromonitor International from International Monetary Fund (IMF), International Financial Statistics and World Economic Outlook/UN/national statistics

Life Expectancy

Romania: Life expectancy 1998-2004

Table: 4.983

As stated

	1998	1999	2000	2001	2002	2003	2004	% change 1998-2004
Life expectancy at birth: total population (years)	71.1	71.1	71.1	71.1	71.5	71.7	71.8	1.04
Life expectancy at birth: total population: year on year growth	0.1	0.0	0.0	0.0	0.6	0.2	0.2	
Healthy life expectancy at birth (years)	62.0			61.0	60.9			
Healthy life expectancy at birth: year on year growth					-0.1			

Source: Euromonitor International from World Bank

Sanitation

Romania: Improved sanitary facilities and water source 2000

Table: 4.984

As stated

	2000
Population with access to improved sanitary facilities (% of population)	53.0
Population with access to improved water source (% of population)	58.0
Population with improved access to sanitation facilities, rural (% of rural population with access)	10.0
Population with improved access to sanitation facilities, urban (% of urban population with access)	86.0

Source: National statistics/World Bank

Health Expenditure

Romania: Public health expenditure 1998-2004

Table: 4.985

As stated

	1998	1999	2000	2001	2002	2003	2004
Share of total health expenditure in GDP (% of total GDP)	6.6	6.8	6.6	6.5	6.3	6.4	6.3
Health expenditure (US$ per capita)	96.0	91.0	96.0	109.0	128.0	136.0	145.0

Source: Euromonitor International from OECD/national statistics

Romania: Private health expenditure 1998-2004

Table: 4.986

As stated

	1998	1999	2000	2001	2002	2003	2004
Consumer expenditure on health goods and medical services (Leu million)	10,444,243.0	14,779,253.6	21,047,227.2	27,934,655.0	35,990,499.6	36,264,981.2	40,762,110.8
Consumer expenditure on health goods and medical services: real growth in national currency: 1990 = 100	86.9	84.3	82.4	81.3	85.5	74.8	75.1
Consumer expenditure on health goods and medical services as a percentage of total consumer expenditure	3.7	3.8	3.8	3.5	3.6	2.7	2.6

Source: *National statistical offices/OECD/Eurostat/Euromonitor International*

Romania: Consumer expenditure on health goods and medical services by sector 1998-2004

Table: 4.987

% of total consumer expenditure on health goods and medical services

	1998	1999	2000	2001	2002	2003	2004
Pharmaceuticals, medical appliances/ equipment	76.1	78.6	79.1	80.1	81.4	81.6	81.6
Outpatient services	22.1	20.1	19.3	18.0	16.7	16.5	16.5
Hospital services	1.8	1.3	1.6	1.9	1.9	1.9	1.9
Total	100.0	100.0	100.0	100.0	100.0	100.0	100.0

Source: *National statistical offices/OECD/Eurostat/Euromonitor International*

Healthcare Infrastructure and Services

Romania: Healthcare infrastructure and services by sector 1998-2004

Table: 4.988

As stated

	1998	1999	2000	2001	2002	2003	2004
Active pharmacists (number)	1,642	1,598	1,588	1,490	1,467	1,426	1,396
Dentists (number)	5,367	5,261	4,983	5,057	5,019	4,940	4,873
Doctors (number)	41,310	42,975	42,371	42,339	42,678	43,170	43,748
Hospital admissions (number)	4,577,841	4,653,375	5,024,995	5,458,747	5,449,589	5,712,762	5,912,313
Hospitals and clinics (number)	414	425	439	442	449	450	452
In-patient beds ('000)	165	164	167	168	169	170	171
In-patient surgical procedures (number)	3,219,472	2,998,207	3,608,080	3,040,326	3,612,944	3,548,069	3,623,804
Nurses (number)	92,055	92,453	92,762				
Out-patient contacts (per capita)	7	6	5	5	6	6	6

Source: *Euromonitor International from national statistics*

Romania: Healthcare infrastructure and services by sector: growth 1998-2004

Table: 4.989

Year on year growth: % change in stated unit

	1998	1999	2000	2001	2002	2003	2004
Active pharmacists (number)	-2.8	-2.7	-0.6	-6.2	-1.5	-2.8	-2.1
Dentists (number)	1.3	-2.0	-5.3	1.5	-0.8	-1.6	-1.4
Doctors (number)	2.3	4.0	-1.4	-0.1	0.8	1.2	1.3
Hospital admissions (number)	-3.0	1.6	8.0	8.6	-0.2	4.8	3.5
Hospitals and clinics (number)	-0.5	2.7	3.3	0.7	1.6	0.2	0.4
In-patient beds (number)	-1.1	-0.2	1.6	0.6	0.7	0.6	0.6
In-patient surgical procedures (number)		-6.9	20.3	-15.7	18.8	-1.8	2.1
Nurses (number)		0.4	0.3				
Out-patient contacts (per capita)	-15.0	-5.9	-20.3	5.9	5.6	-1.8	0.0

Source: *Euromonitor International from national statistics*

Immunisation

Romania: Vaccination rates by disease type 1998-2004

Table: 4.990

%

	1998	1999	2000	2001	2002	2003	2004
Vaccination rate against MMR (measles, mumps, rubella) (%)	97.2	98.2	97.8	97.8	98.2	98.0	99.0
Vaccination rate against polio (%)	97.6	97.6	98.8	98.8	99.0	99.0	99.0

Source: WHO

Infectious Diseases

Romania: Incidence of disease by type 1998-2004

Table: 4.991

Number

	1998	1999	2000	2001	2002	2003	2004
Incidence of AIDS	678	492	490	192	222	72	78
Incidence of diphtheria	0	0	0	0	0		
Incidence of measles	9,547	240	35	10	14		
Incidence of polio	0	0	0	0	0		

Source: WHO

Romania: Incidence of disease by type: growth 1998-2004

Table: 4.992

Year on year growth: %

	1998	1999	2000	2001	2002	2003	2004
Incidence of AIDS	3.7	-27.4	-0.4	-60.8	15.6	-67.6	8.3
Incidence of measles	-59.5	-97.5	-85.4	-71.4	40.0		

Source: WHO

Causes of Death

Romania: Deaths by disease 1998-2004

Table: 4.993

Number per 100,000 inhabitants

	1998	1999	2000	2001	2002	2003	2004
Death by diseases of the circulatory system	737.9	736.0	702.2	712.8	701.9	698.9	697.8
Deaths from heart disease	252.4	256.6	242.6	240.6	235.6	230.5	225.9
Death by malignant neoplasms (cancers)	174.4	176.4	184.1	191.4	194.4	190.8	191.5
Death by diseases of the digestive system	71.6	65.4	64.0	70.9	69.4	67.2	67.7
Death by diseases of the respiratory system	70.8	74.3	66.1	63.1	62.9	60.8	59.7
Deaths from lung cancer	36.0	35.4	37.9	38.3	39.0	39.7	40.7
Deaths from chronic liver disease and cirrhosis	54.8	47.6	46.4	41.5	37.7	34.1	30.5
Deaths from ulcers of the stomach and duodenum	3.6	3.4	4.1	4.2	4.4	4.6	4.8

Source: WHO/Euromonitor International
Notes: Data is ranked in descending order by year 2004

Romania: Deaths by disease: growth 1998-2004

Table: 4.994

% year on year growth

	1998	1999	2000	2001	2002	2003	2004
Deaths from ulcers of the stomach and duodenum	-4.4	-6.7	21.1	2.2	4.8	4.5	3.6
Deaths from lung cancer	1.4	-1.6	7.1	1.0	1.8	1.8	2.5
Death by diseases of the digestive system	-5.0	-8.7	-2.1	10.8	-2.1	-3.2	0.7
Death by malignant neoplasms (cancers)	0.6	1.1	4.4	4.0	1.6	-1.9	0.4
Death by diseases of the circulatory system	-3.0	-0.3	-4.6	1.5	-1.5	-0.4	-0.2
Death by diseases of the respiratory system	-8.6	4.9	-11.0	-4.5	-0.3	-3.3	-1.8
Deaths from heart disease	-2.3	1.7	-5.5	-0.8	-2.1	-2.2	-2.0
Deaths from chronic liver disease and cirrhosis	-5.0	-13.1	-2.5	-10.6	-9.2	-9.5	-10.5

Source: WHO/Euromonitor International
Notes: Data is ranked in descending order by year 2004

Romania: Other selected causes of death: 1998-2004

Table: 4.995

Number per 100,000 inhabitants

	1998	1999	2000	2001	2002	2003	2004
Death by injury and poisoning	72.1	64.3	64.3	63.9	63.1	62.5	61.5

Source: Euromonitor International from national statistics

Romania: Other selected causes of death: growth 1998-2004

Table: 4.996

% year on year growth

	1998	1999	2000	2001	2002	2003	2004
Death by injury and poisoning	-6.0	-10.8	0.0	-0.6	-1.3	-1.0	-1.6

Source: Euromonitor International from national statistics

Smoking

Romania: Smoking prevalence in population aged 15+ 1998-2004

Table: 4.997

% of population aged 15+

	1998	1999	2000	2001	2002	2003	2004
Smoking prevalence in population aged 15+ (% of population aged 15+)			20.8				
Smoking prevalence in male population aged 15+ (% of male population)			32.3				
Smoking prevalence in female population aged 15+ (% of female population)			10.1				

Source: WHO/OECD/Euromonitor International

Nutrition and Obesity

Romania: Nutrition and obesity 1998-2004

Table: 4.998

As stated

	1998	1999	2000	2001	2002	2003	2004
Availability of fruit and vegetables (kg/capita/year)	187.0	197.1	185.8	210.6	210.5	218.3	224.8
Average supply of calories per day (calories per capita)	3,291.8	3,315.2	3,361.8	3,424.4	3,454.6	3,494.3	3,538.4
Average supply of fat per day (grams per capita)	88.7	91.0	93.9	96.7	96.1	96.7	97.5
Average supply of protein per day (grams per capita)	104.5	102.6	101.4	104.5	107.4	109.7	112.3
Microbiological food-borne diseases (per 100000 population)	35.0	17.0	24.0	36.0	31.0	32.0	33.0
Obese population (BMI 30kg/sq m or more) (% of population aged 15+)	22.3	21.7	21.0	20.4	20.0	20.0	19.7

Source: WHO/OECD/Euromonitor International

Over-the-Counter Healthcare

Romania: Trends in OTC healthcare retail sales 1998-2004

Table: 4.999

As stated

	1998	1999	2000	2001	2002	2003	2004
OTC Healthcare (Leu billion)	945.7	1,345.1	1,908.9	2,558.9	3,236.4	3,922.1	4,627.0
OTC Healthcare: real growth in national currency: 1998 = 100	100.0	97.6	95.0	94.7	97.8	102.8	108.8
OTC Healthcare: year on year (% real growth)	-6.2	-2.4	-2.6	-0.3	3.2	5.1	5.8
OTC Healthcare ('000 Leu per capita)	42.0	59.8	85.0	114.1	144.6	175.8	207.9
OTC Healthcare ('000 Leu per capita)	42.0	59.8	85.0	114.1	144.6	175.8	207.9

Source: Euromonitor International from industry sources/national statistics

Romania: OTC healthcare retail sales by sector 1998-2004

Table: 4.1000

% of OTC retail value sales

	1998	1999	2000	2001	2002	2003	2004
Analgesics	25.7	26.8	26.9	26.8	26.7	26.1	25.2
Cough, cold and allergy (hay fever) remedies	14.1	13.4	13.1	12.9	12.6	12.4	12.2
Digestive remedies	17.9	18.3	18.5	17.9	17.3	16.6	15.9
Medicated skin care	6.9	7.1	7.2	7.4	7.6	7.7	7.8
Vitamins and dietary supplements	23.9	23.2	23.5	24.5	26.2	28.7	31.1

Source: Euromonitor International from industry sources/national statistics
Notes: Only selected sectors are shown, so values are not expected to sum to 100

■ **Russia**

Socio-economic Parameters

Russia: Socio-economic parameters 1998-2004

Table: 4.1001

As stated

	1998	1999	2000	2001	2002	2003	2004
Population: national estimates at January 1st ('000)	146,739.4	146,327.6	145,559.2	144,819.1	143,954.4	143,097.0	142,411.2
% aged 0-14 yrs	19.8	19.0	18.3	17.6	16.8	16.2	15.6
% aged 15-64 yrs	67.7	68.4	69.2	69.8	70.3	70.6	70.8
% aged 65 + yrs	12.5	12.5	12.5	12.6	12.9	13.3	13.6
% Male	46.9	46.9	46.9	46.8	46.7	46.7	46.6
% Female	53.1	53.1	53.1	53.2	53.3	53.3	53.4
% Urban	77.0	77.3	77.5	77.8	78.1	78.5	78.8
Occupants per household at January 1st (Number)	2.9	2.9	2.8	2.8	2.7	2.7	2.7
Households ('000)	50,464.0	51,019.5	51,653.3	52,266.3	52,707.0	52,663.4	52,874.6
Annual rates of inflation (% growth)	27.7	85.7	20.8	21.5	15.8	13.7	10.9
GDP (Rb million)	2,629,600.0	4,823,200.0	7,305,600.0	8,943,600.0	10,817,500.0	13,201,100.0	16,778,800.0
GDP (US$ million)	270,950.9	195,906.6	259,715.9	306,618.4	345,072.3	430,115.3	582,320.2
GDP (US$ per capita)	1,846.5	1,338.8	1,784.3	2,117.3	2,397.1	3,005.8	4,089.0

Source: Euromonitor International from International Monetary Fund (IMF), International Financial Statistics and World Economic Outlook/UN/national statistics

Life Expectancy

Russia: Life expectancy 1998-2004

Table: 4.1002

As stated

	1998	1999	2000	2001	2002	2003	2004	% change 1998-2004
Life expectancy at birth: total population (years)	65.6	65.6	65.2	65.2	64.8			
Life expectancy at birth: total population: year on year growth	0.0	0.0	-0.6	0.0	-0.6			
Healthy life expectancy at birth (years)	61.0			56.6	56.7			
Healthy life expectancy at birth: year on year growth					0.1			

Source: Euromonitor International from World Bank

Sanitation

Russia: Improved sanitary facilities and water source 2000

Table: 4.1003

As stated

	2000
Population with access to improved water source (% of population)	99.0
Population with improved access to sanitation facilities, rural (% of rural population with access)	96.0

Source: National statistics/World Bank

Health Expenditure

Russia: Public health expenditure 1998-2004

Table: 4.1004

As stated

	1998	1999	2000	2001	2002	2003	2004
Share of total health expenditure in GDP (% of total GDP)	5.8	5.4	5.3	5.4	5.3	5.2	5.1
Health expenditure (US$ per capita)	112.0	70.0	102.0	128.0	150.0	166.0	180.0

Source: Euromonitor International from OECD/national statistics

Russia: Private health expenditure 1998-2004

Table: 4.1005

As stated

	1998	1999	2000	2001	2002	2003	2004
Consumer expenditure on health goods and medical services (Rb million)	26,496.0	54,029.0	70,128.0	92,169.0	117,502.0	155,858.4	177,287.8
Consumer expenditure on health goods and medical services: real growth in national currency: 1990 = 100	89.4	98.1	105.4	114.1	125.6	146.6	150.4
Consumer expenditure on health goods and medical services as a percentage of total consumer expenditure	1.8	2.2	2.3	2.3	2.3	2.3	2.3

Source: National statistical offices/OECD/Eurostat/Euromonitor International

Russia: Consumer expenditure on health goods and medical services by sector 1998-2004

Table: 4.1006

% of total consumer expenditure on health goods and medical services

	1998	1999	2000	2001	2002	2003	2004
Pharmaceuticals, medical appliances/ equipment	16.3	13.8	12.4	10.8	9.1	9.0	8.1
Outpatient services	72.9	79.4	81.6	83.7	86.8	87.0	87.9
Hospital services	10.8	6.7	6.0	5.6	4.1	4.0	4.0
Total	100.0	100.0	100.0	100.0	100.0	100.0	100.0

Source: National statistical offices/OECD/Eurostat/Euromonitor International

Healthcare Infrastructure and Services

Russia: Healthcare infrastructure and services by sector 1998-2004

Table: 4.1007

As stated

	1998	1999	2000	2001	2002	2003	2004
Dentists (number)	54,400	56,000	56,800	57,200	57,600	57,800	58,100
Doctors (number)	680,000	683,000	680,000	698,000	710,000	720,000	728,000
Hospital admissions (number)	30,184,113	30,458,497	31,724,846	32,296,942	32,559,646	33,127,697	33,680,133
Hospitals and clinics (number)	11,100	10,900	10,700	10,465	10,234	10,063	9,889
In-patient beds ('000)	1,717	1,672	1,672	1,642	1,615	1,592	1,577
In-patient surgical procedures (number)	8,496,236	8,465,013	8,587,019	8,751,012	8,728,731	8,777,914	8,941,622
Midwives (number)	93,800	89,300	85,700	84,200	84,900	85,100	85,600
Nurses (number)	1,621,000	1,612,000	1,564,000	1,618,894	1,674,364	1,732,432	1,780,701
Out-patient contacts (per capita)	9	9	9	10	10	10	10

Source: Euromonitor International from national statistics

Russia: Healthcare infrastructure and services by sector: growth 1998-2004

Table: 4.1008

Year on year growth: % change in stated unit

	1998	1999	2000	2001	2002	2003	2004
Dentists (number)	5.6	2.9	1.4	0.7	0.7	0.3	0.5
Doctors (number)	9.3	0.4	-0.4	2.6	1.7	1.4	1.1
Hospital admissions (number)	0.8	0.9	4.2	1.8	0.8	1.7	1.7
Hospitals and clinics (number)	-3.5	-1.8	-1.8	-2.2	-2.2	-1.7	-1.7
In-patient beds (number)	-2.8	-2.6	0.0	-1.8	-1.6	-1.4	-0.9
In-patient surgical procedures (number)	1.8	-0.4	1.4	1.9	-0.3	0.6	1.9
Midwives (number)	-10.2	-4.8	-4.0	-1.8	0.8	0.2	0.6
Nurses (number)	66.6	-0.6	-3.0	3.5	3.4	3.5	2.8
Out-patient contacts (per capita)	0.0	2.2	1.1	1.1	1.1	4.2	-3.0

Source: Euromonitor International from national statistics

Immunisation

Russia: Vaccination rates by disease type 1998-2004

Table: 4.1009

%

	1998	1999	2000	2001	2002	2003	2004
Vaccination rate against MMR (measles, mumps, rubella) (%)	94.2	96.9	98.0	98.4	97.9	99.0	99.0
Vaccination rate against polio (%)	94.3	97.1	97.0	96.7	97.1	97.0	97.0

Source: WHO

Infectious Diseases

Russia: Incidence of disease by type 1998-2004

Table: 4.1010

Number

	1998	1999	2000	2001	2002	2003	2004
Incidence of AIDS	4,058	19,953	59,257	88,422	50,373	39,505	32,101
Incidence of diphtheria	1,409	838	771	909	778		
Incidence of measles	6,215	7,428	4,800	2,072	580		
Incidence of polio	0	0	0	0	0		

Source: WHO

Russia: Incidence of disease by type: growth 1998-2004

Table: 4.1011

Year on year growth: %

	1998	1999	2000	2001	2002	2003	2004
Incidence of AIDS	-7.0	391.7	197.0	49.2	-43.0	-21.6	-18.7
Incidence of diphtheria	-65.1	-40.5	-8.0	17.9	-14.4		
Incidence of measles	116.2	19.5	-35.4	-56.8	-72.0		

Source: WHO

Causes of Death

Russia: Deaths by disease 1998-2004

Table: 4.1012

Number per 100,000 inhabitants

	1998	1999	2000	2001	2002	2003	2004
Death by diseases of the circulatory system	751.0	818.0	852.0	901.0	948.0	998.0	1,055.2
Deaths from heart disease	349.0	383.5	452.8	497.0	547.0	596.4	650.5
Death by malignant neoplasms (cancers)	201.0	205.0	206.0	209.0	211.0	215.0	218.1
Death by diseases of the respiratory system		65.0	70.7	73.0	75.0	81.0	85.1
Deaths from chronic liver disease and cirrhosis		17.8	20.2	26.5	31.2	36.5	44.4
Deaths from lung cancer	41.0	40.8	40.2	37.3	32.8	26.8	23.6
Deaths from ulcers of the stomach and duodenum	5.7	6.3	6.0	6.0	5.7	5.2	5.0
Death by diseases of the digestive system		42.0	45.0				

Source: WHO/Euromonitor International
Notes: Data is ranked in descending order by year 2004

Russia: Deaths by disease: growth 1998-2004

Table: 4.1013

% year on year growth

	1998	1999	2000	2001	2002	2003	2004
Deaths from chronic liver disease and cirrhosis			13.4	31.0	17.7	17.0	21.7
Deaths from heart disease	-1.0	9.9	18.1	9.8	10.1	9.0	9.1
Death by diseases of the circulatory system	-0.3	8.9	4.2	5.8	5.2	5.3	5.7
Death by diseases of the respiratory system			8.8	3.3	2.7	8.0	5.1
Death by malignant neoplasms (cancers)		2.0	0.5	1.5	1.0	1.9	1.4
Deaths from ulcers of the stomach and duodenum	0.1	9.3	-4.6	0.4	-5.0	-8.8	-4.7
Deaths from lung cancer	-2.3	-0.4	-1.6	-7.2	-12.1	-18.3	-11.8
Death by diseases of the digestive system			7.1				

Source: WHO/Euromonitor International
Notes: Data is ranked in descending order by year 2004

Smoking

Russia: Smoking prevalence in population aged 15+ 1998-2004

Table: 4.1014

% of population aged 15+

	1998	1999	2000	2001	2002	2003	2004
Smoking prevalence in population aged 15+ (% of population aged 15+)	36.0	42.5	42.1	41.7	41.5	41.2	41.5
Smoking prevalence in male population aged 15+ (% of male population)	63.2	62.1	61.5	61.3	60.9	60.8	60.3
Smoking prevalence in female population aged 15+ (% of female population)	9.7	25.8	25.7	25.1	25.2	24.6	25.6

Source: WHO/OECD/Euromonitor International

Nutrition and Obesity

Russia: Nutrition and obesity 1998-2004

Table: 4.1015

As stated

	1998	1999	2000	2001	2002	2003	2004
Availability of fruit and vegetables (kg/capita/year)	113.6	113.7	125.6	131.1	141.6	149.0	159.1
Average supply of calories per day (calories per capita)	2,869.7	2,898.2	2,915.9	3,011.7	3,071.8	3,131.4	3,201.0
Average supply of fat per day (grams per capita)	77.5	75.8	77.4	80.9	83.0	85.4	84.6
Average supply of protein per day (grams per capita)	88.8	87.1	86.0	88.5	91.4	93.6	96.1
Microbiological food-borne diseases (per 100000 population)		21.0					
Obese population (BMI 30kg/sq m or more) (% of population aged 15+)	18.1	18.2	18.0	18.0	17.5	17.5	17.5

Source: WHO/OECD/Euromonitor International

Over-the-Counter Healthcare

Russia: Trends in OTC healthcare retail sales 1998-2004

Table: 4.1016

As stated

	1998	1999	2000	2001	2002	2003	2004
OTC Healthcare (US$ million)	749.2	583.3	654.3	771.8	925.5	1,087.6	1,213.9
OTC Healthcare (US$ per capita)	5.1	4.0	4.5	5.3	6.4	7.6	8.5

Source: Euromonitor International from industry sources/national statistics

Russia: OTC healthcare retail sales by sector 1998-2004

Table: 4.1017

% of OTC retail value sales

	1998	1999	2000	2001	2002	2003	2004
Analgesics	14.9	15.3	15.4	14.6	14.2	13.7	13.9
Cough, cold and allergy (hay fever) remedies	21.7	20.3	19.8	18.7	18.4	19.1	18.5
Digestive remedies	14.4	13.5	13.3	13.1	13.0	12.3	12.2
Medicated skin care	10.1	10.7	10.1	9.9	9.6	9.4	9.2
Vitamins and dietary supplements	27.5	28.1	29.9	32.6	33.9	34.8	35.4

Source: *Euromonitor International from industry sources/national statistics*
Notes: *Only selected sectors are shown, so values are not expected to sum to 100*

Health and Wellness

Russia: Retail sales of packaged foods by health and wellness category 2002-2004

Table: 4.1018

US$ million

	2002	2003	2004
Packaged food: Total	33,716.8	36,940.0	40,548.5
Better for you	1,968.5	2,079.6	2,222.0
For food intolerance	35.1	38.7	42.7
Fortified/functional	51.5	62.9	75.2
Organic	16.2	16.4	17.6

Source: *Euromonitor International from industry sources/national statistics*

Russia: Per capita sales of packaged foods by health and wellness category 2002-2004

Table: 4.1019

US$ per capita

	2002	2003	2004
Better for you	13.7	14.6	15.7
For food intolerance	0.2	0.3	0.3
Fortified/functional	0.4	0.4	0.5
Organic	0.1	0.1	0.1

Source: *Euromonitor International from industry sources/national statistics*

Russia: Retail sales of packaged food by health and wellness category: % share of total packaged food market 2002-2004

Table: 4.1020

% value

	2002	2003	2004
Better for you	5.8	5.6	5.5
For food intolerance	0.1	0.1	0.1
Fortified/functional	0.2	0.2	0.2
Organic	0.0	0.0	0.0

Source: *Euromonitor International from industry sources/national statistics*

Russia: Retail sales of packaged food by health and wellness category: real growth index 2002-2004

Table: 4.1021

2002 = 100

	2002	2003	2004
Better for you	100.00	103.43	103.75
For food intolerance	100.00	108.12	111.95
Fortified/functional	100.00	119.49	134.17
Organic	100.00	98.94	100.02

Source: *Euromonitor International from industry sources/national statistics*

Russia: Retail sales of better-for-you packaged foods by sector 2002-2004

% of total packaged food / as stated

	2002	2003	2004	% real change in value 2002-2004
Reduced fat	2.61	2.54	2.53	16.74
Reduced salt	2.08	1.98	1.90	9.45

Source: Euromonitor International from industry sources/national statistics

Russia: Retail sales of packaged foods for food intolerances by sector 2002-2004

% of total packaged food / as stated

	2002	2003	2004	% real change in value 2002-2004
Diabetic	0.09	0.09	0.09	19.84
Lactose-free	0.01	0.01	0.01	39.96

Source: Euromonitor International from industry sources/national statistics

Russia: Retail sales of naturally healthy packaged foods by sector 2002-2004

% of total packaged food / as stated

	2002	2003	2004	% real change in value 2002-2004
High fibre	0.96	0.94	0.94	16.96
Other naturally healthy food	0.94	0.91	0.87	10.99

Source: Euromonitor International from industry sources/national statistics

■ **Saudi Arabia**

Socio-economic Parameters

Saudi Arabia: Socio-economic parameters 1998-2004

As stated

	1998	1999	2000	2001	2002	2003	2004
Population: national estimates at January 1st ('000)	19,842.4	20,338.4	20,846.9	21,555.7	22,288.6	22,944.0	23,596.7
% aged 0-14 yrs	40.3	40.3	40.3	40.3	40.3	40.0	39.8
% aged 15-64 yrs	56.7	56.7	56.7	56.7	56.7	56.9	57.2
% aged 65+ yrs	3.0	3.0	3.0	3.0	3.0	3.0	3.1
% Male	54.3	54.3	54.3	54.3	54.3	54.2	54.1
% Female	45.7	45.7	45.7	45.7	45.7	45.8	45.9
% Urban	84.5	85.1	85.3	85.7	86.1	86.6	87.1
Occupants per household at January 1st (Number)	6.1	6.1	6.1	6.0	6.0	5.9	5.9
Households ('000)	3,250.0	3,330.0	3,430.0	3,570.0	3,710.0	3,860.0	3,990.0
Annual rates of inflation (% growth)	-0.4	-1.3	-1.1	-1.1	0.2	0.6	0.4
GDP (SR million)	546,648.0	603,588.0	706,657.0	686,296.0	707,067.0	797,175.0	931,803.0
GDP (US$ million)	145,967.4	161,171.7	188,693.5	183,256.6	188,802.9	212,863.8	248,812.6
GDP (US$ per capita)	7,356.3	7,924.5	9,051.4	8,501.5	8,470.8	9,277.5	10,544.4

Source: Euromonitor International from International Monetary Fund (IMF), International Financial Statistics and World Economic Outlook/UN/national statistics

Life Expectancy

Saudi Arabia: Life expectancy 1998-2004

Table: 4.1026

As stated

	1998	1999	2000	2001	2002	2003	2004	% change 1998-2004
Life expectancy at birth: total population (years)	70.2	70.5	70.3	70.5	70.8	71.0	71.2	1.39
Life expectancy at birth: total population: year on year growth	0.4	0.4	-0.3	0.3	0.4	0.3	0.3	
Healthy life expectancy at birth (years)	65.0			59.8	60.0			
Healthy life expectancy at birth: year on year growth					0.3			

Source: Euromonitor International from World Bank

Sanitation

Saudi Arabia: Improved sanitary facilities and water source 2000

Table: 4.1027

As stated

	2000
Population with access to improved sanitary facilities (% of population)	100.0
Population with access to improved water source (% of population)	95.0
Population with improved access to sanitation facilities, rural (% of rural population with access)	100.0
Population with improved access to sanitation facilities, urban (% of urban population with access)	100.0

Source: National statistics/World Bank

Health Expenditure

Saudi Arabia: Public health expenditure 1998-2004

Table: 4.1028

As stated

	1998	1999	2000	2001	2002	2003	2004
Share of total health expenditure in GDP (% of total GDP)	5.2	4.5	4.4	4.6	4.4	4.5	4.4
Health expenditure (US$ per capita)	354.0	313.0	336.0	360.0	345.0	356.0	362.0

Source: Euromonitor International from OECD/national statistics

Saudi Arabia: Private health expenditure 1998-2004

Table: 4.1029

As stated

	1998	1999	2000	2001	2002	2003	2004
Consumer expenditure on health goods and medical services (SR million)	6,174.0	6,880.0	7,049.0	6,993.0	7,520.0	7,856.3	8,378.3
Consumer expenditure on health goods and medical services: real growth in national currency: 1990 = 100	124.8	141.0	146.1	146.5	157.2	163.3	173.5
Consumer expenditure on health goods and medical services as a percentage of total consumer expenditure	2.5	2.8	2.8	2.8	2.9	2.8	2.9

Source: National statistical offices/OECD/Eurostat/Euromonitor International

Saudi Arabia: Consumer expenditure on health goods and medical services by sector 1998-2004

Table: 4.1030

% of total consumer expenditure on health goods and medical services

	1998	1999	2000	2001	2002	2003	2004
Pharmaceuticals, medical appliances/ equipment	66.4	64.2	64.1	63.7	62.7	65.0	65.2
Outpatient services	29.5	31.5	31.3	31.1	31.8	30.0	29.7
Hospital services	4.1	4.3	4.5	5.2	5.6	5.0	5.1
Total	100.0	100.0	100.0	100.0	100.0	100.0	100.0

Source: National statistical offices/OECD/Eurostat/Euromonitor International

Healthcare Infrastructure and Services

Saudi Arabia: Healthcare infrastructure and services by sector 1998-2004

Table: 4.1031

As stated

	1998	1999	2000	2001	2002	2003	2004
Active pharmacists (number)	652	642	661	676	680	690	699
Dentists (number)	201	237	262	278	284	290	293
Doctors (number)	13,807	14,077	13,975	13,876	13,876	13,918	13,922
Hospitals and clinics (number)	182	186	55	55	55	56	57
In-patient beds ('000)	27	28	28	28	28	28	28
Nurses (number)	35,463	36,887	37,614	38,612	39,369	39,965	40,231

Source: Euromonitor International from national statistics

Saudi Arabia: Healthcare infrastructure and services by sector: growth 1998-2004

Table: 4.1032

Year on year growth: % change in stated unit

	1998	1999	2000	2001	2002	2003	2004
Active pharmacists (number)	21.2	-1.5	3.0	2.3	0.6	1.5	1.3
Dentists (number)	10.4	17.9	10.5	6.1	2.2	2.1	1.0
Doctors (number)	-1.6	2.0	-0.7	-0.7	0.0	0.3	0.0
Hospitals and clinics (number)	1.1	2.2	-70.4	0.0	0.0	1.8	1.8
In-patient beds (number)	1.4	1.3	0.7	0.0	0.0	0.0	0.0
Nurses (number)	3.8	4.0	2.0	2.7	2.0	1.5	0.7

Source: Euromonitor International from national statistics

Immunisation

Saudi Arabia: Vaccination rates by disease type 1998-2004

Table: 4.1033

%

	1998	1999	2000	2001	2002	2003	2004
Vaccination rate against DTP (diphtheria, tetanus, pertussis) 1 & 2 (%)				98.7	97.0	95.0	94.0
Vaccination rate against MMR (measles, mumps, rubella) (%)	93.0	92.0	92.0	94.4	96.7	97.0	98.0
Vaccination rate against polio (%)	94.0	93.0	94.0	96.8	94.7	97.0	97.0

Source: WHO

Infectious Diseases

Saudi Arabia: Incidence of disease by type 1998-2004

Table: 4.1034

Number

	1998	1999	2000	2001	2002	2003	2004
Incidence of AIDS	39	24	24	39	48	52	43
Incidence of diphtheria	0	0		0	9		
Incidence of measles	5,519	2,815		155	311		
Incidence of polio	1	0	0	0	0		

Source: WHO

Saudi Arabia: Incidence of disease by type: growth 1998-2004

Table: 4.1035

Year on year growth: %

	1998	1999	2000	2001	2002	2003	2004
Incidence of AIDS	-65.2	-38.5	0.0	62.5	23.1	8.3	-17.3
Incidence of diphtheria	-100.0						
Incidence of measles	38.7	-49.0			100.6		
Incidence of polio		-100.0					

Source: WHO

Smoking

Saudi Arabia: Smoking prevalence in population aged 15+ 1998-2004

Table: 4.1036

% of population aged 15+

	1998	1999	2000	2001	2002	2003	2004
Smoking prevalence in population aged 15+ (% of population aged 15+)	26.4	25.7	27.3	27.3	27.7	28.0	28.4
Smoking prevalence in male population aged 15+ (% of male population)	34.8	35.7	35.6	36.3	36.6	37.2	37.7
Smoking prevalence in female population aged 15+ (% of female population)	15.4	12.6	16.4	15.6	16.2	16.2	16.5

Source: WHO/OECD/Euromonitor International

Nutrition and Obesity

Saudi Arabia: Nutrition and obesity 1998-2004

Table: 4.1037

As stated

	1998	1999	2000	2001	2002	2003	2004
Average supply of calories per day (calories per capita)	2,808.6	2,831.0	2,837.9	2,850.6	2,844.5	2,843.6	2,844.0
Average supply of fat per day (grams per capita)	77.0	79.5	85.0	85.4	86.7	88.6	90.2
Average supply of protein per day (grams per capita)	76.0	78.2	75.6	74.6	73.8	72.7	73.7
Obese population (BMI 30kg/sq m or more) (% of population aged 15+)	26.3	26.4	26.7	27.0	27.4	27.7	28.0

Source: WHO/OECD/Euromonitor International

Over-the-Counter Healthcare

Saudi Arabia: Trends in OTC healthcare retail sales 1998-2004

Table: 4.1038

As stated

	1998	1999	2000	2001	2002	2003	2004
OTC Healthcare (SR million)	1,073.9	1,107.3	1,146.0	1,204.9	1,267.7	1,329.4	1,397.8
OTC Healthcare: real growth in national currency: 1998 = 100	100.0	104.5	109.4	116.3	122.1	127.3	130.6
OTC Healthcare: year on year (% real growth)	4.7	4.5	4.7	6.3	5.0	4.2	2.6
OTC Healthcare (SR per capita)	54.1	54.4	55.0	55.9	56.9	57.9	59.2

Source: Euromonitor International from industry sources/national statistics

Saudi Arabia: OTC healthcare retail sales by sector 1998-2004

Table: 4.1039

% of OTC retail value sales

	1998	1999	2000	2001	2002	2003	2004
Analgesics	18.2	18.4	18.8	19.3	19.6	20.0	20.2
Cough, cold and allergy (hay fever) remedies	27.4	27.4	27.5	27.7	27.7	27.7	27.7
Digestive remedies	18.4	18.3	17.7	16.8	16.2	15.9	15.5
Medicated skin care	17.1	17.1	17.1	17.2	17.1	16.9	16.8
Vitamins and dietary supplements	14.0	14.0	14.1	14.3	14.6	14.8	15.1

Source: Euromonitor International from industry sources/national statistics
Notes: Only selected sectors are shown, so values are not expected to sum to 100

■ Singapore

Socio-economic Parameters

Singapore: Socio-economic parameters 1998-2004

Table: 4.1040

As stated

	1998	1999	2000	2001	2002	2003	2004
Population: national estimates at January 1st ('000)	3,174.8	3,222.0	3,263.2	3,319.4	3,378.2	3,430.0	3,478.2
% aged 0-14 yrs	22.1	21.8	21.5	21.2	21.0	20.6	19.9
% aged 15-64 yrs	71.0	71.1	71.2	71.4	71.5	71.8	72.1
% aged 65+ yrs	6.9	7.1	7.3	7.4	7.5	7.7	8.0
% Male	50.1	50.0	50.0	49.9	49.8	49.8	49.7
% Female	49.9	50.0	50.0	50.1	50.2	50.2	50.3
% Urban	100.0	100.0	100.0	100.0	100.0	100.0	100.0
Occupants per household at January 1st (Number)	3.7	3.6	3.5	3.5	3.5	3.5	3.5
Households ('000)	868.2	896.5	923.3	947.1	968.5	988.8	1,007.2
Annual rates of inflation (% growth)	-0.3	0.0	1.4	1.0	-0.4	0.5	1.7
GDP (S$ million)	137,089.0	139,616.0	159,662.0	154,078.0	158,064.0	159,135.0	180,554.0
GDP (US$ million)	81,912.6	82,371.3	92,613.5	85,994.5	88,274.8	91,342.5	106,822.1
GDP (US$ per capita)	25,800.9	25,565.3	28,381.1	25,906.6	26,130.7	26,630.2	30,712.1

Source: Euromonitor International from International Monetary Fund (IMF), International Financial Statistics and World Economic Outlook/UN/national statistics

Life Expectancy

Singapore: Life expectancy 1998-2004

Table: 4.1041

As stated

	1998	1999	2000	2001	2002	2003	2004	% change 1998-2004
Life expectancy at birth: total population (years)	78.3	78.5	78.4	78.8	79.5	79.9	80.3	2.67
Life expectancy at birth: total population: year on year growth	0.3	0.3	-0.1	0.5	1.0	0.4	0.6	
Healthy life expectancy at birth (years)	69.0			68.5	68.7			
Healthy life expectancy at birth: year on year growth					0.3			

Source: Euromonitor International from World Bank

Sanitation

Singapore: Improved sanitary facilities and water source 2000

Table: 4.1042

As stated

	2000
Population with access to improved sanitary facilities (% of population)	100.0
Population with access to improved water source (% of population)	100.0
Population with improved access to sanitation facilities, urban (% of urban population with access)	100.0

Source: National statistics/World Bank

Health Expenditure

Singapore: Public health expenditure 1998-2004

Table: 4.1043

As stated

	1998	1999	2000	2001	2002	2003	2004
Share of total health expenditure in GDP (% of total GDP)	4.2	4.0	3.6	3.9	4.1	4.1	4.0
Health expenditure (US$ per capita)	900.0	849.0	824.0	816.0	898.0	914.0	944.0

Source: Euromonitor International from OECD/national statistics

Singapore: Private health expenditure 1998-2004

Table: 4.1044

As stated

	1998	1999	2000	2001	2002	2003	2004
Consumer expenditure on health goods and medical services (S$ million)	3,137.2	3,370.6	3,591.5	3,865.2	4,095.7	4,206.1	4,428.2
Consumer expenditure on health goods and medical services: real growth in national currency: 1990 = 100	174.8	187.8	197.4	210.4	223.8	228.7	236.8
Consumer expenditure on health goods and medical services as a percentage of total consumer expenditure	5.6	5.6	5.3	5.8	6.1	6.1	6.2

Source: National statistical offices/OECD/Eurostat/Euromonitor International

Singapore: Consumer expenditure on health goods and medical services by sector 1998-2004

Table: 4.1045

% of total consumer expenditure on health goods and medical services

	1998	1999	2000	2001	2002	2003	2004
Pharmaceuticals, medical appliances/ equipment	29.7	29.0	29.3	29.2	29.1	29.1	29.2
Outpatient services	43.8	43.9	43.5	43.2	43.1	43.0	42.8
Hospital services	26.5	27.1	27.2	27.6	27.9	28.0	28.1
Total	100.0	100.0	100.0	100.0	100.0	100.0	100.0

Source: National statistical offices/OECD/Eurostat/Euromonitor International

Healthcare Infrastructure and Services

Singapore: Healthcare infrastructure and services by sector 1998-2004

Table: 4.1046

As stated

	1998	1999	2000	2001	2002	2003	2004
Active pharmacists (number)	998	1,043	1,098	1,141	1,191	1,236	1,271
Dentists (number)	914	942	1,028	1,087	1,130	1,183	1,224
Doctors (number)	5,148	5,325	5,577	5,922	6,029	6,292	6,487
Hospitals and clinics (number)	23	28	28	28	29	29	29
In-patient beds ('000)	11	12	12	12	12	12	12
Midwives (number)	456	449	437	415	393	371	358
Nurses (number)	11,491	11,765	12,353	12,828	13,308	13,740	14,089

Source: Euromonitor International from national statistics

Singapore: Healthcare infrastructure and services by sector: growth 1998-2004

Table: 4.1047

Year on year growth: % change in stated unit

	1998	1999	2000	2001	2002	2003	2004
Active pharmacists (number)	5.7	4.5	5.3	3.9	4.4	3.8	2.8
Dentists (number)	4.1	3.1	9.1	5.7	4.0	4.7	3.5
Doctors (number)	4.8	3.4	4.7	6.2	1.8	4.4	3.1
Hospitals and clinics (number)	-4.2	21.7	0.0	0.0	3.6	0.0	0.0
In-patient beds (number)	1.0	3.1	0.9	0.7	-1.5	0.8	1.2
Midwives (number)	-3.6	-1.5	-2.7	-5.0	-5.3	-5.6	-3.5
Nurses (number)	5.7	2.4	5.0	3.8	3.7	3.2	2.5

Source: Euromonitor International from national statistics

Immunisation

Singapore: Vaccination rates by disease type 1998-2004

Table: 4.1048

%

	1998	1999	2000	2001	2002	2003	2004
Vaccination rate against MMR (measles, mumps, rubella) (%)	96.0	92.9	90.0	89.0	90.9	92.0	90.0
Vaccination rate against polio (%)	96.0	95.0	93.0	91.0	91.8	90.0	90.0

Source: WHO

Infectious Diseases

Singapore: Incidence of disease by type 1998-2004

Table: 4.1049

Number

	1998	1999	2000	2001	2002	2003	2004
Incidence of AIDS	125	140	143	152	146	143	151
Incidence of diphtheria	0	0	0		0		
Incidence of measles	114	65	141	408	211		
Incidence of polio	0	0	0	0	0		

Source: WHO

Singapore: Incidence of disease by type: growth 1998-2004

Table: 4.1050

Year on year growth: %

	1998	1999	2000	2001	2002	2003	2004
Incidence of AIDS	42.0	12.0	2.1	6.3	-3.9	-2.1	5.6
Incidence of measles	-91.9	-43.0	116.9	189.4	-48.3		

Source: WHO

Causes of Death

Singapore: Deaths by disease 1998-2004

Table: 4.1051

Number per 100,000 inhabitants

	1998	1999	2000	2001	2002	2003	2004
Death by diseases of the circulatory system	145.6	147.1	143.1	134.5	137.9	130.9	126.2
Death by malignant neoplasms (cancers)	104.3	105.5	106.5	105.8	104.3	102.3	101.9
Deaths from heart disease	95.1	96.9	91.3	90.6	88.5	86.4	84.3
Death by diseases of the respiratory system	62.9	59.7	62.3	53.4	57.8	56.0	54.5
Death by diseases of the digestive system	32.4	31.2	29.9	32.5	32.5	30.7	31.0
Deaths from lung cancer	30.1	29.1	27.5	26.4	25.2	23.9	22.9
Deaths from chronic liver disease and cirrhosis	4.2	4.3	3.0	2.7	2.6	2.6	2.5
Deaths from ulcers of the stomach and duodenum	2.2	2.9	1.6	1.6	1.3	1.2	1.1

Source: WHO/Euromonitor International
Notes: Data is ranked in descending order by year 2004

Singapore: Deaths by disease: growth 1998-2004

Table: 4.1052

% year on year growth

	1998	1999	2000	2001	2002	2003	2004
Death by diseases of the digestive system	-5.5	-3.7	-4.2	8.7	0.0	-5.5	1.0
Death by malignant neoplasms (cancers)	-5.3	1.2	0.9	-0.7	-1.4	-1.9	-0.3
Deaths from heart disease	-0.1	1.9	-5.8	-0.8	-2.3	-2.4	-2.4
Death by diseases of the respiratory system	0.0	-5.1	4.4	-14.3	8.2	-3.1	-2.7
Death by diseases of the circulatory system	-2.7	1.0	-2.7	-6.0	2.5	-5.1	-3.6
Deaths from lung cancer	5.5	-3.3	-5.5	-4.1	-4.5	-5.2	-4.3
Deaths from chronic liver disease and cirrhosis	-0.2	3.0	-29.2	-11.0	-3.7	0.0	-4.4
Deaths from ulcers of the stomach and duodenum	-4.4	31.9	-47.0	2.4	-18.8	-7.7	-8.7

Source: WHO/Euromonitor International
Notes: Data is ranked in descending order by year 2004

Singapore: Other selected causes of death: 1998-2004

Table: 4.1053

Number per 100,000 inhabitants

	1998	1999	2000	2001	2002	2003	2004
Death by suicide and self-inflicted injury	9.5	7.8	8.7	7.5	7.7	7.1	6.6
Death by motor traffic accidents	5.9	5.4	5.5	4.5	4.6	4.3	4.0

Source: Euromonitor International from national statistics
Notes: Data is ranked in descending order by year 2004

Singapore: Other selected causes of death: growth 1998-2004

Table: 4.1054

% year on year growth

	1998	1999	2000	2001	2002	2003	2004
Death by suicide and self-inflicted injury	4.4	-17.9	11.5	-13.8	2.7	-7.8	-6.4
Death by motor traffic accidents	-21.3	-8.5	1.9	-18.2	2.2	-6.5	-7.1

Source: Euromonitor International from national statistics
Notes: Data is ranked in descending order by year 2004

Smoking

Singapore: Smoking prevalence in population aged 15+ 1998-2004

Table: 4.1055

% of population aged 15+

	1998	1999	2000	2001	2002	2003	2004
Smoking prevalence in population aged 15+ (% of population aged 15+)	25.8	25.8	26.0	26.0	26.1	26.3	25.9
Smoking prevalence in male population aged 15+ (% of male population)	28.9	28.9	26.9	28.5	28.4	29.5	30.1
Smoking prevalence in female population aged 15+ (% of female population)	22.8	22.8	25.1	23.6	24.0	23.1	21.8

Source: WHO/OECD/Euromonitor International

Nutrition and Obesity

Singapore: Nutrition and obesity 1998-2004

Table: 4.1056

As stated

	1998	1999	2000	2001	2002	2003	2004
Average supply of calories per day (calories per capita)	3,101.7	3,087.5	3,161.2	3,022.0	3,008.2	2,988.7	2,951.9
Average supply of fat per day (grams per capita)	103.5	103.4	108.6	100.6	103.3	104.8	105.0
Average supply of protein per day (grams per capita)	107.5	106.8	106.2	103.2	102.4	101.2	99.8
Obese population (BMI 30kg/sq m or more) (% of population aged 15+)	6.3	6.5	6.5	6.6	6.7	6.7	6.7

Source: WHO/OECD/Euromonitor International

Over-the-Counter Healthcare

Singapore: Trends in OTC healthcare retail sales 1998-2004

Table: 4.1057

As stated

	1998	1999	2000	2001	2002	2003	2004
OTC Healthcare (S$ million)	227.5	238.7	253.1	267.7	279.4	295.8	299.6
OTC Healthcare: real growth in national currency: 1998 = 100	100.0	104.9	109.7	114.9	120.4	126.8	126.2
OTC Healthcare: year on year (% real growth)	4.6	4.9	4.6	4.7	4.8	5.3	-0.5
OTC Healthcare (S$ per capita)	71.7	74.1	77.6	80.6	82.7	86.2	86.1

Source: Euromonitor International from industry sources/national statistics

Singapore: OTC healthcare retail sales by sector 1998-2004

Table: 4.1058

% of OTC retail value sales

	1998	1999	2000	2001	2002	2003	2004
Analgesics	8.2	8.3	8.4	8.4	8.4	8.4	8.7
Cough, cold and allergy (hay fever) remedies	25.7	25.7	25.7	25.7	25.8	25.1	25.6
Digestive remedies	5.1	5.0	4.9	4.8	4.8	4.6	4.7
Medicated skin care	7.7	7.7	7.7	7.6	7.5	7.5	7.4
Vitamins and dietary supplements	50.2	50.1	50.1	50.3	50.4	51.3	50.5

Source: Euromonitor International from industry sources/national statistics
Notes: Only selected sectors are shown, so values are not expected to sum to 100

■ Slovakia

Socio-economic Parameters

Slovakia: Socio-economic parameters 1998-2004

Table: 4.1059

As stated

	1998	1999	2000	2001	2002	2003	2004
Population: national estimates at January 1st ('000)	5,367.7	5,372.4	5,376.7	5,378.8	5,379.0	5,375.3	5,370.8
% aged 0-14 yrs	21.0	20.4	19.8	19.4	18.7	18.1	17.5
% aged 15-64 yrs	67.7	68.3	68.8	69.3	69.9	70.5	71.2
% aged 65+ yrs	11.2	11.3	11.4	11.3	11.4	11.3	11.3
% Male	48.6	48.6	48.6	48.6	48.6	48.6	48.7
% Female	51.4	51.4	51.4	51.4	51.4	51.4	51.3
% Urban	57.2	57.3	57.4	57.6	57.7	58.7	59.2
Occupants per household at January 1st (Number)	2.7	2.7	2.6	2.6	2.6	2.5	2.5
Households ('000)	1,994.3	2,019.6	2,045.4	2,072.0	2,092.4	2,110.7	2,128.5
Annual rates of inflation (% growth)	6.7	10.6	12.0	7.3	3.3	8.6	7.5
GDP (SKK million)	781,437.0	844,108.0	934,079.0	1,009,840.0	1,098,660.0	1,201,200.0	1,325,490.0
GDP (US$ million)	22,178.9	20,407.4	20,290.5	20,884.0	24,238.7	32,665.4	41,091.7
GDP (US$ per capita)	4,132.0	3,798.6	3,773.8	3,882.7	4,506.2	6,077.0	7,651.0

Source: Euromonitor International from International Monetary Fund (IMF), International Financial Statistics and World Economic Outlook/UN/national statistics

Life Expectancy

Slovakia: Life expectancy 1998-2004

Table: 4.1060

As stated

	1998	1999	2000	2001	2002	2003	2004	% change 1998-2004
Life expectancy at birth: total population (years)	72.9	73.0	73.3	73.3	74.0	74.4	74.8	2.66
Life expectancy at birth: total population: year on year growth	0.3	0.2	0.4	0.0	1.0	0.5	0.5	
Healthy life expectancy at birth (years)	67.0			64.1	64.1			
Healthy life expectancy at birth: year on year growth					0.1			

Source: Euromonitor International from World Bank

Sanitation

Slovakia: Improved sanitary facilities and water source 2000

Table: 4.1061

As stated

	2000
Population with access to improved sanitary facilities (% of population)	100.0
Population with access to improved water source (% of population)	100.0
Population with improved access to sanitation facilities, rural (% of rural population with access)	100.0
Population with improved access to sanitation facilities, urban (% of urban population with access)	100.0

Source: National statistics/World Bank

Health Expenditure

Slovakia: Public health expenditure 1998-2004

Table: 4.1062

As stated

	1998	1999	2000	2001	2002	2003	2004
Public expenditure on pharmaceuticals and other medical non-durables (SKK million)		12,638.0	14,488.0	15,814.0	19,665.0	23,637.0	30,264.1
Share of total health expenditure in GDP (% of total GDP)	5.8	5.8	5.7	5.7	5.4	5.6	5.6
Health expenditure (US$ per capita)	235.0	218.0	208.0	216.0	256.0	269.0	282.0

Source: Euromonitor International from OECD/national statistics

Slovakia: Private health expenditure 1998-2004

Table: 4.1063

As stated

	1998	1999	2000	2001	2002	2003	2004
Consumer expenditure on health goods and medical services (SKK million)	4,092.0	5,444.0	6,354.0	7,865.0	8,440.0	10,209.0	11,203.3
Consumer expenditure on health goods and medical services as a percentage of total consumer expenditure	1.0	1.2	1.2	1.4	1.4	1.5	1.5

Source: National statistical offices/OECD/Eurostat/Euromonitor International

Slovakia: Consumer expenditure on health goods and medical services by sector 1998-2004

Table: 4.1064

% of total consumer expenditure on health goods and medical services

	1998	1999	2000	2001	2002	2003	2004
Pharmaceuticals, medical appliances/ equipment	79.8	81.7	76.2	74.6	71.8	74.1	74.1
Outpatient services	18.4	16.8	22.6	24.1	26.6	24.5	24.5
Hospital services	1.8	1.4	1.3	1.3	1.6	1.4	1.4
Total	100.0	100.0	100.0	100.0	100.0	100.0	100.0

Source: National statistical offices/OECD/Eurostat/Euromonitor International

Healthcare Infrastructure and Services

Slovakia: Healthcare infrastructure and services by sector 1998-2004

Table: 4.1065

As stated

	1998	1999	2000	2001	2002	2003	2004
Active pharmacists (number)	2,236	2,253	2,400	2,344	2,420	2,460	2,481
Consultations with GPs (general practitioners) (per capita)	15	15	15	13	13	13	13
Dentists (number)	2,490	2,253	2,400	2,344	2,556	2,586	2,618
Doctors (number)	18,837	19,059	19,303	18,982	18,743	18,784	18,794
Hospital admissions (number)	1,095,175	1,044,213	1,075,208	1,061,996	1,022,339	1,022,981	1,030,511
In-patient beds ('000)	38	38	56	55	54	54	54
In-patient surgical procedures (number)	37,277	34,012	33,388	34,102	33,271	33,416	33,430
Nurses (number)	39,702	40,380	39,428	38,352	38,130	37,935	37,903
Out-patient contacts (per capita)	16	16	16	15	14	13	14

Source: Euromonitor International from national statistics

Slovakia: Healthcare infrastructure and services by sector: growth 1998-2004

Table: 4.1066

Year on year growth: % change in stated unit

	1998	1999	2000	2001	2002	2003	2004
Active pharmacists (number)	2.9	0.8	6.5	-2.3	3.2	1.7	0.9
Consultations with GPs (general practitioners) (per capita)	25.0	0.0	0.0	-13.3	0.0	0.0	0.0
Dentists (number)	3.3	-9.5	6.5	-2.3	9.0	1.2	1.2
Doctors (number)	63.3	1.2	1.3	-1.7	-1.3	0.2	0.1
Hospital admissions (number)	2.3	-4.7	3.0	-1.2	-3.7	0.1	0.7
In-patient beds (number)	-2.2	-0.8	48.2	-2.7	-0.6	-0.4	-0.3
In-patient surgical procedures (number)	-6.0	-8.8	-1.8	2.1	-2.4	0.4	0.0
Nurses (number)	24.7	1.7	-2.4	-2.7	-0.6	-0.5	-0.1
Out-patient contacts (per capita)	21.3	-0.4	-0.7	-10.1	-0.9	-9.5	4.6

Source: Euromonitor International from national statistics

Immunisation

Slovakia: Vaccination rates by disease type 1998-2004

Table: 4.1067

%

	1998	1999	2000	2001	2002	2003	2004
Vaccination rate against DTP (diphtheria, tetanus, pertussis) 1 & 2 (%)				99.4	99.3	99.0	99.0
Vaccination rate against MMR (measles, mumps, rubella) (%)	99.0	99.0	98.6	98.6	98.6	98.0	98.0
Vaccination rate against polio (%)	98.2	99.0	99.0	98.9	98.4	98.0	98.0

Source: WHO

Infectious Diseases

Slovakia: Incidence of disease by type 1998-2004

Table: 4.1068

Number

	1998	1999	2000	2001	2002	2003	2004
Incidence of AIDS	3	2	4	5	2	1	2
Incidence of diphtheria	0	0	0	0	0		
Incidence of measles	530	0	0	0	0		
Incidence of polio	0	0	0	0	0		

Source: WHO

Slovakia: Incidence of disease by type: growth 1998-2004

Table: 4.1069

Year on year growth: %

	1998	1999	2000	2001	2002	2003	2004
Incidence of AIDS	-40.0	-33.3	100.0	25.0	-60.0	-50.0	100.0
Incidence of measles	-14.5	-100.0					

Source: WHO

Causes of Death

Slovakia: Deaths by disease 1998-2004

Table: 4.1070

Number per 100,000 inhabitants

	1998	1999	2000	2001	2002	2003	2004
Death by diseases of the circulatory system	548.7	517.7	512.9	510.7	508.9	507.6	501.3
Deaths from heart disease	266.2	268.8	290.4	299.5	311.9	324.5	336.4
Death by malignant neoplasms (cancers)	223.9	215.8	212.6	211.4	206.2	200.5	197.6
Death by diseases of the respiratory system	44.4	47.5	52.5	56.2	60.2	52.1	51.4
Death by diseases of the digestive system	44.4	47.0	45.9	43.1	43.1	42.6	42.0
Deaths from lung cancer	41.3	40.2	41.6	41.2	41.2	41.0	40.6
Deaths from chronic liver disease and cirrhosis	25.3	26.7	25.9	26.6	26.8	26.9	27.2
Deaths from ulcers of the stomach and duodenum	4.7	4.8	5.0	5.1	5.2	5.3	5.4

Source: WHO/Euromonitor International
Notes: Data is ranked in descending order by year 2004

Slovakia: Deaths by disease: growth 1998-2004

Table: 4.1071

% year on year growth

	1998	1999	2000	2001	2002	2003	2004
Deaths from heart disease	0.4	1.0	8.0	3.1	4.1	4.0	3.7
Deaths from ulcers of the stomach and duodenum	6.1	2.7	3.0	2.8	2.0	1.9	2.7
Deaths from chronic liver disease and cirrhosis	21.5	5.6	-3.1	2.8	0.8	0.4	1.1
Deaths from lung cancer	3.6	-2.7	3.6	-1.1	0.0	-0.5	-0.9
Death by diseases of the circulatory system	3.3	-5.6	-0.9	-0.4	-0.4	-0.3	-1.2
Death by diseases of the respiratory system	-37.2	7.0	10.5	7.0	7.1	-13.5	-1.3
Death by malignant neoplasms (cancers)	7.8	-3.6	-1.5	-0.6	-2.5	-2.8	-1.4
Death by diseases of the digestive system	11.3	5.9	-2.3	-6.1	0.0	-1.2	-1.5

Source: WHO/Euromonitor International
Notes: Data is ranked in descending order by year 2004

Slovakia: Other selected causes of death: 1998-2004

Table: 4.1072

Number per 100,000 inhabitants

	1998	1999	2000	2001	2002	2003	2004
Death by injury and poisoning	59.5	54.5	54.3	53.4	50.9	48.3	46.2
Death by suicide and self-inflicted injury	11.5	11.9	12.4	12.7	13.1	12.8	13.0
Death by motor traffic accidents	19.1	15.2	14.4	13.9	11.5	9.2	7.8

Source: Euromonitor International from national statistics
Notes: Data is ranked in descending order by year 2004

Slovakia: Other selected causes of death: growth 1998-2004

Table: 4.1073

% year on year growth

	1998	1999	2000	2001	2002	2003	2004
Death by suicide and self-inflicted injury	3.6	3.5	4.2	2.4	3.1	-2.3	1.5
Death by injury and poisoning	-10.4	-8.4	-0.4	-1.7	-4.7	-5.1	-4.3
Death by motor traffic accidents	4.9	-20.4	-5.3	-3.5	-17.3	-20.0	-14.7

Source: Euromonitor International from national statistics
Notes: Data is ranked in descending order by year 2004

Smoking

Slovakia: Smoking prevalence in population aged 15+ 1998-2004

Table: 4.1074

% of population aged 15+

	1998	1999	2000	2001	2002	2003	2004
Smoking prevalence in population aged 15+ (% of population aged 15+)	29.0	41.3	42.8	45.8	47.4	48.3	49.6
Smoking prevalence in male population aged 15+ (% of male population)	44.1	53.0	53.0	52.7	53.6	53.8	54.0
Smoking prevalence in female population aged 15+ (% of female population)	14.7	30.5	33.4	39.5	41.6	43.3	45.5

Source: WHO/OECD/Euromonitor International

Nutrition and Obesity

Slovakia: Nutrition and obesity 1998-2004

Table: 4.1075

As stated

	1998	1999	2000	2001	2002	2003	2004
Availability of fruit and vegetables (kg/capita/year)	170.4	169.3	141.7	134.4	123.6	114.8	106.2
Average supply of calories per day (calories per capita)	3,129.2	3,023.8	2,869.3	2,873.9	2,888.9	2,874.7	2,868.3
Average supply of fat per day (grams per capita)	121.2	116.8	101.9	111.2	111.5	111.1	112.5
Average supply of protein per day (grams per capita)	85.6	82.9	77.5	77.0	77.6	77.1	76.8
Microbiological food-borne diseases (per 100000 population)	84.0	96.0	108.0	108.0	78.0	84.0	78.0
Obese population (BMI 30kg/sq m or more) (% of population aged 15+)	15.8	16.8	16.5	16.8	17.0	17.0	17.2

Source: WHO/OECD/Euromonitor International

Over-the-Counter Healthcare

Slovakia: Trends in OTC healthcare retail sales 1998-2004

Table: 4.1076

As stated

	1998	1999	2000	2001	2002	2003	2004
OTC Healthcare (SKK million)	2,537.1	2,686.6	2,841.6	3,010.1	3,186.5	3,375.3	3,568.4
OTC Healthcare: real growth in national currency: 1998 = 100	100.0	95.8	90.4	89.2	91.4	89.2	87.6
OTC Healthcare: year on year (% real growth)	-1.1	-4.2	-5.6	-1.3	2.5	-2.4	-1.8
OTC Healthcare (SKK per capita)	472.7	500.1	528.5	559.6	592.4	627.9	664.4

Source: Euromonitor International from industry sources/national statistics

Slovakia: OTC healthcare retail sales by sector 1998-2004

Table: 4.1077

% of OTC retail value sales

	1998	1999	2000	2001	2002	2003	2004
Analgesics	26.6	26.2	25.6	25.1	24.6	24.2	24.1
Cough, cold and allergy (hay fever) remedies	19.4	18.9	18.4	18.0	17.6	17.3	17.1
Digestive remedies	10.3	10.2	10.1	9.9	9.8	9.7	9.6
Medicated skin care	13.0	12.7	12.4	12.1	11.9	11.7	11.6
Vitamins and dietary supplements	23.8	25.3	26.8	28.3	29.5	30.5	31.0

Source: Euromonitor International from industry sources/national statistics
Notes: Only selected sectors are shown, so values are not expected to sum to 100

■ Slovenia

Socio-economic Parameters

Slovenia: Socio-economic parameters 1998-2004

Table: 4.1078

As stated

	1998	1999	2000	2001	2002	2003	2004
Population: national estimates at January 1st ('000)	1,984.9	1,978.3	1,987.8	1,990.1	1,994.0	1,996.4	1,998.4
% aged 0-14 yrs	17.0	16.6	16.1	15.7	15.4	15.0	14.6
% aged 15-64 yrs	69.7	69.8	70.0	70.1	70.1	70.3	70.5
% aged 65+ yrs	13.2	13.6	13.9	14.1	14.5	14.7	14.8
% Male	48.8	48.7	48.8	48.9	48.9	48.9	48.9
% Female	51.2	51.3	51.2	51.1	51.1	51.1	51.1
% Urban	50.3	50.3	52.5	52.3	52.1	52.0	52.4
Occupants per household at January 1st (Number)	3.0	3.0	3.0	2.9	2.9	2.9	2.9
Households ('000)	662.7	667.1	671.6	676.1	684.8	689.5	694.3
Annual rates of inflation (% growth)	8.0	6.1	8.9	8.4	7.5	5.6	3.6
GDP (Tolars million)	3,464,890.0	3,874,720.0	4,252,310.0	4,761,810.0	5,314,490.0	5,747,170.0	6,191,160.0
GDP (US$ million)	20,856.0	21,316.7	19,098.1	19,616.2	22,120.9	27,748.8	32,181.8
GDP (US$ per capita)	10,507.2	10,775.1	9,607.9	9,856.9	11,093.6	13,899.6	16,103.6

Source: Euromonitor International from International Monetary Fund (IMF), International Financial Statistics and World Economic Outlook/UN/national statistics

© Euromonitor International 2005

Life Expectancy

Slovenia: Life expectancy 1998-2004

Table: 4.1079

As stated

	1998	1999	2000	2001	2002	2003	2004	% change 1998-2004
Life expectancy at birth: total population (years)	75.2	75.4	75.7	75.9	76.7	77.0	77.5	3.12
Life expectancy at birth: total population: year on year growth	0.3	0.3	0.4	0.3	1.0	0.5	0.6	
Healthy life expectancy at birth (years)	68.0			67.5	67.7			
Healthy life expectancy at birth: year on year growth					0.2			

Source: Euromonitor International from World Bank

Sanitation

Slovenia: Improved sanitary facilities and water source 2000

Table: 4.1080

As stated

	2000
Population with access to improved water source (% of population)	100.0
Population with improved access to sanitation facilities, rural (% of rural population with access)	100.0

Source: National statistics/World Bank

Health Expenditure

Slovenia: Public health expenditure 1998-2004

Table: 4.1081

As stated

	1998	1999	2000	2001	2002	2003	2004
Share of total health expenditure in GDP (% of total GDP)	8.3	8.2	8.0	8.4	8.4	8.8	8.5
Health expenditure (US$ per capita)	813.0	829.0	765.0	821.0	922.0	953.0	995.0

Source: Euromonitor International from OECD/national statistics

Slovenia: Private health expenditure 1998-2004

Table: 4.1082

As stated

	1998	1999	2000	2001	2002	2003	2004
Consumer expenditure on health goods and medical services (Tolars million)	46,407.0	51,535.0	58,638.0	65,490.0	73,482.0	84,896.8	89,528.3
Consumer expenditure on health goods and medical services as a percentage of total consumer expenditure	2.5	2.5	2.5	2.5	2.6	2.5	2.5

Source: National statistical offices/OECD/Eurostat/Euromonitor International

Slovenia: Consumer expenditure on health goods and medical services by sector 1998-2004

Table: 4.1083

% of total consumer expenditure on health goods and medical services

	1998	1999	2000	2001	2002	2003	2004
Pharmaceuticals, medical appliances/ equipment	43.3	45.4	46.7	48.6	50.3	49.8	49.7
Outpatient services	37.9	35.2	34.4	32.8	31.2	31.7	31.7
Hospital services	18.8	19.4	19.0	18.6	18.4	18.6	18.7
Total	100.0	100.0	100.0	100.0	100.0	100.0	100.0

Source: National statistical offices/OECD/Eurostat/Euromonitor International

Healthcare Infrastructure and Services

Slovenia: Healthcare infrastructure and services by sector 1998-2004

Table: 4.1084

As stated

	1998	1999	2000	2001	2002	2003	2004
Active pharmacists (number)	887	917	1,079	1,122	1,255	1,272	1,284
Dentists (number)	1,201	1,199	1,188	1,208	1,231	1,242	1,255
Doctors (number)	1,363	1,413	1,417	1,467	1,521	1,564	1,607
Hospital admissions (number)	325,742	328,819	332,601	330,302	327,175	326,933	325,885
Hospitals and clinics (number)	26	26	27	27	27	27	27
In-patient beds ('000)	11	11	11	10	10	10	10
In-patient surgical procedures (number)				109,036	114,855	121,277	127,252
Nurses (number)	13,460	13,120	13,120	13,120	13,341	13,452	13,543
Out-patient contacts (per capita)	7	7	7	7	6	6	6

Source: Euromonitor International from national statistics

Slovenia: Healthcare infrastructure and services by sector: growth 1998-2004

Table: 4.1085

Year on year growth: % change in stated unit

	1998	1999	2000	2001	2002	2003	2004
Active pharmacists (number)	-15.9	3.4	17.7	4.0	11.9	1.4	0.9
Dentists (number)	3.1	-0.2	-0.9	1.7	1.9	0.9	1.0
Doctors (number)	-50.7	3.7	0.3	3.5	3.7	2.8	2.7
Hospital admissions (number)	1.5	0.9	1.2	-0.7	-0.9	-0.1	-0.3
Hospitals and clinics (number)	8.3	0.0	3.8	0.0	0.0	0.0	0.0
In-patient beds (number)	-1.2	-1.2	-2.0	-4.3	-1.4	-0.2	-0.2
In-patient surgical procedures (number)					5.3	5.6	4.9
Nurses (number)		-2.5	0.0	0.0	1.7	0.8	0.7
Out-patient contacts (per capita)	4.4	3.7	-7.2	-2.2	-4.3	-4.5	-4.9

Source: Euromonitor International from national statistics

Immunisation

Slovenia: Vaccination rates by disease type 1998-2004

Table: 4.1086

%

	1998	1999	2000	2001	2002	2003	2004
Vaccination rate against DTP (diphtheria, tetanus, pertussis) 1 & 2 (%)				96.3	97.0	98.0	98.0
Vaccination rate against MMR (measles, mumps, rubella) (%)	93.0	98.0	95.0	94.0	95.0	97.0	98.0
Vaccination rate against polio (%)	90.0	93.0	93.0	92.6	92.0	92.0	91.0

Source: WHO

Infectious Diseases

Slovenia: Incidence of disease by type 1998-2004

Table: 4.1087

Number

	1998	1999	2000	2001	2002	2003	2004
Incidence of AIDS	14	9	7	3	2	2	3
Incidence of diphtheria	0	0		0	0		
Incidence of measles	13	1		0	0		
Incidence of polio	0	0	0		0		

Source: WHO

Slovenia: Incidence of disease by type: growth 1998-2004

Table: 4.1088

Year on year growth: %

	1998	1999	2000	2001	2002	2003	2004
Incidence of AIDS	1,300.0	-35.7	-22.2	-57.1	-33.3	0.0	50.0
Incidence of measles	44.4	-92.3					

Source: WHO

Causes of Death

Slovenia: Deaths by disease 1998-2004

Table: 4.1089

Number per 100,000 inhabitants

	1998	1999	2000	2001	2002	2003	2004
Death by malignant neoplasms (cancers)	241.2	245.7	241.9	241.0	237.6	235.0	230.9
Death by diseases of the circulatory system	398.1	388.3	236.9	234.5	232.5	214.2	205.9
Deaths from heart disease	141.1	132.9	132.6	130.2	127.8	125.4	122.1
Death by diseases of the respiratory system	77.2	79.1	79.0	70.4	71.1	69.1	65.8
Deaths from lung cancer	46.2	49.0	50.2	51.8	53.5	55.2	56.7
Deaths from chronic liver disease and cirrhosis	32.2	34.0	35.5	37.0	38.6	40.2	42.3
Death by diseases of the digestive system	39.2	40.8	42.1	41.3	42.3	41.6	41.2
Deaths from ulcers of the stomach and duodenum	5.0	6.3	6.4	6.9	7.3	7.7	8.1

Source: WHO/Euromonitor International
Notes: Data is ranked in descending order by year 2004

Slovenia: Deaths by disease: growth 1998-2004

Table: 4.1090

% year on year growth

	1998	1999	2000	2001	2002	2003	2004
Deaths from ulcers of the stomach and duodenum	-8.9	26.1	1.2	7.8	5.8	5.5	5.8
Deaths from chronic liver disease and cirrhosis	4.2	5.4	4.5	4.2	4.3	4.1	5.2
Deaths from lung cancer	0.9	6.0	2.5	3.2	3.3	3.2	2.7
Death by diseases of the digestive system	-0.3	4.1	3.2	-1.9	2.4	-1.7	-0.9
Death by malignant neoplasms (cancers)	0.5	1.9	-1.5	-0.4	-1.4	-1.1	-1.8
Deaths from heart disease	2.7	-5.8	-0.3	-1.8	-1.8	-1.9	-2.6
Death by diseases of the circulatory system	-1.3	-2.5	-39.0	-1.0	-0.9	-7.9	-3.9
Death by diseases of the respiratory system	0.8	2.5	-0.1	-10.9	1.0	-2.8	-4.8

Source: WHO/Euromonitor International
Notes: Data is ranked in descending order by year 2004

Slovenia: Other selected causes of death: 1998-2004

Table: 4.1091

Number per 100,000 inhabitants

	1998	1999	2000	2001	2002	2003	2004
Death by suicide and self-inflicted injury	30.8	29.8	29.8	30.3	29.8	29.3	29.3
Death by injury and poisoning			16.0	16.0	16.0	16.1	16.2
Death by motor traffic accidents	17.2	17.9	16.8	16.9	15.8	15.6	15.1

Source: Euromonitor International from national statistics
Notes: Data is ranked in descending order by year 2004

Slovenia: Other selected causes of death: growth 1998-2004

Table: 4.1092

% year on year growth

	1998	1999	2000	2001	2002	2003	2004
Death by injury and poisoning				0.0	0.0	0.6	0.8
Death by suicide and self-inflicted injury	3.4	-3.2	0.0	1.7	-1.7	-1.7	0.1
Death by motor traffic accidents	-9.9	4.1	-6.1	0.6	-6.5	-1.3	-3.4

Source: Euromonitor International from national statistics
Notes: Data is ranked in descending order by year 2004

Smoking

Slovenia: Smoking prevalence in population aged 15+ 1998-2004

Table: 4.1093

% of population aged 15+

	1998	1999	2000	2001	2002	2003	2004
Smoking prevalence in population aged 15+ (% of population aged 15+)	25.3	24.5	23.9	23.7	23.4	23.2	23.1
Smoking prevalence in male population aged 15+ (% of male population)	31.9	30.0	29.0	28.0	27.5	27.3	27.0
Smoking prevalence in female population aged 15+ (% of female population)	20.3	20.3	20.2	20.1	20.1	20.0	19.9

Source: WHO/OECD/Euromonitor International

Nutrition and Obesity

Slovenia: Nutrition and obesity 1998-2004

Table: 4.1094

As stated

	1998	1999	2000	2001	2002	2003	2004
Availability of fruit and vegetables (kg/capita/year)	188.2	199.0	196.7	163.5	150.3	144.2	134.6
Average supply of calories per day (calories per capita)	2,997.4	3,135.3	3,111.1	2,932.5	3,001.4	3,015.9	3,007.3
Average supply of fat per day (grams per capita)	113.2	112.7	107.0	110.7	106.3	103.2	101.1
Average supply of protein per day (grams per capita)	99.1	107.4	104.7	102.5	102.6	101.9	101.1
Microbiological food-borne diseases (per 100000 population)	26.0	24.0	28.0	27.0	41.0	42.0	47.0
Obese population (BMI 30kg/sq m or more) (% of population aged 15+)	10.8	10.8	10.9	11.0	11.1	11.1	11.2

Source: WHO/OECD/Euromonitor International

■ **South Africa**

Socio-economic Parameters

South Africa: Socio-economic parameters 1998-2004

As stated

	1998	1999	2000	2001	2002	2003	2004
Population: national estimates at January 1st ('000)	42,130.0	43,054.0	43,851.7	44,819.7	45,653.9	46,429.8	47,550.5
% aged 0-14 yrs	33.5	33.1	32.6	32.1	31.6	31.3	30.8
% aged 15-64 yrs	61.6	62.0	62.5	63.0	63.4	63.7	64.1
% aged 65 + yrs	4.8	4.8	4.8	4.9	5.0	5.0	5.1
% Male	48.3	48.3	48.1	47.8	47.8	47.7	47.6
% Female	51.7	51.7	51.9	52.2	52.2	52.3	52.4
% Urban	50.0	50.2	50.4	50.6	50.9	51.3	51.7
Occupants per household at January 1st (Number)	4.3	4.2	4.1	4.0	3.9	3.9	3.9
Households ('000)	9,861.7	10,291.1	10,728.5	11,205.7	11,568.2	11,917.5	12,238.4
Annual rates of inflation (% growth)	6.9	5.2	5.3	5.7	9.2	5.9	1.4
GDP (R million)	742,424.0	813,683.0	922,148.0	1,020,007.0	1,164,945.0	1,251,468.0	1,375,258.0
GDP (US$ million)	134,295.7	133,183.7	132,877.6	118,479.0	110,518.8	165,434.2	212,898.5
GDP (US$ per capita)	3,187.6	3,093.4	3,030.2	2,643.5	2,420.8	3,563.1	4,477.3

Source: Euromonitor International from International Monetary Fund (IMF), International Financial Statistics and World Economic Outlook/UN/national statistics

Life Expectancy

South Africa: Life expectancy 1998-2004

As stated

	1998	1999	2000	2001	2002	2003	2004	% change 1998-2004
Life expectancy at birth: total population (years)	54.0	52.2	51.2	49.0	50.7	50.3	50.4	-6.79
Life expectancy at birth: total population: year on year growth	-3.6	-3.4	-1.8	-4.3	3.5	-0.8	0.1	
Healthy life expectancy at birth (years)	40.0			43.0	41.3			
Healthy life expectancy at birth: year on year growth					-3.8			

Source: Euromonitor International from World Bank

Sanitation

South Africa: Improved sanitary facilities and water source 2000

As stated

	2000
Population with access to improved sanitary facilities (% of population)	87.0
Population with access to improved water source (% of population)	86.0
Population with improved access to sanitation facilities, rural (% of rural population with access)	80.0
Population with improved access to sanitation facilities, urban (% of urban population with access)	93.0

Source: National statistics/World Bank

Health Expenditure

South Africa: Public health expenditure 1998-2004

As stated

	1998	1999	2000	2001	2002	2003	2004
Share of total health expenditure in GDP (% of total GDP)	8.7	8.8	8.7	8.6	8.8	8.4	8.3
Health expenditure (US$ per capita)	261.0	266.0	244.0	224.0	206.0	196.0	188.0

Source: Euromonitor International from OECD/national statistics

South Africa: Private health expenditure 1998-2004

Table: 4.1099

As stated

	1998	1999	2000	2001	2002	2003	2004
Consumer expenditure on health goods and medical services (R million)	32,771.0	36,969.0	41,068.0	46,185.0	54,439.0	61,738.9	64,068.4
Consumer expenditure on health goods and medical services: real growth in national currency: 1990 = 100	190.5	204.3	215.5	229.2	247.5	265.2	271.4
Consumer expenditure on health goods and medical services as a percentage of total consumer expenditure	7.0	7.3	7.4	7.6	8.0	8.0	7.9

Source: National statistical offices/OECD/Eurostat/Euromonitor International

South Africa: Consumer expenditure on health goods and medical services by sector 1998-2004

Table: 4.1100

% of total consumer expenditure on health goods and medical services

	1998	1999	2000	2001	2002	2003	2004
Pharmaceuticals, medical appliances/equipment	24.4	24.2	24.2	22.7	22.3	22.5	22.6
Outpatient services	66.5	66.6	65.9	66.5	66.9	66.3	66.0
Hospital services	9.0	9.1	9.9	10.8	10.9	11.3	11.3
Total	100.0	100.0	100.0	100.0	100.0	100.0	100.0

Source: National statistical offices/OECD/Eurostat/Euromonitor International

Healthcare Infrastructure and Services

South Africa: Healthcare infrastructure and services by sector 1998-2004

Table: 4.1101

As stated

	1998	1999	2000	2001	2002	2003	2004
Active pharmacists (number)	9,948	9,959	9,971	9,986	10,003	10,021	10,050
Dentists (number)	4,387	4,412	4,448	4,981	5,100	5,213	5,290
Doctors (number)	29,369	30,521	31,336	31,687	31,614	31,098	31,012
Midwives (number)	229						
Nurses (number)	174,754	174,895	175,126	175,214	175,314	175,388	175,575

Source: Euromonitor International from national statistics

South Africa: Healthcare infrastructure and services by sector: growth 1998-2004

Table: 4.1102

Year on year growth: % change in stated unit

	1998	1999	2000	2001	2002	2003	2004
Active pharmacists (number)	0.0	0.1	0.1	0.2	0.2	0.2	0.3
Dentists (number)	2.1	0.6	0.8	12.0	2.4	2.2	1.5
Doctors (number)	1.2	3.9	2.7	1.1	-0.2	-1.6	-0.3
Midwives (number)	-15.2						
Nurses (number)	-0.5	0.1	0.1	0.1	0.1	0.0	0.1

Source: Euromonitor International from national statistics

Immunisation

South Africa: Vaccination rates by disease type 1998-2004

Table: 4.1103

%

	1998	1999	2000	2001	2002	2003	2004
Vaccination rate against DTP (diphtheria, tetanus, pertussis) 1 & 2 (%)			95.0	87.0	88.0	83.0	80.0
Vaccination rate against MMR (measles, mumps, rubella) (%)	82.0	82.2	95.0	72.0	78.0	76.0	75.0
Vaccination rate against polio (%)		72.1	96.0	80.0	84.0	88.0	90.0

Source: WHO

Infectious Diseases

South Africa: Incidence of disease by type 1998-2004

Table: 4.1104

Number

	1998	1999	2000	2001	2002	2003	2004
Incidence of diphtheria	4	0	2	0	1		
Incidence of measles	977	385	1,459	1,166	1,043		
Incidence of polio	104	4	0	0	0		

Source: WHO

South Africa: Incidence of disease by type: growth 1998-2004

Table: 4.1105

Year on year growth: %

	1998	1999	2000	2001	2002	2003	2004
Incidence of diphtheria	33.3	-100.0		-100.0			
Incidence of measles	-26.9	-60.6	279.0	-20.1	-10.5		
Incidence of polio		-96.2	-100.0				

Source: WHO

Causes of Death

South Africa: Deaths by disease 1998-2004

Table: 4.1106

Number per 100,000 inhabitants

	1998	1999	2000	2001	2002	2003	2004
Deaths from heart disease	29.9	30.3	30.7	31.1	31.4	31.7	31.7
Deaths from chronic liver disease and cirrhosis	9.3	10.6	12.0	13.4	14.9	16.4	18.3
Deaths from lung cancer	9.9	9.7	9.5	9.3	9.0	8.7	8.5
Deaths from ulcers of the stomach and duodenum	2.9	3.0	3.1	3.2	3.3	3.4	3.5

Source: WHO/Euromonitor International
Notes: Data is ranked in descending order by year 2004

South Africa: Deaths by disease: growth 1998-2004

Table: 4.1107

% year on year growth

	1998	1999	2000	2001	2002	2003	2004
Deaths from chronic liver disease and cirrhosis	16.3	14.0	13.2	11.7	11.2	10.1	11.3
Deaths from ulcers of the stomach and duodenum	3.6	3.4	3.3	3.2	3.1	3.0	3.6
Deaths from heart disease	1.4	1.3	1.3	1.3	1.0	1.0	0.1
Deaths from lung cancer	-1.0	-2.0	-2.1	-2.1	-3.2	-3.3	-2.5

Source: WHO/Euromonitor International
Notes: Data is ranked in descending order by year 2004

Smoking

South Africa: Smoking prevalence in population aged 15+ 1998-2004

Table: 4.1108

% of population aged 15+

	1998	1999	2000	2001	2002	2003	2004
Smoking prevalence in population aged 15+ (% of population aged 15+)	34.6	34.8	34.9	35.5	35.8	36.2	36.5
Smoking prevalence in male population aged 15+ (% of male population)	53.9	54.6	55.5	56.1	56.2	57.0	56.7
Smoking prevalence in female population aged 15+ (% of female population)	17.2	17.0	16.5	17.3	17.8	18.0	18.9

Source: WHO/OECD/Euromonitor International

Nutrition and Obesity

South Africa: Nutrition and obesity 1998-2004

Table: 4.1109

As stated

	1998	1999	2000	2001	2002	2003	2004
Average supply of calories per day (calories per capita)	2,820.4	2,843.8	2,886.4	2,909.1	2,956.1	2,999.4	3,039.2
Average supply of fat per day (grams per capita)	72.3	70.9	72.5	75.6	77.5	79.7	82.1
Average supply of protein per day (grams per capita)	71.7	73.2	76.4	75.7	76.2	77.0	76.5
Obese population (BMI 30kg/sq m or more) (% of population aged 15+)	19.3	20.1	20.8	21.5	22.1	23.0	25.4

Source: WHO/OECD/Euromonitor International

Over-the-Counter Healthcare

South Africa: Trends in OTC healthcare retail sales 1998-2004

Table: 4.1110

As stated

	1998	1999	2000	2001	2002	2003	2004
OTC Healthcare (R million)	3,152.7	3,302.6	3,433.9	3,618.6	3,804.1	3,997.9	4,269.0
OTC Healthcare: real growth in national currency: 1998 = 100	100.0	99.6	98.3	98.0	94.4	93.7	97.5
OTC Healthcare: year on year (% real growth)	-2.6	-0.4	-1.3	-0.3	-3.7	-0.7	4.1
OTC Healthcare (R per capita)	74.8	76.7	78.3	80.7	83.3	86.1	89.8

Source: Euromonitor International from industry sources/national statistics

South Africa: OTC healthcare retail sales by sector 1998-2004

Table: 4.1111

% of OTC retail value sales

	1998	1999	2000	2001	2002	2003	2004
Analgesics	28.7	28.6	28.8	28.9	29.1	29.5	29.9
Cough, cold and allergy (hay fever) remedies	30.6	30.5	30.5	30.4	30.2	30.0	29.8
Digestive remedies	8.4	8.3	8.2	8.0	7.9	7.7	7.5
Medicated skin care	16.3	16.2	16.0	15.7	15.6	15.4	15.3
Vitamins and dietary supplements	10.4	10.8	10.9	11.0	11.2	11.3	11.5

Source: Euromonitor International from industry sources/national statistics
Notes: Only selected sectors are shown, so values are not expected to sum to 100

■ **South Korea**

Socio-economic Parameters

South Korea: Socio-economic parameters 1998-2004

Table: 4.1112

As stated

	1998	1999	2000	2001	2002	2003	2004
Population: national estimates at January 1st ('000)	45,434.0	45,714.0	45,985.0	46,253.0	46,542.0	46,819.0	47,085.0
% aged 0-14 yrs	21.0	21.0	21.0	21.0	21.0	20.0	20.0
% aged 15-64 yrs	72.0	72.0	72.0	72.0	72.0	71.0	71.0
% aged 65 + yrs	7.0	7.0	7.0	8.0	8.0	8.0	9.0
% Male	50.0	50.0	50.0	50.0	50.0	50.0	50.0
% Female	50.0	50.0	50.0	50.0	50.0	50.0	50.0
% Urban	80.0	81.0	82.0	82.0	83.0	83.0	84.0
Occupants per household at January 1st (Number)	3.0	3.0	3.0	3.0	3.0	3.0	3.0
Households ('000)	15,173.0	15,442.0	15,765.0	16,081.0	16,489.0	16,756.0	17,035.0
Annual rates of inflation (% growth)	8.0	1.0	2.0	4.0	3.0	4.0	4.0
GDP (Won million)	484,103,000.0	529,500,000.0	578,665,000.0	622,123,000.0	684,263,000.0	724,675,000.0	778,445,000.0
GDP (US$ million)	345,433.0	445,400.0	511,658.0	481,896.0	546,933.0	608,148.0	679,675.0
GDP (US$ per capita)	7,603.0	9,743.0	11,127.0	10,419.0	11,751.0	12,989.0	14,435.0

Source: Euromonitor International from International Monetary Fund (IMF), International Financial Statistics and World Economic Outlook/UN/national statistics

Life Expectancy

South Korea: Life expectancy 1998-2004

Table: 4.1113

As stated

	1998	1999	2000	2001	2002	2003	2004	% change 1998-2004
Life expectancy at birth: total population (years)	74.4	74.6	74.6	74.9	75.5	75.7	75.9	2.08
Life expectancy at birth: total population: year on year growth	0.3	0.3	0.0	0.4	0.8	0.3	0.3	
Healthy life expectancy at birth (years)	65.0			67.2	67.4			
Healthy life expectancy at birth: year on year growth					0.4			

Source: Euromonitor International from World Bank

Sanitation

South Korea: Improved sanitary facilities and water source 2000

Table: 4.1114

As stated

	2000
Population with access to improved sanitary facilities (% of population)	63.0
Population with access to improved water source (% of population)	92.0
Population with improved access to sanitation facilities, rural (% of rural population with access)	4.0
Population with improved access to sanitation facilities, urban (% of urban population with access)	76.0

Source: National statistics/World Bank

Health Expenditure

South Korea: Public health expenditure 1998-2004

Table: 4.1115

As stated

	1998	1999	2000	2001	2002	2003	2004
Public expenditure on pharmaceuticals and other medical non-durables (Won million)	163,300.0	204,170.0	847,860.0	3,785,830.0	3,926,450.0	4,036,390.0	6,700,086.6
Private insurance expenditure (% of total expenditure on health)	2.6	2.7	2.9	2.1	2.4	2.4	2.3
Share of total health expenditure in GDP (% of total GDP)	5.1	5.6	5.9	6.0	6.1	5.9	5.7
Health expenditure (US$ per capita)	328.0	435.0	503.0	528.0	577.0	601.0	617.0

Source: Euromonitor International from OECD/national statistics

South Korea: Private health expenditure 1998-2004

Table: 4.1116

As stated

	1998	1999	2000	2001	2002	2003	2004
Consumer expenditure on health goods and medical services (Won million)	17,796,491.0	19,853,883.0	20,954,850.0	24,403,272.0	26,710,687.0	28,386,655.6	30,396,646.2
Consumer expenditure on health goods and medical services: real growth in national currency: 1990 = 100	172.3	190.7	196.8	220.2	234.7	240.9	249.0
Consumer expenditure on health goods and medical services as a percentage of total consumer expenditure	7.4	7.4	7.1	7.6	7.7	7.7	7.8

Source: National statistical offices/OECD/Eurostat/Euromonitor International

South Korea: Consumer expenditure on health goods and medical services by sector 1998-2004

Table: 4.1117

% of total consumer expenditure on health goods and medical services

	1998	1999	2000	2001	2002	2003	2004
Pharmaceuticals, medical appliances/equipment	24.5	23.7	24.2	24.2	24.5	24.2	24.0
Outpatient services	46.4	46.4	46.1	45.3	45.8	45.2	45.4
Hospital services	29.1	29.8	29.6	30.5	29.8	30.5	30.6
Total	100.0	100.0	100.0	100.0	100.0	100.0	100.0

Source: National statistical offices/OECD/Eurostat/Euromonitor International

Healthcare Infrastructure and Services

South Korea: Healthcare infrastructure and services by sector 1998-2004

Table: 4.1118

As stated

	1998	1999	2000	2001	2002	2003	2004
Active pharmacists (number)	3,131	3,120	2,312	2,607	2,704	2,748	2,772
Consultations with GPs (general practitioners) (per capita)		9	9	10	11	11	11
Dentists (number)	12,070	13,199	13,593	13,814	14,679	15,171	15,430
Doctors (number)	47,387	50,424	49,220	53,189	57,779	60,412	62,861
Hospitals and clinics (number)	38,037	40,244	42,082	43,675	47,430	49,412	51,333
In-patient beds ('000)	236	259	287	289	316	322	323
Midwives (number)	1,268	1,428	1,080	1,227	1,174	1,162	1,147
Nurses (number)	53,954	59,104	59,791	68,013	75,239	76,952	77,399

Source: Euromonitor International from national statistics

South Korea: Healthcare infrastructure and services by sector: growth 1998-2004

Table: 4.1119

Year on year growth: % change in stated unit

	1998	1999	2000	2001	2002	2003	2004
Active pharmacists (number)	4.1	-0.4	-25.9	12.8	3.7	1.6	0.9
Consultations with GPs (general practitioners) (per capita)			4.5	6.5	8.2	1.9	1.9
Dentists (number)	5.3	9.4	3.0	1.6	6.3	3.4	1.7
Doctors (number)	2.1	6.4	-2.4	8.1	8.6	4.6	4.1
Hospitals and clinics (number)	4.8	5.8	4.6	3.8	8.6	4.2	3.9
In-patient beds (number)	6.5	9.6	10.8	0.7	9.4	1.8	0.4
Midwives (number)	-4.3	12.6	-24.4	13.6	-4.3	-1.0	-1.3
Nurses (number)	4.9	9.5	1.2	13.8	10.6	2.3	0.6

Source: Euromonitor International from national statistics

Immunisation

South Korea: Vaccination rates by disease type 1998-2004

Table: 4.1120

%

	1998	1999	2000	2001	2002	2003	2004
Vaccination rate against DTP (diphtheria, tetanus, pertussis) 1 & 2 (%)			96.8	58.9	97.0	98.0	98.0
Vaccination rate against MMR (measles, mumps, rubella) (%)	85.0	90.0	95.0	65.5	97.0	86.0	86.0
Vaccination rate against polio (%)	71.0		99.4	58.5	99.0	99.0	99.0

Source: WHO

Infectious Diseases

South Korea: Incidence of disease by type 1998-2004

Table: 4.1121

Number

	1998	1999	2000	2001	2002	2003	2004
Incidence of AIDS	35	34	32	42	41	40	39
Incidence of diphtheria	0			0			
Incidence of measles	4		32,088	23,044	41		
Incidence of polio	0	0	0	0	0		

Source: WHO

South Korea: Incidence of disease by type: growth 1998-2004

Table: 4.1122

Year on year growth: %

	1998	1999	2000	2001	2002	2003	2004
Incidence of AIDS	6.1	-2.9	-5.9	31.3	-2.4	-2.4	-2.5
Incidence of measles	100.0			-28.2	-99.8		

Source: WHO

Causes of Death

South Korea: Deaths by disease 1998-2004

Table: 4.1123

Number per 100,000 inhabitants

	1998	1999	2000	2001	2002	2003	2004
Death by diseases of the circulatory system	196.7	190.2	183.7	177.2	170.7	173.3	169.6
Death by malignant neoplasms (cancers)	171.9	169.5	167.1	164.7	162.3	161.1	159.6
Death by diseases of the respiratory system	41.7	40.3	38.9	37.5	36.1	36.7	36.1
Deaths from heart disease	16.2	18.5	21.5	24.3	27.4	30.7	34.5
Deaths from lung cancer	20.5	22.1	24.4	26.4	28.6	30.9	33.5
Deaths from chronic liver disease and cirrhosis	24.1	22.0	21.3	19.2	17.2	14.9	13.1
Death by diseases of the digestive system	12.9	12.3	11.9	13.2	13.1	11.5	11.3
Deaths from ulcers of the stomach and duodenum	1.5	1.3	1.5	1.5	1.4	1.4	1.4

Source: WHO/Euromonitor International
Notes: Data is ranked in descending order by year 2004

South Korea: Deaths by disease: growth 1998-2004

Table: 4.1124

% year on year growth

	1998	1999	2000	2001	2002	2003	2004
Deaths from heart disease	18.5	14.4	16.2	13.0	12.8	12.0	12.5
Deaths from lung cancer	-0.6	8.0	10.5	8.1	8.3	8.0	8.4
Death by malignant neoplasms (cancers)	-0.2	-1.4	-1.4	-1.4	-1.5	-0.7	-0.9
Death by diseases of the respiratory system	-1.9	-3.4	-3.5	-3.6	-3.7	1.7	-1.6
Death by diseases of the digestive system	-3.7	-4.7	-3.3	10.9	-0.8	-12.2	-1.9
Death by diseases of the circulatory system	-5.0	-3.3	-3.4	-3.5	-3.7	1.5	-2.1
Deaths from ulcers of the stomach and duodenum	1.3	-9.3	12.3	-0.1	-6.7	0.0	-2.1
Deaths from chronic liver disease and cirrhosis	-1.7	-8.7	-3.5	-9.7	-10.4	-13.4	-11.9

Source: WHO/Euromonitor International
Notes: Data is ranked in descending order by year 2004

South Korea: Other selected causes of death: 1998-2004

Table: 4.1125

Number per 100,000 inhabitants

	1998	1999	2000	2001	2002	2003	2004
Death by injury and poisoning	76.4	73.7	71.0	68.3	65.6	66.8	65.9
Death by motor traffic accidents	34.1	33.0	32.6	32.9	33.2	32.2	31.9
Death by suicide and self-inflicted injury	14.5	14.9	15.3	15.7	16.1	15.4	15.6

Source: Euromonitor International from national statistics
Notes: Data is ranked in descending order by year 2004

South Korea: Other selected causes of death: growth 1998-2004

Table: 4.1126

% year on year growth

	1998	1999	2000	2001	2002	2003	2004
Death by suicide and self-inflicted injury	2.1	2.8	2.7	2.6	2.5	-4.3	1.1
Death by motor traffic accidents	-7.1	-3.2	-1.2	0.9	0.9	-3.0	-1.0
Death by injury and poisoning	-4.0	-3.5	-3.7	-3.8	-4.0	1.8	-1.3

Source: Euromonitor International from national statistics
Notes: Data is ranked in descending order by year 2004

Smoking

South Korea: Smoking prevalence in population aged 15+ 1998-2004

Table: 4.1127

% of population aged 15+

	1998	1999	2000	2001	2002	2003	2004
Smoking prevalence in population aged 15+ (% of population aged 15+)	35.2	35.7	35.3	35.4	35.1	34.9	34.7
Smoking prevalence in male population aged 15+ (% of male population)	64.1	65.1	64.5	64.9	64.4	64.1	64.0
Smoking prevalence in female population aged 15+ (% of female population)	6.9	6.9	6.7	6.5	6.5	6.2	5.9

Source: WHO/OECD/Euromonitor International

Nutrition and Obesity

South Korea: Nutrition and obesity 1998-2004

Table: 4.1128

As stated

	1998	1999	2000	2001	2002	2003	2004
Average supply of calories per day (calories per capita)	2,935.7	3,056.7	3,063.1	3,054.5	3,058.0	3,060.5	3,060.2
Average supply of fat per day (grams per capita)	71.3	72.3	74.9	75.2	77.1	78.9	80.5
Average supply of protein per day (grams per capita)	80.4	88.3	86.4	88.7	89.6	90.2	91.1
Obese population (BMI 30kg/sq m or more) (% of population aged 15+)	2.2	2.5	2.4	2.5	2.5	2.5	2.5

Source: WHO/OECD/Euromonitor International

Over-the-Counter Healthcare

South Korea: Trends in OTC healthcare retail sales 1998-2004

Table: 4.1129

As stated

	1998	1999	2000	2001	2002	2003	2004
OTC Healthcare (Won billion)	2,022.6	2,188.3	2,424.2	2,395.6	2,661.6	2,352.4	2,331.3
OTC Healthcare: real growth in national currency: 1998 = 100	100.0	107.3	116.3	110.4	119.4	101.9	97.3
OTC Healthcare: year on year (% real growth)	-12.1	7.3	8.3	-5.1	8.2	-14.6	-4.5
OTC Healthcare ('000 Won per capita)	44.5	47.9	52.7	51.8	57.2	50.2	49.5

Source: Euromonitor International from industry sources/national statistics

South Korea: OTC healthcare retail sales by sector 1998-2004

Table: 4.1130

% of OTC retail value sales

	1998	1999	2000	2001	2002	2003	2004
Analgesics	7.3	7.2	7.2	7.8	7.3	7.4	7.4
Cough, cold and allergy (hay fever) remedies	9.9	9.5	8.5	8.0	7.3	6.9	5.8
Digestive remedies	15.5	14.8	13.0	9.9	8.9	9.0	7.8
Medicated skin care	8.3	8.1	7.2	6.0	5.4	5.2	5.2
Vitamins and dietary supplements	56.7	58.2	62.1	66.9	69.4	70.0	71.8

Source: Euromonitor International from industry sources/national statistics
Notes: Only selected sectors are shown, so values are not expected to sum to 100

Health and Wellness

South Korea: Retail sales of packaged foods by health and wellness category 2002-2004

Table: 4.1131

Won billion

	2002	2003	2004
Packaged food: Total	18,945.5	19,755.1	20,399.6
Better for you	261.2	276.4	311.7
For food intolerance	0.2	0.3	0.7
Fortified/functional	1,913.2	2,016.4	2,018.1
Organic	57.8	97.5	135.2

Source: Euromonitor International from industry sources/national statistics

South Korea: Per capita sales of packaged foods by health and wellness category 2002-2004

Table: 4.1132

'000 Won per capita

	2002	2003	2004
Better for you	5.4	5.7	6.3
For food intolerance	0.0	0.0	0.0
Fortified/functional	39.7	41.4	40.9
Organic	1.2	2.0	2.7

Source: Euromonitor International from industry sources/national statistics

South Korea: Retail sales of packaged food by health and wellness category: % share of total packaged food market 2002-2004

Table: 4.1133

% value

	2002	2003	2004
Better for you	1.4	1.4	1.5
For food intolerance	0.0	0.0	0.0
Fortified/functional	10.1	10.2	9.9
Organic	0.3	0.5	0.7

Source: Euromonitor International from industry sources/national statistics

South Korea: Retail sales of packaged food by health and wellness category: real growth index 2002-2004

Table: 4.1134

2002 =100

	2002	2003	2004
Better for you	100.00	102.43	112.16
For food intolerance	100.00	142.27	341.77
Fortified/functional	100.00	102.03	99.14
Organic	100.00	163.20	219.81

Source: Euromonitor International from industry sources/national statistics

South Korea: Retail sales of better-for-you packaged foods by sector 2002-2004

Table: 4.1135

% of total packaged food / as stated

	2002	2003	2004	% real change in value 2002-2004
Combination	0.02	0.03	0.11	434.46
Reduced carb	0.04	0.04	0.04	5.29
Reduced fat	1.22	1.22	1.25	3.86
Reduced salt	0.01	0.01	0.01	8.63

Source: Euromonitor International from industry sources/national statistics

South Korea: Retail sales of packaged foods for food intolerances by sector 2002-2004

Table: 4.1136

% of total packaged food / as stated

	2002	2003	2004	% real change in value 2002-2004
Lactose-free	0.00	0.00	0.00	241.77

Source: Euromonitor International from industry sources/national statistics

South Korea: Retail sales of naturally healthy packaged foods by sector 2002-2004

Table: 4.1137

% of total packaged food / as stated

	2002	2003	2004	% real change in value 2002-2004
High fibre	0.21	0.21	0.32	51.70
Other naturally healthy food	0.61	0.77	0.82	36.40
Soy-based dairy alternatives	1.14	1.32	1.29	13.91

Source: Euromonitor International from industry sources/national statistics

■ **Spain**

Socio-economic Parameters

Spain: Socio-economic parameters 1998-2004

Table: 4.1138

As stated

	1998	1999	2000	2001	2002	2003	2004
Population: national estimates at January 1st ('000)	39,387.5	39,519.2	39,733.0	40,121.7	40,409.3	40,592.7	40,748.4
% aged 0-14 yrs	15.4	15.1	14.9	14.7	14.6	14.6	14.6
% aged 15-64 yrs	68.4	68.4	68.4	68.4	68.3	68.4	68.4
% aged 65+ yrs	16.2	16.5	16.8	16.9	17.1	17.0	17.0
% Male	48.9	48.9	48.9	48.9	48.9	49.0	49.0
% Female	51.1	51.1	51.1	51.1	51.1	51.0	51.0
% Urban	77.2	77.4	77.5	77.7	77.9	78.2	78.4
Occupants per household at January 1st (Number)	2.9	2.9	2.9	2.8	2.8	2.7	2.7
Households ('000)	13,383.2	13,635.1	13,930.2	14,270.7	14,562.9	14,815.6	15,037.6
Annual rates of inflation (% growth)	1.8	2.3	3.4	3.6	3.1	3.0	3.0
GDP (EUR million)	527,956.7	565,419.0	609,732.8	653,927.0	698,589.0	744,754.0	798,672.0
GDP (US$ million)	591,839.4	602,389.4	561,758.6	585,164.3	657,464.6	840,547.9	991,689.5
GDP (US$ per capita)	15,026.1	15,243.0	14,138.3	14,584.7	16,270.1	20,706.9	24,336.9

Source: Euromonitor International from International Monetary Fund (IMF), International Financial Statistics and World Economic Outlook/UN/national statistics

Life Expectancy

Spain: Life expectancy 1998-2004

Table: 4.1139

As stated

	1998	1999	2000	2001	2002	2003	2004	% change 1998-2004
Life expectancy at birth: total population (years)	78.6	78.7	78.8	78.9	79.5	79.8	80.2	1.97
Life expectancy at birth: total population: year on year growth	0.2	0.2	0.1	0.1	0.8	0.4	0.4	
Healthy life expectancy at birth (years)	73.0			70.7	70.9			
Healthy life expectancy at birth: year on year growth					0.2			

Source: Euromonitor International from World Bank

Health Expenditure

Spain: Public health expenditure 1998-2004

Table: 4.1140

As stated

	1998	1999	2000	2001	2002	2003	2004
Public expenditure on pharmaceuticals and other medical non-durables (EUR million)	5,999.0	6,600.0	7,110.0	7,680.0	8,412.0	9,162.0	10,254.3
Private insurance expenditure (% of total expenditure on health)	3.7	3.8	3.9	4.0	4.1	4.2	4.3
Share of total health expenditure in GDP (% of total GDP)	7.5	7.5	7.5	7.5	7.7	7.5	7.9
Health expenditure (US$ per capita)	1,112.0	1,139.0	1,028.0	1,063.0	1,196.0	1,215.0	1,246.0

Source: Euromonitor International from OECD/national statistics

Spain: Private health expenditure 1998-2004

Table: 4.1141

As stated

	1998	1999	2000	2001	2002	2003	2004
Consumer expenditure on health goods and medical services (EUR million)	10,762.0	11,683.0	12,601.0	13,696.0	14,651.0	15,447.0	16,250.6
Consumer expenditure on health goods and medical services: real growth in national currency: 1990 = 100	157.6	167.3	174.4	183.0	189.9	194.4	198.5
Consumer expenditure on health goods and medical services as a percentage of total consumer expenditure	3.2	3.3	3.3	3.4	3.4	3.4	3.4

Source: National statistical offices/OECD/Eurostat/Euromonitor International

Spain: Consumer expenditure on health goods and medical services by sector 1998-2004

Table: 4.1142

% of total consumer expenditure on health goods and medical services

	1998	1999	2000	2001	2002	2003	2004
Pharmaceuticals, medical appliances/equipment	32.1	32.1	31.4	31.1	31.1	31.1	31.6
Outpatient services	53.8	53.7	54.2	54.4	54.6	54.7	54.1
Hospital services	14.1	14.3	14.4	14.4	14.3	14.3	14.3
Total	100.0	100.0	100.0	100.0	100.0	100.0	100.0

Source: National statistical offices/OECD/Eurostat/Euromonitor International

Healthcare Infrastructure and Services

Spain: Healthcare infrastructure and services by sector 1998-2004

Table: 4.1143

As stated

	1998	1999	2000	2001	2002	2003	2004
Active pharmacists (number)	28,100	27,100	32,600	41,000	37,400	37,186	37,013
Dentists (number)	16,133	16,891	17,538	18,507	19,292	20,008	20,536
Doctors (number)	111,000	117,200	127,100	124,900	120,200	118,660	118,178
Hospital admissions (number)	4,592,343	4,721,698	4,824,961	4,928,224	5,031,488	5,124,482	5,279,919
In-patient beds ('000)	128	139	147	151	155	156	157
In-patient surgical procedures (number)	2,087,521						
Midwives (number)	6,148	6,102	6,144	6,164	6,236	6,342	6,414
Nurses (number)	243,100	257,600	258,000	269,500	298,800	315,285	328,634
Out-patient contacts (per capita)				9			

Source: Euromonitor International from national statistics

Spain: Healthcare infrastructure and services by sector: growth 1998-2004

Table: 4.1144

Year on year growth: % change in stated unit

	1998	1999	2000	2001	2002	2003	2004
Active pharmacists (number)	10.2	-3.6	20.3	25.8	-8.8	-0.6	-0.5
Dentists (number)	5.5	4.7	3.8	5.5	4.2	3.7	2.6
Doctors (number)	-2.1	5.6	8.4	-1.7	-3.8	-1.3	-0.4
Hospital admissions (number)	1.5	2.8	2.2	2.1	2.1	1.8	3.0
In-patient beds (number)	9.5	8.7	6.0	2.6	2.4	0.7	0.6
In-patient surgical procedures (number)	-1.3						
Midwives (number)	0.9	-0.7	0.7	0.3	1.2	1.7	1.1
Nurses (number)	-2.1	6.0	0.2	4.5	10.9	5.5	4.2

Source: Euromonitor International from national statistics

Immunisation

Spain: Vaccination rates by disease type 1998-2004

Table: 4.1145

%

	1998	1999	2000	2001	2002	2003	2004
Vaccination rate against MMR (measles, mumps, rubella) (%)	93.0	93.0	94.0	95.0	96.6	97.0	97.0
Vaccination rate against polio (%)			95.0	96.0	96.4	97.0	98.0

Source: WHO

Infectious Diseases

Spain: Incidence of disease by type 1998-2004

Table: 4.1146

Number

	1998	1999	2000	2001	2002	2003	2004
Incidence of AIDS	4,222	3,427	2,847	2,942	2,356	1,243	1,189
Incidence of diphtheria	0	0	0		0		
Incidence of measles	446	246	152		67		
Incidence of polio	0	0	0	0	0		

Source: WHO

Spain: Incidence of disease by type: growth 1998-2004

Table: 4.1147

Year on year growth: %

	1998	1999	2000	2001	2002	2003	2004
Incidence of AIDS	-30.3	-18.8	-16.9	3.3	-19.9	-47.2	-4.3
Incidence of measles	-75.8	-44.8	-38.2				

Source: WHO

Causes of Death

Spain: Deaths by disease 1998-2004

Table: 4.1148

Number per 100,000 inhabitants

	1998	1999	2000	2001	2002	2003	2004
Death by diseases of the circulatory system	215.2	203.7	198.8	189.5	181.3	197.3	197.0
Death by malignant neoplasms (cancers)	165.7	164.4	164.1	163.7	163.2	162.4	161.8
Death by diseases of the respiratory system	60.8	69.3	70.4	76.4	77.2	79.5	83.3
Deaths from heart disease	84.9	80.4	73.7	67.3	61.2	55.4	50.4
Deaths from lung cancer	43.7	44.5	45.0	45.3	45.3	45.0	44.9
Death by diseases of the digestive system	32.9	32.0	30.3	29.7	29.0	28.0	27.2
Deaths from chronic liver disease and cirrhosis	15.9	15.1	14.4	13.7	13.0	12.3	11.8
Deaths from ulcers of the stomach and duodenum	2.5	2.3	2.2	2.1	2.0	1.8	1.7

Source: WHO/Euromonitor International
Notes: Data is ranked in descending order by year 2004

Spain: Deaths by disease: growth 1998-2004

Table: 4.1149

% year on year growth

	1998	1999	2000	2001	2002	2003	2004
Death by diseases of the respiratory system	5.9	14.0	1.6	8.5	1.0	3.0	4.8
Death by diseases of the circulatory system	-0.2	-5.3	-2.4	-4.7	-4.3	8.8	-0.2
Deaths from lung cancer	3.5	1.8	1.1	0.7	0.0	-0.7	-0.2
Death by malignant neoplasms (cancers)	-0.2	-0.8	-0.2	-0.2	-0.3	-0.5	-0.3
Death by diseases of the digestive system	-0.3	-2.7	-5.3	-2.0	-2.4	-3.4	-2.9
Deaths from chronic liver disease and cirrhosis	-2.9	-4.8	-4.6	-4.9	-5.1	-5.4	-4.5
Deaths from ulcers of the stomach and duodenum	-1.8	-7.4	-4.3	-4.5	-4.8	-10.0	-6.3
Deaths from heart disease	-14.8	-5.3	-8.3	-8.7	-9.1	-9.5	-9.1

Source: WHO/Euromonitor International
Notes: Data is ranked in descending order by year 2004

Spain: Other selected causes of death: 1998-2004

Table: 4.1150

Number per 100,000 inhabitants

	1998	1999	2000	2001	2002	2003	2004
Death by injury and poisoning	36.6	35.1	35.3	34.4	33.7	35.0	34.9
Death by motor traffic accidents	14.8	14.7	15.3	15.4	15.7	15.2	15.2
Death by suicide and self-inflicted injury	6.9	6.7	6.6	6.4	6.2	6.5	6.4

Source: Euromonitor International from national statistics
Notes: Data is ranked in descending order by year 2004

Spain: Other selected causes of death: growth 1998-2004

Table: 4.1151

% year on year growth

	1998	1999	2000	2001	2002	2003	2004
Death by motor traffic accidents	6.5	-0.7	4.1	0.7	1.9	-3.2	0.0
Death by injury and poisoning	1.4	-4.1	0.6	-2.5	-2.0	3.9	-0.3
Death by suicide and self-inflicted injury	-4.2	-2.9	-1.5	-3.0	-3.1	4.8	-1.0

Source: Euromonitor International from national statistics
Notes: Data is ranked in descending order by year 2004

Smoking

Spain: Smoking prevalence in population aged 15+ 1998-2004

Table: 4.1152

% of population aged 15+

	1998	1999	2000	2001	2002	2003	2004
Smoking prevalence in population aged 15+ (% of population aged 15+)	33.4	33.7	34.2	34.4	34.4	34.6	34.5
Smoking prevalence in male population aged 15+ (% of male population)	42.1	42.1	42.1	42.1	42.1	42.0	42.0
Smoking prevalence in female population aged 15+ (% of female population)	25.6	26.4	26.8	27.2	27.4	27.7	27.9

Source: WHO/OECD/Euromonitor International

Nutrition and Obesity

Spain: Nutrition and obesity 1998-2004

Table: 4.1153

As stated

	1998	1999	2000	2001	2002	2003	2004
Availability of fruit and vegetables (kg/capita/year)	262.1	291.7	274.9	276.8	267.3	257.7	251.3
Average supply of calories per day (calories per capita)	3,297.7	3,337.8	3,369.9	3,349.2	3,370.6	3,385.7	3,396.8
Average supply of fat per day (grams per capita)	149.9	149.0	150.6	149.8	150.9	151.8	152.5
Average supply of protein per day (grams per capita)	111.0	109.9	110.7	110.9	111.7	112.4	113.0
Obese population (BMI 30kg/sq m or more) (% of population aged 15+)	11.7	11.9	12.0	12.0	12.0	12.2	12.4

Source: WHO/OECD/Euromonitor International

Over-the-Counter Healthcare

Spain: Trends in OTC healthcare retail sales 1998-2004

Table: 4.1154

As stated

	1998	1999	2000	2001	2002	2003	2004
OTC Healthcare (EUR million)	919.7	972.9	1,031.0	1,066.8	1,116.9	1,174.3	1,205.2
OTC Healthcare: real growth in national currency: 1998 = 100	100.0	103.4	105.9	105.8	107.5	109.7	109.5
OTC Healthcare: year on year (% real growth)	2.3	3.4	2.4	-0.1	1.6	2.0	-0.2

Source: Euromonitor International from industry sources/national statistics

Spain: OTC healthcare retail sales by sector 1998-2004

Table: 4.1155

% of OTC retail value sales

	1998	1999	2000	2001	2002	2003	2004
Analgesics	18.7	18.4	18.4	18.9	19.2	19.0	19.0
Cough, cold and allergy (hay fever) remedies	28.3	29.1	29.9	28.6	28.3	28.6	27.8
Digestive remedies	17.7	17.1	16.5	16.4	16.0	15.6	15.3
Medicated skin care	10.7	10.6	10.5	11.0	11.1	11.2	11.5
Vitamins and dietary supplements	16.9	16.7	16.4	16.7	16.8	17.0	17.4

Source: Euromonitor International from industry sources/national statistics
Notes: Only selected sectors are shown, so values are not expected to sum to 100

Health and Wellness

Spain: Retail sales of packaged foods by health and wellness category 2002-2004

Table: 4.1156

EUR million

	2002	2003	2004
Packaged food: Total	22,124.0	23,346.5	24,496.4
Better for you	1,313.9	1,389.1	1,462.1
For food intolerance	40.8	43.4	48.9
Fortified/functional	1,034.7	1,200.9	1,340.7
Organic	41.2	46.7	52.6

Source: Euromonitor International from industry sources/national statistics

Spain: Per capita sales of packaged foods by health and wellness category 2002-2004

Table: 4.1157

EUR per capita

	2002	2003	2004
Better for you	33.2	35.1	36.9
For food intolerance	1.0	1.1	1.2
Fortified/functional	26.2	30.4	33.8
Organic	1.0	1.2	1.3

Source: Euromonitor International from industry sources/national statistics

Spain: Retail sales of packaged food by health and wellness category: % share of total packaged food market 2002-2004

Table: 4.1158

% value

	2002	2003	2004
Better for you	5.9	5.9	6.0
For food intolerance	0.2	0.2	0.2
Fortified/functional	4.7	5.1	5.5
Organic	0.2	0.2	0.2

Source: Euromonitor International from industry sources/national statistics

Spain: Retail sales of packaged food by health and wellness category: real growth index 2002-2004

Table: 4.1159

2002 =100

	2002	2003	2004
Better for you	100.00	102.54	105.09
For food intolerance	100.00	103.21	113.34
Fortified/functional	100.00	112.58	122.38
Organic	100.00	109.72	120.51

Source: Euromonitor International from industry sources/national statistics

Spain: Retail sales of better-for-you packaged foods by sector 2002-2004

Table: 4.1160

% of total packaged food / as stated

	2002	2003	2004	% real change in value 2002-2004
Combination	0.26	0.29	0.33	30.49
Reduced carb	0.00	0.00	0.00	6.56
Reduced fat	4.33	4.27	4.22	1.94
Reduced salt	0.17	0.19	0.19	16.01

Source: Euromonitor International from industry sources/national statistics

Spain: Retail sales of packaged foods for food intolerances by sector 2002-2004

Table: 4.1161

% of total packaged food / as stated

	2002	2003	2004	% real change in value 2002-2004
Diabetic	0.10	0.10	0.11	12.37
Gluten-free	0.07	0.07	0.08	13.46
Lactose-free	0.01	0.01	0.01	28.66

Source: Euromonitor International from industry sources/national statistics

Spain: Retail sales of naturally healthy packaged foods by sector 2002-2004

Table: 4.1162

% of total packaged food / as stated

	2002	2003	2004	% real change in value 2002-2004
High fibre	3.05	3.01	2.99	2.68
Other naturally healthy food	4.90	4.81	4.88	4.23
Soy-based dairy alternatives	0.09	0.12	0.17	109.78

Source: Euromonitor International from industry sources/national statistics

■ **Sweden**

Socio-economic Parameters

Sweden: Socio-economic parameters 1998-2004

Table: 4.1163

As stated

	1998	1999	2000	2001	2002	2003	2004
Population: national estimates at January 1st ('000)	8,847.6	8,854.3	8,861.4	8,882.8	8,909.1	8,940.0	8,971.0
% aged 0-14 yrs	18.7	18.6	18.5	18.4	18.2	18.0	17.7
% aged 15-64 yrs	63.9	64.0	64.2	64.4	64.6	64.8	65.1
% aged 65 + yrs	17.4	17.4	17.3	17.2	17.2	17.2	17.2
% Male	49.4	49.4	49.4	49.5	49.5	49.5	49.5
% Female	50.6	50.6	50.6	50.5	50.5	50.5	50.5
% Urban	83.2	83.3	83.3	83.4	83.5	83.6	83.7
Occupants per household at January 1st (Number)	2.2	2.2	2.2	2.2	2.1	2.1	2.1
Households ('000)	4,076.7	4,092.9	4,104.5	4,127.5	4,152.9	4,175.3	4,196.8
Annual rates of inflation (% growth)	-0.3	0.5	0.9	2.4	2.2	1.9	0.4
GDP (SEK million)	1,971,870.0	2,076,520.0	2,194,970.0	2,269,150.0	2,352,940.0	2,438,450.0	2,542,850.0
GDP (US$ million)	248,038.0	251,320.7	239,567.0	219,685.2	241,646.4	301,553.2	346,018.2
GDP (US$ per capita)	28,034.4	28,384.0	27,034.8	24,731.5	27,123.5	33,730.8	38,570.7

Source: Euromonitor International from International Monetary Fund (IMF), International Financial Statistics and World Economic Outlook/UN/national statistics

Life Expectancy

Sweden: Life expectancy 1998-2004

Table: 4.1164

As stated

	1998	1999	2000	2001	2002	2003	2004	% change 1998-2004
Life expectancy at birth: total population (years)	79.6	79.7	79.8	80.0	80.4	80.5	80.7	1.42
Life expectancy at birth: total population: year on year growth	0.2	0.2	0.1	0.3	0.5	0.1	0.2	
Healthy life expectancy at birth (years)	73.0			71.6	71.8			
Healthy life expectancy at birth: year on year growth					0.3			

Source: Euromonitor International from World Bank

Sanitation

Sweden: Improved sanitary facilities and water source 2000

Table: 4.1165

As stated

	2000
Population with access to improved sanitary facilities (% of population)	100.0
Population with access to improved water source (% of population)	100.0
Population with improved access to sanitation facilities, rural (% of rural population with access)	100.0
Population with improved access to sanitation facilities, urban (% of urban population with access)	100.0

Source: National statistics/World Bank

Health Expenditure

Sweden: Public health expenditure 1998-2004

Table: 4.1166

As stated

	1998	1999	2000	2001	2002	2003	2004
Public expenditure on pharmaceuticals and other medical non-durables (SEK million)	15,421.0	17,123.0	17,915.0	18,193.0	19,617.0	20,484.0	21,601.7
Share of total health expenditure in GDP (% of total GDP)	8.3	8.4	8.4	8.7	8.5	8.4	8.1
Health expenditure (US$ per capita)	2,335.0	2,396.0	2,280.0	2,172.0	2,494.0	2,527.0	2,609.0

Source: Euromonitor International from OECD/national statistics

Sweden: Private health expenditure 1998-2004

Table: 4.1167

As stated

	1998	1999	2000	2001	2002	2003	2004
Consumer expenditure on health goods and medical services (SEK million)	22,347.0	23,470.0	25,518.0	27,872.0	29,237.0	30,358.0	30,972.0
Consumer expenditure on health goods and medical services: real growth in national currency: 1990 = 100	128.2	134.1	144.5	154.1	158.2	161.2	163.8
Consumer expenditure on health goods and medical services as a percentage of total consumer expenditure	2.4	2.4	2.5	2.6	2.6	2.7	2.6

Source: National statistical offices/OECD/Eurostat/Euromonitor International

Sweden: Consumer expenditure on health goods and medical services by sector 1998-2004

Table: 4.1168

% of total consumer expenditure on health goods and medical services

	1998	1999	2000	2001	2002	2003	2004
Pharmaceuticals, medical appliances/ equipment	48.1	48.5	47.4	46.3	46.5	46.4	46.3
Outpatient services	47.7	47.6	48.9	50.2	50.2	50.3	50.4
Hospital services	4.1	4.0	3.8	3.5	3.3	3.3	3.3
Total	100.0	100.0	100.0	100.0	100.0	100.0	100.0

Source: National statistical offices/OECD/Eurostat/Euromonitor International

Healthcare Infrastructure and Services

Sweden: Healthcare infrastructure and services by sector 1998-2004

Table: 4.1169

As stated

	1998	1999	2000	2001	2002	2003	2004
Active pharmacists (number)	5,249	5,317					
Consultations with GPs (general practitioners) (per capita)	3	3	3	3	3	3	3
Dentists (number)	7,667	7,837	7,722	7,763	7,856	7,919	7,941
Doctors (number)	24,957	25,428	26,979	27,579	28,405	29,368	30,144
Hospital admissions (number)	1,464,625	1,437,623	1,407,863	1,391,850	1,386,000	1,347,189	1,345,738
In-patient beds ('000)	23	22	22	31	32	33	33
In-patient surgical procedures (number)	544,855	556,828	547,834	550,974	565,825	565,713	563,648
Nurses (number)	73,562	74,657	78,380	95,109	102,337	106,693	109,123

Source: Euromonitor International from national statistics

Sweden: Healthcare infrastructure and services by sector: growth 1998-2004

Table: 4.1170

Year on year growth: % change in stated unit

	1998	1999	2000	2001	2002	2003	2004
Active pharmacists (number)	-13.1	1.3					
Consultations with GPs (general practitioners) (per capita)	3.6	-3.4	3.6	0.0	0.7	0.7	0.7
Dentists (number)	2.0	2.2	-1.5	0.5	1.2	0.8	0.3
Doctors (number)	1.5	1.9	6.1	2.2	3.0	3.4	2.6
Hospital admissions (number)	-0.7	-1.8	-2.1	-1.1	-0.4	-2.8	-0.1
In-patient beds (number)	-4.4	-1.2	-3.4	43.2	3.8	1.2	0.6
In-patient surgical procedures (number)	14.5	2.2	-1.6	0.6	2.7	0.0	-0.4
Nurses (number)	1.3	1.5	5.0	21.3	7.6	4.3	2.3

Source: Euromonitor International from national statistics

Immunisation

Sweden: Vaccination rates by disease type 1998-2004

Table: 4.1171

%

	1998	1999	2000	2001	2002	2003	2004
Vaccination rate against MMR (measles, mumps, rubella) (%)			95.4	94.0	90.5	88.0	86.0
Vaccination rate against polio (%)			98.6	99.0	98.5	99.0	99.0

Source: WHO

Infectious Diseases

Sweden: Incidence of disease by type 1998-2004

Table: 4.1172

Number

	1998	1999	2000	2001	2002	2003	2004
Incidence of AIDS	63	74	54	21	59	26	32
Incidence of diphtheria			0	0	0		
Incidence of measles			59	5	9		
Incidence of polio	0	0	0	0	0		

Source: WHO

Sweden: Incidence of disease by type: growth 1998-2004

Table: 4.1173

Year on year growth: %

	1998	1999	2000	2001	2002	2003	2004
Incidence of AIDS	-18.2	17.5	-27.0	-61.1	181.0	-55.9	23.1
Incidence of measles				-91.5	80.0		

Source: WHO

Causes of Death

Sweden: Deaths by disease 1998-2004

Table: 4.1174

Number per 100,000 inhabitants

	1998	1999	2000	2001	2002	2003	2004
Death by diseases of the circulatory system	259.9	253.4	246.7	246.5	240.1	233.5	228.8
Deaths from heart disease	245.2	239.1	235.0	230.4	225.8	221.3	218.9
Death by malignant neoplasms (cancers)	152.3	151.3	150.8	150.0	149.3	150.6	149.0
Deaths from lung cancer	33.0	33.9	33.8	33.9	34.1	34.2	34.6
Death by diseases of the respiratory system	36.2	38.7	34.5	34.8	33.9	33.6	33.3
Death by diseases of the digestive system	18.5	18.2	17.1	16.9	15.7	15.3	14.7
Deaths from chronic liver disease and cirrhosis	6.5	6.4	7.0	7.4	7.8	8.1	8.5
Deaths from ulcers of the stomach and duodenum	5.2	5.3	5.4	5.6	5.7	5.9	6.1

Source: WHO/Euromonitor International
Notes: Data is ranked in descending order by year 2004

Sweden: Deaths by disease: growth 1998-2004

Table: 4.1175

% year on year growth

	1998	1999	2000	2001	2002	2003	2004
Deaths from chronic liver disease and cirrhosis	18.5	-2.0	10.1	5.7	5.4	3.8	5.3
Deaths from ulcers of the stomach and duodenum	4.0	2.3	2.2	3.7	1.8	3.5	2.6
Deaths from lung cancer	-1.5	2.7	-0.2	0.3	0.6	0.3	1.2
Death by diseases of the respiratory system	-8.1	6.9	-10.9	0.9	-2.6	-0.9	-1.0
Death by malignant neoplasms (cancers)	-2.0	-0.7	-0.3	-0.5	-0.5	0.9	-1.0
Deaths from heart disease	-1.3	-2.5	-1.7	-2.0	-2.0	-2.0	-1.1
Death by diseases of the circulatory system	-1.7	-2.5	-2.6	-0.1	-2.6	-2.7	-2.0
Death by diseases of the digestive system	4.5	-1.6	-6.0	-1.2	-7.1	-2.5	-4.0

Source: WHO/Euromonitor International
Notes: Data is ranked in descending order by year 2004

Sweden: Other selected causes of death: 1998-2004

Table: 4.1176

Number per 100,000 inhabitants

	1998	1999	2000	2001	2002	2003	2004
Death by injury and poisoning	36.8	35.5	35.7	35.0	34.4	35.5	35.3
Death by suicide and self-inflicted injury	11.9	12.0	11.8	11.8	11.7	11.8	11.9
Death by motor traffic accidents	5.6	5.6	5.6	5.7	5.7	5.6	5.6

Source: Euromonitor International from national statistics
Notes: Data is ranked in descending order by year 2004

Sweden: Other selected causes of death: growth 1998-2004

% year on year growth

	1998	1999	2000	2001	2002	2003	2004
Death by suicide and self-inflicted injury	0.0	0.8	-1.7	0.0	-0.8	0.9	0.6
Death by motor traffic accidents	-3.4	0.0	0.0	1.8	0.0	-1.8	-0.1
Death by injury and poisoning	0.5	-3.5	0.6	-2.0	-1.7	3.2	-0.6

Source: Euromonitor International from national statistics
Notes: Data is ranked in descending order by year 2004

Smoking

Sweden: Smoking prevalence in population aged 15+ 1998-2004

% of population aged 15+

	1998	1999	2000	2001	2002	2003	2004
Smoking prevalence in population aged 15+ (% of population aged 15+)	19.1	19.3	18.9	18.9	17.8	18.4	18.0
Smoking prevalence in male population aged 15+ (% of male population)	17.0	19.2	16.8	17.9	16.3	14.9	14.4
Smoking prevalence in female population aged 15+ (% of female population)	21.1	19.4	21.0	19.9	19.3	21.7	21.5

Source: WHO/OECD/Euromonitor International

Nutrition and Obesity

Sweden: Nutrition and obesity 1998-2004

As stated

	1998	1999	2000	2001	2002	2003	2004
Availability of fruit and vegetables (kg/capita/year)	164.3	172.2	170.5	175.8	177.1	179.3	180.9
Average supply of calories per day (calories per capita)	3,084.7	3,166.1	3,089.2	3,131.1	3,185.4	3,217.5	3,255.1
Average supply of fat per day (grams per capita)	125.5	130.0	122.3	123.6	125.6	126.0	127.4
Average supply of protein per day (grams per capita)	100.4	103.1	101.7	104.0	106.6	108.6	107.8
Obese population (BMI 30kg/sq m or more) (% of population aged 15+)	9.8	10.0	10.8	10.9	11.0	11.1	11.1

Source: WHO/OECD/Euromonitor International

Over-the-Counter Healthcare

Sweden: Trends in OTC healthcare retail sales 1998-2004

As stated

	1998	1999	2000	2001	2002	2003	2004
OTC Healthcare (SEK million)	4,564.1	4,664.9	4,823.7	4,949.9	5,226.2	5,406.6	5,623.2
OTC Healthcare: real growth in national currency: 1998 = 100	100.0	101.7	104.3	104.5	108.0	109.6	113.0
OTC Healthcare: year on year (% real growth)	3.7	1.7	2.5	0.2	3.3	1.5	3.1
OTC Healthcare (SEK per capita)	515.9	526.8	544.3	557.3	586.6	604.8	626.8

Source: Euromonitor International from industry sources/national statistics

Sweden: OTC healthcare retail sales by sector 1998-2004

Table: 4.1181

% of OTC retail value sales

	1998	1999	2000	2001	2002	2003	2004
Analgesics	13.6	13.9	14.1	14.5	14.9	15.6	16.3
Cough, cold and allergy (hay fever) remedies	29.2	28.6	28.0	27.2	27.4	27.6	27.3
Digestive remedies	6.9	6.9	7.1	6.9	6.7	6.4	6.3
Medicated skin care	7.9	8.0	8.1	8.1	7.8	7.8	7.8
Vitamins and dietary supplements	30.6	30.6	30.6	30.6	29.6	28.7	28.2

Source: Euromonitor International from industry sources/national statistics
Notes: Only selected sectors are shown, so values are not expected to sum to 100

Health and Wellness

Sweden: Retail sales of packaged foods by health and wellness category 2002-2004

Table: 4.1182

SEK million

	2002	2003	2004
Packaged food: Total	93,804.0	98,397.5	102,331.8
Better for you	10,990.2	12,216.4	13,411.6
For food intolerance	1,095.1	1,290.8	1,456.0
Fortified/functional	1,186.1	1,377.7	1,496.8
Organic	2,380.7	2,745.1	3,104.4

Source: Euromonitor International from industry sources/national statistics

Sweden: Per capita sales of packaged foods by health and wellness category 2002-2004

Table: 4.1183

SEK per capita

	2002	2003	2004
Better for you	1,238.2	1,375.3	1,508.8
For food intolerance	123.4	145.3	163.8
Fortified/functional	133.6	155.1	168.4
Organic	268.2	309.0	349.2

Source: Euromonitor International from industry sources/national statistics

Sweden: Retail sales of packaged food by health and wellness category: % share of total packaged food market 2002-2004

Table: 4.1184

% value

	2002	2003	2004
Better for you	11.7	12.4	13.1
For food intolerance	1.2	1.3	1.4
Fortified/functional	1.3	1.4	1.5
Organic	2.5	2.8	3.0

Source: Euromonitor International from industry sources/national statistics

Sweden: Retail sales of packaged food by health and wellness category: real growth index 2002-2004

Table: 4.1185

2002 =100

	2002	2003	2004
Better for you	100.00	109.51	117.87
For food intolerance	100.00	116.12	128.42
Fortified/functional	100.00	114.44	121.90
Organic	100.00	113.60	125.95

Source: Euromonitor International from industry sources/national statistics

Sweden: Retail sales of better-for-you packaged foods by sector 2002-2004

Table: 4.1186

% of total packaged food / as stated

	2002	2003	2004	% real change in value 2002-2004
Combination	0.18	0.19	0.20	17.69
Reduced carb	0.03	0.03	0.04	59.68
Reduced fat	9.72	10.45	11.13	20.64
Reduced salt	0.34	0.36	0.38	16.23

Source: Euromonitor International from industry sources/national statistics

Sweden: Retail sales of packaged foods for food intolerances by sector 2002-2004

Table: 4.1187

% of total packaged food / as stated

	2002	2003	2004	% real change in value 2002-2004
Diabetic	0.11	0.12	0.12	9.74
Gluten-free	0.48	0.51	0.54	17.83
Lactose-free	0.57	0.69	0.77	40.95

Source: Euromonitor International from industry sources/national statistics

Sweden: Retail sales of naturally healthy packaged foods by sector 2002-2004

Table: 4.1188

% of total packaged food / as stated

	2002	2003	2004	% real change in value 2002-2004
High fibre	1.87	1.98	2.17	21.77
Other naturally healthy food	2.12	2.10	2.06	2.72
Soy-based dairy alternatives	0.11	0.13	0.16	53.82

Source: Euromonitor International from industry sources/national statistics

■ Switzerland

Socio-economic Parameters

Switzerland: Socio-economic parameters 1998-2004

Table: 4.1189

As stated

	1998	1999	2000	2001	2002	2003	2004
Population: national estimates at January 1st ('000)	7,096.5	7,123.5	7,164.4	7,204.1	7,261.2	7,291.7	7,316.2
% aged 0-14 yrs	17.6	17.5	17.4	17.3	17.1	17.0	16.7
% aged 15-64 yrs	67.4	67.3	67.3	67.3	67.4	67.6	67.8
% aged 65+ yrs	15.0	15.2	15.3	15.4	15.5	15.5	15.5
% Male	48.8	48.8	48.9	48.9	48.9	48.9	48.9
% Female	51.2	51.2	51.1	51.1	51.1	51.1	51.1
% Urban	66.9	67.0	67.7	67.8	67.9	68.9	69.3
Occupants per household at January 1st (Number)	2.3	2.3	2.3	2.2	2.2	2.2	2.2
Households ('000)	3,126.6	3,152.0	3,181.6	3,208.0	3,245.7	3,270.4	3,289.3
Annual rates of inflation (% growth)	0.0	0.8	1.5	1.0	0.6	0.6	0.8
GDP (CHF million)	390,191.0	397,894.0	415,529.0	422,485.0	431,064.0	433,366.0	444,642.0
GDP (US$ million)	269,132.5	264,883.0	246,044.0	250,345.2	276,569.5	321,810.4	357,573.0
GDP (US$ per capita)	37,924.9	37,184.2	34,342.4	34,750.6	38,088.6	44,134.0	48,874.2

Source: Euromonitor International from International Monetary Fund (IMF), International Financial Statistics and World Economic Outlook/UN/national statistics

Life Expectancy

Switzerland: Life expectancy 1998-2004

Table: 4.1190

As stated

	1998	1999	2000	2001	2002	2003	2004	% change 1998-2004
Life expectancy at birth: total population (years)	79.8	79.9	79.9	80.2	80.6	80.7	81.0	1.47
Life expectancy at birth: total population: year on year growth	0.1	0.1	0.0	0.4	0.5	0.1	0.3	
Healthy life expectancy at birth (years)	72.0			72.5	72.8			
Healthy life expectancy at birth: year on year growth					0.3			

Source: Euromonitor International from World Bank

Sanitation

Switzerland: Improved sanitary facilities and water source 2000

Table: 4.1191

As stated

	2000
Population with access to improved sanitary facilities (% of population)	100.0
Population with access to improved water source (% of population)	100.0
Population with improved access to sanitation facilities, rural (% of rural population with access)	100.0
Population with improved access to sanitation facilities, urban (% of urban population with access)	100.0

Source: National statistics/World Bank

Health Expenditure

Switzerland: Public health expenditure 1998-2004

Table: 4.1192

As stated

	1998	1999	2000	2001	2002	2003	2004
Public expenditure on pharmaceuticals and other medical non-durables (CHF million)	2,352.0	2,523.0	2,821.0	3,064.0	3,301.0	3,586.0	3,921.9
Private insurance expenditure (% of total expenditure on health)	11.4	10.4	10.5	10.2	9.6	9.2	8.8
Share of total health expenditure in GDP (% of total GDP)	10.6	10.7	10.7	11.0	10.8	10.7	10.5
Health expenditure (US$ per capita)	3,908.0	3,881.0	3,572.0	3,774.0	4,217.0	4,329.0	4,497.0

Source: Euromonitor International from OECD/national statistics

Switzerland: Private health expenditure 1998-2004

Table: 4.1193

As stated

	1998	1999	2000	2001	2002	2003	2004
Consumer expenditure on health goods and medical services (CHF million)	31,040.6	32,052.2	33,500.2	35,068.1	36,379.0	36,545.6	37,165.2
Consumer expenditure on health goods and medical services: real growth in national currency: 1990 = 100	135.9	139.2	143.3	148.5	153.1	152.8	154.2
Consumer expenditure on health goods and medical services as a percentage of total consumer expenditure	13.6	13.6	13.8	14.1	14.4	14.3	14.2

Source: National statistical offices/OECD/Eurostat/Euromonitor International

Switzerland: Consumer expenditure on health goods and medical services by sector 1998-2004

Table: 4.1194

% of total consumer expenditure on health goods and medical services

	1998	1999	2000	2001	2002	2003	2004
Pharmaceuticals, medical appliances/ equipment	16.4	16.6	16.5	16.3	16.5	16.5	16.5
Outpatient services	68.7	68.2	68.1	68.1	67.9	67.9	67.9
Hospital services	14.8	15.2	15.4	15.6	15.6	15.6	15.7
Total	100.0	100.0	100.0	100.0	100.0	100.0	100.0

Source: National statistical offices/OECD/Eurostat/Euromonitor International

Healthcare Infrastructure and Services

Switzerland: Healthcare infrastructure and services by sector 1998-2004

Table: 4.1195

As stated

	1998	1999	2000	2001	2002	2003	2004
Active pharmacists (number)	1,651	1,640	1,658	1,621	1,618	1,618	1,614
Consultations with GPs (general practitioners) (per capita)					3		
Dentists (number)	3,470	3,449	3,468	3,432	3,501	3,514	3,533
Doctors (number)	23,679	24,026	25,216	25,395	25,921	26,569	27,269
Hospital admissions (number)	1,207,203						
In-patient beds ('000)	31	32	30	29	27	26	25
Nurses (number)			77,120	77,232	77		

Source: Euromonitor International from national statistics

Switzerland: Healthcare infrastructure and services by sector: growth 1998-2004

Table: 4.1196

Year on year growth: % change in stated unit

	1998	1999	2000	2001	2002	2003	2004
Active pharmacists (number)	0.0	-0.7	1.1	-2.2	-0.2	0.0	-0.2
Dentists (number)	-2.2	-0.6	0.6	-1.0	2.0	0.4	0.5
Doctors (number)	2.3	1.5	5.0	0.7	2.1	2.5	2.6
Hospital admissions (number)	-2.5						
In-patient beds (number)	-9.3	1.0	-6.8	-3.4	-4.5	-3.4	-4.4
Nurses (number)				0.1	-99.9		

Source: Euromonitor International from national statistics

Immunisation

Switzerland: Vaccination rates by disease type 1998-2004

Table: 4.1197

%

	1998	1999	2000	2001	2002	2003	2004
Vaccination rate against DTP (diphtheria, tetanus, pertussis) 1 & 2 (%)				98.0	98.0	98.0	98.0
Vaccination rate against MMR (measles, mumps, rubella) (%)	81.0	81.0	80.0	81.0	79.0	79.0	79.0
Vaccination rate against polio (%)				92.0	94.0	96.0	98.0

Source: WHO

Infectious Diseases

Switzerland: Incidence of disease by type 1998-2004

Table: 4.1198

Number

	1998	1999	2000	2001	2002	2003	2004
Incidence of AIDS	423	262	257	175	199	282	301
Incidence of diphtheria	0	0	0	0	0		
Incidence of measles	2,000	800		700			
Incidence of polio	0	0	0	0	0		

Source: WHO

Switzerland: Incidence of disease by type: growth 1998-2004

Table: 4.1199

Year on year growth: %

	1998	1999	2000	2001	2002	2003	2004
Incidence of AIDS	-25.1	-38.1	-1.9	-31.9	13.7	41.7	6.7
Incidence of measles	-68.8	-60.0					

Source: WHO

Causes of Death

Switzerland: Deaths by disease 1998-2004

Table: 4.1200

Number per 100,000 inhabitants

	1998	1999	2000	2001	2002	2003	2004
Deaths from heart disease	244.2	241.6	256.4	260.4	284.2	271.2	277.4
Death by diseases of the circulatory system	209.5	204.5	199.5	194.5	189.6	197.6	195.6
Death by malignant neoplasms (cancers)	153.7	150.6	148.7	147.1	146.0	143.5	142.7
Death by diseases of the respiratory system	37.9	38.6	41.1	42.4	43.9	40.4	40.0
Death by diseases of the digestive system	20.6	20.9	22.0	21.9	22.9	21.5	21.3
Deaths from lung cancer	37.5	36.8	32.7	27.0	23.6	19.4	16.4
Deaths from chronic liver disease and cirrhosis	10.3	10.5	8.7	9.1	9.2	8.9	9.0
Deaths from ulcers of the stomach and duodenum	2.7	2.7	1.8	2.1	1.9	2.0	2.1

Source: WHO/Euromonitor International
Notes: Data is ranked in descending order by year 2004

Switzerland: Deaths by disease: growth 1998-2004

Table: 4.1201

% year on year growth

	1998	1999	2000	2001	2002	2003	2004
Deaths from ulcers of the stomach and duodenum	-18.2	3.2	-34.5	16.7	-9.5	5.3	3.2
Deaths from heart disease	55.6	-1.1	6.1	1.6	9.1	-4.6	2.3
Deaths from chronic liver disease and cirrhosis	-4.6	1.9	-17.2	4.6	1.1	-3.3	1.3
Death by malignant neoplasms (cancers)	-1.4	-2.0	-1.3	-1.1	-0.7	-1.7	-0.6
Death by diseases of the circulatory system	-3.9	-2.4	-2.4	-2.5	-2.5	4.2	-1.0
Death by diseases of the respiratory system	0.3	1.8	6.5	3.2	3.5	-8.0	-1.1
Death by diseases of the digestive system	-3.7	1.5	5.3	-0.5	4.6	-6.1	-1.2
Deaths from lung cancer	3.2	-2.1	-11.1	-17.4	-12.6	-17.8	-15.7

Source: WHO/Euromonitor International
Notes: Data is ranked in descending order by year 2004

Switzerland: Other selected causes of death: 1998-2004

Table: 4.1202

Number per 100,000 inhabitants

	1998	1999	2000	2001	2002	2003	2004
Death by injury and poisoning	40.0	38.7	37.8	36.7	35.6	37.4	37.2
Death by suicide and self-inflicted injury	16.5	15.4	14.9	14.0	13.2	14.7	14.6

Source: Euromonitor International from national statistics
Notes: Data is ranked in descending order by year 2004

Switzerland: Other selected causes of death: growth 1998-2004

Table: 4.1203

% year on year growth

	1998	1999	2000	2001	2002	2003	2004
Death by suicide and self-inflicted injury	1.2	-6.7	-3.2	-6.0	-5.7	11.4	-0.3
Death by injury and poisoning	-1.7	-3.2	-2.3	-2.9	-3.0	5.1	-0.7

Source: Euromonitor International from national statistics
Notes: Data is ranked in descending order by year 2004

Smoking

Switzerland: Smoking prevalence in population aged 15+ 1998-2004

Table: 4.1204

% of population aged 15+

	1998	1999	2000	2001	2002	2003	2004
Smoking prevalence in population aged 15+ (% of population aged 15+)	30.2	30.8	30.5	30.2	29.0	29.8	29.6
Smoking prevalence in male population aged 15+ (% of male population)	35.6	35.3	34.7	34.4	34.0	33.6	33.3
Smoking prevalence in female population aged 15+ (% of female population)	25.1	26.6	26.6	26.3	25.0	26.3	26.1

Source: WHO/OECD/Euromonitor International

Nutrition and Obesity

Switzerland: Nutrition and obesity 1998-2004

Table: 4.1205

As stated

	1998	1999	2000	2001	2002	2003	2004
Availability of fruit and vegetables (kg/capita/year)	217.7	183.1	189.1	179.4	180.5	177.4	175.1
Average supply of calories per day (calories per capita)	3,296.6	3,256.2	3,441.0	3,448.9	3,526.2	3,612.0	3,683.8
Average supply of fat per day (grams per capita)	148.4	143.6	149.2	153.0	156.2	160.1	158.4
Average supply of protein per day (grams per capita)	92.4	90.2	94.0	94.6	96.0	97.7	96.8
Microbiological food-borne diseases (per 100000 population)	14.0	12.0	7.0	11.0	11.0	10.0	9.0
Obese population (BMI 30kg/sq m or more) (% of population aged 15+)	6.1	5.4	5.4	5.5	5.5	5.6	5.6

Source: WHO/OECD/Euromonitor International

Over-the-Counter Healthcare

Switzerland: Trends in OTC healthcare retail sales 1998-2004

Table: 4.1206

As stated

	1998	1999	2000	2001	2002	2003	2004
OTC Healthcare (CHF million)	980.2	1,010.8	1,036.0	1,051.4	1,057.1	1,070.1	1,076.4
OTC Healthcare: real growth in national currency: 1998 = 100	100.0	102.3	103.2	103.7	103.6	104.3	104.1
OTC Healthcare: year on year (% real growth)	2.1	2.3	0.9	0.5	-0.1	0.6	-0.1
OTC Healthcare (CHF per capita)	138.1	141.9	144.6	145.9	145.6	146.8	147.1

Source: *Euromonitor International from industry sources/national statistics*

Switzerland: OTC healthcare retail sales by sector 1998-2004

Table: 4.1207

% of OTC retail value sales

	1998	1999	2000	2001	2002	2003	2004
Analgesics	14.1	14.0	14.0	14.2	13.8	14.0	13.5
Cough, cold and allergy (hay fever) remedies	26.4	26.7	27.0	26.6	26.1	26.3	26.6
Digestive remedies	11.7	11.4	11.3	11.2	11.1	10.9	10.9
Medicated skin care	16.1	16.2	16.2	16.2	16.4	16.4	16.6
Vitamins and dietary supplements	17.2	17.2	16.9	16.8	16.9	16.4	16.3

Source: *Euromonitor International from industry sources/national statistics*
Notes: *Only selected sectors are shown, so values are not expected to sum to 100*

Health and Wellness

Switzerland: Retail sales of packaged foods by health and wellness category 2002-2004

Table: 4.1208

CHF million

	2002	2003	2004
Packaged food: Total	14,441.4	14,515.4	14,645.9
Better for you	856.7	876.5	897.6
For food intolerance	69.9	72.6	76.2
Fortified/functional	282.8	296.8	316.4
Organic	541.7	608.0	664.5

Source: *Euromonitor International from industry sources/national statistics*

Switzerland: Per capita sales of packaged foods by health and wellness category 2002-2004

Table: 4.1209

CHF per capita

	2002	2003	2004
Better for you	119.0	121.3	123.7
For food intolerance	9.7	10.0	10.5
Fortified/functional	39.3	41.1	43.6
Organic	75.2	84.1	91.6

Source: *Euromonitor International from industry sources/national statistics*

Switzerland: Retail sales of packaged food by health and wellness category: % share of total packaged food market 2002-2004

Table: 4.1210

% value

	2002	2003	2004
Better for you	5.9	6.0	6.1
For food intolerance	0.5	0.5	0.5
Fortified/functional	2.0	2.0	2.2
Organic	3.8	4.2	4.5

Source: Euromonitor International from industry sources/national statistics

Switzerland: Retail sales of packaged food by health and wellness category: real growth index 2002-2004

Table: 4.1211

2002 =100

	2002	2003	2004
Better for you	100.00	101.90	103.84
For food intolerance	100.00	103.40	108.08
Fortified/functional	100.00	104.53	110.89
Organic	100.00	111.81	121.58

Source: Euromonitor International from industry sources/national statistics

Switzerland: Retail sales of better-for-you packaged foods by sector 2002-2004

Table: 4.1212

% of total packaged food / as stated

	2002	2003	2004	% real change in value 2002-2004
Combination	0.09	0.10	0.10	12.25
Reduced carb	0.00	0.00	0.00	13.26
Reduced fat	4.68	4.75	4.82	3.68
Reduced salt	0.00	0.00	0.00	7.54

Source: Euromonitor International from industry sources/national statistics

Switzerland: Retail sales of packaged foods for food intolerances by sector 2002-2004

Table: 4.1213

% of total packaged food / as stated

	2002	2003	2004	% real change in value 2002-2004
Diabetic	0.36	0.37	0.38	7.53
Gluten-free	0.10	0.10	0.11	12.32
Lactose-free	0.03	0.03	0.03	0.19

Source: Euromonitor International from industry sources/national statistics

Switzerland: Retail sales of naturally healthy packaged foods by sector 2002-2004

Table: 4.1214

% of total packaged food / as stated

	2002	2003	2004	% real change in value 2002-2004
High fibre	1.56	1.58	1.59	2.22
Other naturally healthy food	1.38	1.41	1.43	4.10
Soy-based dairy alternatives	0.07	0.07	0.07	6.49

Source: Euromonitor International from industry sources/national statistics

■ Taiwan

Socio-economic Parameters

Taiwan: Socio-economic parameters 1998-2004

Table: 4.1215

As stated

	1998	1999	2000	2001	2002	2003	2004
Population: national estimates at January 1st ('000)	21,928.6	22,092.4	22,276.7	22,405.6	22,520.8	22,628.0	22,734.4
% aged 0-14 yrs	22.0	21.4	21.1	20.8	20.4	19.9	19.5
% aged 15-64 yrs	69.8	70.1	70.3	70.4	70.6	70.9	71.2
% aged 65+ yrs	8.3	8.4	8.6	8.8	9.0	9.1	9.3
% Male	51.3	51.2	51.1	51.1	51.0	51.0	50.9
% Female	48.7	48.8	48.9	48.9	49.0	49.0	49.1
% Urban	69.2	69.3	77.5	77.7	77.9	72.2	72.4
Occupants per household at January 1st (Number)	3.6	3.5	3.4	3.4	3.3	3.3	3.2
Households ('000)	6,140.9	6,310.1	6,495.0	6,636.7	6,777.9	6,912.3	7,038.1
Annual rates of inflation (% growth)	1.7	0.2	1.3	0.0	-0.2	-0.3	1.1
GDP (NT$ million)	8,938,967.0	9,289,929.0	9,663,388.0	9,447,649.0	9,735,364.0	9,844,203.0	10,205,933.0
GDP (US$ million)	267,400.8	288,301.2	288,489.0	287,597.9	281,615.8	285,649.7	303,791.4
GDP (US$ per capita)	12,194.2	13,049.8	12,950.3	12,836.0	12,504.7	12,623.7	13,362.6

Source: Euromonitor International from International Monetary Fund (IMF), International Financial Statistics and World Economic Outlook/UN/national statistics

Life Expectancy

Taiwan: Life expectancy 1998-2004

Table: 4.1216

As stated

	1998	1999	2000	2001	2002	2003	2004	% change 1998-2004
Life expectancy at birth: total population (years)	72.7	73.0	73.3	73.5	73.8	74.0	74.3	2.24
Life expectancy at birth: total population: year on year growth	1.6	0.4	0.5	0.3	0.4	0.3	0.4	

Source: Euromonitor International from World Bank

Health Expenditure

Taiwan: Public health expenditure 1998-2004

Table: 4.1217

As stated

	1998	1999	2000	2001	2002	2003	2004
Share of total health expenditure in GDP (% of total GDP)	0.3	0.3	0.4	0.4	0.4	0.4	0.4
Health expenditure (US$ per capita)	744.1	842.7	941.3	989.9	1,083.0	1,170.0	1,251.0

Source: Euromonitor International from OECD/national statistics

Taiwan: Private health expenditure 1998-2004

Table: 4.1218

As stated

	1998	1999	2000	2001	2002	2003	2004
Consumer expenditure on health goods and medical services (NT$ million)	439,533.0	482,333.0	525,736.0	546,896.0	577,637.0	591,714.0	614,780.8
Consumer expenditure on health goods and medical services: real growth in national currency: 1990 = 100	224.9	246.3	265.0	275.7	291.8	299.8	308.1
Consumer expenditure on health goods and medical services as a percentage of total consumer expenditure	8.2	8.6	8.8	9.1	9.3	9.5	9.6

Source: National statistical offices/OECD/Eurostat/Euromonitor International

Taiwan: Consumer expenditure on health goods and medical services by sector 1998-2004

Table: 4.1219

% of total consumer expenditure on health goods and medical services

	1998	1999	2000	2001	2002	2003	2004
Pharmaceuticals, medical appliances/ equipment	68.3	68.2	68.0	68.5	68.6	68.8	68.6
Outpatient services	8.7	8.7	8.7	8.0	7.9	8.3	8.6
Hospital services	23.0	23.1	23.3	23.5	23.5	22.9	22.9
Total	100.0	100.0	100.0	100.0	100.0	100.0	100.0

Source: National statistical offices/OECD/Eurostat/Euromonitor International

Healthcare Infrastructure and Services

Taiwan: Healthcare infrastructure and services by sector 1998-2004

Table: 4.1220

As stated

	1998	1999	2000	2001	2002	2003	2004
Active pharmacists (number)	22,763	23,940	24,407	24,895	25,352	26,134	26,789
Dentists (number)	7,895	8,244	8,597	8,940	9,211	9,379	9,454
Doctors (number)	30,629	31,757	33,323	34,548	35,633	36,709	37,312
Hospitals and clinics (number)	17,731	17,770	18,082	18,265	18,228	18,203	18,180
In-patient beds ('000)	125	123	126	128	133	136	139
Midwives (number)	845	889	929	969	1,006	1,039	1,071
Nurses (number)	71,214	75,598	79,176	82,762	89,564	93,120	95,066

Source: Euromonitor International from national statistics

Taiwan: Healthcare infrastructure and services by sector: growth 1998-2004

Table: 4.1221

Year on year growth: % change in stated unit

	1998	1999	2000	2001	2002	2003	2004
Active pharmacists (number)	7.2	5.2	2.0	2.0	1.8	3.1	2.5
Dentists (number)	4.3	4.4	4.3	4.0	3.0	1.8	0.8
Doctors (number)	5.5	3.7	4.9	3.7	3.1	3.0	1.6
Hospitals and clinics (number)	1.9	0.2	1.8	1.0	-0.2	-0.1	-0.1
In-patient beds (number)	2.5	-1.3	2.9	1.0	4.5	2.1	2.4
Midwives (number)	4.8	5.2	4.5	4.3	3.8	3.3	3.1
Nurses (number)	2.2	6.2	4.7	4.5	8.2	4.0	2.1

Source: Euromonitor International from national statistics

Infectious Diseases

Taiwan: Incidence of disease by type 1998-2004

Table: 4.1222

Number

	1998	1999	2000	2001	2002	2003	2004
Incidence of AIDS	151	175	221	236	267	289	172

Source: WHO

Taiwan: Incidence of disease by type: growth 1998-2004

Table: 4.1223

Year on year growth: %

	1998	1999	2000	2001	2002	2003	2004
Incidence of AIDS	13.5	15.9	26.3	6.8	13.1	8.2	-40.5

Source: WHO

Causes of Death

Taiwan: Deaths by disease 1998-2004

Table: 4.1224

Number per 100,000 inhabitants

	1998	1999	2000	2001	2002	2003	2004
Death by malignant neoplasms (cancers)	134.0	135.3	135.7	136.1	136.4	135.9	136.6
Death by diseases of the circulatory system	50.5	51.3	52.2	52.9	52.7	50.1	49.9
Deaths from heart disease	36.6	35.1	39.8	38.4	38.6	37.7	36.8
Death by diseases of the digestive system	19.2	18.9	20.7	18.9	18.5	19.1	18.7
Deaths from lung cancer	18.1	18.0	17.6	17.1	16.9	16.5	16.3
Deaths from ulcers of the stomach and duodenum	19.2	18.9	20.7	18.9	18.5	17.2	16.1
Death by diseases of the respiratory system	9.1	8.2	8.0	7.8	7.5	7.6	7.5
Deaths from chronic liver disease and cirrhosis	6.0	5.7	5.4	5.2	5.0	4.8	4.6

Source: WHO/Euromonitor International
Notes: Data is ranked in descending order by year 2004

Taiwan: Deaths by disease: growth 1998-2004

Table: 4.1225

% year on year growth

	1998	1999	2000	2001	2002	2003	2004
Death by malignant neoplasms (cancers)	-0.1	1.0	0.3	0.3	0.2	-0.4	0.5
Death by diseases of the circulatory system	1.6	1.6	1.8	1.3	-0.4	-4.9	-0.5
Death by diseases of the respiratory system	1.1	-9.9	-2.4	-2.5	-3.8	1.3	-0.8
Deaths from lung cancer	-14.6	-0.6	-2.2	-2.8	-1.2	-2.4	-1.4
Death by diseases of the digestive system	-9.0	-1.6	9.5	-8.7	-2.1	3.2	-2.1
Deaths from heart disease	-7.3	-4.1	13.4	-3.5	0.5	-2.3	-2.3
Deaths from chronic liver disease and cirrhosis	-3.2	-5.0	-5.3	-3.7	-3.8	-4.0	-4.7
Deaths from ulcers of the stomach and duodenum	-9.0	-1.6	9.5	-8.7	-2.1	-7.0	-6.5

Source: WHO/Euromonitor International
Notes: Data is ranked in descending order by year 2004

Taiwan: Other selected causes of death: 1998-2004

Table: 4.1226

Number per 100,000 inhabitants

	1998	1999	2000	2001	2002	2003	2004
Death by suicide and self-inflicted injury	10.0	10.4	10.4	10.5	10.6	10.4	10.4
Death by motor traffic accidents	11.6	11.0	10.4	9.7	9.7	9.6	9.4

Source: Euromonitor International from national statistics
Notes: Data is ranked in descending order by year 2004

Taiwan: Other selected causes of death: growth 1998-2004

Table: 4.1227

% year on year growth

	1998	1999	2000	2001	2002	2003	2004
Death by suicide and self-inflicted injury	0.0	4.0	0.0	1.0	1.0	-1.9	0.2
Death by motor traffic accidents	-9.4	-5.2	-5.5	-6.7	0.0	-1.0	-1.8

Source: Euromonitor International from national statistics
Notes: Data is ranked in descending order by year 2004

Smoking

Taiwan: Smoking prevalence in population aged 15+ 1998-2004

% of population aged 15+

	1998	1999	2000	2001	2002	2003	2004
Smoking prevalence in population aged 15+ (% of population aged 15+)	35.2	35.1	34.8	34.7	34.4	34.1	33.7
Smoking prevalence in male population aged 15+ (% of male population)	55.8	55.0	54.5	53.9	53.6	53.1	52.7
Smoking prevalence in female population aged 15+ (% of female population)	13.8	14.4	14.4	15.0	14.5	14.6	14.2

Source: WHO/OECD/Euromonitor International

Nutrition and Obesity

Taiwan: Nutrition and obesity 1998-2004

As stated

	1998	1999	2000	2001	2002	2003	2004
Average supply of calories per day (calories per capita)	3,170.6	3,151.2	3,197.1	3,255.6	3,274.7	3,306.8	3,342.4
Average supply of fat per day (grams per capita)	151.9	159.5	148.7	147.1	142.9	138.4	134.6
Average supply of protein per day (grams per capita)	102.0	105.0	102.2	104.9	105.2	105.3	105.9
Obese population (BMI 30kg/sq m or more) (% of population aged 15+)	6.1	6.1	6.2	6.0	5.9	5.8	5.7

Source: WHO/OECD/Euromonitor International

Over-the-Counter Healthcare

Taiwan: Trends in OTC healthcare retail sales 1998-2004

As stated

	1998	1999	2000	2001	2002	2003	2004
OTC Healthcare (NT$ million)	29,775.1	31,461.0	33,320.4	35,340.6	37,125.4	38,836.0	40,720.7
OTC Healthcare: real growth in national currency: 1998 = 100	100.0	105.5	110.3	116.9	123.1	129.1	133.9
OTC Healthcare: year on year (% real growth)	3.5	5.5	4.6	6.1	5.3	4.9	3.7
OTC Healthcare (NT$ per capita)	1,357.8	1,424.1	1,495.8	1,577.3	1,648.5	1,716.3	1,791.1

Source: Euromonitor International from industry sources/national statistics

Taiwan: OTC healthcare retail sales by sector 1998-2004

% of OTC retail value sales

	1998	1999	2000	2001	2002	2003	2004
Analgesics	5.1	5.1	5.1	5.0	4.6	4.3	4.1
Cough, cold and allergy (hay fever) remedies	11.0	10.7	10.5	10.2	9.9	9.0	8.4
Digestive remedies	3.9	4.2	4.2	4.3	4.1	3.9	3.7
Medicated skin care	5.7	5.9	6.0	5.9	5.8	5.8	5.7
Vitamins and dietary supplements	73.2	73.0	73.2	73.7	74.7	76.1	77.2

Source: Euromonitor International from industry sources/national statistics
Notes: Only selected sectors are shown, so values are not expected to sum to 100

Health and Wellness

Taiwan: Retail sales of packaged foods by health and wellness category 2002-2004

Table: 4.1232

NT$ million

	2002	2003	2004
Packaged food: Total	195,062.5	196,119.1	199,715.0
Better for you	10,450.2	10,870.1	11,133.5
For food intolerance	143.4	142.5	161.1
Fortified/functional	7,243.3	7,426.0	8,051.0
Organic	34.1	38.3	222.5

Source: *Euromonitor International from industry sources/national statistics*

Taiwan: Per capita sales of packaged foods by health and wellness category 2002-2004

Table: 4.1233

NT$ per capita

	2002	2003	2004
Better for you	463.0	477.4	484.8
For food intolerance	6.4	6.3	7.0
Fortified/functional	320.9	326.2	350.6
Organic	1.5	1.7	9.7

Source: *Euromonitor International from industry sources/national statistics*

Taiwan: Retail sales of packaged food by health and wellness category: % share of total packaged food market 2002-2004

Table: 4.1234

% value

	2002	2003	2004
Better for you	5.4	5.5	5.6
For food intolerance	0.1	0.1	0.1
Fortified/functional	3.7	3.8	4.0
Organic	0.0	0.0	0.1

Source: *Euromonitor International from industry sources/national statistics*

Taiwan: Retail sales of packaged food by health and wellness category: real growth index 2002-2004

Table: 4.1235

2002 =100

	2002	2003	2004
Better for you	100.00	103.91	105.59
For food intolerance	100.00	99.29	111.31
Fortified/functional	100.00	102.42	110.16
Organic	100.00	112.05	645.61

Source: *Euromonitor International from industry sources/national statistics*

Taiwan: Retail sales of better-for-you packaged foods by sector 2002-2004

Table: 4.1236

% of total packaged food / as stated

	2002	2003	2004	% real change in value 2002-2004
Reduced fat	4.57	4.75	4.78	6.05
Reduced salt	0.08	0.09	0.10	33.12

Source: *Euromonitor International from industry sources/national statistics*

Taiwan: Retail sales of packaged foods for food intolerances by sector 2002-2004

Table: 4.1237

% of total packaged food / as stated

	2002	2003	2004	% real change in value 2002-2004
Lactose-free	0.07	0.07	0.08	11.31

Source: *Euromonitor International from industry sources/national statistics*

Taiwan: Retail sales of naturally healthy packaged foods by sector 2002-2004

Table: 4.1238

% of total packaged food / as stated

	2002	2003	2004	% real change in value 2002-2004
High fibre	0.44	0.46	0.50	13.87
Other naturally healthy food	0.66	0.66	0.66	0.65
Soy-based dairy alternatives	0.99	0.98	1.00	1.86

Source: *Euromonitor International from industry sources/national statistics*

▪ Thailand

Socio-economic Parameters

Thailand: Socio-economic parameters 1998-2004

Table: 4.1239

As stated

	1998	1999	2000	2001	2002	2003	2004
Population: national estimates at January 1st ('000)	58,085.7	58,797.4	58,875.9	59,362.2	59,891.3	60,579.7	61,249.0
% aged 0-14 yrs	23.8	23.5	23.3	23.0	22.6	22.4	22.1
% aged 15-64 yrs	70.4	70.4	70.6	70.6	70.7	70.8	70.9
% aged 65 + yrs	5.8	6.0	6.1	6.4	6.6	6.9	7.1
% Male	49.7	49.5	49.5	49.5	49.4	49.4	49.4
% Female	50.3	50.5	50.5	50.5	50.6	50.6	50.6
% Urban	21.0	21.3	21.6	21.9	22.3	22.8	23.4
Occupants per household at January 1st (Number)	3.8	3.8	3.8	3.7	3.7	3.7	3.6
Households ('000)	15,099.6	15,480.6	15,662.3	15,953.4	16,249.2	16,578.9	16,895.6
Annual rates of inflation (% growth)	8.1	0.3	1.6	1.6	0.6	1.8	2.8
GDP (Bt million)	4,626,450.0	4,637,080.0	4,922,730.0	5,133,500.0	5,446,040.0	5,930,360.0	6,576,030.0
GDP (US$ million)	111,859.7	122,629.6	122,725.2	115,536.4	126,769.7	142,953.3	163,491.7
GDP (US$ per capita)	1,925.8	2,085.6	2,084.5	1,946.3	2,116.7	2,359.8	2,669.3

Source: *Euromonitor International from International Monetary Fund (IMF), International Financial Statistics and World Economic Outlook/UN/national statistics*

Life Expectancy

Thailand: Life expectancy 1998-2004

Table: 4.1240

As stated

	1998	1999	2000	2001	2002	2003	2004	% change 1998-2004
Life expectancy at birth: total population (years)	68.3	68.5	68.8	68.9	69.3	69.6	69.9	2.37
Life expectancy at birth: total population: year on year growth	0.4	0.4	0.3	0.2	0.6	0.4	0.4	
Healthy life expectancy at birth (years)	60.0			58.6	58.6			
Healthy life expectancy at birth: year on year growth					0.0			

Source: Euromonitor International from World Bank

Sanitation

Thailand: Improved sanitary facilities and water source 2000

Table: 4.1241

As stated

	2000
Population with access to improved sanitary facilities (% of population)	96.0
Population with access to improved water source (% of population)	84.0
Population with improved access to sanitation facilities, rural (% of rural population with access)	96.0
Population with improved access to sanitation facilities, urban (% of urban population with access)	96.0

Source: National statistics/World Bank

Health Expenditure

Thailand: Public health expenditure 1998-2004

Table: 4.1242

As stated

	1998	1999	2000	2001	2002	2003	2004
Share of total health expenditure in GDP (% of total GDP)	3.9	3.7	3.6	3.7	3.5	3.6	3.4
Health expenditure (US$ per capita)	73.0	75.0	72.0	66.0	90.0	93.0	98.0

Source: Euromonitor International from OECD/national statistics

Thailand: Private health expenditure 1998-2004

Table: 4.1243

As stated

	1998	1999	2000	2001	2002	2003	2004
Consumer expenditure on health goods and medical services (Bt million)	218,033.0	220,880.0	230,027.0	245,148.0	253,655.0	267,545.9	283,956.5
Consumer expenditure on health goods and medical services: real growth in national currency: 1990 = 100	119.1	120.3	123.3	129.3	133.0	137.8	142.3
Consumer expenditure on health goods and medical services as a percentage of total consumer expenditure	8.1	7.9	7.7	7.8	7.7	7.7	7.8

Source: National statistical offices/OECD/Eurostat/Euromonitor International

Thailand: Consumer expenditure on health goods and medical services by sector 1998-2004

Table: 4.1244

% of total consumer expenditure on health goods and medical services

	1998	1999	2000	2001	2002	2003	2004
Pharmaceuticals, medical appliances/ equipment	22.7	23.7	24.1	25.8	26.1	25.9	25.9
Outpatient services	47.4	46.3	45.6	43.4	43.1	43.1	43.0
Hospital services	29.9	30.0	30.2	30.8	30.8	31.0	31.1
Total	100.0	100.0	100.0	100.0	100.0	100.0	100.0

Source: National statistical offices/OECD/Eurostat/Euromonitor International

Healthcare Infrastructure and Services

Thailand: Healthcare infrastructure and services by sector 1998-2004

Table: 4.1245

As stated

	1998	1999	2000	2001	2002	2003	2004
Active pharmacists (number)	5,911	6,062	6,384	6,823	7,080	7,326	7,434
Dentists (number)	3,917	4,026	4,141	4,299	4,470	4,625	4,769
Doctors (number)	17,955	18,140	18,025	18,779	19,392	19,790	20,297
Hospitals and clinics (number)	3,608	3,627	3,682	3,712	3,773	3,821	3,822
In-patient beds ('000)	366	370	410	414	430	442	447
Nurses (number)	63,708	68,008	70,978	77,008	80,174	81,391	81,820

Source: Euromonitor International from national statistics

Thailand: Healthcare infrastructure and services by sector: growth 1998-2004

Table: 4.1246

Year on year growth: % change in stated unit

	1998	1999	2000	2001	2002	2003	2004
Active pharmacists (number)	-0.5	2.6	5.3	6.9	3.8	3.5	1.5
Dentists (number)	14.7	2.8	2.9	3.8	4.0	3.5	3.1
Doctors (number)	8.4	1.0	-0.6	4.2	3.3	2.1	2.6
Hospitals and clinics (number)	2.3	0.5	1.5	0.8	1.6	1.3	0.0
In-patient beds (number)	1.0	0.9	10.8	1.0	3.9	2.8	1.1
Nurses (number)	13.0	6.7	4.4	8.5	4.1	1.5	0.5

Source: Euromonitor International from national statistics

Immunisation

Thailand: Vaccination rates by disease type 1998-2004

Table: 4.1247

%

	1998	1999	2000	2001	2002	2003	2004
Vaccination rate against DTP (diphtheria, tetanus, pertussis) 1 & 2 (%)			98.5	98.5	98.5	99.0	99.0
Vaccination rate against MMR (measles, mumps, rubella) (%)		96.0	94.2	94.2	94.2	93.0	93.0
Vaccination rate against polio (%)		96.6	96.6	96.6	96.6	97.0	97.0

Source: WHO

Infectious Diseases

Thailand: Incidence of disease by type 1998-2004

Table: 4.1248

Number

	1998	1999	2000	2001	2002	2003	2004
Incidence of AIDS	27,485	27,010	26,114	24,042	21,650	13,585	12,621
Incidence of diphtheria	43	52	15	11			
Incidence of measles	13,734	3,167	4,074	7,319			
Incidence of polio	31	24	20	0			

Source: WHO

Thailand: Incidence of disease by type: growth 1998-2004

Table: 4.1249

Year on year growth: %

	1998	1999	2000	2001	2002	2003	2004
Incidence of AIDS	2.0	-1.7	-3.3	-7.9	-9.9	-37.3	-7.1
Incidence of diphtheria	13.2	20.9	-71.2	-26.7			
Incidence of measles	-9.2	-76.9	28.6	79.7			
Incidence of polio	63.2	-22.6	-16.7	-100.0			

Source: WHO

Causes of Death

Thailand: Deaths by disease 1998-2004

Table: 4.1250

Number per 100,000 inhabitants

	1998	1999	2000	2001	2002	2003	2004
Deaths from heart disease	42.3	44.4	47.9	44.0	45.7	43.7	42.6
Deaths from lung cancer	28.9	31.2	29.4	31.0	31.0	31.9	33.0
Death by diseases of the digestive system	18.7	17.1	18.9	16.4	15.5	14.6	13.3
Deaths from ulcers of the stomach and duodenum	18.7	17.1	18.9	16.4	15.5	13.7	12.4
Deaths from chronic liver disease and cirrhosis	9.7	9.6	9.5	9.4	9.1	8.9	8.7

Source: WHO/Euromonitor International
Notes: Data is ranked in descending order by year 2004

Thailand: Deaths by disease: growth 1998-2004

Table: 4.1251

% year on year growth

	1998	1999	2000	2001	2002	2003	2004
Deaths from lung cancer	18.0	8.0	-5.8	5.4	0.0	2.9	3.6
Deaths from heart disease	15.6	5.0	7.9	-8.1	3.9	-4.4	-2.4
Deaths from chronic liver disease and cirrhosis	0.0	-1.0	-1.0	-1.1	-3.2	-2.2	-2.4
Death by diseases of the digestive system	-10.1	-8.6	10.5	-13.2	-5.5	-5.8	-9.0
Deaths from ulcers of the stomach and duodenum	-10.1	-8.6	10.5	-13.2	-5.5	-11.6	-9.3

Source: WHO/Euromonitor International
Notes: Data is ranked in descending order by year 2004

Smoking

Thailand: Smoking prevalence in population aged 15+ 1998-2004

Table: 4.1252

% of population aged 15+

	1998	1999	2000	2001	2002	2003	2004
Smoking prevalence in population aged 15+ (% of population aged 15+)	31.3	31.1	31.1	31.2	31.4	30.8	30.8
Smoking prevalence in male population aged 15+ (% of male population)	48.3	48.1	47.9	48.1	46.8	46.5	46.0
Smoking prevalence in female population aged 15+ (% of female population)	14.9	14.9	15.1	15.0	16.7	15.9	16.3

Source: WHO/OECD/Euromonitor International

Nutrition and Obesity

Thailand: Nutrition and obesity 1998-2004

Table: 4.1253

As stated

	1998	1999	2000	2001	2002	2003	2004
Average supply of calories per day (calories per capita)	2,453.8	2,442.8	2,435.3	2,455.8	2,467.3	2,476.1	2,488.0
Average supply of fat per day (grams per capita)	51.4	50.8	50.3	50.4	51.1	51.5	51.9
Average supply of protein per day (grams per capita)	56.9	56.4	56.1	56.7	57.0	57.3	57.7
Obese population (BMI 30kg/sq m or more) (% of population aged 15 +)	3.6	3.7	3.8	3.8	3.6	3.6	3.7

Source: WHO/OECD/Euromonitor International

Over-the-Counter Healthcare

Thailand: Trends in OTC healthcare retail sales 1998-2004

Table: 4.1254

As stated

	1998	1999	2000	2001	2002	2003	2004
OTC Healthcare (Bt million)	11,531.6	11,783.2	12,237.6	12,799.3	13,524.3	14,330.5	15,148.3
OTC Healthcare: real growth in national currency: 1998 = 100	100.0	101.9	104.2	107.2	112.6	117.2	120.6
OTC Healthcare: year on year (% real growth)	-7.7	1.9	2.3	2.9	5.0	4.1	2.9
OTC Healthcare (Bt per capita)	198.5	200.4	207.9	215.6	225.8	236.6	247.3

Source: Euromonitor International from industry sources/national statistics

Thailand: OTC healthcare retail sales by sector 1998-2004

Table: 4.1255

% of OTC retail value sales

	1998	1999	2000	2001	2002	2003	2004
Analgesics	14.9	14.6	14.4	14.5	14.5	14.5	14.6
Cough, cold and allergy (hay fever) remedies	23.8	24.2	24.3	23.6	23.7	23.6	23.6
Digestive remedies	5.6	5.7	5.6	5.6	5.6	5.6	5.6
Medicated skin care	10.6	10.6	10.4	10.1	9.9	9.8	9.8
Vitamins and dietary supplements	41.4	41.5	41.9	42.8	42.9	43.0	42.8

Source: Euromonitor International from industry sources/national statistics
Notes: Only selected sectors are shown, so values are not expected to sum to 100

Health and Wellness

Thailand: Retail sales of packaged foods by health and wellness category 2002-2004

Table: 4.1256

Bt million

	2002	2003	2004
Packaged food: Total	154,746.2	164,028.1	173,921.0
Better for you	3,744.8	3,976.5	4,424.5
For food intolerance	279.0	307.8	341.2
Fortified/functional	11,888.7	12,730.4	13,830.8
Organic	988.9	1,098.6	1,287.7

Source: Euromonitor International from industry sources/national statistics

Thailand: Per capita sales of packaged foods by health and wellness category 2002-2004

Table: 4.1257

Bt per capita

	2002	2003	2004
Better for you	60.2	63.3	69.9
For food intolerance	4.5	4.9	5.4
Fortified/functional	191.0	202.8	218.5
Organic	15.9	17.5	20.3

Source: Euromonitor International from industry sources/national statistics

Thailand: Retail sales of packaged food by health and wellness category: % share of total packaged food market 2002-2004

Table: 4.1258

% value

	2002	2003	2004
Better for you	2.4	2.4	2.5
For food intolerance	0.2	0.2	0.2
Fortified/functional	7.7	7.8	8.0
Organic	0.6	0.7	0.7

Source: Euromonitor International from industry sources/national statistics

Thailand: Retail sales of packaged food by health and wellness category: real growth index 2002-2004

Table: 4.1259

2002 = 100

	2002	2003	2004
Better for you	100.00	104.72	116.40
For food intolerance	100.00	108.80	120.48
Fortified/functional	100.00	105.60	114.61
Organic	100.00	109.55	128.29

Source: Euromonitor International from industry sources/national statistics

Thailand: Retail sales of better-for-you packaged foods by sector 2002-2004

Table: 4.1260

% of total packaged food / as stated

	2002	2003	2004	% real change in value 2002-2004
Combination	0.01	0.01	0.06	372.33
Reduced carb	0.00	0.00	0.00	6.67
Reduced fat	1.81	1.82	1.88	15.16
Reduced salt			0.01	

Source: Euromonitor International from industry sources/national statistics

Thailand: Retail sales of packaged foods for food intolerances by sector 2002-2004

Table: 4.1261

% of total packaged food / as stated

	2002	2003	2004	% real change in value 2002-2004
Lactose-free	0.18	0.19	0.20	20.48

Source: Euromonitor International from industry sources/national statistics

Thailand: Retail sales of naturally healthy packaged foods by sector 2002-2004

Table: 4.1262

% of total packaged food / as stated

	2002	2003	2004	% real change in value 2002-2004
High fibre	0.36	0.37	0.39	17.26
Other naturally healthy food	0.23	0.22	0.23	9.66
Soy-based dairy alternatives	2.24	2.24	2.22	10.07

Source: *Euromonitor International from industry sources/national statistics*

■ **Tunisia**

Socio-economic Parameters

Tunisia: Socio-economic parameters 1998-2004

Table: 4.1263

As stated

	1998	1999	2000	2001	2002	2003	2004
Population: national estimates at January 1st ('000)	9,248.0	9,357.6	9,464.6	9,570.4	9,675.3	9,779.4	9,883.6
% aged 0-14 yrs	32.5	31.6	30.7	29.8	29.0	28.1	27.3
% aged 15-64 yrs	62.2	62.9	63.7	64.5	65.2	66.0	66.7
% aged 65 + yrs	5.4	5.5	5.6	5.7	5.8	5.9	6.0
% Male	50.4	50.4	50.4	50.4	50.4	50.4	50.3
% Female	49.6	49.6	49.6	49.6	49.6	49.6	49.7
% Urban	64.1	64.8	65.5	66.0	66.6	67.2	67.7
Occupants per household at January 1st (Number)	4.8	4.7	4.7	4.6	4.6	4.5	4.5
Households ('000)	1,910.9	1,971.2	2,026.8	2,077.0	2,124.0	2,167.8	2,210.1
Annual rates of inflation (% growth)	3.1	2.7	2.9	2.0	2.7	2.7	3.6
GDP (TND million)	22,561.0	24,672.0	26,650.0	28,760.0	29,930.0	32,210.0	35,100.0
GDP (US$ million)	19,812.6	20,798.8	19,442.9	19,990.1	21,051.8	24,998.8	28,182.1
GDP (US$ per capita)	2,142.4	2,222.7	2,054.3	2,088.7	2,175.8	2,556.3	2,851.4

Source: *Euromonitor International from International Monetary Fund (IMF), International Financial Statistics and World Economic Outlook/UN/national statistics*

Life Expectancy

Tunisia: Life expectancy 1998-2004

Table: 4.1264

As stated

	1998	1999	2000	2001	2002	2003	2004	% change 1998-2004
Life expectancy at birth: total population (years)	70.5	70.8	70.9	71.1	71.6	72.0	72.3	2.52
Life expectancy at birth: total population: year on year growth	0.4	0.4	0.2	0.3	0.7	0.6	0.4	
Healthy life expectancy at birth (years)	61.0			61.1	61.3			
Healthy life expectancy at birth: year on year growth					0.2			

Source: *Euromonitor International from World Bank*

Sanitation

Tunisia: Improved sanitary facilities and water source 2000

Table: 4.1265

As stated

	2000
Population with access to improved sanitary facilities (% of population)	84.0
Population with access to improved water source (% of population)	80.0
Population with improved access to sanitation facilities, rural (% of rural population with access)	62.0
Population with improved access to sanitation facilities, urban (% of urban population with access)	96.0

Source: *National statistics/World Bank*

Health Expenditure

Tunisia: Public health expenditure 1998-2004

Table: 4.1266

As stated

	1998	1999	2000	2001	2002	2003	2004
Share of total health expenditure in GDP (% of total GDP)	6.3	6.3	6.2	6.4	6.6	6.7	6.5
Health expenditure (US$ per capita)	126.0	124.0	115.0	120.0	126.0	127.0	129.0

Source: Euromonitor International from OECD/national statistics

Tunisia: Private health expenditure 1998-2004

Table: 4.1267

As stated

	1998	1999	2000	2001	2002	2003	2004
Consumer expenditure on health goods and medical services (TND million)	1,167.7	1,282.0	1,394.8	1,512.1	1,633.0	1,791.8	1,907.7
Consumer expenditure on health goods and medical services: real growth in national currency: 1990 = 100	156.2	167.0	176.5	187.6	197.1	210.4	216.2
Consumer expenditure on health goods and medical services as a percentage of total consumer expenditure	8.8	8.9	8.9	8.9	9.0	8.9	9.0

Source: National statistical offices/OECD/Eurostat/Euromonitor International

Tunisia: Consumer expenditure on health goods and medical services by sector 1998-2004

Table: 4.1268

% of total consumer expenditure on health goods and medical services

	1998	1999	2000	2001	2002	2003	2004
Pharmaceuticals, medical appliances/ equipment	23.0	24.6	24.9	26.4	26.8	26.7	26.7
Outpatient services	6.1	5.5	4.5	3.9	3.3	3.6	3.5
Hospital services	70.9	69.9	70.5	69.7	69.9	69.7	69.8
Total	100.0	100.0	100.0	100.0	100.0	100.0	100.0

Source: National statistical offices/OECD/Eurostat/Euromonitor International

Healthcare Infrastructure and Services

Tunisia: Healthcare infrastructure and services by sector 1998-2004

Table: 4.1269

As stated

	1998	1999	2000	2001	2002	2003	2004
Active pharmacists (number)	1,623	1,690	1,951	1,998	2,050	2,101	2,130
Dentists (number)	1,276	1,301	1,315	1,380	1,394	1,427	1,462
Doctors (number)	6,819	7,149	7,444	7,761	7,964	8,095	8,143
Hospitals and clinics (number)	163	164	167	167	168	170	172
In-patient beds ('000)	16	16	17	17	17	17	17

Source: Euromonitor International from national statistics

Tunisia: Healthcare infrastructure and services by sector: growth 1998-2004

Table: 4.1270

Year on year growth: % change in stated unit

	1998	1999	2000	2001	2002	2003	2004
Active pharmacists (number)	3.6	4.1	15.4	2.4	2.6	2.5	1.4
Dentists (number)	6.3	2.0	1.1	4.9	1.0	2.4	2.5
Doctors (number)	5.5	4.8	4.1	4.3	2.6	1.6	0.6
Hospitals and clinics (number)	0.6	0.6	1.8	0.0	0.6	1.2	1.2
In-patient beds (number)	0.4	1.5	2.5	0.0	1.2	1.3	0.9

Source: Euromonitor International from national statistics

Immunisation

Tunisia: Vaccination rates by disease type 1998-2004

Table: 4.1271

%

	1998	1999	2000	2001	2002	2003	2004
Vaccination rate against DTP (diphtheria, tetanus, pertussis) 1 & 2 (%)			94.2	96.0	96.0	97.0	98.0
Vaccination rate against MMR (measles, mumps, rubella) (%)	94.0	99.0	84.6	92.2	94.0	96.0	98.0
Vaccination rate against polio (%)	96.0	99.0	96.0	98.0	96.0	96.0	95.0

Source: WHO

Infectious Diseases

Tunisia: Incidence of disease by type 1998-2004

Table: 4.1272

Number

	1998	1999	2000	2001	2002	2003	2004
Incidence of AIDS	44	42	48	43	39	37	41
Incidence of diphtheria	0	0	0	0	0		
Incidence of measles	123	101	47	231	98		
Incidence of polio	0	0	0	0	0		

Source: WHO

Tunisia: Incidence of disease by type: growth 1998-2004

Table: 4.1273

Year on year growth: %

	1998	1999	2000	2001	2002	2003	2004
Incidence of AIDS	-29.0	-4.5	14.3	-10.4	-9.3	-5.1	10.8
Incidence of measles	-66.8	-17.9	-53.5	391.5	-57.6		

Source: WHO

Smoking

Tunisia: Smoking prevalence in population aged 15+ 1998-2004

Table: 4.1274

% of population aged 15+

	1998	1999	2000	2001	2002	2003	2004
Smoking prevalence in population aged 15+ (% of population aged 15+)	37.4	36.9	36.9	36.7	36.4	36.2	36.0
Smoking prevalence in male population aged 15+ (% of male population)	61.6	62.1	62.3	62.4	61.8	61.9	61.7
Smoking prevalence in female population aged 15+ (% of female population)	13.2	11.8	11.5	11.1	11.0	10.5	10.3

Source: WHO/OECD/Euromonitor International

Nutrition and Obesity

Tunisia: Nutrition and obesity 1998-2004

Table: 4.1275

As stated

	1998	1999	2000	2001	2002	2003	2004
Average supply of calories per day (calories per capita)	3,333.1	3,397.9	3,303.9	3,272.2	3,237.8	3,218.8	3,185.9
Average supply of fat per day (grams per capita)	94.6	103.6	98.8	96.6	95.0	96.4	97.2
Average supply of protein per day (grams per capita)	90.6	91.8	90.9	90.9	87.0	88.6	90.2
Obese population (BMI 30kg/sq m or more) (% of population aged 15+)	5.5	5.0	5.1	5.2	5.0	5.0	4.9

Source: WHO/OECD/Euromonitor International

Over-the-Counter Healthcare

Tunisia: Trends in OTC healthcare retail sales 1998-2004

Table: 4.1276

As stated

	1998	1999	2000	2001	2002	2003	2004
OTC Healthcare (US$ million)	10.8	11.1	10.8	11.1	12.3	14.7	15.6
OTC Healthcare (US$ per capita)	1.2	1.2	1.1	1.2	1.3	1.5	1.6

Source: Euromonitor International from industry sources/national statistics

Tunisia: OTC healthcare retail sales by sector 1998-2004

Table: 4.1277

% of OTC retail value sales

	1998	1999	2000	2001	2002	2003	2004
Analgesics	15.1	14.7	14.3	13.9	13.5	13.2	13.0
Cough, cold and allergy (hay fever) remedies	21.8	21.6	21.4	21.1	21.0	20.9	20.6
Digestive remedies	10.8	11.0	11.2	11.4	11.5	11.6	11.9
Medicated skin care	17.2	17.6	18.1	18.5	18.8	18.9	18.9
Vitamins and dietary supplements	28.7	28.8	28.9	29.0	29.1	29.3	29.5

Source: Euromonitor International from industry sources/national statistics
Notes: Only selected sectors are shown, so values are not expected to sum to 100

■ Turkey

Socio-economic Parameters

Turkey: Socio-economic parameters 1998-2004

Table: 4.1278

As stated

	1998	1999	2000	2001	2002	2003	2004
Population: national estimates at January 1st ('000)	65,157.0	66,288.0	67,419.0	68,527.0	69,625.0	70,712.0	71,790.0
% aged 0-14 yrs	30.6	30.3	30.0	29.7	29.6	29.4	29.2
% aged 15-64 yrs	64.1	64.4	64.7	64.8	64.9	65.0	65.1
% aged 65+ yrs	5.2	5.3	5.4	5.4	5.5	5.6	5.7
% Male	50.5	50.5	50.5	50.5	50.5	50.5	50.5
% Female	49.5	49.5	49.5	49.5	49.5	49.5	49.5
% Urban	72.9	74.1	74.3	75.2	76.1	77.0	78.0
Occupants per household at January 1st (Number)	4.8	4.8	4.8	4.8	4.8	4.8	4.7
Households ('000)	13,476.7	13,761.2	14,034.8	14,304.0	14,582.6	14,862.3	15,133.9
Annual rates of inflation (% growth)	84.6	64.9	54.9	54.4	45.0	25.3	8.6
GDP (TL billion)	52,224,900.0	77,415,300.0	124,583,000.0	178,412,000.0	276,003,000.0	359,763,000.0	430,511,000.0
GDP (US$ million)	200,307.2	184,857.8	199,263.3	145,572.3	183,119.4	239,699.8	301,998.5
GDP (US$ per capita)	3,074.2	2,788.7	2,955.6	2,124.3	2,630.1	3,389.8	4,206.7

Source: Euromonitor International from International Monetary Fund (IMF), International Financial Statistics and World Economic Outlook/UN/national statistics

Life Expectancy

Turkey: Life expectancy 1998-2004

As stated

	1998	1999	2000	2001	2002	2003	2004	% change 1998-2004
Life expectancy at birth: total population (years)	68.3	68.6	68.9	69.0	70.0	70.5	71.1	4.10
Life expectancy at birth: total population: year on year growth	0.5	0.4	0.4	0.2	1.4	0.8	0.8	
Healthy life expectancy at birth (years)	63.0			59.7	59.8			
Healthy life expectancy at birth: year on year growth					0.2			

Source: Euromonitor International from World Bank

Sanitation

Turkey: Improved sanitary facilities and water source 2000

As stated

	2000
Population with access to improved sanitary facilities (% of population)	90.0
Population with access to improved water source (% of population)	82.0
Population with improved access to sanitation facilities, rural (% of rural population with access)	70.0
Population with improved access to sanitation facilities, urban (% of urban population with access)	97.0

Source: National statistics/World Bank

Health Expenditure

Turkey: Public health expenditure 1998-2004

As stated

	1998	1999	2000	2001	2002	2003	2004
Public expenditure on pharmaceuticals and other medical non-durables (TL million)		710,590,000.0	1,278,710,000.0	1,982,010,000.0	2,973,020,000.0	3,711,270,000.0	4,777,370,141.0
Private insurance expenditure (% of total expenditure on health)		4.2	4.4	4.3	4.7	4.9	5.1
Share of total health expenditure in GDP (% of total GDP)	4.8	4.9	5.0	5.0	5.1	5.2	5.0
Health expenditure (US$ per capita)	149.0	179.0	196.0	137.0	172.0	180.0	187.0

Source: Euromonitor International from OECD/national statistics

Turkey: Private health expenditure 1998-2004

As stated

	1998	1999	2000	2001	2002	2003	2004
Consumer expenditure on health goods and medical services (TL million)	2,027,635,884.0	3,384,576,160.0	5,393,663,096.0	7,803,359,742.0	11,477,218,035.0	15,613,393,086.9	17,735,664,949.7
Consumer expenditure on health goods and medical services: real growth in national currency: 1990 = 100	276.7	280.1	288.1	270.0	273.9	297.4	311.1
Consumer expenditure on health goods and medical services as a percentage of total consumer expenditure	5.4	5.9	5.9	5.9	6.1	6.3	6.4

Source: National statistical offices/OECD/Eurostat/Euromonitor International

Turkey: Consumer expenditure on health goods and medical services by sector 1998-2004

% of total consumer expenditure on health goods and medical services

	1998	1999	2000	2001	2002	2003	2004
Pharmaceuticals, medical appliances/ equipment	35.6	38.6	39.1	40.2	41.8	42.1	42.2
Outpatient services	60.0	57.1	56.3	55.2	53.6	53.3	53.3
Hospital services	4.4	4.3	4.6	4.6	4.6	4.6	4.5
Total	100.0	100.0	100.0	100.0	100.0	100.0	100.0

Source: National statistical offices/OECD/Eurostat/Euromonitor International

Healthcare Infrastructure and Services

Turkey: Healthcare infrastructure and services by sector 1998-2004

As stated

	1998	1999	2000	2001	2002	2003	2004
Active pharmacists (number)	21,441	22,065	23,266	22,922	22,500	22,423	22,403
Consultations with GPs (general practitioners) (per capita)	2	2	3	3	4	4	4
Dentists (number)	13,421	14,226	16,002	15,866	16,000	16,285	16,556
Doctors (number)	77,344	81,988	85,117	90,757	91,000	91,224	91,278
Hospital admissions (number)	4,640,357	4,864,134	5,075,170	5,290,024	5,508,263	5,732,650	5,888,445
Hospitals and clinics (number)	19,441	19,474	18,631	18,750	18,668	18,484	18,266
In-patient beds ('000)	140	143	146	147	150	153	156
In-patient surgical procedures (number)	1,438,179	1,494,629	1,638,098	1,875,851	2,053,651	2,177,180	2,333,223
Midwives (number)	41,059	41,271	41,590	42,447	43,032	43,656	44,321
Nurses (number)	110,305	111,541	113,190	117,037	117,838	119,960	122,397
Out-patient contacts (per capita)	2	2	2	3	3	3	3

Source: Euromonitor International from national statistics

Turkey: Healthcare infrastructure and services by sector: growth 1998-2004

Year on year growth: % change in stated unit

	1998	1999	2000	2001	2002	2003	2004
Active pharmacists (number)	4.3	2.9	5.4	-1.5	-1.8	-0.3	-0.1
Consultations with GPs (general practitioners) (per capita)	5.0	0.0	19.0	4.0	50.0	2.6	0.0
Dentists (number)	5.4	6.0	12.5	-0.8	0.8	1.8	1.7
Doctors (number)	5.0	6.0	3.8	6.6	0.3	0.2	0.1
Hospital admissions (number)	5.3	4.8	4.3	4.2	4.1	4.1	2.7
Hospitals and clinics (number)	1.0	0.2	-4.3	0.6	-0.4	-1.0	-1.2
In-patient beds (number)	2.9	2.4	1.6	1.0	2.0	2.0	2.0
In-patient surgical procedures (number)	6.2	3.9	9.6	14.5	9.5	6.0	7.2
Midwives (number)	2.1	0.5	0.8	2.1	1.4	1.5	1.5
Nurses (number)	2.6	1.1	1.5	3.4	0.7	1.8	2.0
Out-patient contacts (per capita)	5.0	0.0	14.3	9.6	10.3	3.4	6.7

Source: Euromonitor International from national statistics

Immunisation

Turkey: Vaccination rates by disease type 1998-2004

%

	1998	1999	2000	2001	2002	2003	2004
Vaccination rate against DTP (diphtheria, tetanus, pertussis) 1 & 2 (%)			92.0	95.0	82.0	80.0	75.0
Vaccination rate against MMR (measles, mumps, rubella) (%)	80.0	82.0	86.0	90.0	82.0	88.0	89.0
Vaccination rate against polio (%)	76.0		85.0	88.0	78.0	77.0	73.0

Source: WHO

Infectious Diseases

Turkey: Incidence of disease by type 1998-2004

Table: 4.1287

Number

	1998	1999	2000	2001	2002	2003	2004
Incidence of AIDS	29	28	46	27	44	27	22
Incidence of diphtheria	6	4	4	5	2		
Incidence of measles	27,120	16,329	16,244	30,509	7,823		
Incidence of polio	26	0	0	0	0		

Source: WHO

Turkey: Incidence of disease by type: growth 1998-2004

Table: 4.1288

Year on year growth: %

	1998	1999	2000	2001	2002	2003	2004
Incidence of AIDS	-23.7	-3.4	64.3	-41.3	63.0	-38.6	-18.5
Incidence of diphtheria	200.0	-33.3	0.0	25.0	-60.0		
Incidence of measles	19.0	-39.8	-0.5	87.8	-74.4		
Incidence of polio	333.3	-100.0					

Source: WHO

Causes of Death

Turkey: Deaths by disease 1998-2004

Table: 4.1289

Number per 100,000 inhabitants

	1998	1999	2000	2001	2002	2003	2004
Deaths from heart disease	82.2	77.9	74.7	78.6	76.6	78.5	79.9
Deaths from lung cancer	41.6	40.3	38.5	39.6	39.5	40.2	40.4
Deaths from ulcers of the stomach and duodenum	36.0	32.4	33.4	35.5	35.6	37.1	38.8
Death by diseases of the digestive system	36.0	32.4	33.4	35.5	35.6	35.2	35.7
Deaths from chronic liver disease and cirrhosis	8.5	8.1	7.8	8.5	8.2	8.6	9.0

Source: WHO/Euromonitor International
Notes: Data is ranked in descending order by year 2004

Turkey: Deaths by disease: growth 1998-2004

Table: 4.1290

% year on year growth

	1998	1999	2000	2001	2002	2003	2004
Deaths from ulcers of the stomach and duodenum	-0.6	-10.0	3.1	6.3	0.3	4.2	4.5
Deaths from chronic liver disease and cirrhosis	-2.3	-4.7	-3.7	9.0	-3.5	4.9	4.1
Deaths from heart disease	-4.8	-5.2	-4.1	5.2	-2.5	2.5	1.8
Death by diseases of the digestive system	-0.6	-10.0	3.1	6.3	0.3	-1.1	1.6
Deaths from lung cancer	-3.9	-3.1	-4.5	2.9	-0.3	1.8	0.4

Source: WHO/Euromonitor International
Notes: Data is ranked in descending order by year 2004

Smoking

Turkey: Smoking prevalence in population aged 15+ 1998-2004

Table: 4.1291

% of population aged 15+

	1998	1999	2000	2001	2002	2003	2004
Smoking prevalence in population aged 15+ (% of population aged 15+)	48.8	49.3	50.1	50.4	51.1	51.8	52.5
Smoking prevalence in male population aged 15+ (% of male population)	67.9	67.9	68.2	68.7	68.4	68.4	68.3
Smoking prevalence in female population aged 15+ (% of female population)	29.5	30.4	31.8	31.9	33.6	35.0	36.5

Source: WHO/OECD/Euromonitor International

Nutrition and Obesity

Turkey: Nutrition and obesity 1998-2004

Table: 4.1292

As stated

	1998	1999	2000	2001	2002	2003	2004
Availability of fruit and vegetables (kg/capita/year)	341.1	351.0	349.0	330.3	321.8	313.9	299.6
Average supply of calories per day (calories per capita)	3,375.3	3,336.7	3,371.8	3,346.5	3,357.0	3,364.3	3,368.4
Average supply of fat per day (grams per capita)	87.5	86.2	91.9	87.6	91.6	90.6	90.2
Average supply of protein per day (grams per capita)	97.2	97.0	96.4	95.3	95.4	95.7	95.8
Obese population (BMI 30kg/sq m or more) (% of population aged 15+)	13.1	12.9	12.9	12.9	13.0	13.0	13.1

Source: WHO/OECD/Euromonitor International

Over-the-Counter Healthcare

Turkey: Trends in OTC healthcare retail sales 1998-2004

Table: 4.1293

As stated

	1998	1999	2000	2001	2002	2003	2004
OTC Healthcare (US$ million)	786.0	832.1	894.3	807.4	956.4	1,181.6	1,335.2
OTC Healthcare (US$ per capita)	12.1	12.6	13.3	11.8	13.7	16.7	18.6

Source: Euromonitor International from industry sources/national statistics

Turkey: OTC healthcare retail sales by sector 1998-2004

Table: 4.1294

% of OTC retail value sales

	1998	1999	2000	2001	2002	2003	2004
Analgesics	32.3	32.7	32.4	30.9	29.2	28.0	28.3
Cough, cold and allergy (hay fever) remedies	28.4	27.8	26.8	25.4	26.4	28.6	28.4
Digestive remedies	7.8	7.7	9.2	10.4	10.7	10.9	10.4
Medicated skin care	9.2	9.4	9.3	8.9	8.4	7.4	7.1
Vitamins and dietary supplements	8.5	8.7	8.7	8.5	8.5	9.0	9.3

Source: Euromonitor International from industry sources/national statistics
Notes: Only selected sectors are shown, so values are not expected to sum to 100

■ **Turkmenistan**

Socio-economic Parameters

Turkmenistan: Socio-economic parameters 1998-2004

Table: 4.1295

As stated

	1998	1999	2000	2001	2002	2003	2004
Population: national estimates at January 1st ('000)	4,439.5	4,522.9	4,603.1	4,681.0	4,756.3	4,829.6	4,902.5
% aged 0-14 yrs	38.3	37.5	36.8	36.0	35.1	34.2	33.3
% aged 15-64 yrs	57.5	58.2	58.9	59.7	60.4	61.2	62.0
% aged 65 + yrs	4.2	4.3	4.3	4.4	4.5	4.6	4.7
% Male	49.5	49.5	49.5	49.5	49.5	49.5	49.5
% Female	50.5	50.5	50.5	50.5	50.5	50.5	50.5
% Urban	44.7	44.7	44.8	45.0	45.1	45.7	46.1
Occupants per household at January 1st (Number)	3.7	3.7	3.6	3.6	3.6	3.5	3.4
Households ('000)	1,185.0	1,223.1	1,266.6	1,287.9	1,337.4	1,387.7	1,438.7
Annual rates of inflation (% growth)	16.8	23.5	8.0	11.6	8.8	5.6	5.9
GDP (TMM million)	13,995,000.0	20,056,000.0	25,648,000.0	35,119,000.0	45,240,000.0	55,709,000.0	63,480,000.0
GDP (US$ million)	2,861.9	3,856.9	4,932.3	6,753.7	8,700.0	10,713.3	12,272.2
GDP (US$ per capita)	644.6	852.8	1,071.5	1,442.8	1,829.2	2,218.2	2,503.3

Source: Euromonitor International from International Monetary Fund (IMF), International Financial Statistics and World Economic Outlook/UN/national statistics

Life Expectancy

Turkmenistan: Life expectancy 1998-2004

Table: 4.1296

As stated

	1998	1999	2000	2001	2002	2003	2004	% change 1998-2004
Life expectancy at birth: total population (years)	61.8	62.1	62.4	62.5	62.7	63.1	63.3	2.50
Life expectancy at birth: total population: year on year growth	0.6	0.6	0.5	0.1	0.3	0.6	0.3	
Healthy life expectancy at birth (years)	54.0			50.2	50.3			
Healthy life expectancy at birth: year on year growth					0.2			

Source: Euromonitor International from World Bank

Sanitation

Turkmenistan: Improved sanitary facilities and water source 2000

Table: 4.1297

As stated

	2000
Population with access to improved sanitary facilities (% of population)	100.0

Source: National statistics/World Bank

Health Expenditure

Turkmenistan: Public health expenditure 1998-2004

Table: 4.1298

As stated

	1998	1999	2000	2001	2002	2003	2004
Share of total health expenditure in GDP (% of total GDP)	5.0	5.0	4.0	4.1	4.3	4.3	4.5
Health expenditure (US$ per capita)	27.0	29.0	46.0	58.0	79.0	87.0	94.0

Source: Euromonitor International from OECD/national statistics

Turkmenistan: Private health expenditure 1998-2004

Table: 4.1299

As stated

	1998	1999	2000	2001	2002	2003	2004
Consumer expenditure on health goods and medical services (TMM million)	178,009.6	231,860.0	298,032.6	407,847.0	506,974.0	676,079.2	728,234.8
Consumer expenditure on health goods and medical services as a percentage of total consumer expenditure	4.1	3.8	3.8	3.8	4.0	4.0	4.0

Source: National statistical offices/OECD/Eurostat/Euromonitor International

Turkmenistan: Consumer expenditure on health goods and medical services by sector 1998-2004

Table: 4.1300

% of total consumer expenditure on health goods and medical services

	1998	1999	2000	2001	2002	2003	2004
Pharmaceuticals, medical appliances/ equipment	58.3	51.5	50.7	47.9	48.2	48.5	49.2
Outpatient services	36.3	44.7	45.9	48.8	49.1	48.8	48.1
Hospital services	5.4	3.8	3.4	3.3	2.7	2.7	2.6
Total	100.0	100.0	100.0	100.0	100.0	100.0	100.0

Source: National statistical offices/OECD/Eurostat/Euromonitor International

Healthcare Infrastructure and Services

Turkmenistan: Healthcare infrastructure and services by sector 1998-2004

Table: 4.1301

As stated

	1998	1999	2000	2001	2002	2003	2004
Dentists (number)	883	896	904	915	924	931	933
Doctors (number)	12,691						
Hospitals and clinics (number)	323	310	296	280	270	265	259
In-patient beds ('000)	36	35	34	33	32	31	30
Midwives (number)	3,611	3,575	3,439	3,370	3,260	3,136	3,044
Nurses (number)	22,879	22,412	22,355	22,025	21,873	21,783	21,680

Source: Euromonitor International from national statistics

Turkmenistan: Healthcare infrastructure and services by sector: growth 1998-2004

Table: 4.1302

Year on year growth: % change in stated unit

	1998	1999	2000	2001	2002	2003	2004
Dentists (number)	1.4	1.5	0.9	1.2	1.0	0.8	0.2
Doctors (number)	4.7						
Hospitals and clinics (number)	-2.4	-4.0	-4.5	-5.4	-3.6	-1.9	-2.3
In-patient beds (number)	8.5	-3.0	-2.9	-3.1	-2.0	-3.1	-3.2
Midwives (number)	-3.0	-1.0	-3.8	-2.0	-3.3	-3.8	-2.9
Nurses (number)	1.8	-2.0	-0.3	-1.5	-0.7	-0.4	-0.5

Source: Euromonitor International from national statistics

Immunisation

Turkmenistan: Vaccination rates by disease type 1998-2004

Table: 4.1303

%

	1998	1999	2000	2001	2002	2003	2004
Vaccination rate against DTP (diphtheria, tetanus, pertussis) 1 & 2 (%)			97.2	96.0	98.8	99.0	100.0
Vaccination rate against MMR (measles, mumps, rubella) (%)	99.0	97.2	96.5	97.6	88.0	90.0	92.0
Vaccination rate against polio (%)	99.0	98.2	98.0	94.3	99.0	99.0	99.0

Source: WHO

Infectious Diseases

Turkmenistan: Incidence of disease by type 1998-2004

Table: 4.1304

Number

	1998	1999	2000	2001	2002	2003	2004
Incidence of diphtheria	18	49	30	2	1		
Incidence of measles	1,035	452	113	9	11		
Incidence of polio	0	0	0	0	0		

Source: WHO

Turkmenistan: Incidence of disease by type: growth 1998-2004

Table: 4.1305

Year on year growth: %

	1998	1999	2000	2001	2002	2003	2004
Incidence of diphtheria	-52.6	172.2	-38.8	-93.3	-50.0		
Incidence of measles	174.5	-56.3	-75.0	-92.0	22.2		

Source: WHO

Causes of Death

Turkmenistan: Deaths by disease 1998-2004

Table: 4.1306

Number per 100,000 inhabitants

	1998	1999	2000	2001	2002	2003	2004
Deaths from heart disease	146.5	123.3	112.1	98.5	98.6	87.5	80.3
Death by diseases of the digestive system	33.1	29.8	28.2	29.7	30.0	30.9	31.6
Deaths from lung cancer	4.2	3.6	2.9	2.3	2.2	2.5	2.4
Deaths from ulcers of the stomach and duodenum	2.4	2.3	2.2	2.0	1.8	1.7	1.6

Source: WHO/Euromonitor International
Notes: Data is ranked in descending order by year 2004

Turkmenistan: Deaths by disease: growth 1998-2004

Table: 4.1307

% year on year growth

	1998	1999	2000	2001	2002	2003	2004
Death by diseases of the digestive system	4.7	-10.0	-5.4	5.3	1.0	3.0	2.2
Deaths from lung cancer	-21.6	-14.0	-19.4	-20.7	-4.3	13.6	-5.8
Deaths from heart disease	-7.7	-15.8	-9.1	-12.1	0.1	-11.3	-8.2
Deaths from ulcers of the stomach and duodenum	22.2	-5.0	-4.3	-9.1	-10.0	-5.6	-8.4

Source: WHO/Euromonitor International
Notes: Data is ranked in descending order by year 2004

Smoking

Turkmenistan: Smoking prevalence in population aged 15+ 1998-2004

Table: 4.1308

% of population aged 15+

	1998	1999	2000	2001	2002	2003	2004
Smoking prevalence in population aged 15+ (% of population aged 15+)	25.7	26.3	26.1	26.5	27.6	27.0	27.5
Smoking prevalence in male population aged 15+ (% of male population)	37.5	40.0	39.8	40.0	40.0	40.5	40.6
Smoking prevalence in female population aged 15+ (% of female population)	14.4	13.3	13.0	13.6	15.8	14.1	15.0

Source: WHO/OECD/Euromonitor International

Nutrition and Obesity

Turkmenistan: Nutrition and obesity 1998-2004

Table: 4.1309

As stated

	1998	1999	2000	2001	2002	2003	2004
Availability of fruit and vegetables (kg/capita/year)	123.0	116.3	115.0	115.6	115.9	115.5	114.8
Average supply of calories per day (calories per capita)	2,770.5	2,728.3	2,711.5	2,702.8	2,741.6	2,762.7	2,781.5
Average supply of fat per day (grams per capita)	73.5	74.2	72.4	64.9	62.9	60.3	57.3
Average supply of protein per day (grams per capita)	79.4	78.5	77.6	79.2	79.4	79.6	80.0
Obese population (BMI 30kg/sq m or more) (% of population aged 15+)	4.3	4.2	4.2	4.3	4.2	4.3	4.3

Source: WHO/OECD/Euromonitor International

■ Ukraine

Socio-economic Parameters

Ukraine: Socio-economic parameters 1998-2004

Table: 4.1310

As stated

	1998	1999	2000	2001	2002	2003	2004
Population: national estimates at January 1st ('000)	50,245.2	49,850.9	49,456.1	49,052.7	48,240.9	47,787.7	47,339.4
% aged 0-14 yrs	19.2	18.5	17.8	17.2	16.5	15.7	15.1
% aged 15-64 yrs	66.8	67.6	68.3	68.8	69.1	69.1	69.2
% aged 65+ yrs	14.0	13.9	13.8	14.0	14.5	15.2	15.7
% Male	46.5	46.5	46.5	46.4	46.3	46.2	46.2
% Female	53.5	53.5	53.5	53.6	53.7	53.8	53.8
% Urban	67.8	67.9	72.1	71.6	71.0	69.9	70.3
Occupants per household at January 1st (Number)	2.6	2.6	2.5	2.5	2.5	2.4	2.4
Households ('000)	19,412.0	19,546.6	19,640.1	19,750.7	19,668.2	19,730.9	19,763.8
Annual rates of inflation (% growth)	10.6	22.7	28.2	12.0	0.8	5.2	9.0
GDP (Hr million)	102,593.0	130,442.0	170,070.0	204,190.0	220,932.0	263,407.0	345,943.0
GDP (US$ million)	41,882.6	31,580.7	31,261.5	38,008.9	41,477.0	49,394.8	65,036.9
GDP (US$ per capita)	833.6	633.5	632.1	774.9	859.8	1,033.6	1,373.8

Source: Euromonitor International from International Monetary Fund (IMF), International Financial Statistics and World Economic Outlook/UN/national statistics

Life Expectancy

Ukraine: Life expectancy 1998-2004

Table: 4.1311

As stated

	1998	1999	2000	2001	2002	2003	2004	% change 1998-2004
Life expectancy at birth: total population (years)	67.7	67.7	67.8	67.7	67.2	67.2	66.9	-1.14
Life expectancy at birth: total population: year on year growth	0.0	0.0	0.1	-0.1	-0.7	-0.1	-0.4	
Healthy life expectancy at birth (years)	63.0			57.5	57.4			
Healthy life expectancy at birth: year on year growth					-0.1			

Source: *Euromonitor International from World Bank*

Sanitation

Ukraine: Improved sanitary facilities and water source 2000

Table: 4.1312

As stated

	2000
Population with access to improved sanitary facilities (% of population)	99.0
Population with access to improved water source (% of population)	98.0
Population with improved access to sanitation facilities, rural (% of rural population with access)	98.0
Population with improved access to sanitation facilities, urban (% of urban population with access)	100.0

Source: *National statistics/World Bank*

Health Expenditure

Ukraine: Public health expenditure 1998-2004

Table: 4.1313

As stated

	1998	1999	2000	2001	2002	2003	2004
Share of total health expenditure in GDP (% of total GDP)	5.0	4.3	4.2	4.3	4.5	4.7	4.7
Health expenditure (US$ per capita)	41.0	27.0	26.0	34.0	40.0	43.0	47.0

Source: *Euromonitor International from OECD/national statistics*

Ukraine: Private health expenditure 1998-2004

Table: 4.1314

As stated

	1998	1999	2000	2001	2002	2003	2004
Consumer expenditure on health goods and medical services (Hr million)	472.0	619.0	736.0	879.0	987.0	1,072.9	1,215.1
Consumer expenditure on health goods and medical services as a percentage of total consumer expenditure	0.8	0.9	0.8	0.8	0.9	0.8	0.8

Source: *National statistical offices/OECD/Eurostat/Euromonitor International*

Ukraine: Consumer expenditure on health goods and medical services by sector 1998-2004

Table: 4.1315

% of total consumer expenditure on health goods and medical services

	1998	1999	2000	2001	2002	2003	2004
Pharmaceuticals, medical appliances/ equipment	28.2	31.5	34.5	37.3	38.6	36.9	37.6
Outpatient services	48.7	46.4	44.4	42.7	42.5	42.4	42.3
Hospital services	23.1	22.1	21.1	20.0	18.9	20.8	20.0
Total	100.0	100.0	100.0	100.0	100.0	100.0	100.0

Source: National statistical offices/OECD/Eurostat/Euromonitor International

Healthcare Infrastructure and Services

Ukraine: Healthcare infrastructure and services by sector 1998-2004

Table: 4.1316

As stated

	1998	1999	2000	2001	2002	2003	2004
Dentists (number)	19,595						
Doctors (number)	227,000	226,000	226,000	226,000	226,664	227,829	228,863
Hospital admissions (number)	9,606,114	9,536,600	9,557,970	9,686,347	9,575,106	9,570,653	9,637,147
Hospitals and clinics (number)	3,300	3,200	3,086	2,976	2,860	2,740	2,644
In-patient beds ('000)	483	469	461	453	449	447	445
In-patient surgical procedures (number)			2,445,841	2,439,699	2,478,257	2,467,119	2,515,739
Nurses (number)	557,000	549,000	548,451	547,902	552,234	558,921	564,798
Out-patient contacts (per capita)	10	10	10	10	10	11	10

Source: Euromonitor International from national statistics

Ukraine: Healthcare infrastructure and services by sector: growth 1998-2004

Table: 4.1317

Year on year growth: % change in stated unit

	1998	1999	2000	2001	2002	2003	2004
Doctors (number)	0.0	-0.4	0.0	0.0	0.3	0.5	0.5
Hospital admissions (number)	-0.3	-0.7	0.2	1.3	-1.1	0.0	0.7
Hospitals and clinics (number)	-2.9	-3.0	-3.6	-3.6	-3.9	-4.2	-3.5
In-patient beds (number)	-4.0	-2.9	-1.7	-1.7	-0.9	-0.4	-0.4
In-patient surgical procedures (number)				-0.3	1.6	-0.4	2.0
Nurses (number)	-1.7	-1.4	-0.1	-0.1	0.8	1.2	1.1
Out-patient contacts (per capita)	5.4	0.0	3.1	1.0	2.0	1.9	-1.9

Source: Euromonitor International from national statistics

Immunisation

Ukraine: Vaccination rates by disease type 1998-2004

Table: 4.1318

%

	1998	1999	2000	2001	2002	2003	2004
Vaccination rate against DTP (diphtheria, tetanus, pertussis) 1 & 2 (%)				96.4	96.8	97.0	98.0
Vaccination rate against MMR (measles, mumps, rubella) (%)	96.0	99.0	98.8	98.8	98.9	99.0	99.0
Vaccination rate against polio (%)	98.0	98.0	98.9	99.0	99.0	99.0	99.0

Source: WHO

Infectious Diseases

Ukraine: Incidence of disease by type 1998-2004

Table: 4.1319

Number

	1998	1999	2000	2001	2002	2003	2004
Incidence of AIDS	287	580	648	361	1,353	1,915	1,528
Incidence of diphtheria	706	375	365	283	285		
Incidence of measles	5,107	1,389	817	16,970	7,587		
Incidence of polio	0	0	0	0	0		

Source: WHO

Ukraine: Incidence of disease by type: growth 1998-2004

Table: 4.1320

Year on year growth: %

	1998	1999	2000	2001	2002	2003	2004
Incidence of AIDS	48.7	102.1	11.7	-44.3	274.8	41.5	-20.2
Incidence of diphtheria	-48.2	-46.9	-2.7	-22.5	0.7		
Incidence of measles	-27.0	-72.8	-41.2	1,977.1	-55.3		

Source: WHO

Causes of Death

Ukraine: Deaths by disease 1998-2004

Table: 4.1321

Number per 100,000 inhabitants

	1998	1999	2000	2001	2002	2003	2004
Deaths from heart disease	538.7	573.4	607.6	642.6	677.7	713.2	755.4
Deaths from lung cancer	38.6	37.9	38.2	37.3	36.4	35.3	34.3
Death by diseases of the digestive system	30.4	31.2	31.8	30.2	30.2	29.2	28.3
Deaths from ulcers of the stomach and duodenum	4.3	4.1	4.2	4.1	4.0	3.9	3.8

Source: WHO/Euromonitor International
Notes: Data is ranked in descending order by year 2004

Ukraine: Deaths by disease: growth 1998-2004

Table: 4.1322

% year on year growth

	1998	1999	2000	2001	2002	2003	2004
Deaths from heart disease	-1.9	6.4	6.0	5.8	5.5	5.2	5.9
Deaths from ulcers of the stomach and duodenum	-3.2	-4.4	3.7	-2.8	-2.4	-2.5	-2.9
Deaths from lung cancer	0.6	-1.8	0.7	-2.3	-2.4	-3.0	-3.0
Death by diseases of the digestive system	-8.2	2.6	1.9	-5.0	0.0	-3.3	-3.1

Source: WHO/Euromonitor International
Notes: Data is ranked in descending order by year 2004

Smoking

Ukraine: Smoking prevalence in population aged 15+ 1998-2004

Table: 4.1323

% of population aged 15+

	1998	1999	2000	2001	2002	2003	2004
Smoking prevalence in population aged 15+ (% of population aged 15+)	37.5	37.1	34.0	33.8	33.6	33.5	33.4
Smoking prevalence in male population aged 15+ (% of male population)	55.2	57.7	58.0	61.5	61.9	61.2	61.4
Smoking prevalence in female population aged 15+ (% of female population)	22.8	19.9	14.0	14.0	13.8	13.7	13.8

Source: WHO/OECD/Euromonitor International

Nutrition and Obesity

Ukraine: Nutrition and obesity 1998-2004

Table: 4.1324

As stated

	1998	1999	2000	2001	2002	2003	2004
Availability of fruit and vegetables (kg/capita/year)	122.8	118.7	132.8	134.9	144.7	153.6	116.6
Average supply of calories per day (calories per capita)	2,824.3	2,781.5	2,897.9	3,003.2	3,053.6	3,128.1	3,205.4
Average supply of fat per day (grams per capita)	73.2	73.6	74.3	76.2	81.7	83.4	80.2
Average supply of protein per day (grams per capita)	81.3	78.9	80.2	82.9	84.1	85.6	87.3
Microbiological food-borne diseases (per 100000 population)	55.0	55.0	46.0	48.0	47.0	45.0	43.0
Obese population (BMI 30kg/sq m or more) (% of population aged 15+)	12.2	12.3	12.3	12.4	12.5	12.7	12.7

Source: WHO/OECD/Euromonitor International

Over-the-Counter Healthcare

Ukraine: Trends in OTC healthcare retail sales 1998-2004

Table: 4.1325

As stated

	1998	1999	2000	2001	2002	2003	2004
OTC Healthcare (Hr million)	487.7	566.1	753.2	913.9	1,072.6	1,233.3	1,382.4
OTC Healthcare: real growth in national currency: 1998 = 100	100.0	94.6	98.2	106.4	123.9	135.5	140.2
OTC Healthcare: year on year (% real growth)	7.8	-5.4	3.8	8.4	16.5	9.3	3.5
OTC Healthcare (Hr per capita)	9.7	11.4	15.2	18.6	22.2	25.8	29.2

Source: Euromonitor International from industry sources/national statistics

Ukraine: OTC healthcare retail sales by sector 1998-2004

Table: 4.1326

% of OTC retail value sales

	1998	1999	2000	2001	2002	2003	2004
Analgesics	12.9	12.9	12.0	11.6	11.2	10.6	10.1
Cough, cold and allergy (hay fever) remedies	29.9	30.5	32.8	33.9	33.6	34.0	34.3
Digestive remedies	15.6	15.6	14.6	13.8	13.4	12.9	12.6
Medicated skin care	7.4	7.4	7.3	7.5	7.7	7.7	7.7
Vitamins and dietary supplements	19.8	20.1	21.5	22.1	23.7	25.1	26.1

Source: Euromonitor International from industry sources/national statistics
Notes: Only selected sectors are shown, so values are not expected to sum to 100

■ **United Arab Emirates**

Socio-economic Parameters

United Arab Emirates: Socio-economic parameters 1998-2004

Table: 4.1327

As stated

	1998	1999	2000	2001	2002	2003	2004
Population: national estimates at January 1st ('000)	2,834.0	3,033.0	3,247.0	3,488.0	3,754.0	3,966.4	4,180.1
% aged 0-14 yrs	25.7	25.6	25.4	25.3	25.2	25.0	24.9
% aged 15-64 yrs	73.3	73.4	73.6	73.7	73.9	74.0	74.2
% aged 65 + yrs	1.0	1.0	1.0	1.0	1.0	1.0	0.9
% Male	67.1	67.2	67.4	67.6	67.7	67.8	67.9
% Female	32.9	32.8	32.6	32.4	32.3	32.2	32.1
% Urban	85.1	85.5	85.6	85.9	86.2	86.5	86.8
Occupants per household at January 1st (Number)	6.0	6.0	6.1	6.2	6.4	6.4	6.4
Households ('000)	476.0	505.2	536.0	559.0	584.9	618.5	652.2
Annual rates of inflation (% growth)	2.0	2.1	1.4	2.8	3.1	2.8	3.8
GDP (AED million)	170,666.0	202,698.0	257,991.0	255,408.0	263,359.0	295,361.0	351,535.0
GDP (US$ million)	46,471.3	55,193.5	70,249.4	69,546.1	71,711.1	80,425.1	95,720.9
GDP (US$ per capita)	16,397.8	18,197.7	21,635.1	19,938.7	19,102.6	20,276.6	22,898.9

Source: Euromonitor International from International Monetary Fund (IMF), International Financial Statistics and World Economic Outlook/UN/national statistics

Life Expectancy

United Arab Emirates: Life expectancy 1998-2004

Table: 4.1328

As stated

	1998	1999	2000	2001	2002	2003	2004	% change 1998-2004
Life expectancy at birth: total population (years)	72.3	72.4	71.6	71.7	72.5	72.7	73.0	1.01
Life expectancy at birth: total population: year on year growth	0.2	0.2	-1.1	0.1	1.1	0.3	0.4	
Healthy life expectancy at birth (years)	65.0			62.4	62.5			
Healthy life expectancy at birth: year on year growth					0.1			

Source: Euromonitor International from World Bank

Health Expenditure

United Arab Emirates: Public health expenditure 1998-2004

Table: 4.1329

As stated

	1998	1999	2000	2001	2002	2003	2004
Share of total health expenditure in GDP (% of total GDP)	4.0	3.7	3.5	3.5	3.6	3.7	3.7
Health expenditure (US$ per capita)	724.0	704.0	787.0	824.0	802.0	835.0	851.0

Source: Euromonitor International from OECD/national statistics

United Arab Emirates: Private health expenditure 1998-2004

Table: 4.1330

As stated

	1998	1999	2000	2001	2002	2003	2004
Consumer expenditure on health goods and medical services (AED million)	2,807.0	2,805.0	2,795.0	2,867.0	2,983.0	3,254.3	3,415.0
Consumer expenditure on health goods and medical services: real growth in national currency: 1990 = 100	166.2	162.7	159.8	159.5	161.3	170.7	171.2
Consumer expenditure on health goods and medical services as a percentage of total consumer expenditure	3.1	3.2	3.3	3.2	3.3	3.3	3.3

Source: National statistical offices/OECD/Eurostat/Euromonitor International

United Arab Emirates: Consumer expenditure on health goods and medical services by sector 1998-2004

Table: 4.1331

% of total consumer expenditure on health goods and medical services

	1998	1999	2000	2001	2002	2003	2004
Pharmaceuticals, medical appliances/ equipment	32.5	32.2	31.7	31.6	31.3	31.8	32.4
Outpatient services	59.5	59.3	59.4	58.8	58.6	58.1	57.4
Hospital services	8.0	8.5	8.9	9.6	10.1	10.2	10.3
Total	100.0	100.0	100.0	100.0	100.0	100.0	100.0

Source: National statistical offices/OECD/Eurostat/Euromonitor International

Healthcare Infrastructure and Services

United Arab Emirates: Healthcare infrastructure and services by sector 1998-2004

Table: 4.1332

As stated

	1998	1999	2000	2001	2002	2003	2004
Dentists (number)	838	880	750	784	1,071	1,127	1,160
Doctors (number)	5,664	5,235	5,222	6,003	6,328	6,540	6,633
Hospitals and clinics (number)	59	60	59	62	65	67	69
In-patient beds ('000)	8	7	7	8	8	8	8
Nurses (number)	12,288	10,390	10,762	12,280	13,211	13,764	13,966

Source: Euromonitor International from national statistics

United Arab Emirates: Healthcare infrastructure and services by sector: growth 1998-2004

Table: 4.1333

Year on year growth: % change in stated unit

	1998	1999	2000	2001	2002	2003	2004
Dentists (number)	104.9	5.0	-14.8	4.5	36.6	5.2	2.9
Doctors (number)	33.3	-7.6	-0.2	15.0	5.4	3.4	1.4
Hospitals and clinics (number)	5.4	1.7	-1.7	5.1	4.8	3.1	3.0
In-patient beds (number)	26.0	-16.4	1.2	6.7	4.2	1.5	0.0
Nurses (number)	29.5	-15.4	3.6	14.1	7.6	4.2	1.5

Source: Euromonitor International from national statistics

Immunisation

United Arab Emirates: Vaccination rates by disease type 1998-2004

Table: 4.1334

%

	1998	1999	2000	2001	2002	2003	2004
Vaccination rate against DTP (diphtheria, tetanus, pertussis) 1 & 2 (%)			96.0	96.0	96.0	96.0	96.0
Vaccination rate against MMR (measles, mumps, rubella) (%)	95.0	96.0	94.0	94.0	94.0	94.0	93.0
Vaccination rate against polio (%)	94.0	94.0	94.0	94.0	94.0	94.0	94.0

Source: WHO

Infectious Diseases

United Arab Emirates: Incidence of disease by type 1998-2004

Number

	1998	1999	2000	2001	2002	2003	2004
Incidence of AIDS	1	2	3	2	4	1	2
Incidence of diphtheria	0	1	0	0	0		
Incidence of measles	296	117	69	30	53		
Incidence of polio	0	0	0	0	0		

Source: WHO

United Arab Emirates: Incidence of disease by type: growth 1998-2004

Year on year growth: %

	1998	1999	2000	2001	2002	2003	2004
Incidence of AIDS	0.0	100.0	50.0	-33.3	100.0	-75.0	100.0
Incidence of diphtheria			-100.0				
Incidence of measles	21.8	-60.5	-41.0	-56.5	76.7		

Source: WHO

Smoking

United Arab Emirates: Smoking prevalence in population aged 15+ 1998-2004

% of population aged 15+

	1998	1999	2000	2001	2002	2003	2004
Smoking prevalence in population aged 15+ (% of population aged 15+)	26.2	26.0	25.7	25.9	25.1	25.4	25.6
Smoking prevalence in male population aged 15+ (% of male population)	25.0	25.5	26.2	26.3	25.9	26.1	26.5
Smoking prevalence in female population aged 15+ (% of female population)	29.5	27.2	24.3	24.7	22.8	23.7	23.4

Source: WHO/OECD/Euromonitor International

Nutrition and Obesity

United Arab Emirates: Nutrition and obesity 1998-2004

As stated

	1998	1999	2000	2001	2002	2003	2004
Average supply of calories per day (calories per capita)	3,150.3	3,173.8	3,166.9	3,205.2	3,224.7	3,241.6	3,262.2
Average supply of fat per day (grams per capita)	103.1	102.2	94.4	95.4	97.8	98.3	99.2
Average supply of protein per day (grams per capita)	98.4	101.7	99.6	100.2	101.0	101.3	101.7
Obese population (BMI 30kg/sq m or more) (% of population aged 15+)	26.3	26.4	26.7	26.7	26.8	26.8	26.8

Source: WHO/OECD/Euromonitor International

Over-the-Counter Healthcare

United Arab Emirates: Trends in OTC healthcare retail sales 1998-2004

Table: 4.1339

As stated

	1998	1999	2000	2001	2002	2003	2004
OTC Healthcare (US$ million)	5.1	5.5	6.3	6.9	7.1	7.1	7.7
OTC Healthcare (US$ per capita)	1.8	1.8	1.9	2.0	1.9	1.8	1.8

Source: Euromonitor International from industry sources/national statistics

United Arab Emirates: OTC healthcare retail sales by sector 1998-2004

Table: 4.1340

% of OTC retail value sales

	1998	1999	2000	2001	2002	2003	2004
Analgesics	13.0	13.2	13.5	13.7	14.2	14.4	14.5
Cough, cold and allergy (hay fever) remedies	21.6	21.6	21.6	21.5	21.9	21.9	21.8
Digestive remedies	6.0	6.0	5.9	5.9	5.9	5.9	5.8
Medicated skin care	15.0	15.0	15.0	15.0	13.3	13.2	13.1
Vitamins and dietary supplements	40.1	40.0	39.7	39.8	40.6	40.5	40.7

Source: Euromonitor International from industry sources/national statistics
Notes: Only selected sectors are shown, so values are not expected to sum to 100

■ United Kingdom

Socio-economic Parameters

United Kingdom: Socio-economic parameters 1998-2004

Table: 4.1341

As stated

	1998	1999	2000	2001	2002	2003	2004
Population: national estimates at January 1st ('000)	58,305.3	58,481.1	58,643.2	59,050.8	59,229.0	59,427.4	59,612.6
% aged 0-14 yrs	19.4	19.3	19.1	18.8	18.6	18.3	18.1
% aged 15-64 yrs	64.7	64.9	65.0	65.4	65.5	65.7	65.8
% aged 65+ yrs	15.9	15.8	15.8	15.9	15.9	16.0	16.1
% Male	48.6	48.6	48.6	48.8	48.8	48.8	48.9
% Female	51.4	51.4	51.4	51.2	51.2	51.2	51.1
% Urban	89.4	89.4	89.5	89.5	89.6	89.7	89.7
Occupants per household at January 1st (Number)	2.4	2.4	2.4	2.4	2.4	2.4	2.4
Households ('000)	24,093.5	24,286.1	24,469.4	24,761.7	24,929.0	25,095.7	25,262.7
Annual rates of inflation (% growth)	3.4	1.6	2.9	1.8	1.6	2.9	3.0
GDP (£ million)	859,436.0	903,167.0	950,561.0	994,309.0	1,044,145.0	1,101,144.0	1,160,339.0
GDP (US$ million)	1,423,322.0	1,461,300.5	1,438,215.2	1,431,371.0	1,564,911.6	1,797,868.3	2,124,462.6
GDP (US$ per capita)	24,411.6	24,987.6	24,524.8	24,239.6	26,421.4	30,253.2	35,637.8

Source: Euromonitor International from International Monetary Fund (IMF), International Financial Statistics and World Economic Outlook/UN/national statistics

Life Expectancy

United Kingdom: Life expectancy 1998-2004

Table: 4.1342

As stated

	1998	1999	2000	2001	2002	2003	2004	% change 1998-2004
Life expectancy at birth: total population (years)	77.0	77.2	77.0	77.5	78.2	78.5	78.9	2.52
Life expectancy at birth: total population: year on year growth	0.3	0.3	-0.2	0.6	0.8	0.4	0.6	
Healthy life expectancy at birth (years)	72.0			69.2	69.6			
Healthy life expectancy at birth: year on year growth					0.6			

Source: Euromonitor International from World Bank

Sanitation

United Kingdom: Improved sanitary facilities and water source 2000

Table: 4.1343

As stated

	2000
Population with access to improved sanitary facilities (% of population)	100.0
Population with access to improved water source (% of population)	100.0
Population with improved access to sanitation facilities, rural (% of rural population with access)	100.0
Population with improved access to sanitation facilities, urban (% of urban population with access)	100.0

Source: National statistics/World Bank

Health Expenditure

United Kingdom: Public health expenditure 1998-2004

Table: 4.1344

As stated

	1998	1999	2000	2001	2002	2003	2004
Public expenditure on pharmaceuticals and other medical non-durables (£ million)	5,896.0	6,298.0	6,914.0	7,649.0	8,809.0	9,711.0	10,984.2
Private insurance expenditure (% of total expenditure on health)							
Share of total health expenditure in GDP (% of total GDP)	6.9	7.2	7.3	7.6	7.6	7.8	7.6
Health expenditure (US$ per capita)	1,688.0	1,781.0	1,784.0	1,837.0	2,031.0	2,114.0	2,224.0

Source: Euromonitor International from OECD/national statistics

United Kingdom: Private health expenditure 1998-2004

Table: 4.1345

As stated

	1998	1999	2000	2001	2002	2003	2004
Consumer expenditure on health goods and medical services (£ million)	8,081.0	8,529.0	8,987.0	9,502.0	10,383.0	11,638.0	12,465.6
Consumer expenditure on health goods and medical services: real growth in national currency: 1990 = 100	141.2	146.7	150.2	156.0	167.7	182.7	190.0
Consumer expenditure on health goods and medical services as a percentage of total consumer expenditure	1.5	1.5	1.5	1.5	1.6	1.7	1.7

Source: National statistical offices/OECD/Eurostat/Euromonitor International

United Kingdom: Consumer expenditure on health goods and medical services by sector 1998-2004

Table: 4.1346

% of total consumer expenditure on health goods and medical services

	1998	1999	2000	2001	2002	2003	2004
Pharmaceuticals, medical appliances/ equipment	58.1	58.5	58.6	60.7	58.0	61.5	61.2
Outpatient services	24.8	24.5	24.2	23.2	25.6	23.1	23.3
Hospital services	17.1	16.9	17.2	16.1	16.4	15.3	15.6
Total	100.0	100.0	100.0	100.0	100.0	100.0	100.0

Source: National statistical offices/OECD/Eurostat/Euromonitor International

Healthcare Infrastructure and Services

United Kingdom: Healthcare infrastructure and services by sector 1998-2004

Table: 4.1347

As stated

	1998	1999	2000	2001	2002	2003	2004
Active pharmacists (number)	33,724	31,964	29,751	28,136	27,000	26,348	26,437
Consultations with GPs (general practitioners) (per capita)	5	5	5	5	4	4	4
Dentists (number)	24,174	24,785	25,234	25,914	26,490	27,179	27,900
Doctors (number)	112,889	115,089	117,579	120,912	123,236	126,113	129,439
Hospital admissions (number)	8,964,200	9,064,867	9,155,867	9,246,867	9,337,867	9,438,296	9,443,708
In-patient beds ('000)	230	230	230	230	230	232	234
Nurses (number)	490,000	515,000	515,000	530,000	545,000	561,109	576,091
Out-patient contacts (per capita)	5	5	5	5	5	4	4

Source: Euromonitor International from national statistics

United Kingdom: Healthcare infrastructure and services by sector: growth 1998-2004

Table: 4.1348

Year on year growth: % change in stated unit

	1998	1999	2000	2001	2002	2003	2004
Active pharmacists (number)	-4.8	-5.2	-6.9	-5.4	-4.0	-2.4	0.3
Consultations with GPs (general practitioners) (per capita)	-6.9	-5.6	-3.9	-7.1	-3.3	0.0	-2.3
Dentists (number)	3.2	2.5	1.8	2.7	2.2	2.6	2.7
Doctors (number)	2.7	1.9	2.2	2.8	1.9	2.3	2.6
Hospital admissions (number)	0.7	1.1	1.0	1.0	1.0	1.1	0.1
In-patient beds (number)	0.0	0.0	0.0	0.0	0.0	0.9	0.9
Nurses (number)	4.3	5.1	0.0	2.9	2.8	3.0	2.7
Out-patient contacts (per capita)	-7.7	-2.3	-4.5	-4.7	-0.1	-12.5	-7.1

Source: Euromonitor International from national statistics

Immunisation

United Kingdom: Vaccination rates by disease type 1998-2004

Table: 4.1349

%

	1998	1999	2000	2001	2002	2003	2004
Vaccination rate against MMR (measles, mumps, rubella) (%)	91.0	90.0	88.1	84.7	83.0	82.0	80.0
Vaccination rate against polio (%)	93.0		92.4	94.2	91.0	91.0	90.0

Source: WHO

Infectious Diseases

United Kingdom: Incidence of disease by type 1998-2004

Table: 4.1350

Number

	1998	1999	2000	2001	2002	2003	2004
Incidence of AIDS	963	790	737	824	807	810	803
Incidence of diphtheria	0		2	4	6		
Incidence of measles	74		104	73	314		
Incidence of polio	0	0	0		0		

Source: WHO

United Kingdom: Incidence of disease by type: growth 1998-2004

Table: 4.1351

Year on year growth: %

	1998	1999	2000	2001	2002	2003	2004
Incidence of AIDS	-30.1	-18.0	-6.7	11.8	-2.1	0.4	-0.9
Incidence of diphtheria				100.0	50.0		
Incidence of measles	-98.5			-29.8	330.1		

Source: WHO

Causes of Death

United Kingdom: Deaths by disease 1998-2004

Table: 4.1352

Number per 100,000 inhabitants

	1998	1999	2000	2001	2002	2003	2004
Death by diseases of the circulatory system	276.2	265.4	256.1	255.0	246.2	236.4	231.8
Deaths from heart disease	234.2	221.9	215.6	208.0	200.4	193.0	185.8
Death by malignant neoplasms (cancers)	188.8	184.7	182.4	181.5	179.1	176.1	174.9
Death by diseases of the respiratory system	100.4	108.5	108.5	114.0	115.1	107.5	107.6
Deaths from lung cancer	59.0	57.5	57.0	56.1	55.2	54.3	53.1
Death by diseases of the digestive system	27.6	28.4	28.1	28.8	28.4	28.1	27.9
Deaths from chronic liver disease and cirrhosis	9.1	9.6	10.2	10.7	11.1	11.6	12.0
Deaths from ulcers of the stomach and duodenum	7.3	7.4	7.4	7.4	7.4	7.4	7.3

Source: WHO/Euromonitor International
Notes: Data is ranked in descending order by year 2004

United Kingdom: Deaths by disease: growth 1998-2004

Table: 4.1353

% year on year growth

	1998	1999	2000	2001	2002	2003	2004
Deaths from chronic liver disease and cirrhosis	8.9	5.1	6.4	4.9	3.7	4.5	3.4
Death by diseases of the respiratory system	-2.7	8.1	0.0	5.1	1.0	-6.6	0.1
Death by malignant neoplasms (cancers)	-0.5	-2.2	-1.2	-0.5	-1.3	-1.7	-0.7
Death by diseases of the digestive system	2.6	2.9	-1.1	2.5	-1.4	-1.1	-0.7
Deaths from ulcers of the stomach and duodenum	-1.1	1.8	-0.6	0.0	0.0	0.0	-1.0
Death by diseases of the circulatory system	-2.0	-3.9	-3.5	-0.4	-3.5	-4.0	-2.0
Deaths from lung cancer	-0.1	-2.5	-0.9	-1.6	-1.6	-1.6	-2.2
Deaths from heart disease	-1.4	-5.2	-2.8	-3.5	-3.7	-3.7	-3.7

Source: WHO/Euromonitor International
Notes: Data is ranked in descending order by year 2004

United Kingdom: Other selected causes of death: 1998-2004

Table: 4.1354

Number per 100,000 inhabitants

	1998	1999	2000	2001	2002	2003	2004
Death by injury and poisoning	27.4	27.7	27.5	27.7	27.7	27.2	27.1
Death by suicide and self-inflicted injury	6.9	6.9	7.1	7.2	7.3	7.0	7.0
Death by motor traffic accidents	5.8	5.8	5.6	5.5	5.4	5.3	5.2

Source: Euromonitor International from national statistics
Notes: Data is ranked in descending order by year 2004

United Kingdom: Other selected causes of death: growth 1998-2004

Table: 4.1355

% year on year growth

	1998	1999	2000	2001	2002	2003	2004
Death by injury and poisoning	-1.8	1.1	-0.7	0.7	0.0	-1.8	-0.3
Death by suicide and self-inflicted injury	6.2	0.0	2.9	1.4	1.4	-4.1	-0.5
Death by motor traffic accidents	-7.9	0.0	-3.4	-1.8	-1.8	-1.9	-2.6

Source: Euromonitor International from national statistics
Notes: Data is ranked in descending order by year 2004

Smoking

United Kingdom: Smoking prevalence in population aged 15+ 1998-2004

Table: 4.1356

% of population aged 15+

	1998	1999	2000	2001	2002	2003	2004
Smoking prevalence in population aged 15+ (% of population aged 15+)	27.0	27.0	27.0	27.0	26.6	25.4	24.8
Smoking prevalence in male population aged 15+ (% of male population)	28.0	28.5	29.0	28.0	25.4	25.1	24.6
Smoking prevalence in female population aged 15+ (% of female population)	26.0	25.6	25.0	26.0	27.7	25.7	25.0

Source: WHO/OECD/Euromonitor International

Nutrition and Obesity

United Kingdom: Nutrition and obesity 1998-2004

Table: 4.1357

As stated

	1998	1999	2000	2001	2002	2003	2004
Availability of fruit and vegetables (kg/capita/year)	172.4	172.6	167.9	180.9	183.0	187.4	191.4
Average supply of calories per day (calories per capita)	3,344.9	3,395.6	3,357.6	3,420.7	3,412.2	3,411.5	3,418.7
Average supply of fat per day (grams per capita)	142.0	143.3	142.2	142.5	138.9	137.4	136.2
Average supply of protein per day (grams per capita)	98.9	99.6	99.4	102.1	102.4	103.0	104.0
Obese population (BMI 30kg/sq m or more) (% of population aged 15+)	19.3	19.9	20.3	22.3	23.0	24.5	25.9

Source: WHO/OECD/Euromonitor International

Over-the-Counter Healthcare

United Kingdom: Trends in OTC healthcare retail sales 1998-2004

Table: 4.1358

As stated

	1998	1999	2000	2001	2002	2003	2004
OTC Healthcare (£ million)	1,909.2	2,058.2	2,184.4	2,272.2	2,325.2	2,405.1	2,473.7
OTC Healthcare: real growth in national currency: 1998 = 100	100.0	106.2	109.5	111.8	112.6	113.2	114.6
OTC Healthcare: year on year (% real growth)	1.5	6.2	3.1	2.2	0.7	0.5	1.2
OTC Healthcare (£ per capita)	32.7	35.2	37.2	38.5	39.3	40.5	41.5

Source: Euromonitor International from industry sources/national statistics

United Kingdom: OTC healthcare retail sales by sector 1998-2004

Table: 4.1359

% of OTC retail value sales

	1998	1999	2000	2001	2002	2003	2004
Analgesics	20.9	21.1	21.4	21.2	21.2	21.1	20.2
Cough, cold and allergy (hay fever) remedies	25.3	26.0	25.7	25.2	24.5	24.0	23.1
Digestive remedies	111,051.3	104,604.5	100,135.0	96,916.6	94,418.2	91,365.8	89,452.7
Digestive remedies	11.7	11.3	11.2	11.1	11.3	11.3	11.6
Medicated skin care	14.5	14.4	14.5	15.0	15.5	15.8	16.0
Vitamins and dietary supplements	19.9	19.2	19.0	18.4	17.8	16.9	17.9

Source: Euromonitor International from industry sources/national statistics
Notes: Only selected sectors are shown, so values are not expected to sum to 100

Health and Wellness

United Kingdom: Retail sales of packaged foods by health and wellness category 2002-2004

Table: 4.1360

£ million

	2002	2003	2004
Packaged food: Total	41,359.4	42,929.2	44,014.8
Better for you	3,781.1	3,965.1	4,171.1
For food intolerance	62.2	76.4	85.6
Fortified/functional	672.8	728.4	780.5
Organic	640.9	698.4	760.9

Source: Euromonitor International from industry sources/national statistics

United Kingdom: Per capita sales of packaged foods by health and wellness category 2002-2004

Table: 4.1361

£ per capita

	2002	2003	2004
Better for you	63.5	66.4	69.7
For food intolerance	1.0	1.3	1.4
Fortified/functional	11.3	12.2	13.0
Organic	10.8	11.7	12.7

Source: Euromonitor International from industry sources/national statistics

United Kingdom: Retail sales of packaged food by health and wellness category: % share of total packaged food market 2002-2004

Table: 4.1362

% value

	2002	2003	2004
Better for you	9.1	9.2	9.5
For food intolerance	0.2	0.2	0.2
Fortified/functional	1.6	1.7	1.8
Organic	1.5	1.6	1.7

Source: Euromonitor International from industry sources/national statistics

United Kingdom: Retail sales of packaged food by health and wellness category: real growth index 2002-2004

Table: 4.1363

2002 = 100

	2002	2003	2004
Better for you	100.00	102.01	104.69
For food intolerance	100.00	119.57	130.63
Fortified/functional	100.00	105.32	110.10
Organic	100.00	106.01	112.67

Source: Euromonitor International from industry sources/national statistics

United Kingdom: Retail sales of better-for-you packaged foods by sector 2002-2004

Table: 4.1364

% of total packaged food / as stated

	2002	2003	2004	% real change in value 2002-2004
Combination	0.26	0.25	0.24	-4.22
Reduced carb	0.00	0.01	0.03	693.25
Reduced fat	8.33	8.41	8.57	3.92
Reduced salt	0.02	0.02	0.04	147.26

Source: Euromonitor International from industry sources/national statistics

United Kingdom: Retail sales of packaged foods for food intolerances by sector 2002-2004

Table: 4.1365

% of total packaged food / as stated

	2002	2003	2004	% real change in value 2002-2004
Diabetic	0.03	0.03	0.03	-2.10
Gluten-free	0.08	0.10	0.12	53.65
Lactose-free	0.04	0.05	0.05	11.70

Source: Euromonitor International from industry sources/national statistics

United Kingdom: Retail sales of naturally healthy packaged foods by sector 2002-2004

Table: 4.1366

% of total packaged food / as stated

	2002	2003	2004	% real change in value 2002-2004
High fibre	2.15	2.16	2.17	2.34
Other naturally healthy food	0.70	0.71	0.71	2.99
Soy-based dairy alternatives	0.14	0.15	0.17	22.21

Source: Euromonitor International from industry sources/national statistics

■ **USA**

Socio-economic Parameters

USA: Socio-economic parameters 1998-2004

Table: 4.1367

As stated

	1998	1999	2000	2001	2002	2003	2004
Population: national estimates at January 1st ('000)	270,248.0	272,690.8	275,135.2	277,504.2	279,807.3	282,068.0	284,322.1
% aged 0-14 yrs	21.5	21.4	21.3	21.2	21.1	21.0	20.9
% aged 15-64 yrs	65.8	65.9	66.1	66.3	66.5	66.7	66.9
% aged 65 + yrs	12.7	12.7	12.6	12.5	12.4	12.3	12.3
% Male	48.9	48.9	48.9	48.9	48.9	48.9	49.0
% Female	51.1	51.1	51.1	51.1	51.1	51.1	51.0
% Urban	76.8	77.0	77.1	77.3	77.5	77.8	78.1
Occupants per household at January 1st (Number)	2.7	2.7	2.6	2.6	2.6	2.6	2.6
Households ('000)	101,139.0	102,191.3	105,780.1	107,049.9	108,297.4	109,282.8	110,242.3
Annual rates of inflation (% growth)	1.6	2.2	3.4	2.8	1.6	2.3	2.7
GDP (US$ million)	8,746,970.0	9,268,420.0	9,816,970.0	10,127,950.0	10,486,975.0	11,004,050.0	11,733,475.0
GDP (US$ per capita)	32,366.5	33,988.8	35,680.5	36,496.6	37,479.3	39,012.0	41,268.3

Source: Euromonitor International from International Monetary Fund (IMF), International Financial Statistics and World Economic Outlook/UN/national statistics

Life Expectancy

USA: Life expectancy 1998-2004

Table: 4.1368

As stated

	1998	1999	2000	2001	2002	2003	2004	% change 1998-2004
Life expectancy at birth: total population (years)	76.4	76.6	76.8	77.0	77.3	77.4	77.6	1.62
Life expectancy at birth: total population: year on year growth	0.3	0.3	0.3	0.3	0.4	0.1	0.3	
Healthy life expectancy at birth (years)	70.0			67.4	67.6			
Healthy life expectancy at birth: year on year growth					0.2			

Source: Euromonitor International from World Bank

Sanitation

USA: Improved sanitary facilities and water source 2000

Table: 4.1369

As stated

	2000
Population with access to improved sanitary facilities (% of population)	100.0
Population with access to improved water source (% of population)	100.0
Population with improved access to sanitation facilities, rural (% of rural population with access)	100.0
Population with improved access to sanitation facilities, urban (% of urban population with access)	100.0

Source: National statistics/World Bank

Health Expenditure

USA: Public health expenditure 1998-2004

Table: 4.1370

As stated

	1998	1999	2000	2001	2002	2003	2004
Public expenditure on pharmaceuticals and other medical non-durables (US$ million)	19,627.0	23,390.0	27,978.0	32,962.0	37,833.0	43,923.0	52,385.9
Private insurance expenditure (% of total expenditure on health)	33.9	34.4	35.1	35.7	36.2	36.5	37.0
Share of total health expenditure in GDP (% of total GDP)	13.0	13.0	13.1	13.9	13.7	13.9	13.8
Health expenditure (US$ per capita)	4,096.0	4,298.0	4,538.0	4,869.0	5,267.0	5,590.0	5,941.0

Source: Euromonitor International from OECD/national statistics

USA: Private health expenditure 1998-2004

Table: 4.1371

As stated

	1998	1999	2000	2001	2002	2003	2004
Consumer expenditure on health goods and medical services (US$ million)	997,757.0	1,054,725.0	1,134,365.0	1,233,583.0	1,341,520.0	1,457,272.0	1,558,943.4
Consumer expenditure on health goods and medical services: real growth in national currency: 1990 = 100	135.2	139.8	145.5	153.8	164.7	174.9	182.3
Consumer expenditure on health goods and medical services as a percentage of total consumer expenditure	17.0	16.9	16.9	17.6	18.3	18.9	19.1

Source: National statistical offices/OECD/Eurostat/Euromonitor International

USA: Consumer expenditure on health goods and medical services by sector 1998-2004

Table: 4.1372

% of total consumer expenditure on health goods and medical services

	1998	1999	2000	2001	2002	2003	2004
Pharmaceuticals, medical appliances/ equipment	14.8	16.1	16.9	17.3	17.4	17.6	17.6
Outpatient services	41.5	40.9	40.6	40.4	40.2	40.1	40.2
Hospital services	43.7	43.0	42.5	42.3	42.3	42.3	42.2
Total	100.0	100.0	100.0	100.0	100.0	100.0	100.0

Source: National statistical offices/OECD/Eurostat/Euromonitor International

Healthcare Infrastructure and Services

USA: Healthcare infrastructure and services by sector 1998-2004

Table: 4.1373

As stated

	1998	1999	2000	2001	2002	2003	2004
Active pharmacists (number)	190,900	193,400	196,100	199,852	203,016	206,198	209,155
Consultations with GPs (general practitioners) (per capita)	10	10	9	9	9	9	9
Dentists (number)	151,300	152,200	155,200	157,571	160,197	162,506	164,778
Doctors (number)	777,900	797,600	813,800	836,200	858,128	882,246	905,292
Hospitals and clinics (number)	6,021	5,890	5,810	5,801	5,731	5,764	5,716
In-patient beds ('000)	842	831	825	823	817	814	812
Nurses (number)	2,180,040	2,201,810	2,249,440	2,262,020	2,291,851	2,322,901	2,356,334

Source: Euromonitor International from national statistics

USA: Healthcare infrastructure and services by sector: growth 1998-2004

Table: 4.1374

Year on year growth: % change in stated unit

	1998	1999	2000	2001	2002	2003	2004
Active pharmacists (number)	1.5	1.3	1.4	1.9	1.6	1.6	1.4
Consultations with GPs (general practitioners) (per capita)	1.0	3.0	-14.4	1.1	-1.1	0.4	0.0
Dentists (number)	2.4	0.6	2.0	1.5	1.7	1.4	1.4
Doctors (number)	2.8	2.5	2.0	2.8	2.6	2.8	2.6
Hospitals and clinics (number)	-1.2	-2.2	-1.4	-0.2	-1.2	0.6	-0.8
In-patient beds (number)	-1.5	-1.3	-0.7	-0.3	-0.7	-0.4	-0.2
Nurses (number)	1.0	1.0	2.2	0.6	1.3	1.4	1.4

Source: Euromonitor International from national statistics

Immunisation

USA: Vaccination rates by disease type 1998-2004

Table: 4.1375

%

	1998	1999	2000	2001	2002	2003	2004
Vaccination rate against DTP (diphtheria, tetanus, pertussis) 1 & 2 (%)			99.0	98.0	97.4	97.0	96.0
Vaccination rate against MMR (measles, mumps, rubella) (%)	92.0	92.0	91.0	91.0	91.3	91.0	91.0
Vaccination rate against polio (%)	91.0	90.0	90.0	89.0	89.8	89.0	89.0

Source: WHO

Infectious Diseases

USA: Incidence of disease by type 1998-2004

Table: 4.1376

Number

	1998	1999	2000	2001	2002	2003	2004
Incidence of AIDS	43,894	46,143	42,156	43,265	42,786	42,135	41,895
Incidence of diphtheria	1	1	2	2	1		
Incidence of measles	100	100	85	116	37		
Incidence of polio	0	0	0		0		

Source: WHO

USA: Incidence of disease by type: growth 1998-2004

Table: 4.1377

Year on year growth: %

	1998	1999	2000	2001	2002	2003	2004
Incidence of AIDS	-12.2	5.1	-8.6	2.6	-1.1	-1.5	-0.6
Incidence of diphtheria	-80.0	0.0	100.0	0.0	-50.0		
Incidence of measles	-27.5	0.0	-15.0	36.5	-68.1		

Source: WHO

Causes of Death

USA: Deaths by disease 1998-2004

Table: 4.1378

Number per 100,000 inhabitants

	1998	1999	2000	2001	2002	2003	2004
Deaths from heart disease	170.1	194.2	199.7	210.2	220.9	231.9	245.2
Death by diseases of the circulatory system	264.7	261.0	253.5	248.8	243.4	239.0	236.7
Death by malignant neoplasms (cancers)	174.8	174.7	171.9	170.9	169.6	168.0	166.6
Death by diseases of the respiratory system	67.5	64.5	65.6	64.0	63.1	63.3	61.9
Deaths from lung cancer	57.2	55.8	55.1	53.9	52.5	50.8	49.0
Death by diseases of the digestive system	24.0	24.7	24.5	24.9	25.1	24.0	24.0
Deaths from chronic liver disease and cirrhosis	9.3	10.7	11.1	11.7	12.4	13.1	13.8
Deaths from ulcers of the stomach and duodenum	1.7	1.7	1.5	1.4	1.2	1.0	0.9

Source: WHO/Euromonitor International
Notes: Data is ranked in descending order by year 2004

USA: Deaths by disease: growth 1998-2004

Table: 4.1379

% year on year growth

	1998	1999	2000	2001	2002	2003	2004
Deaths from heart disease	-2.3	14.2	2.8	5.3	5.1	5.0	5.7
Deaths from chronic liver disease and cirrhosis	-0.9	14.3	4.2	5.4	6.0	5.6	5.4
Death by diseases of the digestive system	-1.6	2.9	-0.8	1.6	0.8	-4.4	-0.2
Death by malignant neoplasms (cancers)	-1.5	-0.1	-1.6	-0.6	-0.8	-0.9	-0.9
Death by diseases of the circulatory system	-3.0	-1.4	-2.9	-1.9	-2.2	-1.8	-1.0
Death by diseases of the respiratory system	2.1	-4.4	1.7	-2.4	-1.4	0.3	-2.2
Deaths from lung cancer	-0.2	-2.4	-1.3	-2.2	-2.6	-3.2	-3.5
Deaths from ulcers of the stomach and duodenum	-9.1	-3.6	-10.4	-6.7	-14.3	-16.7	-11.9

Source: WHO/Euromonitor International
Notes: Data is ranked in descending order by year 2004

USA: Other selected causes of death: 1998-2004

Table: 4.1380

Number per 100,000 inhabitants

	1998	1999	2000	2001	2002	2003	2004
Death by injury and poisoning	51.0	51.4	50.7	50.7	50.5	49.6	48.8
Death by motor traffic accidents	15.5	16.2	15.9	16.3	16.5	15.7	15.6
Death by suicide and self-inflicted injury	10.7	10.1	9.9	9.5	9.1	9.6	9.5

Source: Euromonitor International from national statistics
Notes: Data is ranked in descending order by year 2004

USA: Other selected causes of death: growth 1998-2004

Table: 4.1381

% year on year growth

	1998	1999	2000	2001	2002	2003	2004
Death by motor traffic accidents	-1.9	4.5	-1.9	2.5	1.2	-4.8	-0.6
Death by suicide and self-inflicted injury	-0.9	-5.6	-2.0	-4.0	-4.2	5.5	-0.6
Death by injury and poisoning	-1.2	0.8	-1.4	0.0	-0.4	-1.8	-1.6

Source: Euromonitor International from national statistics
Notes: Data is ranked in descending order by year 2004

Smoking

USA: Smoking prevalence in population aged 15+ 1998-2004

Table: 4.1382

% of population aged 15+

	1998	1999	2000	2001	2002	2003	2004
Smoking prevalence in population aged 15+ (% of population aged 15+)	20.3	19.9	19.1	19.0	18.6	18.1	17.7
Smoking prevalence in male population aged 15+ (% of male population)	21.6	20.6	21.0	20.5	20.2	19.7	19.4
Smoking prevalence in female population aged 15+ (% of female population)	19.1	19.2	17.3	17.6	17.2	16.7	16.1

Source: WHO/OECD/Euromonitor International

Nutrition and Obesity

USA: Nutrition and obesity 1998-2004

As stated

	1998	1999	2000	2001	2002	2003	2004
Average supply of calories per day (calories per capita)	3,664.3	3,705.3	3,813.7	3,795.6	3,774.1	3,774.0	3,768.0
Average supply of fat per day (grams per capita)	143.6	147.5	155.8	157.8	156.5	157.4	158.0
Average supply of protein per day (grams per capita)	112.3	114.7	114.4	114.1	114.0	113.9	113.8
Obese population (BMI 30kg/sq m or more) (% of population aged 15 +)	26.2	27.1	27.6	28.3	30.9	32.3	33.7

Source: WHO/OECD/Euromonitor International

Over-the-Counter Healthcare

USA: Trends in OTC healthcare retail sales 1998-2004

As stated

	1998	1999	2000	2001	2002	2003	2004
OTC Healthcare (US$ million)	26,718.9	27,637.9	27,929.3	28,037.6	28,714.8	31,030.7	32,216.7
OTC Healthcare: real growth in national currency: 1998 = 100	100.0	101.2	99.0	96.6	97.4	102.9	103.7
OTC Healthcare: year on year (% real growth)	4.1	1.2	-2.2	-2.4	0.8	5.7	0.8
OTC Healthcare (US$ per capita)	98.9	101.4	101.5	101.0	102.6	110.0	113.3

Source: Euromonitor International from industry sources/national statistics

USA: OTC healthcare retail sales by sector 1998-2004

% of OTC retail value sales

	1998	1999	2000	2001	2002	2003	2004
Analgesics	13.9	13.7	13.5	13.5	13.3	12.3	11.8
Cough, cold and allergy (hay fever) remedies	13.7	14.2	14.0	14.4	14.6	16.3	15.8
Digestive remedies	11.3	11.2	11.1	11.0	10.9	10.4	10.8
Medicated skin care	10.1	10.1	10.3	10.5	10.5	10.0	9.7
Vitamins and dietary supplements	44.1	43.9	44.0	43.4	43.3	44.2	45.3

Source: Euromonitor International from industry sources/national statistics
Notes: Only selected sectors are shown, so values are not expected to sum to 100

Health and Wellness

USA: Retail sales of packaged foods by health and wellness category 2002-2004

US$ million

	2002	2003	2004
Packaged food: Total	276,691.6	284,885.5	292,283.5
Better for you	37,561.8	39,130.3	41,787.1
For food intolerance	1,543.6	1,680.7	1,922.5
Fortified/functional	4,455.6	4,828.2	5,215.8
Organic	4,314.8	5,013.3	5,646.6

Source: Euromonitor International from industry sources/national statistics

USA: Per capita sales of packaged foods by health and wellness category 2002-2004

Table: 4.1387

US$ per capita

	2002	2003	2004
Better for you	134.6	139.0	147.1
For food intolerance	5.5	6.0	6.8
Fortified/functional	16.0	17.1	18.4
Organic	15.5	17.8	19.9

Source: *Euromonitor International from industry sources/national statistics*

USA: Retail sales of packaged food by health and wellness category: % share of total packaged food market 2002-2004

Table: 4.1388

% value

	2002	2003	2004
Better for you	13.6	13.7	14.3
For food intolerance	0.6	0.6	0.7
Fortified/functional	1.6	1.7	1.8
Organic	1.6	1.8	1.9

Source: *Euromonitor International from industry sources/national statistics*

USA: Retail sales of packaged food by health and wellness category: real growth index 2002-2004

Table: 4.1389

2002 =100

	2002	2003	2004
Better for you	100.00	102.03	107.56
For food intolerance	100.00	106.64	120.42
Fortified/functional	100.00	106.13	113.18
Organic	100.00	113.80	126.53

Source: *Euromonitor International from industry sources/national statistics*

USA: Retail sales of better-for-you packaged foods by sector 2002-2004

Table: 4.1390

% of total packaged food / as stated

	2002	2003	2004	% real change in value 2002-2004
Combination	0.21	0.23	0.26	26.22
Reduced carb	0.21	0.48	0.94	357.88
Reduced fat	11.78	11.63	11.63	0.80
Reduced salt	0.45	0.44	0.43	-1.05

Source: *Euromonitor International from industry sources/national statistics*

USA: Retail sales of packaged foods for food intolerances by sector 2002-2004

Table: 4.1391

% of total packaged food / as stated

	2002	2003	2004	% real change in value 2002-2004
Diabetic	0.02	0.03	0.06	162.83
Gluten-free	0.05	0.06	0.06	20.29
Lactose-free	0.48	0.50	0.53	13.23

Source: *Euromonitor International from industry sources/national statistics*

USA: Retail sales of naturally healthy packaged foods by sector 2002-2004

Table: 4.1392

% of total packaged food / as stated

	2002	2003	2004	% real change in value 2002-2004
High fibre	1.60	1.61	1.62	3.81
Other naturally healthy food	0.40	0.42	0.43	11.31
Soy-based dairy alternatives	0.26	0.29	0.33	30.26

Source: *Euromonitor International from industry sources/national statistics*

■ **Venezuela**

Socio-economic Parameters

Venezuela: Socio-economic parameters 1998-2004

Table: 4.1393

As stated

	1998	1999	2000	2001	2002	2003	2004
Population: national estimates at January 1st ('000)	23,083.0	23,561.0	24,038.0	24,514.0	24,988.0	25,462.0	25,933.0
% aged 0-14 yrs	35.0	35.0	34.0	34.0	33.0	33.0	32.0
% aged 15-64 yrs	61.0	61.0	61.0	62.0	62.0	63.0	63.0
% aged 65 + yrs	4.0	4.0	4.0	5.0	5.0	5.0	5.0
% Male	50.0	50.0	50.0	50.0	50.0	50.0	50.0
% Female	50.0	50.0	50.0	50.0	50.0	50.0	50.0
% Urban	86.0	87.0	87.0	87.0	88.0	88.0	88.0
Occupants per household at January 1st (Number)	5.0	5.0	5.0	5.0	5.0	5.0	5.0
Households ('000)	4,836.0	4,982.0	5,132.0	5,261.0	5,398.0	5,530.0	5,661.0
Annual rates of inflation (% growth)	36.0	24.0	16.0	13.0	22.0	31.0	22.0
GDP (Bs million)	52,482,500.0	62,577,000.0	82,450,700.0	91,324,800.0	110,782,000.0	135,566,824.0	202,666,582.0
GDP (US$ million)	95,849.0	103,311.0	121,258.0	126,197.0	95,424.0	84,362.0	107,156.0
GDP (US$ per capita)	4,152.0	4,385.0	5,044.0	5,148.0	3,819.0	3,313.0	4,132.0

Source: *Euromonitor International from International Monetary Fund (IMF), International Financial Statistics and World Economic Outlook/UN/national statistics*

Life Expectancy

Venezuela: Life expectancy 1998-2004

Table: 4.1394

As stated

	1998	1999	2000	2001	2002	2003	2004	% change 1998-2004
Life expectancy at birth: total population (years)	73.1	73.3	73.4	73.6	73.9	74.1	74.3	1.67
Life expectancy at birth: total population: year on year growth	0.3	0.3	0.2	0.2	0.4	0.3	0.3	
Healthy life expectancy at birth (years)	65.0			60.9	61.1			
Healthy life expectancy at birth: year on year growth					0.3			

Source: *Euromonitor International from World Bank*

Sanitation

Venezuela: Improved sanitary facilities and water source 2000

Table: 4.1395

As stated

	2000
Population with access to improved sanitary facilities (% of population)	68.0
Population with access to improved water source (% of population)	83.0
Population with improved access to sanitation facilities, rural (% of rural population with access)	48.0
Population with improved access to sanitation facilities, urban (% of urban population with access)	71.0

Source: *National statistics/World Bank*

Health Expenditure

Venezuela: Public health expenditure 1998-2004

Table: 4.1396

As stated

	1998	1999	2000	2001	2002	2003	2004
Share of total health expenditure in GDP (% of total GDP)	5.4	5.6	5.9	6.0	6.2	6.4	6.3
Health expenditure (US$ per capita)	220.0	254.0	300.0	261.0	184.0	176.0	162.0

Source: Euromonitor International from OECD/national statistics

Venezuela: Private health expenditure 1998-2004

Table: 4.1397

As stated

	1998	1999	2000	2001	2002	2003	2004
Consumer expenditure on health goods and medical services (Bs million)	1,085,144.0	1,083,447.0	1,185,297.0	1,337,179.0	1,605,821.0	2,484,476.6	3,183,969.9
Consumer expenditure on health goods and medical services: real growth in national currency: 1990 = 100	177.0	143.0	134.6	134.9	132.4	156.2	164.4
Consumer expenditure on health goods and medical services as a percentage of total consumer expenditure	3.0	2.6	2.4	2.3	2.3	2.3	2.3

Source: National statistical offices/OECD/Eurostat/Euromonitor International

Venezuela: Consumer expenditure on health goods and medical services by sector 1998-2004

Table: 4.1398

% of total consumer expenditure on health goods and medical services

	1998	1999	2000	2001	2002	2003	2004
Pharmaceuticals, medical appliances/ equipment	63.0	63.1	63.5	63.9	63.8	63.7	63.6
Outpatient services	15.8	15.6	15.5	15.3	15.4	15.5	15.5
Hospital services	21.2	21.2	21.0	20.8	20.8	20.9	20.9
Total	100.0	100.0	100.0	100.0	100.0	100.0	100.0

Source: National statistical offices/OECD/Eurostat/Euromonitor International

Healthcare Infrastructure and Services

Venezuela: Healthcare infrastructure and services by sector 1998-2004

Table: 4.1399

As stated

	1998	1999	2000	2001	2002	2003	2004
Doctors (number)	40,355	34,905	35,454	35,424	36,132	36,439	36,760
Hospitals and clinics (number)	561	563	567	567	567	566	564
In-patient beds ('000)	44	49	49	49	49	49	49

Source: Euromonitor International from national statistics

Venezuela: Healthcare infrastructure and services by sector: growth 1998-2004

Table: 4.1400

Year on year growth: % change in stated unit

	1998	1999	2000	2001	2002	2003	2004
Doctors (number)	42.4	-13.5	1.6	-0.1	2.0	0.8	0.9
Hospitals and clinics (number)	0.2	0.4	0.7	0.0	0.0	-0.2	-0.4
In-patient beds (number)	-15.8	10.6	0.8	-0.6	0.2	0.2	0.2

Source: Euromonitor International from national statistics

Immunisation

Venezuela: Vaccination rates by disease type 1998-2004

Table: 4.1401

%

	1998	1999	2000	2001	2002	2003	2004
Vaccination rate against DTP (diphtheria, tetanus, pertussis) 1 & 2 (%)			92.1	84.6	77.1	70.0	62.0
Vaccination rate against MMR (measles, mumps, rubella) (%)	94.0	82.0	84.2	49.1	62.4	70.0	72.0
Vaccination rate against polio (%)	64.0	87.0	86.0	88.2	88.0	89.0	89.0

Source: WHO

Infectious Diseases

Venezuela: Incidence of disease by type 1998-2004

Table: 4.1402

Number

	1998	1999	2000	2001	2002	2003	2004
Incidence of AIDS	0						
Incidence of diphtheria	0	0	0	0	0		
Incidence of measles	4	0	22	115	2,392		
Incidence of polio	0	0	0	0	0		

Source: WHO

Venezuela: Incidence of disease by type: growth 1998-2004

Table: 4.1403

Year on year growth: %

	1998	1999	2000	2001	2002	2003	2004
Incidence of AIDS	-100.0						
Incidence of measles	-85.2	-100.0		422.7	1,980.0		

Source: WHO

Causes of Death

Venezuela: Deaths by disease 1998-2004

Table: 4.1404

Number per 100,000 inhabitants

	1998	1999	2000	2001	2002	2003	2004
Deaths from heart disease	64.8	64.0	65.0	64.7	64.8	64.9	65.1
Death by diseases of the digestive system	33.9	32.4	31.6	33.9	33.3	34.1	35.2
Deaths from lung cancer	8.4	8.9	8.7	9.0	9.1	9.3	9.5
Deaths from chronic liver disease and cirrhosis	7.5	7.8	8.0	8.2	8.4	8.7	8.9
Deaths from ulcers of the stomach and duodenum	2.0	2.1	1.8	1.8	1.7	1.6	1.5

Source: WHO/Euromonitor International
Notes: Data is ranked in descending order by year 2004

Venezuela: Deaths by disease: growth 1998-2004

Table: 4.1405

% year on year growth

	1998	1999	2000	2001	2002	2003	2004
Death by diseases of the digestive system	12.6	-4.4	-2.5	7.3	-1.8	2.4	3.2
Deaths from chronic liver disease and cirrhosis	5.1	3.6	2.5	3.1	2.4	3.6	2.6
Deaths from lung cancer	-2.9	5.2	-1.7	3.3	1.1	2.2	2.6
Deaths from heart disease	3.6	-1.3	1.6	-0.4	0.2	0.2	0.3
Deaths from ulcers of the stomach and duodenum	18.1	3.3	-11.5	-1.3	-5.6	-5.9	-5.2

Source: WHO/Euromonitor International
Notes: Data is ranked in descending order by year 2004

Venezuela: Other selected causes of death: 1998-2004

Table: 4.1406

Number per 100,000 inhabitants

	1998	1999	2000	2001	2002	2003	2004
Death by suicide and self-inflicted injury	0.2	0.3	0.2	0.2	0.2	0.2	0.2

Source: Euromonitor International from national statistics

Venezuela: Other selected causes of death: growth 1998-2004

Table: 4.1407

% year on year growth

	1998	1999	2000	2001	2002	2003	2004
Death by suicide and self-inflicted injury	-33.3	50.0	-33.3	0.0	0.0	0.0	0.0

Source: Euromonitor International from national statistics

Smoking

Venezuela: Smoking prevalence in population aged 15+ 1998-2004

Table: 4.1408

% of population aged 15+

	1998	1999	2000	2001	2002	2003	2004
Smoking prevalence in population aged 15+ (% of population aged 15+)	35.1	36.6	37.6	37.9	38.9	39.7	40.6
Smoking prevalence in male population aged 15+ (% of male population)	45.2	45.9	46.5	47.2	48.3	49.0	49.3
Smoking prevalence in female population aged 15+ (% of female population)	25.0	27.3	28.7	28.6	29.5	30.4	31.9

Source: WHO/OECD/Euromonitor International

Nutrition and Obesity

Venezuela: Nutrition and obesity 1998-2004

Table: 4.1409

As stated

	1998	1999	2000	2001	2002	2003	2004
Average supply of calories per day (calories per capita)	2,312.8	2,281.9	2,348.2	2,370.4	2,336.3	2,327.8	2,320.7
Average supply of fat per day (grams per capita)	59.7	59.1	60.7	63.7	63.6	64.3	65.3
Average supply of protein per day (grams per capita)	62.6	60.8	62.1	64.5	63.8	64.0	64.4
Obese population (BMI 30kg/sq m or more) (% of population aged 15+)	13.3	13.0	12.9	12.7	12.5	12.3	12.1

Source: WHO/OECD/Euromonitor International

Over-the-Counter Healthcare

Venezuela: Trends in OTC healthcare retail sales 1998-2004

Table: 4.1410

As stated

	1998	1999	2000	2001	2002	2003	2004
OTC Healthcare (Bs billion)	148.8	204.6	262.2	337.3	379.7	599.5	741.9
OTC Healthcare: real growth in national currency: 1998 = 100	100.0	111.3	122.7	140.3	129.0	155.4	155.4
OTC Healthcare: year on year (% real growth)	3.4	11.3	10.2	14.3	-8.1	20.4	0.0
OTC Healthcare ('000 Bs per capita)	6.4	8.7	10.9	13.8	15.2	23.5	28.6

Source: Euromonitor International from industry sources/national statistics

Venezuela: OTC healthcare retail sales by sector 1998-2004

Table: 4.1411

% of OTC retail value sales

	1998	1999	2000	2001	2002	2003	2004
Analgesics	18.0	16.6	15.0	13.4	13.7	9.3	8.3
Cough, cold and allergy (hay fever) remedies	27.9	28.9	32.6	33.2	34.5	24.6	22.6
Digestive remedies	19.4	15.9	14.2	14.3	13.9	10.0	9.5
Medicated skin care	12.1	13.1	12.1	11.1	10.8	10.2	9.9
Vitamins and dietary supplements	19.8	22.8	23.7	24.5	23.8	42.7	46.5

Source: Euromonitor International from industry sources/national statistics
Notes: Only selected sectors are shown, so values are not expected to sum to 100

■ Vietnam

Socio-economic Parameters

Vietnam: Socio-economic parameters 1998-2004

Table: 4.1412

As stated

	1998	1999	2000	2001	2002	2003	2004
Population: national estimates at January 1st ('000)	75,580.0	76,598.0	77,620.0	78,666.0	79,736.0	80,827.0	81,928.0
% aged 0-14 yrs	35.0	35.0	34.0	33.0	32.0	31.0	31.0
% aged 15-64 yrs	60.0	60.0	61.0	62.0	62.0	63.0	64.0
% aged 65 + yrs	5.0	5.0	5.0	5.0	5.0	5.0	5.0
% Male	50.0	50.0	50.0	50.0	50.0	50.0	50.0
% Female	50.0	50.0	50.0	50.0	50.0	50.0	50.0
% Urban	20.0	20.0	20.0	20.0	20.0	20.0	21.0
Occupants per household at January 1st (Number)	4.0	4.0	4.0	4.0	3.0	3.0	3.0
Households ('000)	20,070.0	20,707.0	21,629.0	22,071.0	22,950.0	23,803.0	24,674.0
Annual rates of inflation (% growth)	8.0	4.0	-2.0	0.0	4.0	3.0	6.0
GDP (VND million)	361,016,000.0	399,942,000.0	441,646,000.0	481,295,000.0	535,762,000.0	613,443,000.0	713,071,948.0
GDP (US$ million)	27,210.0	28,684.0	31,173.0	32,685.0	35,064.0	39,552.0	43,921.0
GDP (US$ per capita)	360.0	374.0	402.0	415.0	440.0	489.0	536.0

Source: Euromonitor International from International Monetary Fund (IMF), International Financial Statistics and World Economic Outlook/UN/national statistics

Life Expectancy

Vietnam: Life expectancy 1998-2004

Table: 4.1413

As stated

	1998	1999	2000	2001	2002	2003	2004	% change 1998-2004
Life expectancy at birth: total population (years)	68.3	68.7	69.1	69.3	69.6	70.0	70.3	2.90
Life expectancy at birth: total population: year on year growth	0.6	0.6	0.6	0.3	0.4	0.5	0.4	
Healthy life expectancy at birth (years)	58.0			58.5	58.6			
Healthy life expectancy at birth: year on year growth					0.2			

Source: Euromonitor International from World Bank

Sanitation

Vietnam: Improved sanitary facilities and water source 2000

Table: 4.1414

As stated

	2000
Population with access to improved sanitary facilities (% of population)	47.0
Population with access to improved water source (% of population)	77.0
Population with improved access to sanitation facilities, rural (% of rural population with access)	38.0
Population with improved access to sanitation facilities, urban (% of urban population with access)	82.0

Source: National statistics/World Bank

Health Expenditure

Vietnam: Public health expenditure 1998-2004

Table: 4.1415

As stated

	1998	1999	2000	2001	2002	2003	2004
Share of total health expenditure in GDP (% of total GDP)	4.9	4.9	5.2	5.1	5.0	4.9	4.8
Health expenditure (US$ per capita)	18.0	18.0	21.0	21.0	23.0	24.0	25.0

Source: Euromonitor International from OECD/national statistics

Vietnam: Private health expenditure 1998-2004

Table: 4.1416

As stated

	1998	1999	2000	2001	2002	2003	2004
Consumer expenditure on health goods and medical services (VND million)	19,615,054.0	21,140,581.0	22,306,834.0	23,972,931.0	26,446,459.0	28,218,085.0	30,477,524.6
Consumer expenditure on health goods and medical services: real growth in national currency: 1990 = 100	82.3	85.1	91.3	98.5	104.5	108.0	110.1
Consumer expenditure on health goods and medical services as a percentage of total consumer expenditure	7.7	7.7	7.7	7.7	7.7	7.5	7.6

Source: National statistical offices/OECD/Eurostat/Euromonitor International

Vietnam: Consumer expenditure on health goods and medical services by sector 1998-2004

Table: 4.1417

% of total consumer expenditure on health goods and medical services

	1998	1999	2000	2001	2002	2003	2004
Pharmaceuticals, medical appliances/ equipment	29.4	29.1	29.0	28.6	28.4	28.5	28.6
Outpatient services	48.1	47.9	48.1	48.0	47.9	47.8	47.6
Hospital services	22.5	23.0	22.9	23.4	23.7	23.7	23.7
Total	100.0	100.0	100.0	100.0	100.0	100.0	100.0

Source: *National statistical offices/OECD/Eurostat/Euromonitor International*

Healthcare Infrastructure and Services

Vietnam: Healthcare infrastructure and services by sector 1998-2004

Table: 4.1418

As stated

	1998	1999	2000	2001	2002	2003	2004
Active pharmacists (number)	12,800	12,900	13,700	14,600	15,679	16,533	17,171
Doctors (number)	34,200	37,100	39,600	41,200	46,323	48,025	49,072
Hospitals and clinics (number)	1,944	1,857					
In-patient beds ('000)	199	196	198	204	213	217	221
Midwives (number)	13,100	13,631	13,900	14,300	15,619	16,354	17,033
Nurses (number)	46,500	45,454	45,000	45,400	50,569	51,712	52,351

Source: *Euromonitor International from national statistics*

Vietnam: Healthcare infrastructure and services by sector: growth 1998-2004

Table: 4.1419

Year on year growth: % change in stated unit

	1998	1999	2000	2001	2002	2003	2004
Active pharmacists (number)	4.9	0.8	6.2	6.6	7.4	5.4	3.9
Doctors (number)	4.0	8.5	6.7	4.0	12.4	3.7	2.2
Hospitals and clinics (number)	0.7	-4.5					
In-patient beds (number)	0.6	-1.6	1.1	2.8	4.8	1.7	1.8
Midwives (number)	2.3	4.1	2.0	2.9	9.2	4.7	4.2
Nurses (number)	0.6	-2.2	-1.0	0.9	11.4	2.3	1.2

Source: *Euromonitor International from national statistics*

Immunisation

Vietnam: Vaccination rates by disease type 1998-2004

Table: 4.1420

%

	1998	1999	2000	2001	2002	2003	2004
Vaccination rate against DTP (diphtheria, tetanus, pertussis) 1 & 2 (%)			96.9	99.0	85.3	82.0	76.0
Vaccination rate against MMR (measles, mumps, rubella) (%)	96.0	93.0	96.6	97.0	95.7	96.0	96.0
Vaccination rate against polio (%)	94.0	93.0	96.0	97.4	91.6	94.0	94.0

Source: *WHO*

Infectious Diseases

Vietnam: Incidence of disease by type 1998-2004

Table: 4.1421

Number

	1998	1999	2000	2001	2002	2003	2004
Incidence of AIDS	953	970	1,164	742	783	764	738
Incidence of diphtheria	130	81	113	133	105		
Incidence of measles	11,690	14,134	16,512	12,058	6,755		
Incidence of polio	0	0	0	0	0		

Source: WHO

Vietnam: Incidence of disease by type: growth 1998-2004

Table: 4.1422

Year on year growth: %

	1998	1999	2000	2001	2002	2003	2004
Incidence of AIDS	38.5	1.8	20.0	-36.3	5.5	-2.4	-3.4
Incidence of diphtheria	-14.5	-37.7	39.5	17.7	-21.1		
Incidence of measles	79.7	20.9	16.8	-27.0	-44.0		
Incidence of polio	-100.0						

Source: WHO

Causes of Death

Vietnam: Deaths by disease 1998-2004

Table: 4.1423

Number per 100,000 inhabitants

	1998	1999	2000	2001	2002	2003	2004
Deaths from heart disease	41.3	39.9	39.0	39.8	40.4	41.0	41.8
Deaths from lung cancer	20.6	20.5	22.6	20.6	20.3	18.9	17.9
Death by diseases of the digestive system	21.8	19.4	20.1	19.2	18.3	17.9	17.2
Deaths from ulcers of the stomach and duodenum	21.8	19.4	20.1	19.2	18.3	17.4	16.5
Deaths from chronic liver disease and cirrhosis	8.3	8.0	7.8	7.6	7.5	7.3	7.2

Source: WHO/Euromonitor International
Notes: Data is ranked in descending order by year 2004

Vietnam: Deaths by disease: growth 1998-2004

Table: 4.1424

% year on year growth

	1998	1999	2000	2001	2002	2003	2004
Deaths from heart disease	0.7	-3.4	-2.3	2.1	1.5	1.5	2.0
Deaths from chronic liver disease and cirrhosis	-2.4	-3.6	-2.5	-2.6	-1.3	-2.7	-1.3
Death by diseases of the digestive system	19.8	-11.0	3.6	-4.5	-4.7	-2.2	-3.7
Deaths from ulcers of the stomach and duodenum	19.8	-11.0	3.6	-4.5	-4.7	-4.9	-5.5
Deaths from lung cancer	4.6	-0.5	10.2	-8.8	-1.5	-6.9	-5.5

Source: WHO/Euromonitor International
Notes: Data is ranked in descending order by year 2004

Smoking

Vietnam: Smoking prevalence in population aged 15+ 1998-2004

Table: 4.1425

% of population aged 15+

	1998	1999	2000	2001	2002	2003	2004
Smoking prevalence in population aged 15+ (% of population aged 15+)	38.8	39.0	39.7	39.9	40.1	40.5	41.5
Smoking prevalence in male population aged 15+ (% of male population)	69.9	69.5	69.7	69.6	69.2	69.2	68.4
Smoking prevalence in female population aged 15+ (% of female population)	8.5	9.4	10.5	10.8	11.7	12.5	15.2

Source: WHO/OECD/Euromonitor International

Nutrition and Obesity

Vietnam: Nutrition and obesity 1998-2004

Table: 4.1426

As stated

	1998	1999	2000	2001	2002	2003	2004
Average supply of calories per day (calories per capita)	2,472.8	2,499.8	2,534.5	2,566.2	2,566.2	2,577.5	2,589.9
Average supply of fat per day (grams per capita)	37.6	40.0	40.2	42.7	45.5	48.0	50.8
Average supply of protein per day (grams per capita)	58.8	59.4	60.4	61.7	62.3	63.1	64.0
Obese population (BMI 30kg/sq m or more) (% of population aged 15+)	4.1	4.2	4.2	4.2	4.3	4.2	4.3

Source: WHO/OECD/Euromonitor International

Over-the-Counter Healthcare

Vietnam: Trends in OTC healthcare retail sales 1998-2004

Table: 4.1427

As stated

	1998	1999	2000	2001	2002	2003	2004
OTC Healthcare (VND billion)	1,218.1	1,334.1	1,550.4	1,748.8	1,836.3	1,951.8	2,091.9
OTC Healthcare: real growth in national currency: 1998 = 100	100.0	105.1	124.1	140.6	141.9	146.2	147.8
OTC Healthcare: year on year (% real growth)	0.4	5.1	18.1	13.3	1.0	3.0	1.1
OTC Healthcare ('000 VND per capita)	16.1	17.4	20.0	22.2	23.0	24.1	25.5

Source: Euromonitor International from industry sources/national statistics

Vietnam: OTC healthcare retail sales by sector 1998-2004

Table: 4.1428

% of OTC retail value sales

	1998	1999	2000	2001	2002	2003	2004
Analgesics	16.3	16.0	14.7	14.2	14.3	14.5	14.5
Cough, cold and allergy (hay fever) remedies	23.6	22.7	20.7	19.2	19.3	19.4	19.3
Digestive remedies	17.9	16.8	15.0	18.9	18.6	18.5	18.5
Medicated skin care	7.9	8.1	8.2	8.5	8.5	8.7	8.8
Vitamins and dietary supplements	23.1	25.1	30.7	28.7	28.6	27.9	28.0

Source: Euromonitor International from industry sources/national statistics
Notes: Only selected sectors are shown, so values are not expected to sum to 100

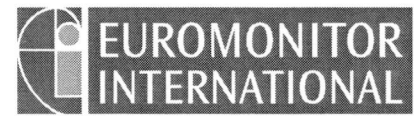

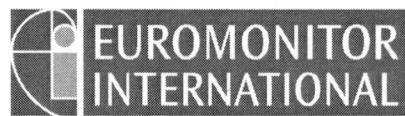

Also available

Country Data

Country data is essential background information when writing business proposals and reports. Using Euromonitor's research it is easy to build a detailed profile of a country. We have data back to 1977 so you can analyse historic as well as recent trends.

Asian Marketing Data and Statistics
www.euromonitor.com/amdas

European Marketing Data and Statistics
www.euromonitor.com/emdas

International Marketing Data and Statistics
www.euromonitor.com/imdas

Latin American Marketing Data and Statistics
www.euromonitor.com/lamdas

World Economic Factbook
www.euromonitor.com/factbook

World Economic Prospects
www.euromonitor.com/worldeconomicprospects

The Enlarged European Union: A Statistical Handbook
www.euromonitor.com/neweu

The Future Demographic: Global Population Trends and Forecasts
www.euromonitor.com/futuredemographic

Lifestyle Data

It is important when researching a new market to understand national habits and lifestyle choices. Euromonitor can help because we research a huge range of lifestyle statistics for 71 countries, including eating and drinking habits, home ownership patterns, income and earning trends, employment, and travel and tourism.

World Consumer Lifestyles Databook: Key Trends
www.euromonitor.com/lifestylesdata

World Consumer Spending
www.euromonitor.com/expenditure

World Income Distribution
www.euromonitor.com/income

Market Size Data and Forecasts

Euromonitor's consumer market directories provide an excellent starting point to investigate international markets. They enable you to understand consumer trends in 52 countries by providing up-to-date market size statistics for more than 330 consumer products. It is easy to identify the largest markets, those forecast to grow, which are static and which are in decline.

Consumer Western Europe
www.euromonitor.com/consumereuroope

Consumer USA
www.euromonitor.com/consumerusa

Consumer Asia
www.euromonitor.com/consumerasia

Consumer Latin America
www.euromonitor.com/consumerlatinamerica

Consumer Middle East
www.euromonitor.com/consumermiddleeast

Consumer Eastern Europe
www.euromonitor.com/consumereasterneurope

Consumer International
www.euromonitor.com/consumerinternational

Consumer China
www.euromonitor.com/consumerchina

European Marketing Forecasts
www.euromonitor.com/europeanforecasts

International Marketing Forecasts
www.euromonitor.com/internationalforecasts

Retail Trade International
www.euromonitor.com/retailtradeinternational

World Retail Data and Statistics
www.euromonitor.com/retailstatistics

Company Directories

Euromonitor's company directories allow you to identify the top players in the food, drinks, household and personal care industries on a national, regional and international level, based on their market share ranking. Our profiles are much more detailed than traditional company directories, you can understand who owns the leading brands in a market, identify the ultimate parent company and learn about a company's key strategies for success

Global Market Share Planner
www.euromonitor.com/globalmarketshareplanner

Market Share Tracker
Www.euromonitor.com/marketsharetracker

Major Performance Rankings
www.euromonitor.com/performancerankings

World Leading Global Brand Owners
www.euromonitor.com/globalbrandowners

Major Market Share Companies: Americas
www.euromonitor.com/companiesamericas

Major Market Share Companies: Asia-Pacific
www.euromonitor.com/companiesasia

Major Market Share Companies: Western Europe
www.euromonitor.com/companieswe

Major Market Share Companies: Eastern Europe, Middle East & Africa
www.euromonitor.com/companiesee_me_a

World Cosmetics and Toiletries Marketing Directory
www.euromonitor.com/cosmeticsdirectory

World Drinks Marketing Directory
www.euromonitor.com/drinksdirectory

World Food Marketing Directory
www.euromonitor.com/fooddirectory

World Retail Directory and Sourcebook
www.euromonitor.com/retaildirectory

Information Source Directories

Euromonitor analysts carry out thousands of research projects every year and consequently have a huge database of business information sources, ranging from trade associations and government departments to online databases and industry journals. Buy one of our directories and you can have access to the same information sources that Euromonitor researchers use when starting new research projects. They are an invaluable reference for librarians who receive requests for information across a broad range of subjects

World Directory of Business Information Libraries
www.euromonitor.com/businesslibraries

World Directory of Business Information Websites
www.euromonitor.com/businesswebsites

World Directory of Non-official Statistical Sources
www.euromonitor.com/nonofficialsources

World Directory of Trade and Business Associations
www.euromonitor.com/tradeassociations

World Directory of Trade and Business Journals
www.euromonitor.com/businessjournals

World Directory of Marketing Information Sources
www.euromonitor.com/marketinginfosources